Lippincott's
Review Series

Medical-Surgical Nursing

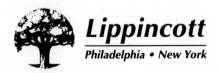

Lippincott

Philadelphia • New York

*Lippincott's
Review Series*

SECOND EDITION

Medical-Surgical Nursing

Ray A. Hargrove-Huttel, RN, PhD
Instructor
Trinity Valley Community College
Kaufman, Texas

Acquisitions Editor: **Susan Glover, RN, MSN**
Sponsoring Editor: **Deedie McMahon**
Project Editor: **Sandra Cherrey Scheinin**
Production Manager: **Helen Ewan**
Design Coordinator: **Doug Smock**
Indexer: **Lynne Mahan**

2nd Edition

Library of Congress Cataloging in Publication Data
Medical surgical nursing.—2nd ed. / [edited by] Ray A. Hargrove
  –Huttel.
      p.   cm.—(Lippincott's review series)
    Includes bibliographical references and index.
    ISBN 0-397-55212-2
    1. Nursing—Outlines, syllabi, etc.   2. Surgical nursing—
  Outlines, syllabi, etc.   3. Nursing—Examinations, questions, etc.
  4. Surgical nursing—Examinations, questions, etc.   I. Hargrove
  –Huttel, Ray A.   II. Series.
    [DNLM: 1. Nursing Care—examination questions.   2. Nursing Care—
  outlines.   3. Surgical Nursing—examination questions.   4. Surgical
  Nursing—outlines.   WY 18.2 M489 1996]
  RT52.L57   1996
  610.73′076—dc20
  DNLM/DLC
  for Library of Congress   95-25024
                                                                        CIP

9 8 7 6 5 4 3 2 1

CONTRIBUTORS TO THE FIRST AND SECOND EDITIONS

Leonard Ative

Martha Bogart, RN, MS

Jan E. Carter, RN, MN, OCN

Barbara Clancy, RN, EdD

Shirley Cudney, RN,C, MA, GNP

Mary Ersek, RN, MN
Assistant Professor
School of Nursing
Seattle University
Seattle, Washington

Joan Farrell, RN, PhD

Pamela Gotch, RN, MSN, CDE

Jacquelyn Grinde, RN, MS, MSC
Staff Nurse
United Hospital
St. Paul, Minnesota

Peggi Guenter, RN, MSN, CNSN

Deborah Kenny, RN, MSN, EdM

Melva Kravitz, RN, PhD

Larry Lancaster, RN, MSN, EdD
Associate Professor
Vanderbilt University School of Nursing
Nashville, Tennessee

Joan LeSage, RN, PhD

Barbara Martin, RN, MS, CS
Professor of Nursing
The University of Tulsa
College of Nursing and Applied Health Sciences
Tulsa, Oklahoma

Jewel McKay, RN, MSN
Manager
Discharge Planning and Utilization Review
Montclair Baptist Medical Center
Birmingham, Alabama

Linda Pachucki-Hyde, RN, MS, CDE

Pam Patterson, RN, MS

Jill Pendarvis, RNC, MA

Sharon B. Roth, RN, MS

Mariah Snyder, RN, PhD, FAAN
Professor, School of Nursing
University of Minnesota
Minneapolis, Minnesota

Judith Sweeney, RN, MSN
Assistant Professor
Vanderbilt University School of Nursing
Nashville, Tennessee

Lydia L. Tordecilla, RN, MS

Kuei-Shen Tu, RN, MSN
Assistant Professor, School of Nursing
University of Alabama at Birmingham
Birmingham, Alabama

Nancy B. Williamson, RN, PhD
Director, Rural Health Outreach Program
Medical College of Georgia
Augusta, Georgia

Jean Winter, RN, EdD

Mary Young, RN, MAN

Neoma Youtsey, RN, MN, CNOR
Assistant Professor
St. Luke's College
Kansas City, Missouri

REVIEWERS
OF THE FIRST AND
SECOND EDITIONS

Martha Banyon, RN, EdD

Diane M. Billings, RN, EdD, FAAN
  Professor and Assistant Dean of Learning Resources
  Indiana University School of Nursing
  Indianapolis, Indiana

Rebecca E. Boehne, RN, MSN

Karen M. Brubakken, RN, MS, CS
  Clinical Nurse Specialist—Surgical/Oncology
  Community Memorial Hospital
  Menomonee Falls, Wisconsin

Betty Chang, RN, DNSc

Barbara Erickson, RN, PhD, CCRN

Mary Fitzgerald, RN, MSN

Ruth H. Franklin, RN, PhD, MPH

Deanna E. Grimes, RN, DrPH, CS
  Associate Professor,
  School of Nursing
  University of Texas Health Science Center
    at Houston
  Houston, Texas

Donna D. Ignatavicius, RN, MS
  MacQueen Gibbs Willis Memorial School
    of Nursing
  Easton, Maryland

Marguerite R. Kinney, RN, DNSc, FAAN

Jane Lancour, RN, MSN

Pamela D. Larsen, RN, MS, CRRN

Patricia P. Lillis, RN, DSN
  Associate Professor
  Medical College of Georgia
  School of Nursing
  Augusta, Georgia

Marilyn Lowe, RNC, MSN
  Perinatal Clinical Specialist
  Methodist Hospital
  Omaha, Nebraska

Kenneth P. Miller, RN, PhD
  Director, Clinical Nursing Research
  National Naval Medical Center
  Bethesda, Maryland

Patricia Gonce Morton, RN, PhD

Ayda G. Nambayan, RN, MEd, OCN

Mary Oberg, RN, MN, CS, CCM, ARNP
*Medical-Surgical Geriatric Clinical Nurse
    Specialist
Shawnee Mission Medical Center
Shawnee Mission, Kansas*

Joyce Olson, RN, MS, CDE
*Pediatric Clinical Nurse Specialist
University of Kansas Medical Center
Kansas City, Kansas*

Linda Pachucki-Hyde, RN, MS, CDE

Catherine Paradiso, RN, CCRN, MSN
*Clinical Nurse Specialist
Mobile Health Unit Coordinator
The Visiting Nurse Association of America
Home Care of Staten Island, Lake Avenue Office
Staten Island, New York*

Phyllis M. C. Patterson, RN, MS, CS, OCN
*Clinical Nurse Specialist—Hematology
University Hospital
University of Michigan
Ann Arbor, Michigan*

Jeanne Salyer, RN, PhD
*Assistant Professor
School of Nursing
Virginia Commonwealth University
Richmond, Virginia*

Linda Sarna, RN, DNSc, FAAN
*Assistant Professor, School of Nursing
University of California at Los Angeles
Los Angeles, California*

Suzanne Shaffer, RN, MN, OCN

Deborah Wright Shpritz, RN, PhD
*Assistant Professor
Department of Acute and Long-term Care
School of Nursing, University of Maryland
Baltimore, Maryland*

Gail W. Snyder, RN, MSN

Clare Marie Tack, RN, MSN, CCRN
*Nurse Educator—Staff Development
Frankford Hospital, Torresdale Division
Philadelphia, Pennsylvania*

Rose Utley, RN, MS, CEN

Connie A. Walleck, RN, MS, CNRN

ACKNOWLEDGMENTS

Many people are responsible for the completion of this book. I would like to thank the Lippincott-Raven staff: Donna Hilton, for giving me an opportunity to pursue a new direction in my nursing career; Susan Keneally, for her encouraging words; and Deedie McMahon, for guiding, supporting, and believing in me.

I want to acknowledge and thank the faculty and staff of Trinity Valley Community College Health Science Center. I am honored to work with such a fine group of nursing educators. A special thanks to Mary Hardy, Judy Toy, Judy Candler, and Helen Reid for being there from the beginning.

This endeavor could not have been completed without the support and encouragement of my family. I would like to dedicate this book to my father, the late T/Sgt Leo R. Hargrove, whose values and standards made me what I am today. I want to thank my mother, Nancy; my sisters, Gail and Debbie; and Paula, for all of their love, encouragement, and support in everything I do in my life. I want to thank my daughter, Teresa, for her editorial assistance; my son, Aaron, for his understanding when Mom had to work on her book; and my husband, Bill, for always being "just me."

INTRODUCTION

Lippincott's Review Series is designed to help you in your study of the key subject areas in nursing. The series consists of six books, one in each core nursing subject area:

Medical-Surgical Nursing   *Mental Health and Psychiatric Nursing*
Pediatric Nursing   *Pathophysiology*
Maternal-Newborn Nursing   *Fluids and Electrolytes*

Each book contains a comprehensive outline content review, chapter study questions and answer keys with rationales for correct and incorrect responses, and a comprehensive examination and answer key with rationales for correct and incorrect responses.

Lippincott's Review Series was planned and developed in response to your requests for outline review books that address each major subject area and also contain a self-test mechanism. These books meet the need for comprehensive subject review books that will also assist you in identifying your strong and weak areas of knowledge. Each book is a complete source for review and self-assessment of a single core subject—all six together provide an excellent comprehensive review of entry-level nursing.

Each book is all-inclusive of the content addressed in major textbooks. The content outline review uses a consistent nursing process format throughout and addresses nursing care for well and ill clients. Also included are necessary teaching and other concepts such as growth and development, nutrition, pharmacology, and body structures, functions, and pathophysiology. Special features of each book are Key Concepts and Nursing Alerts, which are identified by distinctive icons. Key Concepts ☀ are basic facts the nurse needs to know to perform his or her job with ease and efficiency. Nursing Alerts 𝕟 are fundamental guidelines the nurse can follow to ensure safe and effective care.

You can use the books in this series in several different ways. Overall, you can use them as subject reviews to augment general study throughout your basic nursing program and as a review to prepare for the National Council Licensure Examination (NCLEX-RN). How you use each book depends on your individual needs and preferences, and on whether you review each chapter systematically or concentrate only on those chapters whose subject areas are particularly problematic or challenging. You may instead choose to use the comprehensive examination as a self-assessment opportunity to evaluate your knowledge base before you review the content outline.

Likewise, you can use the study questions for pre- or post-testing after study, followed by the comprehensive examination as a means of evaluating your knowledge and competencies of an entire subject area.

Regardless of how you use the books, one of the strengths of the series is the self-assessment opportunity it offers in addition to guidance in studying and reviewing content. The chapter study questions and comprehensive examination questions have been carefully developed to cover all topics in the outline review. Most important, each question is categorized according to the components of the National Council of State Boards of Nursing Licensing Examination (NCLEX).

► Cognitive Level: Knowledge, Comprehension, Application, or Analysis
► Client Need: Safe, Effective Care Environment (Safe care); Physiological Integrity (Physiologic); Psychosocial Integrity (Psychosocial); and Health Promotion and Maintenance (Health promotion)
► Phase of the Nursing Process: Assessment, Analysis (Dx), Planning, Implementation, Evaluation

For those questions not related to a client need or to a phase of the nursing process, NA (not applicable) will be used, as in questions that text knowledge of a basic science.

Unlike the NCLEX examination that tests the cumulative knowledge needed for safe practice by an entry-level nurse, these practice tests systematically evaluate the knowledge base that serves as the building block for the entire nursing educational process. In this way, you can prepare for the NCLEX examination throughout your course of study. Good study habits throughout your educational program are not only the best way to ensure ongoing success, but also will prove the most beneficial way to prepare for the licensing examination.

Keep in mind that these books are not intended to replace formal learning. They cannot substitute for textbook reading, discussion with instructors, or class attendance. Every effort has been made to provide accurate and current information, but class attendance and interaction with an instructor will provide invaluable information not found in books. Used correctly, these books will help you increase understanding, improve comprehension, evaluate strengths and weaknesses in areas of knowledge, increase productive study time, and, as a result, help you improve your grades.

MONEY BACK GUARANTEE—Lippincott's Review Series will help you study more effectively during coursework throughout your educational program, and help you prepare for quizzes and tests, including the NCLEX exam. If you buy and use any of the six volumes in Lippincott's Review Series and fail the NCLEX exam, simply send us verification of your exam results and your copy of the review book to the address below. We will promptly send you a check for our suggested list price.

Lippincott's Review Series
Marketing Department
Lippincott-Raven Publishers
227 East Washington Square
Philadelphia, PA 19106-3780

CONTENTS

Lippincott's
Review Series

Medical-
Surgical
Nursing

Nursing Process
and Health Assessment

I. Overview of nursing and the nursing process

A. Definitions

1. The American Nurses Association defines nursing as "the diagnosis and treatment of human responses to actual or potential health problems." Humans are biopsychosocial beings and human responses are interrelated, interdependent, and of equal importance. Altered human responses involve:

   a. **Self-care limitations**

   b. **Impaired functioning in areas such as sleep, ventilation, activity, elimination, sexuality**

   c. **Pain and discomfort**

   d. **Emotional problems related to illness and treatment, life-threatening or daily events**

   e. **Deficiencies in decision making ability**

   f. **Distortion of interpersonal and intellectual processes, such as delusions**

   g. **Self-image changes**

  2. The *nursing process* is a problem-identification and problem-solving approach developed to meet the health care and nursing needs of clients.

 B. Steps of the nursing process

  1. *Assessment* involves collecting and organizing data about a client's health status.

  2. *Nursing diagnosis* encompasses identifying, delineating, and validating the client's responses to health situations (problems or strengths) that lie within the scope of nursing practice.

  3. *Outcome identification* refers to defining goals (outcomes) which are individualized to the client.

  4. *Planning* involves establishing expected outcomes (goals and objectives) and developing ways to address the client's problems or support his or her strengths.

  5. *Implementation* refers to carrying out the plan of care and achieving the expected outcomes.

  6. *Evaluation* involves comparing the client's responses to nursing care with the expected outcomes.

II. **Overview of nursing health assessment**

 A. **Definition**

  1. Assessment, the first step of the nursing process, refers to systematic appraisal of all factors relevant to a client's health.

  2. Health assessment components include:

   a. **Collecting information through health history, physical examination, and records and reports**

   b. Analyzing information: comparing client data with baseline data

   c. Synthesizing information from all sources to form a complete clinical picture and discover relationships among data

 B. **Purposes**

  1. Surveying the client's health status and risk factors for particular health problems

  2. Identifying latent or occult (undetected) disease

      3. Screening for a specific disease (e.g., diabetes or hypertension [case finding])

      4. Identifying risks for particular health problems

      5. Determining functional impact of disease (human response to actual or potential health problem)

      6. Evaluating the effectiveness of the health care plan

III. Health history overview

A. Purposes

      1. Through the health history, the nurse elicits a detailed, accurate, and chronologic health record as seen from the client's perspective.

      2. The health history also helps the nurse connect with a client and develop good rapport.

      3. It also helps focus and guide subsequent physical examination.

      4. Health history information provides insight into the client's functional status.

B. Data collection techniques

      1. Provide privacy and comfort for the client.

      2. Greet the client and introduce yourself.

      3. Establish a verbal contract with the client that delineates the purpose of the history-taking session, the client's role, and a time limit for the interview.

      4. Ask open-ended questions to explore problem areas (e.g., "Tell me about any problems you may have with your breathing.").

      5. Ask progressively more specific questions after identifying a particular problem (symptom analysis).

      6. Guide the interview to obtain essential information without discouraging the client's discussion.

IV. Health history components

A. Biographic information (*Note:* If this information already is in the client's record, do not repeat it.)

      1. Date and time of interview

      2. Client's name, address, telephone number, and Social Security number

      3. Name, address, and telephone number of person to contact in case of emergency or other situation

      4. Gender, race, ethnic origin, and religious preference

      5. Age, birthdate, birthplace, and marital status

      6. Occupation and level of education

      7. Health insurance, usual source of health care, and source of referral

B. Reliability of data

      1. This component involves a description of client behaviors that lead the interviewer to believe that the client is a reliable, par-

tially reliable, or unreliable source of information (e.g., "Responded promptly to all questions; maintained eye contact; dates consistent. Client reliable.").

2. Reliability may come into question in clients who change their minds about their history, cannot recall certain events, do not know why they take certain medications, and are generally uncertain about their responses.

C. **Health and illness patterns**

1. The client's reason for seeking health care, including:

 a. **Brief statement, usually in the client's own words, of the overriding problem for which he or she is seeking help. This is called the chief complaint.**

    b. Onset and duration of the problem

2. Current health status or chief complaint: details of the client's reason for seeking health care, including:

    a. A detailed chronologic statement of the problem, beginning with when the client last felt well and ending with a description of the current condition

    b. An individual description of each health problem (in cases of multiple problems)

    c. A symptom analysis of each problem that includes bodily location (e.g., pain in lower right abdomen), quality (e.g., sharp), quantity (e.g., "The pain is about a 6 on a 10-point scale."), chronology (onset, duration, constant or intermittent, etc.), setting (precipitating circumstances, place, activity, persons present, etc.), aggravating and alleviating factors (e.g., "When I stand up straight, the pain is worse; when I curl up, it goes away."), and associated manifestations (e.g., vomiting, headache)

    d. Information on possible exposure or incubation period in case of acute infections

    e. Observations of whether and when the client stopped working or went to bed, whether illness is acute or chronic

    f. The client's perception of whether the problem is getting better or worse

    g. Information on previous treatments, including medications (prescribed and over the counter), the prescribing practitioner, treatment setting (e.g., hospital, clinic)

    h. Information on current medications status including prescription drugs and over-the-counter remedies

3. Past health status: health information not specifically associated with the current problem; usually considered to be any problem occurring more than 6 months to 1 year previously and includes:

    a.   General health and strength compared to 1 year ago: stability of weight, appetite

    b.   Past illnesses: childhood illnesses, acute infectious diseases, illnesses not requiring hospitalization, illness requiring hospitalization or surgery

    c.   Accidents and injuries

    d.   Sexual history: sexual performance, sexual preference (heterosexual, homosexual, bisexual), menstrual history, pregnancies (*Note:* This information also may appear in the review of systems.)

    e.   Immunizations

    f.   Allergies, including eczema, hives, and itching (with description of reaction); treatments

    g.   Geographic exposure: areas of residence, foreign travel

    h.   Psychiatric history: history of "nervous breakdown," anxiety, depression

4. Status of physiologic systems: subjective information on the client's perceptions of major body system functions, including current status and any related past symptoms (positives), or lack of symptoms (negatives), with a symptom analysis of any positive findings:

    a.   General: weakness, fatigue, malaise, fever, chills, recent weight loss or gain

    b.   Integument: pruritus, pigmentary and other color changes, bleeding and bruising tendencies, lesions, excessive dryness, change in texture or character of hair or nails, use of hair dyes or any possibly toxic agents

    c.   Head: headache, head injury, syncope, dizziness

    d.   Eyes: pain, recent change in appearance or vision, eyeglasses or contact lenses and recent change in prescription, diplopia, photophobia, blind spots, itching, burning, discharge, conjunctivitis, infection, glaucoma, cataracts, diabetes, hypertension

    e.   Ears: hearing acuity, earaches, tinnitus, vertigo, discharge, infection, mastoiditis

    f.   Nose and sinuses: sense of smell, sinus pain, epistaxis, nasal obstruction, discharge, postnasal drip, frequency of head colds, sneezing, use of nose drops or sprays

    g.   Oral cavity: toothache, recent extractions, state of dental repair; dry mouth, soreness or bleeding of lips, gums, mouth, tongue, or throat; disturbed taste sensation; hoarseness; tonsillectomy

    h.   Neck: pain, limitation of motion, thyroid enlargement

    i.   Lymph nodes: tenderness or enlargement of neck, axillary, epitrochlear, or inguinal nodes; duration and progress of abnormality

j. Breasts: pain, lumps, nipple discharge, surgery, any change in appearance of breast, mammography and breast self-examination, and timing with regard to menstrual cycle, estrogen replacement therapy

k. Respiratory: chest pain (and its relationship to respirations), pleurisy, frequent sneezing, cough, sputum production (character and amount), hemoptysis, wheezing (and its location in the chest), stridor, asthma, bronchitis, pneumonia, tuberculosis or contact therewith, night sweats, date of recent chest radiograph, smoking history

l. Cardiovascular: precordial or retrosternal pain or discomfort, palpitations, dyspnea (and how it relates to exertion), orthopnea (assessing the number of pillows the client needs under his or her head to sleep comfortably), paroxysmal nocturnal dyspnea, edema, cyanosis; history of heart murmur, rheumatic fever (and its manifestations), hypertension (and usual blood pressure, if known), or coronary artery disease; most recent electrocardiogram (ECG) and results

m. Gastrointestinal: appetite, food intolerances, dysphagia (with solids, liquids, or both), heartburn, postprandial pain or distress, biliary colic, jaundice, other abdominal pain or distress, belching, nausea, vomiting, hematemesis or flatulence; change in character or color of stools (bleeding, melena, clay colored, diarrhea, constipation) or change in bowel habits; use of laxatives (type, frequency); rectal conditions (pruritus, hemorrhoids, fissures, fistula); ulcers; gallbladder disease; hepatitis; appendicitis; colitis; parasites; hernia; radiographs (where and when obtained, results)

n. Renal and urinary: renal colic, frequency of urination, nocturia, polyuria, oliguria, urine retention, hesitancy, urgency, dysuria, narrowing of urine stream, dribbling, incontinence, hematuria, albuminuria, pyuria, kidney disease, facial edema, renal calculi, and results of cystoscopy if indicated

o. Male reproductive: testicular pain, change in scrotum; puberty (onset, voice change, erections, emissions); libido and satisfaction with sexual relations

p. Female reproductive: menstrual history (menarche, last period, cycle and duration, amount of flow, premenstrual pain, dysmenorrhea, and intermenstrual bleeding), vaginal discharge, dyspareunia, obstetric history (gravida/para, miscarriages, abortions, complications), menopause and associated symptoms, contraceptive methods used, libido and satisfaction with sexual relations

q. Venereal: gonorrhea, syphilis, herpes, AIDS (date of onset, treatments and their effectiveness, any complications)

r. Peripheral vascular: intermittent claudication, varicose veins, thrombophlebitis

s. Musculoskeletal: joint pain, stiffness, swelling (location, migratory nature, relation to known cardiac involvement); rheumatoid arthritis, gout, bursitis; limitations in function or range of motion; flat feet, osteomyelitis, fractures; muscle pain, cramps; back pain (location and radiation, especially to extremities), stiffness, limitation of motion, sciatica or disk disease

t. Neurologic: loss of consciousness, convulsions, meningitis, encephalitis, stroke, seizures, or other neurologic problems; use of medication for seizure control; cognitive disturbances (recent or remote memory loss, hallucinations, disorientation, speech and language dysfunction, or inability to concentrate); change in sleep pattern; motor problems (gait, balance, coordination), tics, twitching, tremors; muscle weakness, spasms; paralysis, muscle wasting, activity intolerance; sensory disturbances (pain, insensitivity to temperature or touch, paresthesias); neuralgic pain (head, neck, trunk, extremities)

u. Hematopoietic and immune systems: bleeding tendencies of skin or mucous membranes; anemia; blood type, transfusions and reaction; blood dyscrasias, low platelet count, exposure to toxic agents or radiation; unexplained systemic infections and lymph node swelling

v. Endocrine and metabolic: nutritional and growth history; thyroid dysfunction (e.g., goiter), adrenal problems, or diabetes; changes in tolerance to heat and cold; relationship between appetite and weight; excessive voiding or excessive thirst; changes in skin (e.g., pigmentation, texture); changes in body contour, hair distribution, shoe or glove size; unexplained weakness

5. Family health status, covering grandparents, parents, brothers, sisters, spouse, and children, and including:

a. Age and health status or age at death and cause of death (blood relatives, not adopted)

b. History of heart disease, hypertension, stroke, diabetes, gout, kidney disease or calculi, thyroid disease, asthma or other allergic disorders, blood problems, cancer, epilepsy, mental illness, arthritis, alcoholism, obesity

c. Hereditary diseases such as hemophilia or sickle cell disease

d. Family history presented as a genogram or diagram of the

"family tree" with added notations regarding family negatives (diseases not present in the family)

6. Developmental considerations: overview of the client's growth history, including pertinent physical and cognitive developmental milestones and factors

7. Functional history

   a. Status of client's mobility in relationship to activities and demands of daily living (e.g., Shanas' Index of Incapacity: "Can you go out of doors? Can you walk up and down stairs? Can you get out of the house? Can you wash and bathe yourself? Can you dress yourself? Can you put on your shoes? Can you cut your toenails?")

   b. Client's preferred lifestyle (e.g., "Is there anything you cannot do now compared with last year? Do you travel now? Did you in the past? Where did you travel?")

   c. The client's home and neighborhood environment (e.g., "Who buys and carries the groceries? Who cooks? Who does the housekeeping? Do you feel safe in and around your home?")

D. Health promotion and protection patterns

1. Health beliefs, encompassing:

   a. Expectations of health care

   b. Promotive, preventive, and restorative practices (e.g., breast self-examination, seat belt use)

   c. What illness means to the client

   d. Cultural implications of health and illness

2. Personal habits, including:

   a. Use of tobacco, alcohol, street drugs

   b. Use of prescribed and over-the-counter medications

   c. Use of caffeine

   d. Hygiene

   e. Elimination patterns

3. Sleep and wake patterns

4. Exercise and activity

5. Recreation

6. Nutrition, including:

   a. Height, weight, and anthropometric measurements

   b. 24-hour dietary recall, including number of portions and portion sizes

7. Stress and coping patterns

8. Socioeconomic status, encompassing:

   a. Educational level

   b. Financial status

9. Environmental health patterns, including:

   a. Home conditions: living arrangements, housing, others in

home including family and nonrelatives, health of others in the home

    b. General environmental conditions: neighborhood, region

  10. Occupational health patterns, covering:

    a. Exact nature of work, or of previous work if retired

    b. Exposure to toxic agents, fatigue, abnormal surroundings

E. Role and relationship patterns

  1. Self-concept, including:

    a. Self-expectations (short- and long-range goals)

    b. Perceived strengths and weaknesses

  2. Cultural influences

  3. Spiritual and religious influences

  4. Family role and relationship patterns

  5. Sexuality and reproductive patterns, including:

    a. Menstrual history and puberty history

    b. Sexual activity (past and present)

    c. Pregnancies (miscarriages, live births)

  6. Social support patterns (family, friends, agencies)

  7. Emotional health status

F. Conclusion: Complete the health history by asking "Is there anything else you'd like to tell me?" This allows the client to end the interview by discussing feelings and concerns.

V. Physical examination

A. General principles

  1. Physical examination is the second component of a complete nursing health assessment.

  2. Perform a complete or partial physical examination after obtaining a careful comprehensive or problem-related history; history findings help focus the physical examination.

  3. Examine the client in a quiet, warm, well-lit room; consider privacy and comfort needs.

  4. Explain what you plan to do, what the client can expect to feel, and what you expect from the client.

  5. Use appropriate draping for examination, exposing only the portions of the body being examined.

  6. Always compare body sides for symmetry and, where appropriate, compare distal to proximal areas; the client's body can serve as its own control.

  7. Visualize underlying structures and organs when performing the examination.

  8. Use anatomical landmarks to locate specific structures and to report significant findings (e.g., thorax, heart, abdomen).

  9. When possible, examine the client while standing at his or her right side.

B.   Assessment techniques

1.   The nurse uses four basic techniques in physical assessment: inspection, auscultation, palpation, and percussion.

2.   Inspection: The most important of all techniques (but the most commonly slighted), inspection starts at the initial client encounter. The nurse begins each portion of an examination with inspection, using the eyes and other senses as appropriate.

3.   Auscultation: This technique involves listening (usually through a stethoscope) to sounds produced in the body, particularly in the heart, lungs, blood vessels, stomach, and intestines.

4.   Palpation: In this technique, the nurse uses different parts of the hand to detect characteristics of pulsations, vibrations, texture, shape, temperature, and movement. Palpation can confirm and amplify findings observed during inspection.

5.   Percussion: Sharply tapping the body surface with the fingers or hands produces sounds that vary in quality depending on the density of underlying structures (e.g., organ borders, fluid, or gas). This technique is used to elicit tenderness and to assess reflexes. Sometimes, a rubber reflex hammer is used.

C.   Vital signs

1.   Normal ranges for temperature, pulse and respiratory rates, and blood pressure vary depending on the situation and the particular health care institution (see Table 1-1).

TABLE 1-1.
Normal Vital Signs in Adults

SIGN	RANGE
Pulse rate	60–80 beats/min (regular, full, strong)
Respiratory rate	12–20 breaths/min
Blood pressure	Under 140/85 mmHg
Systolic blood pressure*	Normal: Under 140 mmHg (when diastolic is under 90 mmHg) Borderline: 140–159 mmHg Hypertension: 160 mmHg and higher
Diastolic blood pressure*	Normal: Under 85 mmHg High normal: 85–89 mmHg Mild hypertension: 90–104 mmHg Moderate hypertension: 105–114 mmHg Severe hypertension: 115 mmHg and higher
Temperature	35.8–37.3°C (96.4–99.1°F) *Note:* Subnormal readings are common in elderly clients.

*Values defined by the American Heart Association Report of the Joint National Committee on Detection, Evaluation and Treatment of High Blood Pressure, 1988.
1988 Report of the Joint National Committee on Detection, Evaluation and Treatment of High Blood Pressure (NIH Publication #88-1088)

2. In blood pressure measurements, several distinctions are common:
    a. A difference of 5 to 10 mmHg between arms is common; systolic pressure usually is 10 mmHg higher in legs than in arms.
    b. Changing positions from recumbent to standing can cause a 10 to 15 mmHg drop in systolic pressure and a slight rise (5 mmHg or so) in diastolic pressure.
    c. In elderly clients, check blood pressure in the lying, sitting, and standing positions to detect excessive postural hypotension related to antihypertensive drugs or age-related physiologic changes.
3. When assessing a client's vital signs, keep in mind that they normally may vary somewhat with the time of day; for example:
    a. Diurnal body temperature varies from 0.5 to 2°F; lowest during sleep and highest from noon to early evening.
    b. Blood pressure may decrease during sleep and fluctuate throughout the day with no predictable pattern.
    c. Pulse rate may decrease during sleep and increase during the day in response to activity and stress.

D. Height and weight
1. Weight is related to body frame size: small, medium, or large.
2. Adipose tissue measurements (e.g., triceps skinfold thickness) help determine body fat percentage.
3. Aging clients, particularly females, commonly lose height due to osteoporotic kyphosis.

E. General appearance
1. Race
2. Sex
3. General physical development
4. Nutritional status
5. Mental alertness
6. Evidence of pain, restlessness
7. Body position
8. Apparent age
9. Clothing, hygiene, grooming

F. Integument
1. Inspection
    a. Color of skin and mucous membranes (complexion, jaundice, cyanosis, erythema), clubbing of fingers or toes
    b. Pigmentation
    c. Lesions and scars (distribution, type, configuration, size), superficial vascularity
    d. Moisture
    e. Edema

      f.   Hair distribution

      g.   Nails

  2. Palpation

      a.   Temperature

      b.   Texture and consistency, elasticity, turgor, mobility

      c.   Tenderness

  3. Normal findings

      a.   No lesions or rashes

      b.   Skin warm, slightly moist, smooth, finely textured, with elastic skin turgor

      c.   Hair distribution characteristic for gender and age

      d.   Nails present and smooth

      e.   Mucous membranes moist and pink

  4. Gerontologic considerations: common age-related differences in elderly clients include:

      a.   Skin wrinkled, drier (loss of subcutaneous fat and diminished sweat gland activity), and increasingly fragile

      b.   Turgor decreased (cannot be used to assess level of hydration)

      c.   Hair grayer, sparser on head, axilla, extremities, and pubic area; increased facial hair in women; bristly hair in nose and ears of men

      d.   Mucous membranes possibly drier and paler

      e.   Nails possibly horny and tough in response to decreased peripheral circulation

      f.   Common benign lesions: senile lentigines ("age" or "liver spots"); seborrheic keratoses (yellowish or brownish wart-like lesions with oily scale); cherry angiomas (small bright or dark red papules)

G. **Head**

  1. Inspection

      a.   Skull size and shape

      b.   Symmetry of face

      c.   Scalp: flaking, lesions, masses, deformities, swelling, tenderness

      d.   Hair color, distribution, nits on hair shafts

  2. Palpation

      a.   Hair texture

      b.   Scalp

      c.   Skull shape: bony overgrowths, symmetry

  3. Normal findings

      a.   Skull normocephalic

      b.   Face symmetric

      c.   Scalp clear

      d.   No alopecia or foreign bodies in hair

4. Gerontologic considerations: Nose and ears commonly appear larger in proportion to head size.

H. **Eyes and vision**

1. Vision testing
   a. Test visual acuity with a Snellen chart; test a client wearing corrective lenses with and without the lenses.
   b. Test visual peripheral fields.
2. Inspection
   a. Globes: Observe for protrusion.
   b. Palpebral fissures: Assess symmetry and width.
   c. Lid margins: Observe for scaling, secretions, erythema, position of lashes.
   d. Conjunctivae: Inspect for congestion; note color.
   e. Sclerae and irises: Observe color.
   f. Pupils: Note size, shape, symmetry, reaction to light and accommodation.
   g. Eye movement: Assess extraocular movements; note nystagmus or convergence.
3. Palpation
   a. Evaluate strength of the upper lids by attempting to open the client's closed lids against his or her resistance.
   b. Assess tenderness and tension of eyeballs.
4. Funduscopic examination (with an ophthalmoscope)
   a. Locate the red reflex.
   b. Check the transparency of the anterior and posterior chambers, cornea, and lens.
   c. Examine the retina (color, pigmentation, hemorrhages, and exudates); optic disk (color, distinction of margins, pigmentation, degree of elevation, cupping); macula (color); and blood vessels (diameter, atriovenous [AV] ratio, origin and course, venous-arterial crossings).
5. Normal findings
   a. Central vision 20/20 OU (both eyes), visual fields unrestricted
   b. No ptosis or lid lag
   c. Eyes move in conjugate fashion
   d. Anterior and posterior chambers, lens and cornea transparent; sclera and conjunctiva clear
   e. Lacrimal system unobstructed
   f. Pupils equal, round, and reactive to light and accommodation (PERRLA)
   g. Red reflex present bilaterally
   h. Bilateral well-marginated discs revealed on funduscopic examination
   i. C–D ratio 1:4, vessels to all four quadrants

    j. AV ratio 2:3

    k. No arterial narrowing, venous engorgement, AV nicking, hemorrhages, or exudate

  6. Gerontologic considerations

    a. Assess for entropion, ectropion, lens opacity, and eye dryness.

    b. Entropion in elderly clients can cause discomfort and damage to the eye.

    c. Funduscopic examination may be difficult in an elderly client because the pupil commonly is small (3 cm), with limited ability to dilate without a medicinal dilator.

I. Ears and hearing

  1. Hearing assessment

    a. Test gross hearing acuity with whispered words or a watch.

    b. With a tuning fork (512 to 1024 Hz), perform the Weber (bone conduction) and Rinne (air conduction to bone conduction ratio) tests.

  2. Inspection

    a. Pinna: Assess size, shape, placement on head, and color; note any lesions or masses.

    b. External canal: With an otoscope, check for discharge, impacted cerumen, inflammation, masses, and foreign bodies.

    c. Tympanic membrane: With an otoscope inserted inferiorly into the distal portion of the tympanic canal, assess color, luster, shape, position, transparency, and integrity; note any scarring; locate landmarks (cone of light, umbo, handle and short process of malleus, pars flaccida, and pars tensa).

  3. Palpation: Examine pinna for tenderness, consistency of cartilage, swelling, and pain.

  4. Normal findings

    a. Weber test not referred (or lateralized)

    b. Rinne test positive (air conduction greater than bone conduction)

    c. External ear appearance normal

    d. Canals clear without discharge

    e. Tympanic membranes pearly gray and intact, with landmarks visible

  5. Gerontologic considerations: Moderate hearing loss (especially of high-frequency sounds) and difficulty discriminating sounds are common in elderly clients.

J. Nose and sinuses

  1. Inspection

    a. Observe position of the nose on the face.

    b. Note any discharge.

    c.   Assess airway patency; note any nasal obstruction.

    d.   Perform a speculum examination of interior structures: nasal septum (assessing position, noting any bleeding or perforation), mucous membranes (noting hydration and color), and turbinates (assess color, note any swelling).

2.   Palpation: Apply fingertip pressure to the frontal and maxillary sinuses to assess for tenderness.

3.   Normal findings

    a.   Nose symmetrically placed on face

    b.   Nasal passages patent with septum in midline

    c.   Mucous membrane moist and dark pink without perforation or bleeding

    d.   Sinuses nontender

4.   Gerontologic considerations: Elderly clients commonly exhibit pale nasal mucosa.

K. **Mouth and pharynx**

    1.   Inspection (*Note:* Use a penlight and tongue depressor when examining inside the client's mouth.)

        a.   Lips: Observe color, moisture; note abnormal pigmentation, masses, ulcerations, or fissures.

        b.   Teeth: Note number, arrangement, and general condition.

        c.   Gingivae: Assess color and texture; note discharge, swelling, retraction, or bleeding.

        d.   Buccal mucosa: Assess for discoloration, vesicles, ulcerations, or masses.

        e.   Pharynx: Note any inflammation, exudate, or masses.

        f.   Tongue (both at rest and protruded): Assess size, color, moisture, and symmetry; note any lesions, deviations from midline, fasciculations, or tremors.

        g.   Salivary glands: Assess patency.

        h.   Uvula: Assess position on phonation; should be midline.

        i.   Soft palate: Observe symmetry on phonation, intactness.

        j.   Tonsils: Note presence or absence, size, ulcerations, exudate, or inflammation.

        k.   Note breath odor.

        l.   Assess voice volume; note any hoarseness.

        m. Check the client's ability to swallow.

    2.   Palpation (*Note:* Wear gloves when putting your fingers inside the client's mouth.)

        a.   Oral cavity: Palpate for masses and ulcerations.

        b.   Tongue: Grasp the tongue with a gauze sponge to retract and palpate it and to inspect its undersurface and the floor of the oral cavity.

        c.   Gag reflex: Attempt to elicit bilaterally.

3. Normal findings
  a. No lesions of lips, gums, tongue, or buccal mucosa
  b. Tongue pink, moist, well papillated, and in midline, both at rest and on protrusion
  c. Salivary glands unobstructed
  d. Pharynx not injected
  e. Tonsils nonobstructing
  f. Uvula in midline
  g. Palate elevating symmetrically on phonation
  h. Gag reflex present bilaterally
  i. Teeth present with no caries
  j. Gums clear
4. Gerontologic considerations
  a. Assess hydration status by observing for a small saliva pool under the tongue.
  b. If the client wears dentures, be sure he or she removes them before you examine the mouth.

L. Neck

1. Inspection
  a. All areas of neck anteriorly and posteriorly: Assess muscle symmetry and range of motion; note any masses, unusual swelling, or pulsations.
  b. Thyroid: Observe for enlargement.
  c. External jugular veins: Note distention.
2. Palpation
  a. Cervical nodes and salivary glands: Palpate for enlargement, tenderness.
  b. Trachea: Note deviation from midline.
  c. Thyroid: Palpate for nodules, masses, or irregularities.
  d. Carotid arteries: Note amplitude and symmetry of pulsations.
3. Auscultation: Listen for bruits over the carotid arteries and the thyroid.
4. Normal findings
  a. Neck symmetric with no tenderness or limitation of movement
  b. Trachea in midline
  c. Thyroid nonpalpable
  d. No bruits auscultated
5. Gerontologic considerations: Elderly clients are at risk for heart irregularities (reflex drop in pulse rate or blood pressure if carotid arteries are palpated at level of carotid sinuses); to prevent this, palpate well below the upper border of the thyroid cartilage.

M. **Lymph nodes**

    1. Inspection: Note observable nodes.

    2. Palpation

        a. Feel for palpable nodes: Assess size, shape, mobility, and consistency; note tenderness or inflammation.

        b. Locations to palpate: cervical, supra, and infraclavicular; axillary central, lateral, subscapular, and pectoral groups; inguinal (horizontal and vertical); and epitrochlear.

    3. Normal findings: no palpable or tender nodes

    4. Gerontologic considerations: Elderly clients may exhibit shotty nodes in inguinal areas.

N. **Female breasts**

    1. Inspection

        a. With the client sitting and her arms at her side, inspect the nipples and areolae for position, pigmentation, inversion, discharge, crusting, and masses; note any supernumerary nipples.

        b. Observe the size, shape, color, symmetry, surface contour, skin characteristics, and level of breasts; note any retraction or dimpling of skin or nipples, new pigmentation, engorged veins, swelling, or any tendency of a breast to cling to the thorax.

        c. Repeat these observations with the client's hands above or behind her head, with her hands pressed firmly on her hips, with the client leaning forward from the hips, and with the client supine.

    2. Palpation

        a. Palpate the breasts with the client in both sitting and supine positions; when the client is supine, and for a client with large breasts, place a pad under the ipsilateral scapula of the breast being palpated, and raise the arm on that side over the client's head.

        b. Palpate one breast at a time, using the palmar aspects of your fingers in a rotating motion and moving in concentric circles from the periphery of the breast to the nipple. Assess skin texture, moisture, and temperature; note any masses. Be sure to include the tail of Spence (breast tissue extending into the axillary region in the upper outer quadrant of the breast).

        c. Gently squeeze, milk, and then invert the nipple to check for any expressible discharge and to detect any mass beneath the nipple.

        d. Repeat these steps for the other breast, and compare findings on both sides.

        e. Conclude by applying lotion for lubrication, then—using

the palmar surface of the fingers—sweeping both breasts superiorly to inferiorly, compressing them against the thorax; note any masses.

3. Normal findings
   a. Nipples symmetric with no erosion, discharge, or recent inversion
   b. Breasts symmetric although possibly varying in size
   c. Tissue soft, lobular, and homogenous
4. Gerontologic considerations
   a. In postmenopausal women, the breasts may feel nodular or stringy on palpation.
   b. Breast tissue is denser in younger women. Breast tissue thins with age.

O. Male breasts (*Note:* Although this examination is brief, it should not be omitted.)
   1. Inspection: Observe the nipples and areolae for ulceration, nodules, swelling, or discharge.
   2. Palpation: Palpate the areolae, noting nodules and tenderness.
   3. Normal findings
      a. Nipples symmetric with no erosion or discharge
      b. No masses, discharge, or tenderness

P. Thorax and lungs
   1. Inspection
      a. Posterior chest: With the client seated, observe spine for mobility and structural deformity; symmetry, posture, mobility of thorax, and intercostal spaces (bulges or retraction) on respiration; anteroposterior diameter in relation to lateral diameter of chest.
      b. Anterior chest: With the client supine, inspect for structural deformities; assess the width of the costal angle; note rate and rhythm of breathing; observe for respiratory abnormalities (e.g., bulging or retraction of intercostal spaces, use of accessory muscles), and asymmetry.
   2. Palpation
      a. Posterior chest: With the client seated, palpate the ribs and costal margins for symmetry, mobility, and tenderness, and the spine for tenderness and vertebral position. Assess respiratory excursion (note the distance that your thumbs part) and symmetry of motion and fremitus with the client's arms crossed and scapulae separated.
      b. Anterior chest: With the client supine, assess as for the posterior chest, comparing symmetric areas and gently displacing female breasts if necessary.
   3. Percussion
      a. Posterior chest: With the client seated with his or her arms

across the chest and the scapulae separated, percuss symmetric areas, comparing sides (Fig. 1-1). Begin across the top of each shoulder and proceed downward between the scapulae and then under the scapulae, both medially and laterally in axillary lines; note and localize abnormal percussion sounds (Table 1-2). Percuss for diaphragmatic excursion on complete exhalation and inhalation, marking points where resonance changes to dullness; note symmetry and levels.

b. Anterior chest: With the client supine with his or her arms at sides, percuss from just below the clavicles along the midclavicular line (displacing female breasts as necessary), then move laterally. Note intercostal spaces where you detected hepatic dullness on the right side and cardiac dullness and gastric air bubble tympany on the left side.

4. Auscultation

a. Posterior chest: With the client seated as for percussion, ask him or her to breathe somewhat more deeply than

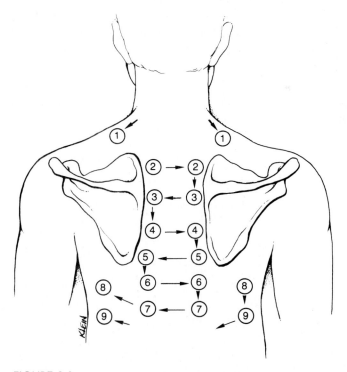

FIGURE 1-1.
Percuss the posterior chest progressively, from the shoulder tops to the costal margins at the midclavicular lines. (Adapted from Bates, B.A. [1991]. *A guide to physical examination and history taking* [5th ed.]. Philadelphia: J.B. Lippincott.)

TABLE 1-2.
Review of Percussion Sounds

SOUND	DESCRIPTION
Flat	Soft, high-pitched, short duration (e.g., thigh)
Dull	Medium intensity, pitch, and duration (e.g., liver)
Resonant	Loud, low-pitched, long duration (normal lung)
Hyperresonant	Very loud, lower pitched, longer duration (e.g., emphysematous lung)
Tympanic	Loud, musical (e.g., gastric air bubble, intestine)

normal with mouth open. With a stethoscope, listen over the same areas and in the same pattern as for percussion, comparing from side to side and moving from apices to lung bases (see Fig. 1-1).

b. Anterior chest: Auscultate over the same areas and in the same pattern as for percussion, comparing sides and proceeding from lung apices to bases. Note the distribution of vesicular and bronchovesicular sounds, both posteriorly and anteriorly (Table 1-3).

5. Normal findings
   a. Respiratory rate 16 to 20 breaths per minute
   b. Thorax symmetric; costal angle less than 90 degrees; transverse diameter 1:2 to 5:7; expansion 3 to 5 cm, symmetric, free and easy; no bulges or retractions in intercostal spaces
   c. Diaphragm position and excursion 3 to 6 cm
   d. Fremitus felt throughout lung fields, diminishing near periphery
   e. Percussion resonant over symmetric areas of lung to expected lung borders (fifth intercostal space [ICS] anteriorly, seventh ICS laterally, T_{10} posteriorly); dullness between the third and fifth left intercostal spaces (LICS)
   f. No adventitious sounds (crackles, gurgles, wheezes, or friction rubs), enhanced voiced sounds (egophony, bronchophony, or whispered pectoriloquy), or bronchial breath sounds

6. Gerontologic considerations
   a. Elderly clients may have "barrel chest" (AP-transverse diameter ratio of 1:1) in the absence of emphysema due to skeletal changes.
   b. In elderly clients, crackles may be auscultated at the lung bases in the absence of congestive heart failure. Such crackles should clear with deep breathing or coughing;

TABLE 1-3.
Review of Lung Sounds

SOUND	DESCRIPTION
Breath sounds	
Vesicular	Longer on inspiration than expiration; low pitch, soft intensity on expiration; heard over most of the peripheral lung
Bronchovesicular	Equal duration on inspiration and expiration; medium pitch and intensity on expiration; heard near the mainstem bronchi (anteriorly, below the clavicle at sternal borders to near the level of the second intercostal space; posteriorly, between the clavicles and between T1 and T4)
Bronchial	Shorter on inspiration than expiration; high pitched and loud intensity on expiration; heard over the trachea. (Bronchial sounds over a lung are always abnormal.)
Adventitious sounds	
Crackles	Formerly called rales or crepitations; discrete noncontinuous sounds usually heard on inspiration in dependent right and left lung bases; may clear on coughing; two types: fine crackles (soft, short, high pitched), coarse crackles (louder, longer, lower pitched)
Gurgles	Loud gurgling, bubbling; heard during inspiration and expiration; may result from secretions in the trachea and large bronchi
Wheezes	Continuous, lengthy, musical; heard during inspiration or expiration
Pleural rub	Loud, low pitched; confined to small area of chest wall; result from inflamed pleura
Altered vocal sounds (sound transformed through airless lung tissue)	
Bronchophony	Unusually loud and clear voiced sound (e.g., "99")
Egophony	Nasal bleating quality: "ee" sounds like "ay"
Whispered pectoriloquy	Unusually loud and clear whispered sounds (e.g., "1, 2, 3")

however, elderly adults tend not to breathe as deeply or cough as productively as younger adults due to decreased rib mobility and reduced vital capacity.

Q. Heart

　1. Inspection
　　　a. Precordium: Look for lifts, heaves, thrusts, or pulsations.
　　　b. Apical impulse: Observe for visible palpations (occur in about 50% of clients).
　2. Palpation
　　　a. Using the palms, palpate all auscultatory areas, noting vibrations or thrills.
　　　b. Locate the apical impulse, and assess the rate and strength of pulsations.

3. Percussion: Percuss the heart's borders in the 3rd to 5th LICS, noting areas of cardiac dullness.
4. Auscultation
   a. Listen with the stethoscope's diaphragm (best for high-pitched sounds) and bell (best for low-pitched sounds) in each auscultatory area.
   b. Identify S1 and S2 (lub-dub).
   c. Determine which sound is louder. (Normally, S2 is loudest in the aortic and pulmonic areas, S1 is louder than or equal to S2 in the tricuspid area, and S1 is loudest in the mitral area.)
   d. Listen for physiologic split in S2.
   e. Determine systolic phase (between S1 and S2) and diastolic phase (between S2 and S1): diastolic should be longer than systolic at a heart rate of 120 beats per minute or less.
   f. Note extra sounds or murmurs.
   g. Determine heart rate and rhythm.
5. Normal findings
   a. AP rate 60 to 90 beats per minute, regular
   b. No thrills, heaves, or abnormal pulsations
   c. Apical impulse 5 LICS at or medial to the midclavicular line (palpated within one ICS and no more than 1 to 2 cm wide; 7 to 9 cm from the sternal border)
   d. Left cardiac border dullness 9 to 12 cm from the sternal border
   e. S1 and S2 heard in expected locations with expected intensities (S2 split common in supine position on inspiration); no extra sounds or murmurs
6. Gerontologic considerations
   a. Arrhythmias become more common with aging; they may or may not indicate stenosis or myocardial insufficiency.
   b. Stiffened valves may cause murmurs or S4 ("Ten-nes-see").
   c. S3 ("Ken-tuck-y") in elderly clients usually is pathologic.

R. **Peripheral circulation**
   1. Inspection
      a. Jugular veins: With the client supine, observe the neck for internal jugular venous pulsations; if present, note their characteristics and relationship to inspiration. With the client sitting, observe for distended jugular veins.
      b. Carotid arteries: Observe for pulsations (timed with apical impulse).
      c. Extremities (arterial): Observe color, noting pallor or rubor; hair distribution, noting abnormal absence; and

skin characteristics, noting shiny or thin skin and any circumscribed lesions on feet and toes.

    d. Extremities (venous): Observe color, noting abnormal brown pigmentation; look for skin lesions on the lower legs, varicosities, and edema.

  2. Palpation

    a. Extremities (arterial): Assess the temperature of the skin. Palpate pulses (radial, femoral, posterior tibial, dorsalis pedis), comparing sides. Check capillary refill times in fingernails and toenails. Perform Allen's test to determine arterial patency by having the client make a fist, compressing the radial and ulnar arteries at the wrist with the (nurse's) thumbs to block blood flow, releasing the thumb over the ulnar artery and watching for the palm to flush, then repeating the procedure for the radial artery.

    b. Extremities (venous): Palpate the skin over the tibia and at the medial malleoli for pitting edema. Compress the calf between your two hands placed anteriorly and posteriorly; note any pain that this maneuver elicits.

  3. Auscultation: Listen over the carotid, abdominal, and femoral arteries for bruits.

  4. Normal findings

    a. Jugular veins soft and undulating, decreasing on inspiration when supine; not observable when sitting

    b. Carotid artery pulsations synchronous with apical impulse

    c. In extremities, skin warm with no discoloration, lesions, varicosities, or edema

    d. Pulses 2+ bilaterally on a scale of 0 to 3+

    e. Capillary refill less than 3 seconds; hands pink immediately in response to Allen's test

    f. No calf tenderness elicited

    g. No bruits auscultated over the carotid, abdominal, or femoral artery

  5. Gerontologic considerations

    a. Elderly persons commonly experience thickening, hardening, and loss of elasticity in vessel walls.

    b. Gradual pink or purple discoloration on the toes and feet is common in elderly persons.

S. Abdomen

  1. Inspection

    a. Skin: scars, striae, and rashes

    b. General contour and symmetry

    c. Visible peristalsis, aortic pulsations, and hernias (umbilical, inguinal, and incisional)

  2. Auscultation (*Note:* Auscultate the abdomen before percussing

and palpating to avoid stimulating intestinal activity and altering bowel sounds.)

    a.   Bowel sounds: Listen in all quadrants; note frequency, pitch, and duration.

    b.   Auscultate for bruits over abdominal aorta and the renal, iliac, and femoral arteries.

3.   Percussion

    a.   Percuss in all quadrants; note areas of tympany or dullness.

    b.   Percuss along the right midclavicular line, starting below the umbilicus and moving upward, to locate the liver borders.

    c.   Percuss in the left upper quadrant for gastric air bubble.

    d.   With the client sitting, strike the back at the costovertebral angles (CVA); note tenderness or pain.

4.   Palpation

    a.   Abdomen: Palpate lightly in all quadrants; follow with deep palpation. Assess organ location and abdominal muscle tone; note unusual masses, pulsations, tenderness, or pain.

    b.   Kidney: Palpate kidneys bimanually slightly below the umbilicus; note size, shape, and any tenderness.

    c.   Abdominal aorta: Palpate for contour and pulsations.

    d.   Lymph nodes: Palpate inguinal and femoral areas bilaterally; note enlargement.

5.   Normal findings

    a.   No scars; abdominal wall flat and symmetric; no incisional, umbilical, or inguinal hernias

    b.   Bowel sounds intermittent (every 5 to 35 seconds) and gurgling with no hyperactive or tinkling sounds; rushing sounds over the ileocecal valve (in the right lower quadrant) 4 to 7 hours after eating; no bruits

    c.   Liver dullness 6 to 12 cm at right midclavicular line (RMCL); tympany of gastric air bubble over left anterior lower border of thorax; tympany in all quadrants

    d.   No CVA tenderness

    e.   Muscle tone normal; abdomen soft with no masses or tenderness

    f.   Aorta width 2.5 to 4 cm; soft, pulsatile

    g.   Pole of right kidney may be palpable

6.   Gerontologic considerations

    a.   Elderly clients commonly exhibit diminished peristalsis.

    b.   In elderly clients, the liver may be 1 to 2 cm below the right costal margin due to an enlarged lung field.

T. **Male genitalia and hernias** (*Note:* **Wear gloves during examination.**)

    1. Inspection
        a. Pubic hair: Assess distribution; note any nits or lice.
        b. Penis: Retract the foreskin, if present. Note any ulcerations, masses, or scarring on the glans penis. Inspect the urethral meatus for location, lesions, and discharge.
        c. Scrotum: Inspect anterior and posterior aspects, assessing size, contour, and symmetry; note ulcerations, masses, redness, or swelling.
        d. Inguinal areas: Look for bulges, with and without the client bearing down, or when raising his head off the bed.

    2. Palpation
        a. Penis: Palpate the shaft for lesions, nodules, or masses; if present, note tenderness, contour, size, and degree of induration.
        b. Scrotum: Palpate each testis and epididymis, assessing size, shape, and consistency. Note any masses of unusual tenderness. Also note any nodules or tenderness of the spermatic cord and vas deferens.
        c. Inguinal and femoral areas: Assess for hernias.

    3. Normal findings
        a. Normal male pubic hair distribution with no infestations
        b. No penile lesions, masses, or discharge
        c. Testes symmetric without masses or undue tenderness; the left testis may be slightly larger and hang lower than the right testis
        d. No inguinal or femoral hernias

    4. Gerontologic considerations
        a. In elderly men, pubic hair commonly thins and scrotal skin loses tone, causing the scrotum to appear more pendulous.
        b. Some degree of testicular atrophy and softening commonly occurs with aging.

U. **Female genitalia** (*Note:* **Wear gloves during examination.**)

    1. Inspection and palpation (performed almost simultaneously)
        a. Place the client in lithotomy position; drape properly.
        b. Assess pubic hair distribution; note any nits or lice.
        c. Inspect the labia majora, mons pubis, and perineum; note skin color and integrity.
        d. Separate the labia majora, and inspect the clitoris, urethral meatus, and vaginal opening; note abnormal color, ulcerations, swelling, nodules, or discharge.

    2. Normal findings
        a. Normal female pubic hair distribution with no infestations

      b.   Outlet, vagina, and perineum free of masses, edema, tenderness, nodules, lesions, and discharge

  3. Gerontologic considerations

      a.   In elderly women, pubic hair becomes gray, more sparse, and brittle.

      b.   External genitalia typically atrophy somewhat.

      c.   Weakened muscle tone with aging increases the likelihood of cystocele.

V. **Rectum (*Note:* Wear gloves during examination.)**

  1. Inspection

      a.   With the client lying in left Sims' position and properly draped, spread the buttocks and examine the anus and the perianal and sacral regions. Note any inflammation, nodules, scars, lesions, ulcerations, rashes, bleeding, fissures, or hemorrhoids.

      b.   Check for bulges when the client bears down.

      c.   If necessary, use an alternative position for examination: for a male client, standing and bent over the table; for a female client, the lithotomy position.

  2. Palpation

      a.   Ask the client to bear down; slowly insert your lubricated index finger of gloved hand through the anal sphincter; assess sphincter tone. Then, gently rotate your index finger to palpate the rectum and rectal walls anteriorly and posteriorly; note any nodules, masses, or tenderness.

      b.   Palpate for fecal impaction.

      c.   In a male client, anteriorly palpate the two lateral lobes of the prostate gland for irregularities, nodules, swelling, or tenderness.

      d.   Withdraw your finger gently; test any fecal material on the glove for occult blood.

  3. Normal findings

      a.   Sphincter closes around finger

      b.   Wall of rectum smooth and moist; soft stool may be present

      c.   No hemorrhoids, fissures, or fistulas

      d.   Stool guaiac test negative

      e.   Male prostate 2.5 to 4 cm in size with a small groove separating the lobes; feels firm, smooth, nonmovable, nontender, and rubbery

  4. Gerontologic considerations: Most older men exhibit some degree of prostatic enlargement.

W. **Musculoskeletal system**

  1. Inspection

      a.   Observe the client's ability to perform functional tasks of daily living (e.g., grasping objects, performing personal hygiene, bathing, dressing, bending, sitting, rising from sitting to standing, and walking up and down stairs as well as on a level surface).

    b.   Note any pain the client experiences while performing functions or being examined.

    c.   Examine the arms and legs; note size, symmetry, muscle mass, and any deformities.

    d.   Assess the spine for range of motion (flexion, extension, lateral flexion, and rotation) and lateral or anterior-posterior curvature.

    e.   Assess all major joints, noting any limitations to active range of motion, swelling, or redness.

    f.   Neck: Assess flexion, extension, lateral rotation.

    g.   Shoulders: Assess flexion, extension, and rotation.

    h.   Elbows: Assess flexion, extension, supination, and pronation.

    i.   Wrists: Assess flexion, extension, and ulnar and radial deviation.

    j.   Fingers: Assess flexion, extension, abduction, and adduction.

    k.   Hips: Assess flexion, extension, and rotation.

    l.   Knees: Assess flexion and extension.

    m.   Ankles: Assess dorsiflexion, plantar flexion, inversion, and eversion.

    n.   Toes: Assess flexion, extension, abduction, and adduction.

2.   Palpation

    a.   Palpate the joints of the neck and upper and lower extremities, noting tenderness, swelling, temperature, limitations to passive range of motion, and crepitation.

    b.   Palpate muscles to assess size, tone, and any tenderness.

    c.   Palpate the spine, noting bony deformities and crepitation.

3.   Percussion: Directly percuss the spine with the ulnar surface of the fist from the cervical to lumbar region; note any pain or tenderness.

4.   Normal findings

    a.   No limitation to function

    b.   No gross deformities or abnormal postures

    c.   Range of joint motion unrestricted in extremities and spine

    d.   Muscle mass symmetric with no hypertrophy or atrophy; tone normal

    e.   No joint pain, crepitus, bony overgrowths, or tenderness in extremities or spine

5. Gerontologic considerations
a. Elderly clients commonly exhibit diminished joint flexibility and decreased muscle mass and strength.
b. Other common age-related musculoskeletal problems include degenerative joint changes, mild scoliosis or kyphosis, stooped body posture, and some degree of functional limitation.

X. Neurologic system

1. Components of neurologic examination include:
a. Mental status
b. Cranial nerve function
c. Cerebellar function
d. Motor function
e. Sensory function
f. Reflexes

2. Mental status: Observed during history taking, includes:
a. State of consciousness: alert, somnolent, stuporous, comatose
b. Orientation to person, place, and time
c. Memory: immediate, recent, remote
d. Cognition: calculations, current events, response to proverbs
e. Judgment and problem-solving ability
f. Emotion: mood, affect, congruence of responses

3. Cranial nerve (CN) function
a. Olfactory (CN I): With the client's eyes closed, present various odors, occluding one nostril at a time. Note the client's ability to identify the odors.
b. Optic (CN II): Test visual acuity and visual fields, and examine the optic disc with an ophthalmoscope.
c. Oculomotor (CN III), trochlear (CN IV), and abducens (CN VI): Assess extraocular motion by evaluating the six cardinal positions of gaze (parallelism, nystagmus), performing the cover-uncover test (movement of eye when uncovered or opposite eye when contralateral eye covered), and corneal light reflex (symmetry of reflection of light on pupil); check size and shape of pupils and pupillary reaction to light and accommodation (PERRLA).
d. Trigeminal (CN V): Motor—Assess the client's ability to chew, assess strength of bite. Sensory—Assess the client's ability to distinguish light touch and pain when you lightly stroke his or her face with a cotton wisp and gently prick the skin with a sterile pin or toothpick on forehead (to assess the ophthalmic branch), cheek (to assess the maxillary branch), and chin (to assess the mandibular branch).

e. Facial (CN VII): Motor—Assess symmetry of facial movements as the client smiles, frowns, grimaces, clenches his or her teeth, and so forth. Sensory—Ask the client to identify various distinct flavors placed on the anterior two thirds of the tongue.

f. Acoustic (CN VIII): Cochlear branch—Assess hearing acuity. Vestibular branch—Perform the Romberg test to evaluate equilibrium. Have the client stand with feet together and eyes closed for 20 to 30 seconds without support. Normally, only minimal swaying occurs.

g. Glossopharyngeal (CN IX): Test for the gag reflex by gently touching the posterior pharyngeal wall with a tongue blade.

h. Vagus (CN X): As the client speaks, check movement of the uvula (noting any deviation from midline) and palate (noting asymmetric elevation).

i. Spinal accessory (CN XI): Assess strength of the sternocleidomastoid (SCM) and upper trapezius muscles by asking the client to move the head against resistance of your hand. Also observe and palpate contraction of SCM muscle on the opposite side; ask the client to shrug the shoulders against resistance of your hands.

j. Hypoglossal (CN XII): Test strength and articulation of the tongue by having the client push the tongue to the side of the mouth against resistance applied to the cheek. Ask the client to stick out the tongue and then return it to the mouth while you observe for deviation, asymmetry, tremors, and fasciculations.

4. Cerebellar function (coordination and balance)
   a. Assess posture, gait, and balance; have the client walk forward and backward in a straight line.
   b. Perform the Romberg test; stand close to the client to provide support if necessary.
   c. Assess coordination in the upper extremities by having the client perform the finger-to-nose test.
   d. Assess coordination in the lower extremities by having the client tap the toes and slide the heel down the contralateral shin.

5. Motor function
   a. Muscle mass: Assess symmetry and distribution distally and proximally, and circumference of extremities bilaterally.
   b. Tone: Evaluate resistance of muscles in response to passive motion during flexion and extension of extremities.
   c. Strength: Assess hand squeeze and evaluate muscle strength in each extremity against resistance during flexion

and extension (also abduction and adduction where appropriate), comparing bilaterally.

    d.   Observe for involuntary movements (tics, fasciculations, tremors, or twitching) and abnormal postures (e.g., fetal, decorticate, decerebrate).

6.   Sensory function: With the client's eyes closed, assess:

    a.   Light touch: Have the client indicate response to cotton wisp lightly stroked on skin at representative dermatomes (i.e., backs of hands, forearms and upper arms, torso, thigh, tibia, and dorsal portion of foot); compare bilaterally and distal to proximal.

    b.   Pain: Repeat the pattern of light touch assessment, using a sterile safety pin to elicit sharp sensation; alternate with the pin's rounded end for contrast.

    c.   Vibration: Place a vibrating low-pitched tuning fork (128 Hz) over the sternum, then quickly on the distal interphalangeal joint of a finger; ask the client to identify whether vibration sensation in the finger is 100%, 75%, 50%, or 25% of that felt in the sternum, and to indicate when vibration is no longer felt. Repeat this procedure in a great toe. If vibration sense is impaired in the finger or toe, proceed to assessment in more proximal bony prominences (wrist and elbow or medial malleolus, patella, anterior iliac spine, and spinous processes).

    d.   Position sense: With your fingers placed on the lateral surface of the client's digit (finger, great toe), move it up or down; ask the client which direction the digit is pointing.

    e.   Stereognosis: Ask the client to identify small objects placed in his or her hand, one hand at a time.

    f.   Graphesthesia: Ask the client to identify a number that you trace in his or her palm with your fingertip.

7.   Deep tendon reflexes: Striking with a reflex hammer, compare reflex amplitude bilaterally, grading on scale of 0 to 4+ (4+ = hyperactive; 2+ or 3+ = average; 1+ = diminished; 0 = no response).

    a.   Brachioradialis (C5, C6): Strike the radius tendon about 1 to 2 inches above the wrist; observe for flexion and supination of the forearm.

    b.   Biceps (C5, C6): Place your thumb or forefinger at the base of the biceps tendon and strike it; observe for flexion of the arm at the elbow.

    c.   Triceps (C7, C8): Strike the triceps tendon, just above the elbow; observe for slight elbow extension.

    d.   Patellar or quadriceps (L2, L3, L4): Sharply strike the patellar tendon; observe for extension of knee.

    e.   Achilles or ankle jerk (S1, S2): Support the client's foot in the dorsiflexed position; tap the Achilles tendon, and observe for plantar flexion.

8. Superficial cutaneous reflexes
   a. Abdominal: Stroke the abdomen above (T8, T9, T10) and below (T10, T11, T12) the umbilicus bilaterally; observe for contraction of abdominal muscles and deviation of the umbilicus toward the stimulus.
   b. Cremasteric (L1, L2): In a male client, stroke the inner surface of the thigh; observe for prompt elevation of the testis on the ipsilateral side.
   c. Plantar (L4, L5, S1, S2): Extend the client's legs with the feet relaxed; stroke the lateral aspect of the sole from the heel to the ball of the foot, curving medially across the ball; observe for flexion of toes.

9. Normal findings
   a. Mental status: alert, quiet, able to follow three-step instructions; oriented to person, place, and time; judgment and intellectual performance within normal limits
   b. Cranial nerve function: CN I through XII grossly normal
   c. Cerebellar function: Romberg test negative, no clumsiness of movement, coordination normal
   d. Motor: no atrophy, tremors, or weakness
   e. Muscle tone: no flaccidity, rigidity, or spasticity
   f. Muscle strength: +5 (on a scale of 0 to +5)
   g. Sensory function: light touch, pain, vibration and position sense normal; stereognosis and graphesthesia normal bilaterally
   h. Reflexes: deep tendon reflexes +2 (on a scale of 0 to +4) (brachioradialis, biceps, triceps, patella, ankle); superficial reflexes present (abdominal, cremasteric); plantar reflexes normal (toes flex)

10. Gerontologic considerations
    a. Many elderly clients exhibit moderate recent memory loss.
    b. The sense of smell tends to become less keen with aging.
    c. Common age-related vision changes include diminished peripheral vision, color discrimination (especially greens and blues), pupil size, accommodation, and upward gaze.
    d. Many elderly clients experience moderate hearing loss (particularly of high-frequency sounds) and diminished ability for sound discrimination. These changes may interfere with the ability to follow instructions associated with testing; the elderly client may need more time to respond or react to verbal stimuli.
    e. Age-related changes in cerebellar function may include drifting during the Romberg test; wide-based, slowed

gait; and diminished sense of equilibrium, especially when moving rapidly.

    f. Elderly clients commonly exhibit some degree of muscle atrophy and decreased muscle strength.

    g. Age-related sensory changes may include diminished pain perception and diminished sense of touch, temperature, vibration, and position.

    h. Reflexes commonly diminish or subside.

VI. Laboratory studies: The third part of a complete health assessment, laboratory study results fall into three basic categories: urinalysis, hematology, and blood chemistry. Normal value ranges may vary according to a health care institution's policies and standards.

A. Urinalysis

    1. Protein

        a. Normal values in young adults range from 0 to 5 mg/100 mL.

        b. Normal values rise slightly with aging.

    2. Glucose

        a. Normal values in young adults range from 0 to 15 mg/100 mL.

        b. Normal values decline slightly with aging.

    3. Specific gravity

        a. Normal value in young adults is 0.032.

        b. Normal value declines to 1.024 by age 80.

B. Hematology

    1. Hemoglobin (Hgb)

        a. Normal values: men, 13 to 18 g/100 mL; women, 12 to 16 g/100 mL

        b. Normal value drops by 1 to 2 g/100 mL in elderly men; no change documented in elderly women.

    2. Hematocrit (Hct)

        a. Normal values: men, 45% to 52%; women, 37% to 48%

        b. Specific changes in elderly are not documented to date; a slight decline has been hypothesized.

    3. Leukocytes (white blood cells [WBC])

        a. Normal values in young adults range from 4300 to 10,800/mm^3.

        b. Total count drops to 3100 to 9000/mm^3 with aging.

    4. Lymphocytes

        a. Normal values in young adults: T-lymphocytes, 500 to 2400/mL; B-lymphocytes, 50 to 200/mL

        b. Both T- and B-lymphocyte counts drop somewhat in elderly clients.

5. Platelets
   a. Normal values range from 150,000 to 350,000/mm^3.
   b. No changes in platelet number have been detected in elderly clients, but changes in platelet characteristics have been documented.
6. Prothrombin time (PT)
   a. Normal time ranges from 11 to 15 seconds.
   b. No change has been identified in healthy elderly clients.

C. Blood chemistry

1. Albumin
   a. Normal values range from 3.5 to 5.0 g/100 mL; before age 65, the level tends to be higher in men than in women.
   b. After age 65, values equalize and decline at the same rate; however, this rate of decline has not been documented.
2. Beta globulin
   a. Normal values range from 2.3 to 3.5 g/100 mL.
   b. Normal values increase slightly with aging.
3. Total serum protein
   a. Normal values range from 6.0 to 8.4 g/100 mL.
   b. No change has been identified in elderly clients; increased beta globulin balances decreased albumin.
4. Sodium
   a. Normal values range from 135 to 145 mEq/L.
   b. No change has been identified in elderly clients.
5. Potassium
   a. Normal values range from 3.5 to 5.5 mEq/L.
   b. Normal value increases slightly in elderly clients.
6. Carbon dioxide
   a. Normal values range from 24 to 30 mEq/L.
   b. No change has been identified in elderly clients.
7. Chloride
   a. Normal values range from 100 to 106 mEq/L.
   b. No change has been identified in elderly clients.
8. Blood urea nitrogen (BUN)
   a. Normal values: men, 10 to 25 mg/100 mL; women, 8 to 20 mg/100 mL
   b. Values increase in elderly clients; sometimes as high as 69 mg/100 mL.
9. Creatinine
   a. Normal values range from 0.6 to 1.5 mg/100 mL.
   b. Increases in elderly men sometimes as high as 1.9 mg/100 mL.
10. Creatinine clearance
    a. Normal values range from 104 to 125 mL/min.

      b.   Formula for calculating age-referenced interval in men: 140 minus age times body weight (in kg), divided by 72 times serum creatinine; in women, age-referenced interval is 85% of this figure.

11.   Glucose tolerance
    a.   Normal findings: 1 hour, < 170 mg/100 mL; 2 hours, < 125 mg/100 mL; 3 hours, fasting level
    b.   In elderly clients, the fasting plasma glucose level rises more quickly in the first 2 hours, then drops to baseline more slowly.

12.   Triglycerides
    a.   Normal values in younger adults range from 40 to 150 mg/100 mL.
    b.   Normal values in elderly clients range from 20 to 200 mg/100 mL.

13.   Cholesterol
    a.   Normal values range from 120 to 220 mg/100 mL.
    b.   In men, values tend to increase up to age 50, then decrease. In women, values tend to be lower than those in men until age 50, then higher up to to age 70; values decrease after age 70.

14.   High-density lipoproteins (HDL)
    a.   Normal values range from 80 to 310 mg/100 mL; values are consistently higher in women than in men.
    b.   This difference diminishes with aging.

15.   Thyroxine (T_4)
    a.   Normal values range from 4.5 to 13.5 mcg/100 mL.
    b.   Values decrease by about 25% in elderly clients.

16.   Triiodothyronine (T_3)
    a.   Normal values range from 90 to 230 mg/100 mL.
    b.   Values decrease by about 25% in elderly clients.

17.   Thyroid-stimulating hormone (TSH)
    a.   Normal values range from 0.5 to 5.0 mcg U/mL.
    b.   Values increase slightly in elderly clients.

18.   Alkaline phosphatase
    a.   Normal values range from 13 to 39 IU/L.
    b.   Values increase by 8 to 10 IU/L in elderly clients.

19.   Acid phosphatase
    a.   Normal values: young men, 0.13 to 0.63 U/mL; young women, 0.01 to 0.56 U/mL
    b.   No age-related changes have been identified.

20.   Aspartate aminotransferase (ALT), formerly SGOT
    a.   Normal values range from 0 to 40 U/L.
    b.   No age-related changes have been identified.

21. Creatinine kinase (CK)
  a. Normal values range from 17 to 148 U/L.
  b. Values increases slightly in elderly clients.

22. Lactate dehydrogenase (LDH)
  a. Normal values range from 45 to 90 U/L.
  b. Values increase slightly in elderly clients.

Bibliography

American Nurses Association. (1991). *Standards of nursing practice.* Kansas City, MO: American Nurses Association.

Bates, B. (1995). *A guide to physical examination and history taking* (6th ed.). Philadelphia: J. B. Lippincott.

Bolander, V. R. (1994). *Sorensen & Luckmann's basic nursing: A psychophysiologic approach* (3rd ed.). Philadelphia: W. B. Saunders.

Carnevali, D. L., & Patrick, M. (1993). *Nursing management for the elderly* (3rd ed.). Philadelphia: J. B. Lippincott.

Malasanos, L., Barkauskas, V., & Stoltenberg-Allen, K. (1990). *Health assessment* (4th ed.). St. Louis: C. V. Mosby.

Nettina, S. (1996). *The Lippincott manual of nursing practice* (6th ed.). Philadelphia: Lippincott-Raven Publishers.

Smeltzer, S. C., & Bare, B. G. (1996). *Brunner and Suddarth's textbook of medical-surgical nursing* (8th ed.). Philadelphia: Lippincott-Raven Publishers.

U.S. Department of Health and Human Services, Public Health Service, National Institutes of Health. (1988). *Report of the Joint National Committee on Detection, Evaluation, and Treatment of High Blood Pressure.* NIH Publication No. 88-1088.

STUDY QUESTIONS

1. To give accountable care that meets the needs of the individual client, the nurse uses a problem-solving method that includes which of the following steps?
   a. assessment, planning, nursing action, evaluation
   b. planning, intervention, evaluation, reassessment
   c. assessment, analysis and diagnosis, planning, implementation, evaluation
   d. analysis, diagnosis, planning, implementation, evaluation

2. A client has come to the nursing clinic for a comprehensive health assessment. Which of the following statements would be the best way to end the history interview?
   a. "What brought you to the clinic today?"
   b. "Would you describe your overall health as good?"
   c. "Do you understand what is happening?"
   d. "Is there anything else you would like to tell me?"

3. A client has come to the nursing clinic for a blood pressure check. Based on readings of 150/86 mmHg, how would you classify the client's blood pressure?
   a. systolic borderline; diastolic normal
   b. systolic normal; diastolic high normal
   c. systolic hypertensive; diastolic high normal
   d. systolic borderline; diastolic high normal

4. After examining the client's mouth and pharynx, the nurse records the following assessment data: "No lesions of lips, gums, tongue, or buccal mucosa. Pharynx not injected (congested); tonsils nonobstructing; uvula in midline; palate elevates symmetrically on phonation." Which of the following statements represents the best critique of this summary?
   a. It is a complete, concise recording.
   b. It lacks important data.
   c. It is biased.
   d. It uses inappropriate terminology.

5. Documentation of skin assessment for an 80-year-old male client reads as follows: "Brownish, oily, wartlike lesions 1 cm or smaller interspersed with dark red papules scattered over anterior and posterior torso. Skin dry with poor turgor. Hair distribution over extremities sparse with bristly hairs in ears and nose. Nails horny. Mucous membranes pale." Which of the following statements provides the best analysis of this data?
   a. The client's skin characteristics are common in men aged 80.
   b. The client is dehydrated and anemic.
   c. The description of the lesions is highly indicative of malignancy.
   d. Descriptions of hair and nails do not belong in a skin assessment.

6. When performing a routine blood pressure check in an elderly man, the nurse measures blood pressure with the client in which position(s)?
   a. lying down
   b. sitting
   c. lying down and sitting
   d. lying down, sitting, and standing

7. When teaching breast self-examination to a woman, the nurse should stress which of the following points?
   a. Half of all breast cancer deaths occur in women between ages 35 and 45.
   b. The "tail of Spence" area must be included in self-examination.
   c. The position of choice for the breast self-examination is supine.
   d. The woman should place a pad under the contralateral scapula of the breast being palpated.

8. A client has come to the nursing clinic for a routine health assessment. To prevent discomfort and injury during otoscopic examination, which of the following should be avoided?
   a. tipping her head away from the examiner and pulling her ear up and back
   b. inserting the otoscope inferiorly into the distal portion of the external canal
   c. inserting the otoscope superiorly into the proximal two thirds of the external canal
   d. bracing the examiner's hand against the client's head

9. To avoid a reflex drop in pulse rate or blood pressure in a 40-year-old client, where should the nurse assess the carotid pulse?
   a. at the suprasternal notch
   b. at the angle of the jaw
   c. lateral to the esophagus
   d. well below the upper border of the thyroid cartilage

10. Which of the following examinations requires the nurse to wear gloves?
    a. oral
    b. ophthalmic
    c. breast
    d. integument

11. To ensure a client's safety during the Romberg test, which of the following measures should the nurse take?
    a. Stand close to provide support if the client loses balance.
    b. Allow the client to keep eyes open.
    c. Allow the client to brace himself or herself by spreading the feet apart.
    d. Instruct the client to hang on to a piece of furniture.

12. During abdominal examination, the nurse performs the four physical examination techniques in what sequence?
    a. auscultation immediately after inspection and before palpation and percussion
    b. percussion, then follow with inspection, auscultation, and palpation
    c. palpate first, then inspect, percuss, and auscultate
    d. the standard sequence—inspection, palpation, percussion, and auscultation

13. A 75-year-old client was hospitalized with a diagnosis of presumptive pneumonia. Which of the following data would the nurse be most concerned with when completing the nursing assessment?
    a. The client is alert and oriented to date, time, and place.
    b. The client has clear breath sounds and nonproductive cough.
    c. The client has buccal cyanosis and capillary refill greater than 3 seconds.
    d. The client has Hgb 13 g/100 mL; Hct 46%: and leukocyte count of 4300/mL.

14. During the nursing assessment, which of the following data represents information concerning health beliefs?
    a. use of prescribed and over-the-counter medications
    b. promotive, preventive, and restorative health practices
    c. educational level and financial status
    d. family role and relationship patterns

15. A 45-year-old client is admitted for a total knee replacement. Which of the following abnormal laboratory data would the nurse report to the physician?
    a. WBC count 14,000/mm^3
    b. Hct 45%
    c. platelets 175,000/mm^3
    d. potassium 3.7 mEq/L

ANSWER KEY

1. **Correct response: c**
   The five steps of the nursing process represent the most recent evolution in the definition of the nursing process and are the framework used for organizing the NCLEX-RN test. Some experts still define the nursing process in four steps: assessment, planning, implementation, and evaluation.
   a, b, and d. These responses do not include all steps of the nursing process.
   Knowledge/Safe care/Assessment

2. **Correct response: d**
   This allows the client to end the interview by discussing feelings and concerns.
   a. This is an ambiguous question to which the client might answer, "my car" or any similarly disingenuous reply.
   b. This is a leading question that puts words in the client's mouth.
   c. This is a yes/no question that can elicit little information from the client.
   Application/Psychosocial/Assessment

3. **Correct response: d**
   The Joint National Committee on High Blood Pressure uses the following guidelines to classify blood pressure:
   ▶ Diastolic: normal pressure, below 85 mmHg; high normal pressure, 85 to 89 mmHg; mild hypertension, 90 to 104 mmHg; moderate hypertension, 105 to 114 mmHg; severe hypertension, 115 mmHg or above
   ▶ Systolic (when diastolic is below 90 mmHg): normal, below 140 mmHg; borderline isolated systolic hypertension, 140 to 159 mmHg; isolated systolic hypertension, 160 mmHg or above.
   Comprehension/Health promotion/Implementation

4. **Correct response: b**
   This summary lacks data about the tongue surface, whether the tongue has tremors at rest or with protrusion, salivary gland condition, condition of teeth, and presence or absence of the gag reflex.
   a. The summary is not complete.
   c. It is not biased because the data listed are presented objectively.
   d. The terminology used is appropriate.
   Analysis/Physiologic/Assessment

5. **Correct response: a**
   All these findings are normal in elderly men.
   b. Because poor turgor and pale mucous membranes are normal age-related changes, they do not necessarily indicate dehydration and anemia.
   c. The lesions described (seborrheic keratoses and cherry angiomas) are benign and commonly seen on aging skin.
   d. Skin assessment includes hair, nails, and mucous membranes.
   Analysis/Physiologic/Assessment

6. **Correct response: d**
   Elderly clients should have blood pressure checked when lying, sitting, and standing to detect excessive postural hypotension, a common age-related manifestation.
   Comprehension/Health promotion/Implementation

7. **Correct response: b**
   The tail of Spence, an extension of the upper outer quadrant of breast tissue, can develop breast tumors.
   a. Half of breast cancer deaths occur in women over age 65.
   c. The correct position for breast self-examination is not limited to just the supine position; the sitting position with hands at sides, above head, and on hips is also recommended.
   d. A pad is placed under the ipsilateral (same side) scapula of the breast being palpated.
   Knowledge/Health promotion/Implementation

8. *Correct response: c*
In the superior position, the speculum of the otoscope is nearest the tympanic membrane, and the most sensitive portion of the external canal is the proximal two thirds. Therefore, it is important to avoid these structures in the examination.
a, b, and d. All other techniques listed are safe and appropriate.
Application/Safe care/Assessment

9. *Correct response: d*
By palpating well below the upper border of the thyroid cartilage, the carotid sinus will be avoided.
a, b, and c. The suprasternal notch, jaw, and esophagus are not landmarks associated with locating the carotid artery.
Application/Physiologic/Assessment

10. *Correct response: a*
Oral, rectal, and genital examinations require gloves because these examinations involve contact with body fluids.
b, c, and d. These examinations normally do not involve contact with the client's body fluids and thus do not require the nurse to wear gloves for protection. If there are areas of skin breakdown or drainage the nurse should use gloves.
Application/Safe care/Assessment

11. *Correct response: a*
During the Romberg test, the client is asked to stand with feet together and eyes shut and still maintain balance with a minimum of sway. Should the client lose his or her balance, having your arm close around the shoulder will prevent a fall.
b, c, and d. These actions all would interfere with the proper execution of the test.
Application/Self care/Assessment

12. *Correct response: a*
In abdominal assessment, auscultating before palpating and percussing avoids altering bowel sounds through manipulation.
b. Although the bladder should be empty for an abdominal examination, percussion does not precede inspection and auscultation; therefore, this answer is incorrect.
c. This answer is incorrect because tender areas are always palpated last.
d. This answer is incorrect because the usual sequence of examination is altered in an abdominal assessment.
Application/Physiologic/Assessment

13. *Correct response: c*
Buccal cyanosis and capillary refill greater than 3 seconds are indicative of decreased oxygen to the tissues, which requires immediate intervention.
a, b, and d. These are all normal data and do not require nursing intervention.
Application/Physiologic/Evaluation

14. *Correct response: b*
The health beliefs assessment includes expectations of health care; promotive, preventive, and restorative practices such as breast self-examination, testicular examination, and seat belt use; and how the client perceives illness.
a, c, and d. These data assess personal habits and role and relationship patterns.
Comprehension/Health promotion/Assessment

15. *Correct response: a*
Normal leukocyte, or white blood cell (WBC), count is 4300–10,800/mm^3. A WBC of 14,000/mm^3 indicates an infection which would need to be evaluated before a client undergoes elective total knee replacement surgery.
b, c, and d. All of these data are within normal limits for a 45-year-old client.
Application/Physiologic/Planning

Client Education

I. Essential concepts

A. Philosophy

1. Client education is an ongoing process of assisting a person to incorporate learned health-related behaviors into his or her lifestyle.

2. Client education is an integral component of comprehensive health care.

3. Teaching is a form of communication directed toward providing instruction and imparting knowledge.

4. Learning involves gaining knowledge or skills that can modify behavior.

5. All interactions between health care providers and clients and their families or significant others contribute to the process and objectives of teaching and learning.

6. Effective teaching incorporates:
   a. Recognizing clients' and families' or significant others' perceptions of learning needs
   b. Setting priorities for learning
   c. Addressing quality of life issues

 7. **The 1991 American Nurses Association *Standards of Nursing Practice* defines health education as an essential component of nursing care directed toward promotion, maintenance, and restoration of health and adaptation to residual effects of illness.**

8. Nurse practice acts have clarified professional responsibility to provide client education.

 9. **Basic standards of nursing practice encompass:**
   a. **Commitment to client care and well-being**
   b. **Broad knowledge and experiential base in both wellness and illness**
   c. **Integration of education into a total approach to client care**
   d. **Promotion of health in individuals, families, and communities**

10. The Patient's Bill of Rights, developed by the American Hospital Association, established standards for health care, including recognition of clients' right to information and promotion of their participation in health care.

11. Mounting evidence indicates that clients' health knowledge may be instrumental in decreasing length of hospital stays and frequency of readmission for the same condition.

B. **Trends in client education**
   1. Milestones in the health promotion movement include the following:
      a. Halbert Dunn's 1959 Theory of High Level Wellness stated that there is more than one optimal level of wellness; each person has the potential to achieve his or her own personal level of wellness.
      b. The World Health Organization, in 1974, defined health as a state of complete physical, mental, and social well-being, not merely as the absence of disease or infirmity.
      c. Over the past two decades in the United States, the focus of public health policy has shifted from disease treatment to disease prevention and health promotion.
      d. Published in 1980 by the Office of the Surgeon General, *Promoting Health/Preventing Disease: Objectives for the Nation* focused on health promotion, health protection, and preventive health services.

e. Published in 1991, *Healthy People 2000* proposed a set of national goals for improving the health of Americans in the 21st century.

2. Wellness programs now are promoted throughout the country in both community and corporate settings.

3. Self-responsibility for health is increasingly promoted in the media as more links are established between lifestyle and disease.

4. Today's better-informed health care consumer expects more sophisticated care and health education.

5. Increased longevity expands the population needing health education.

6. The advent of the current prospective payment system (diagnosis-related groups [DRGs]) has resulted in higher acuity of hospitalized clients and earlier discharge, leading to changes in home care and education needs.

7. Advances in self-testing and self-monitoring equipment and treatment modalities available for home use require more extensive education of clients and family members.

8. More complex testing (e.g., MRI, CT) necessitates increasingly detailed client education and preparation.

C. Health education needs

1. Health education needs vary according to client population.

2. Needs of the well population include information on:
   a. Health maintenance
   b. Promoting a higher level of wellness
   c. Illness prevention
   d. Recognizing early warning signs of illness
   e. Treatment for medical emergencies
   f. Recognizing and treating tobacco, alcohol, and/or drug abuse
   g. Proper nutritional habits
   h. Weight control
   i. A regular exercise program
   j. Stress management
   k. Breast self-examination or testicular self-examination
   l. Over-the-counter and "street" drugs

3. Needs of the episodically ill or acutely ill population include information on:
   a. Pathophysiology and cause of the condition and ways to prevent or minimize recurrence
   b. Self-care measures, including use of prescription and over-the-counter medications
   c. Necessary procedures and treatments, including purpose and expectations

          d.   Expectations for convalescence (e.g., length of hospitaliza-tion, schedule for resuming normal activities)
          e.   Possible long-term effects of illness, likelihood of recurrence
          f.   Follow-up care
          g.   Appropriate items listed under well population education needs above

    4.   Needs of the chronically ill population include information on:
          a.   Management of illness
          b.   Promotion of optimal level of functioning; necessary lifestyle modifications
          c.   Pathophysiology and cause of disease, its treatment, and preventive measures
          d.   Disease complications
          e.   Measures to prevent acute episodes
          f.   Appropriate items listed under well population education needs above

D. **Characteristics of adult learners**
    1.   Assumptions about adult learners, based on the "andragogy" theory of adult learners (Knowles et al., 1984), include the fol-lowing:
          a.   They are self-directed.
          b.   They enter educational activity with more and different experiences than younger learners.
          c.   They are ready to learn when they need information to perform more effectively in some aspect of life, to cope more effectively in some aspect of life, or to cope more ef-fectively with a situation.
          d.   They enter educational activities with a life-centered (task-centered, problem-centered) orientation to learning.
          e.   They are motivated by internal needs (e.g., self-esteem, increased job satisfaction, better quality of life, greater self-confidence, self-actualization).
    2.   Elements important to adult education include:
          a.   A climate conducive to learning: a comfortable physical environment, mutual respect and trust, collaborativeness, supportiveness and humanness, openness and authenticity
          b.   Learner involvement in identifying learning needs
          c.   Learner involvement in formulating learning objectives
          d.   Learner involvement in designing learning plans
          e.   Teacher assistance in carrying out learning plans
          f.   Learner involvement in evaluating learning

II. **Learning process**
  A. **Readiness for learning**
    1.   A client's readiness for learning depends on physical and emo-tional adaptation to illness, recognition of needs, and level of cognition.

2. **Basic physical needs (e.g., food, sleep, comfort) *must* be met before learning can occur.**

3. Learning is reduced when the environment is not conducive to focusing on tasks (e.g., sensory underload or overload).

4. Emotional needs must be recognized and addressed, such as anxiety, fear, distrust, anger, depression.

5. Learning readiness also depends on mastery of emotional, physical, and psychologic tasks essential for development.

6. Emotional maturity is measured by Erikson's developmental stages, which outline tasks specific to each maturation period. Tasks that are not completed at each stage may affect the individual's adjustment to life crises and ability to learn. The developmental tasks are:

   a. Infant: trust vs. mistrust
   b. Toddler: autonomy vs. shame and doubt
   c. Preschooler: initiative vs. guilt
   d. School-aged child: industry vs. inferiority
   e. Adolescent: identity vs. role confusion
   f. Young adult: intimacy vs. isolation
   g. Middle-aged adult: generativity vs. stagnation
   h. Older adult: integrity vs. despair

7. The stress of hospitalization may result in regression to an earlier developmental stage.

8. Jean Piaget, another developmental theorist, proposed two stages of cognition necessary for adults to accommodate and assimilate new information:

   a. The *concrete stage* (approximately first grade to early adolescence), during which the person develops the ability to think abstractly and make rational judgments; concrete objects or observable phenomena must be within sight for this process to occur

   b. The *formal operations stage* (adolescence), during which hypothetical and deductive reasoning develops

B. Motivation for learning

1. Various theories explain the motivations for learning:

   a. *Needs theory:* Maslow's hierarchy of needs implicates the drive to satisfy personal needs ranging from basic survival to self-actualization.

   b. *Cognitive dissonance theory:* Inconsistency experienced in ideas or beliefs creates a tendency to seek resolution of disagreement.

   c. *Attribution theory:* Success or failure is attributed to internal or external, stable or unstable, controllable or uncontrollable factors; locus of control concept is central to the theory.

           d.   *Competence theory:* Persons have a general tendency to strive toward certain types of goals by developing skills or acquiring knowledge.

    2.   The *health belief model* asserts that motivation for learning depends on the person's perception of his or her susceptibility to disease and of disease severity. According to this theory, a person becomes motivated to learn if he or she:

           a.   Believes that he or she is susceptible to the disease in question

           b.   Believes that this disease would have serious effects on his or her life

           c.   Is aware of certain actions to take and believes that these actions may reduce the likelihood of contracting the disease or may reduce disease severity

           d.   Believes that the threat of taking action is not as great as the threat of the disease

C.   Learning styles

    1.   Learning styles refer to a person's preferred method for learning, as influenced by:

           a.   Educational training

           b.   Intelligence

           c.   Personal preferences

    2.   Learning styles can be broadly classified as visual, auditory, and tactile.

    3.   Visual learners learn by:

           a.   Seeing tasks performed

           b.   Reading informational material

           c.   Looking at pictures

    4.   Auditory learners learn by listening to spoken information.

    5.   Tactile learners learn by:

           a.   Performing tasks

           b.   Touching and taking apart or putting together equipment or models

    6.   The nurse can identify a client's learning style by:

           a.   Observing the client's behavior

           b.   Asking the client about his or her preferred methods for learning

           c.   Experimenting with different learning tools

D.   Learning domains

    1.   Learning behaviors fall into three broad *learning domains:* cognitive, psychomotor, and affective.

    2.   Categorizing what a client needs to learn into these domains helps the nurse develop teaching plans and evaluate learning.

3. Tasks to be learned require certain abilities and actions that fall into one, two, or all three of the learning domains. Each domain has specific characteristics necessary for learning.
4. The cognitive domain reflects:
   a. Intellectual ability
   b. Abstract thinking
   c. Knowledge acquisition
   d. Concept development
5. The psychomotor domain includes:
   a. Physical activity
   b. Use of motor skills
   c. Proficiency performance
6. The affective domain incorporates:
   a. Expression of feelings
   b. Expression of attitudes
   c. Expression of beliefs

E. Learning enhancements
1. Ensure optimal learning by arranging for personal pacing, moving at the client's pace and being flexible.
2. Compensate for altered ability to learn in older adults, such as:
   a. Decline in recent recall memory capacity: Use the client's experiences and knowledge from the past as a reference point for addition of new knowledge.
   b. Increased difficulty organizing complex material: Allow the client more time to absorb material; use a stepped approach to learning.
   c. Reduced ability to discriminate between stimuli: Eliminate extraneous stimuli.
3. Clarify structure through such strategies as:
   a. Presenting information in a way that applies to present lifestyle
   b. Creating memorable encounters to reinforce learning
   c. Progressing from basic or easy concepts to more difficult ones
4. Vary the teaching resources used, for example:
   a. Use the client's preferred resources.
   b. Incorporate group discussions to draw on peers' knowledge and experiences.
5. Provide prompt feedback that includes:
   a. Emphasizing abilities
   b. Reinforcing positive learning
   c. Focusing on behaviors, not on progress or personalities
   d. Offering specific suggestions for behavior changes
6. Consider the client's preferred learning style.

F. **Barriers to learning**
1. A low literacy level interferes with a client's ability to read and comprehend written materials.
2. Physical disabilities can hinder learning, including:
   a. Visual impairment
   b. Hearing impairment
   c. Motor deficits
   d. Pain
   e. Chronic illness
3. Socioeconomic or cultural factors that impede learning include:
   a. Beliefs about health and wellness
   b. Cultural and religious beliefs
   c. Support systems and home environment
   d. Financial concerns
4. Communication barriers to learning may include:
   a. Socioeconomic and cultural factors
   b. Inappropriate use of medical or nursing jargon by health care professionals
   c. Language barrier
5. Other barriers to learning may include:
   a. Client fatigue or sleep deprivation resulting from frequently interrupted rest
   b. Overfrequency of scheduled activities
   c. Anxiety resulting from stress of illness
   d. Fear of the unknown (e.g., surgery, diagnosis)
   e. Excessive volume of learning material

III. Teaching process
A. **General principles**

1. **Establish a good teacher-learner rapport by:**
   a. **Developing a trusting relationship**
   b. **Using effective communication techniques (e.g., asking open-ended questions)**
   c. **Understanding the client's unique cultural or ethnic needs**
2. Plan the best time for teaching by:
   a. Recognizing the client's "most teachable" moments
   b. Scheduling teaching sessions to allow the client adequate periods of uninterrupted rest
   c. Controlling the teaching environment

3. **Use the nursing process in client teaching by:**
   a. **Assessing learning needs, beginning with what the client knows**
   b. **Developing nursing diagnoses to address learning needs**

    c.   **Involving the client and family or significant other in defining outcomes**

    d.   **Planning and implementing the teaching plan**

    e.   **Evaluating learning and teaching**

B.   **Teaching methods**

    1.   For maximum effectiveness, the nurse should match teaching methods to the client's primary learning style (e.g., visual, auditory, tactile)

    2.   Effective teaching methods for a visual learner may include:

        a.   Demonstration

        b.   Role playing

    3.   Effective teaching methods for an auditory learner may include:

        a.   Discussion (individual or group)

        b.   Lectures

        c.   Case studies

    4.   Effective teaching methods for a tactile learner may include:

        a.   Return demonstration

        b.   Practice of learned skills

C.   **Teaching tools**

    1.   The nurse should use teaching tools appropriate to the client's primary learning style.

    2.   Visual tools may include:

        a.   Printed materials

        b.   Transparencies

        c.   Slides and filmstrips

        d.   Videotapes

        e.   Closed-circuit TV

        f.   Physical models

        g.   Computer-assisted instruction

    3.   Auditory tools include audiocassette tapes.

    4.   Psychomotor tools include:

        a.   Physical models

        b.   Disease-specific self-treatment or self-monitoring equipment

        c.   Computer-assisted instruction

D.   **Barriers to teaching**

    1.   Teaching may be impeded by insufficient time resulting from:

        a.   Lack of supervisory support

        b.   Overly heavy workload

        c.   Inadequate staffing

    2.   Another barrier may be the teacher's lack of knowledge and ineffective teaching strategies resulting from:

        a.   Inadequate knowledge base

        b.   Inadequate preparation

        c.   Improper development of teaching objectives

           d.   Overly ambitious presentation
           e.   Lack of family (or others') involvement
           f.   No evaluation of learning outcomes
    3.   Poor communication within healthcare team can cause:
           a.   Improperly coordinated teaching
           b.   Duplication or gaps in material presented
           c.   Inadequate reporting of learning needs and progress
    4.   Communication barriers affecting teaching are similar to those affecting learning.

IV.   Applying the nursing process to client education

    A. **Assessment**

        1.   The nurse assesses the client's readiness for learning by evaluating:
           a.   Personal learning goals
           b.   Stages in adaptation to illness
           c.   Emotional maturity
           d.   Past life experiences with health and illness
        2.   The nurse assesses the client's motivation for learning by evaluating:
           a.   Health beliefs
           b.   Religious and sociocultural practices
           c.   Perception of learning needs; the gap between what the client knows and what he or she wants to know
        3.   The nurse assesses the client's ability to learn by evaluating:
           a.   Physical condition
           b.   Intellectual abilities
           c.   Barriers to learning
           d.   Learning styles
        4.   The nurse collects data by interviewing the client or, if appropriate, family members or significant others.
        5.   Principles of conducting a successful assessment include:
           a.   Setting the stage: Providing privacy, if possible, in a quiet, relaxed environment; minimizing interruptions
           b.   Listening attentively
           c.   Observing the client's nonverbal cues
           d.   Asking open-ended questions
           e.   Evaluating the client's use of terms to help guide the level of teaching
           f.   Having a self-awareness of attitudes and beliefs

    B. **Nursing diagnoses (related to learning)**

        1.   Anxiety
        2.   Impaired Verbal Communication
        3.   Ineffective Individual Coping
        4.   Ineffective Family Coping: Compromised
        5.   Ineffective Family Coping: Disabling

      6.   Decisional Conflict
      7.   Fatigue
      8.   Fear
      9.   Anticipatory Grieving
   10.   Altered Health Maintenance
   11.   Health Seeking Behaviors
   12.   Hopelessness
   13.   Knowledge Deficit
   14.   Noncompliance
   15.   Pain
   16.   Powerlessness
   17.   Altered Role Performance
   18.   Self Esteem Disturbance
   19.   Sleep Pattern Disturbance
   20.   Social Isolation
   21.   Altered Thought Processes

C. Outcome identification

    1.   Formulate learning outcomes.
    2.   Involve the client and family members or significant others in developing outcomes.
    3.   Facilitate realistic outcome identification.
    4.   Use behavioral objectives—measurable statements of expectations.
    5.   Include the three learning domains (cognitive, psychomotor, affective).

D. Planning and implementation

    1.   Develop a teaching plan.
        a.   Base teaching content on learning outcomes.
        b.   Base teaching strategies and tools on the client's primary learning styles.
        c.   Incorporate the client's learning strengths into the plan.
        d.   Involve family members or significant others and members of the health care team in planning.
        e.   Determine teaching priorities; teach survival information, including correct method for medication administration, before discharge from the hospital.
        f.   Develop a contract with the client to achieve learning outcomes.
    2.   Determine teaching content.
        a.   Include what the client needs to know for surviving, maintaining health, and preventing disease.
        b.   Include information about the disorder, its causes, complications, and treatments.
        c.   Include information about tests to be performed.

   d. Include discharge information necessary for self-care and for reporting signs and symptoms of complications.

  3. Implement the teaching plan.

   a. Reinforce positive learning.

   b. Redirect teaching to meet the client's changing needs as teaching progresses.

   c. Promote compliance.

   d. Involve the client and family members or significant others in teaching.

  4. Refer the client and family members or significant others to appropriate agencies or resources for more information and support, as necessary.

E. **Evaluation**

  1. Evaluation involves ongoing assessment of the client's and family members' or significant others' learning.

  2. Purposes of evaluation

   a. To reinforce desirable behavior

   b. To redirect undesirable behavior

   c. To measure the client's progress in achieving learning goals

   d. To provide direction in restructuring teaching strategies

   e. To provide necessary documentation and accountability for quality education

   f. To identify effective and ineffective teaching strategies

  3. Evaluation should determine expected outcomes to be measured in terms of client behavior.

  4. The client's evaluation should cover:

   a. Knowledge

   b. Application of learning

   c. Attitude

   d. Compliance

  5. The teacher's evaluation should cover:

   a. Knowledge

   b. Use of teaching strategies

   c. Use of teaching tools

   d. Effectiveness of teaching

  6. Methods of evaluation include:

   a. Interviews

   b. Direct observation and anecdotal notes

   c. Tests (written or oral)

   d. Checklists

   e. Situation simulation

V. **Documentation**

 A. **Nursing implications**

  1. Enhances interdisciplinary communication

    2.   Identifies teaching content, learning outcomes, client understanding, response to teaching, client progress, and ongoing needs

    3.   Records teaching activity

B. **Healthcare implications**

    1.   Fulfills requirements of the Joint Commission for Accreditation of Healthcare Organizations (JCAHO) and other accrediting, professional, and reimbursing bodies

    2.   Constitutes a legal record of professional care

    3.   Fulfills requirements for quality assurance in health care facilities

Bibliography

American Nurses Association. (1991). *Standards of nursing practice.* Kansas City, MO: American Nurses Association.

Bolander, V. R. (1994). *Sorensen & Luckmann's basic nursing: A psychophysiologic approach* (3rd ed.). Philadelphia: W. B. Saunders.

Knowles, M., et al. (1984). *Andragogy in action: Applying modern principles of adult learning.* San Francisco: Jossey Bass.

Nettina, S. (1996). *The Lippincott manual of nursing practice* (6th ed.). Philadelphia: Lippincott-Raven Publishers.

Rankin, S., and Stallings, K. (1990). *Patient education: Issues, principles, and practices.* Philadelphia: J. B. Lippincott.

Redman, B. (1993). *The process of patient education* (7th ed.). St. Louis: C. V. Mosby.

Smeltzer, S. C., & Bare, B. G. (1996). *Brunner & Suddarth's textbook of medical-surgical nursing* (8th ed.). Philadelphia: Lippincott-Raven Publishers.

Springhouse Corp. (1992). *Patient teaching.* Spring House, PA: Springhouse Corp.

U.S. Department of Health and Human Services, Public Health Service. (1991). *Healthy people 2000: National health promotion and disease prevention objectives.* DHHS Publication No. (PHS) 91-50213.

U.S. Department of Health and Human Services, Public Health Service, National Institutes of Health. (1988). *Report of the Joint National Committee on Detection, Evaluation, and Treatment of High Blood Pressure.*

STUDY QUESTIONS

1. When teaching varied client populations, the education plans are based on specific health education needs. In the teaching plan, the inclusion of which of the following distinguishes the episodically or acutely ill or the chronically ill from the well population?
   a. maintenance of health
   b. promotion of higher level of wellness
   c. discussion of pathophysiology or cause of disease
   d. recognition of early warning signs of illness

2. According to Knowles' andragogy theory of adult learners, the nurse assumes that the adult learner
   a. enters educational activity with fewer and less similar experiences than younger learners
   b. is motivated by external needs
   c. is not self-directed
   d. enters educational activities with a life-centered orientation to learning

3. In which of the following settings is the nurse most likely to teach a client with an acute exacerbation of chronic obstructive pulmonary disease (COPD) about the correct administration of theophylline?
   a. hospital
   b. ambulatory clinic
   c. home
   d. community health clinic

4. In assessing a client's learning needs about in-home oxygen therapy for treating COPD, the nurse first needs to evaluate which of the following parameters?
   a. religious and sociocultural practices
   b. dietary habits
   c. pathophysiology of COPD
   d. comfort level

5. Recognizing that physiologic changes in older adults can affect learning, the nurse should modify client teaching to enhance learning specifically for a 75-year-old client in which of the following ways?
   a. Create memorable encounters to reinforce learning.
   b. Progress from basic to more difficult concepts.
   c. Use resources that are preferred by the client.
   d. Reduce input that requires discrimination between stimuli.

6. For an interview to be successful, the nurse must include which of the following?
   a. evaluation of the client's use of language to guide the level of teaching
   b. closed-ended questions
   c. an active and stimulating environment for learning
   d. attentive listening and close observation for verbal cues only

7. A 75-year-old diabetic client who lives alone must understand at a cognitive level and perform at a psychomotor level well enough to read a glucometer. Which of the following nursing diagnoses would prohibit safe performance?
   a. Impaired Gas Exchange
   b. Sensory Perceptual Alterations: Visual
   c. Anticipatory Grieving
   d. Activity Intolerance

8. The nurse has determined that the client must learn by performing the task. This type of learning is characteristic of which learning style?
   a. visual
   b. auditory
   c. tactile
   d. cognitive

9. When the nurse is assessing physical ability, motor skills, and performance proficiency, which of the learning domains is the nurse assessing?
   a. cognitive
   b. psychomotor
   c. affective
   d. attitude

10. Which of the following needs of the client is most important and must be met before learning can occur?
   a. basic physical needs
   b. emotional needs
   c. psychosocial needs
   d. environmental needs

11. When completing the nursing assessment, the nurse identifies which of the following as a barrier to learning?
   a. high literacy level
   b. financial concerns
   c. English as the primary language
   d. no visual or hearing impairment

12. In evaluating the client's response to a discussion about health beliefs, the nurse recognizes the use of abstract thinking. Which of the following categories does this behavior demonstrate?
   a. attribution motivation theory
   b. cognitive learning domain
   c. generativity
   d. psychomotor learning domain

13. When evaluating the client's learning progress, the teacher's evaluation should include
   a. application of learning
   b. use of teaching tools
   c. client's compliance
   d. ability to redirect undesirable behavior

14. In evaluating documentation of client teaching, the nurse should check that documentation includes which of the following?
   a. assessment of progress toward learning goals
   b. resolution of underlying disease progress
   c. progression of physical therapy activities
   d. ability to perform activities of daily living

ANSWER KEY

1. **Correct response: c**
   This answer is appropriate to a specific illness. To include it in general education of a well population is not appropriate because perception of need to know would not be present.
   a, b, and d. These areas are appropriate for both well and ill populations.
   Comprehension/Physiologic/Planning

2. **Correct response: d**
   According to Knowles' adult learning theory, adults enter educational activities with a life-centered (task-centered, problem-centered) orientation to learning.
   a, b, and c. The adult learner has more and different experiences than younger learners, is motivated by internal needs, and is self-directed.
   Knowledge/Safe care/Implementation

3. **Correct response: a**
   A client with an acute exacerbation of COPD would be hospitalized possibly because of improper medication administration. Teaching in the hospital setting should incorporate survival measures which include proper medication administration techniques.
   Comprehension/Health promotion/Implementation

4. **Correct response: d**
   This assessment evaluates the client's ability to learn at this specific time. If the client is in pain or uncomfortable, learning will not take place.
   a, b, and c. Even though these factors are important in overall assessment, it is more important to determine whether the client is physiologically able to listen and comprehend. Pain and discomfort will affect this ability.
   Analysis/Safe care/Assessment

5. **Correct response: d**
   Older adults often have decreased ability to discriminate between stimuli.

   a, b, and c. These factors are important to the enhancement of learning but are not specific to the older adult.
   Application/Physiologic/Implementation

6. **Correct response: a**
   Components of a successful interview include teaching at the client's level of knowledge. Therefore, the nurse must evaluate the client's language ability.
   b, c, and d. The nurse should ask open-ended questions; provide a quiet, nonstimulating, and relaxed environment; listen attentively; and always observe for nonverbal cues.
   Comprehension/Health promotion/Implementation

7. **Correct response: b**
   If the client cannot see the glucometer clearly, he or she cannot safely perform the glucometer reading needed to administer a correct insulin dose.
   a, c, and d. These factors all have the potential to influence understanding or performance; they do not prohibit or preclude safe performance.
   Analysis/Safe care/Analysis (Dx)

8. **Correct response: c**
   Tactile learners learn by performing tasks, for example, by touching and taking apart or putting together equipment or models.
   a. Visual learners learn by seeing the tasks performed, for example, by reading or by looking at pictures.
   b. Auditory learners learn by listening to spoken information.
   d. Cognitive learning is a learning domain, not learning style.
   Comprehension/Health promotion/Evaluation

9. **Correct response: b**
   Of the three learning domains, the psychomotor domain refers to physical

ability, the use of motor skills, and performance proficiency.

a. The cognitive domain reflects intellectual ability, abstract thinking, knowledge acquisition, and concept development.

c. The affective domain reflects expression of feelings, attitudes, and beliefs.

d. Attitude is not a domain.

Knowledge/Health promotion/ Evaluation

10. *Correct response: a*

Basic physical needs (e.g., food, sleep, comfort) *must* be met before learning can occur.

b, c, and d. These needs should be included when assessing the client's readiness for learning but they are not the most important. In some situations, these needs may not be met but learning can still take place.

Knowledge/Health promotion/ Evaluation

11. *Correct response: b*

Barriers to learning include low literacy level, certain physical disabilities, socioeconomic or cultural factors, communication barriers, and poor timing. Financial concerns are major components of socioeconomic factors.

a, c, and d. These are not considered barriers to learning. High literacy level, English as a primary language in an English-speaking region, and no visual or hearing impairments are positive attributes when teaching a client.

Knowledge/Health promotion/ Evaluation

12. *Correct response: b*

Abstract thinking occurs in the cognitive learning domain.

a. This is an inappropriate answer.

c. Generativity is a developmental stage that is a measure of emotional maturity.

d. This is a learning domain that does not include abstract thinking.

Application/Physiologic/Evaluation

13. *Correct response: b*

The evaluation of the teacher should include the use of teaching strategies and teaching tools and the effectiveness of teaching.

a and c. The evaluation of the client's learning should cover knowledge, application of learning, attitude, and compliance. The client's compliance should not be directly related to the teaching.

d. Ability to redirect undesirable behavior is a purpose of evaluation.

Knowledge/Health promotion/ Evaluation

14. *Correct response: a*

This is an appropriate area in which to document supportive teaching and learning that has occurred.

b, c, and d. These are all important points to be documented but do not address evaluation of client teaching.

Application/Health promotion/ Evaluation

Homeostasis

I. Essential concepts

A. Cellular composition

1. **The nurse must be aware of cellular structure, composition, and function to understand the body's reaction to cell injury and the body's ability to maintain homeostasis.**

2. Cells are composed of protoplasm (75% water, electrolytes, proteins, lipids, and carbohydrates).

3. A cell has three major parts (Fig. 3-1):

   a. Nucleus: the control center for the cell; contains deoxyribonucleic acid (DNA), which constitutes chromosomes.

   b. Cytoplasm: surrounds the nucleus and is where the work of the cells takes place; embedded in the cytoplasm are organelles (ribosomes, endoplasmic reticulum, Golgi complex, mitochondria, lysosomes, microtubules, and filaments)

   c. Cell membrane: a semipermeable structure that separates intracellular and extracellular environments, provides receptors for hormones and other chemical messengers that regulate cellular activity, participates in the electrical events that occur in nerve and muscle cells, and aids in regulating cell growth and proliferation

B. Principles of homeostasis

1. **Homeostasis refers to the state of equilibrium in the body's internal environment—the cells, tissues, organs, and fluids.**

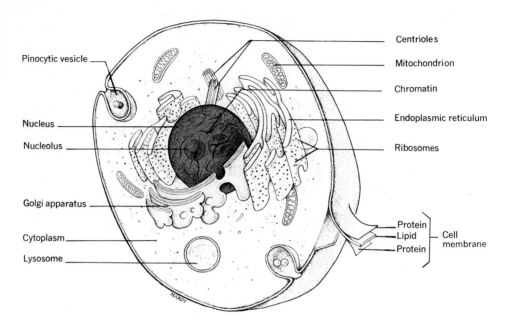

Pinocytic vesicle

Nucleus

Nucleolus

Golgi apparatus

Cytoplasm

Lysosome

Centrioles

Mitochondrion

Chromatin

Endoplasmic reticulum

Ribosomes

Protein
Lipid — Cell
Protein   membrane

FIGURE 3-1.
Cell composite representing the various components of the nucleus and cytoplasm. (From Porth, C.M. [1994]. *Pathophysiology: Concepts of altered health states* [4th ed.]. Philadelphia: J.B. Lippincott.)

2. Maintenance of homeostasis (also called steady state) depends primarily on normal cellular function.
3. Cellular activities related to homeostasis include:
   a. Energy production
   b. Reproduction
   c. Intracellular digestion
4. The control of substances moving in and out of cells is central to maintaining homeostasis.
5. Normal organ function depends on the collective action of the cells that comprise it.

 6. **Homeostasis is constantly being threatened by physical, psychological, and environmental stress. Health represents successful adaptation to that stress.**

C. Cellular repair
   1. During times of stress the cell undergoes changes that permit survival, maintenance of function, and maintenance of homeostasis. Mechanisms of cellular repair include:
      a. Cellular adaptation, which means that cells may adapt by undergoing changes in size, number, and type; adaptation is

the desired outcome in managing actual or perceived stress to reestablish equilibrium

b. Regenerative healing, which occurs when damaged cells and tissues are replaced by new cells and tissues identical to the damaged cells and tissues (e.g., gastrointestinal mucosal cells, epithelial cells of the skin, liver and renal tubule cells after injury)

c. Replacement healing, which occurs with replacement cells such as connective tissue, resulting in scar formation

2. Factors affecting cellular repair include:

a. Age: Elderly clients may have decreased blood flow to skin, organ atrophy and diminished function, and altered immunity; these effects slow cellular repair and increase the risk of infection.

b. Nutritional status: Adequate protein and caloric intake is essential to optimal cellular repair; a person with cellular injury has greater protein and calorie needs.

c. Infection slows cellular repair.

d. Chronic illness: Various chronic conditions can predispose a client to cellular injury (e.g., uncontrolled diabetes mellitus).

e. Nature of wound: Incisional wounds made under aseptic conditions are less prone to infection than traumatic wounds, which typically involve microorganism invasion.

f. Extent of wound and associated blood loss: The greater the extent, the slower the healing process in most cases.

g. Tissue involved: Tissues with good blood supply heal faster (e.g., wounds of the hands and head tend to heal more quickly than those of adipose tissue or lower extremities).

h. Psychosocial factors (e.g., stress, fatigue): These factors can impair healing.

II. Cellular dysfunction

A. Pathophysiology

1. Stress is defined as a state resulting from a change in the environment that is perceived as threatening to homeostasis.

2. A stimulus that evokes this state is known as a stressor.

3. Psychosocial sources of stress include:

a. Daily stressors (e.g., traffic jams, arguments, school difficulties)

b. Major complex occurrences involving large groups or nations; includes events such as war, terrorism, and economic depression

c. Major life events (e.g., death, marriage, birth, divorce, retirement)

4. Physiologic sources of stress include:

a. Hypoxia (inadequate cellular oxygenation): This leading

cause of cell death may result from diminished blood supply to tissue, reduced oxygen-carrying capacity of blood (i.e., hemoglobin), or ventilation-perfusion problems.

b. Temperature extremes (heat or cold): Extreme heat increases metabolic activity of cells, subsequently destroying enzymes and coagulating cytoplasmic protein; cold causes vasoconstriction, which decreases blood supply to tissues, and blood stasis, which may lead to thrombus formation.

c. Trauma: Wounds can disrupt cells and tissues; the outcome of wound healing is related to the type and extent of injury, tissue involved, and mechanism of injury (e.g., blunt vs. penetrating wound).

d. Radiation: Exposure to ionizing radiation can cause cell mutation, damage enzymes, and interrupt cell division.

e. Chemical agents: Various chemicals can injure or destroy cells; damage depends on the nature of the exposure and on cellular susceptibility to the chemical.

f. Infectious agents: Viruses, bacteria, rickettsiae, mycoplasma, fungi, and protozoa may cause disease.

g. Nutritional imbalances: Deficiency or excess of one or more essential nutrients increases stress on cells and tissues.

h. Immune system dysfunction: Immunodeficiency occurs with hypoactivity; hypersensitivity, with hyperactivity.

5. Insults at either the cellular or organ level may result in pathologic (disease) processes.

6. Responses of the internal environment to diseases are termed pathophysiologic processes.

7. The inflammatory response occurs when limits of adaptive capability are exceeded or when no adaptive response is possible; may be reversible or irreversible if cell death occurs.

8. Transient vasoconstriction occurs immediately after injury, followed by vasodilation.

9. Blood flow is increased to the injury site, resulting in local heat and redness.

10. As vascular permeability increases, plasma leaks into inflamed tissues, producing swelling.

11. Swelling causes pressure on nerve endings or possibly direct irritation of nerve endings by chemical mediators such as histamines or kinins.

12. Loss of function usually is attributed to pain and swelling.

13. Plasma elements left in tissue include white blood cells, platelets, and red blood cells.

14. White blood cells (leukocytes) migrate to the injury site; their primary purpose is phagocytosis (engulfing organisms and removing cellular debris).

15. Fibrinogen from leaked plasma coagulates, forming a fibrin wall that helps prevent the spread of infection.

16. Systemic responses to cellular injury include:
  a. Temperature elevation, caused by endogenous pyrogens released from neutrophils and macrophages
  b. Leukocytosis
  c. Malaise, loss of appetite, aching, and weakness

17. Response to cellular injury is either acute or chronic:
  a. Acute responses usually last less than 2 weeks and are characterized by vascular congestion with inflammatory exudate.
  b. Chronic responses, which usually last weeks to months, are characterized by proliferative exudate; a continued cycle of cellular infiltration, necrosis, and fibrosis may cause scarring.

18. Pathologic cellular adaptation results from excessive physiologic stress or pathologic stimuli in effort to preserve the cell; types of maladaptation include:
  a. Atrophy: Cell size shrinks through loss of cell substances; predisposing factors include aging, inadequate nutrition, and diminished workload, such as will occur in paralysis and loss of neural innervation.
  b. Hypertrophy: Cell size increases, resulting in increased organ size; predisposing factors include increased functional demand, as with hypertension, in which the heart muscle enlarges in effort to pump blood more efficiently through vasoconstricted or atherosclerotic arterioles.
  c. Hyperplasia: Number of cells increases in organ or tissue; predisposing factors are related to hormonal influences and tissue removal or destruction (e.g., breast changes in a pregnant female, regeneration of liver cells).
  d. Metaplasia: A reversible change occurs in which one adult cell type (epithelial or mesenchymal) is replaced by another cell type; predisposing factors include stress to highly specialized cells, as occurs with changes in epithelial cells of trachea and bronchi in a habitual cigarette smoker.

B. Assessment
  1. Nursing health history focusing on factors predisposing the client to cellular injury, such as:
  a. Age
  b. Stress
  c. Chronic disease
  d. Current medications and treatments
  e. Nutritional status
  f. Psychosocial status (e.g., ask "Is your household income adequate to secure basic needs such as housing, health care, food, and transportation? Do you have an adequate support network?")

g.   Completion and currency of immunizations

h.   Recent exposures to illness; type of illness and causative agent

i.   Recent travel (In certain areas of the world, particular disorders are endemic.)

j.   Contact with any animal or insect bites

k.   List of drug allergies

2.   *Physical examination* focusing on the following:

    a.   Local inflammation: heat, redness, swelling, pain at injury site, loss of function, or any involuntary cessation of movement

    b.   Systemic inflammation: fever (with agitation, restlessness, diaphoresis, chills); elevated heart and expiratory rate; anorexia and weight loss; malaise and generalized weakness; enlarged lymph nodes

    c.   Nature of wound

    d.   Systems review: abnormal discharge from body openings, skin lesions; changes in normal body functions; characteristics of purulent drainage

    e.   Specific diseases or disorders: for example, in suspected acquired immunodeficiency syndrome (AIDS), assessment would include inspection for signs of Kaposi's sarcoma (typically purple or brown vascular lesions), *Pneumocystis carinii* pneumonia (coughing and shortness of breath at rest), and other opportunistic infections, such as thrush caused by *Candida*

3.   *Supportive diagnostic findings* including:

    a.   Complete blood count (CBC)

    b.   Culture and sensitivity, to determine growth of any microorganisms and evaluate appropriate antibiotic therapy

    c.   Human immunodeficiency virus (HIV) assay

    d.   Electrolytes, blood urea nitrogen (BUN), creatinine levels

C.   Nursing diagnoses

    1.   Activity Intolerance

    2.   Risk for Altered Body Temperature

    3.   Diarrhea

    4.   Impaired Gas Exchange

    5.   Risk for Infection

    6.   Knowledge Deficit

    7.   Altered Nutrition: Less than body requirements

    8.   Pain

    9.   Impaired Skin Integrity

    10.   Social Isolation

D.   Planning and implementation

    1.   Help client avoid infection.

        a.   Use and promote correct handwashing technique (the most important procedure in preventing the spread of microorganisms); wash hands properly after any contact with urine, feces, blood, or other potential infection sources.

b. Wear masks, gowns, gloves, and goggles to prevent the spread of microorganisms.

c. Maintain aseptic technique for all surgical wounds and all indwelling catheters.

d. Monitor for signs and symptoms of inflammation and infection.

e. Administer antibiotics as prescribed.

n ▸ **Assess for allergies.**
  ▸ **After first dose, watch client closely for allergic reaction; after several doses assess for signs of superinfection (thrush, diarrhea, vaginal discharge).**

2. Provide pain relief.
   a. Administer analgesics or narcotics as prescribed.

n ▸ **Assess type, level, and location of pain; rule out complications that require physician's intervention.**
  ▸ **Administer appropriate medication, and institute safety measures.**
  ▸ **Evaluate for effectiveness 30 minutes after medication administration.**

   b. Administer antiinflammatory agents as prescribed.

n ▸ **Administer agent with food to decrease GI distress.**

   c. Position the client to promote comfort.
   d. Teach the client to splint the wound as appropriate.
   e. Elevate the injured area to promote venous return.
   f. After an injury, apply cool packs to the site first, then warm packs, to reduce swelling.

3. Promote adequate nutritional intake.

n a. **Ensure a diet high in protein and calories with vitamin supplements as needed to optimize tissue repair.**
   b. Monitor dietary intake to detect deficiencies.
   c. Monitor serum albumin and total protein levels to identify any nutritional deficits.
   d. Provide nutritional supplementation as necessary.

4. Maintain normothermia.
   a. Monitor vital signs every 4 hours and as needed.
   b. Implement measures to decrease temperature, such as administering antipyretics, reducing the room temperature, and providing tepid baths and cool compresses. (Extreme temperature elevations may necessitate using a cooling blanket.)

      c.   Encourage increased oral fluid intake to compensate for insensible losses (e.g., diaphoresis) as appropriate.

n   **d.**   **Obtain cultures as ordered before administering antibiotics.**

  5.   Maintain skin integrity.

      a.   Promote adequate blood supply to the injury area; avoiding tourniquets and tight dressings.

      b.   Elevate the injured area to increase venous return to the heart, aid wound drainage, and decrease the risk of thrombus formation.

      c.   Prevent pressure points on bony prominences through frequent client repositioning.

      d.   Keep the client's skin clean and dry.

n   **e.**   **Assess the skin every shift for signs of breakdown.**

  6.   Promote adequate rest.

      a.   Cluster necessary activities to allow uninterrupted periods of rest.

      b.   Teach the client energy conservation techniques, such as maintaining good posture and avoiding overactivity.

      c.   Provide bed rest and limit physical activity.

      d.   Limit visitors and long conversations.

  7.   Promote gas exchange.

n   **a.**   **Have the client cough, turn, and do deep-breathing exercises every 2 hours.**

      b.   Have the client ambulate as tolerated.

      c.   Auscultate lung sounds every shift and as needed.

      d.   Assess respiratory rate and pattern and cough.

      e.   Evaluate the color, odor, amount, and consistency of any sputum.

      f.   Monitor arterial blood gas (ABG) values.

      g.   Suction as necessary to clear secretions.

      h.   Monitor capillary refill time, buccal and peripheral cyanosis, and level of consciousness.

  8.   Maintain normal bowel function.

      a.   Assess the usual frequency, character, amount, and consistency of stool.

      b.   Assess for fluid volume deficit.

      c.   Keep the perineal area clean and dry to prevent skin breakdown.

n   **d.**   **Reinforce the principles of handwashing (after each bowel movement).**

      e.   Send stool specimens to the laboratory, maintaining enteric precautions.

      f.   Assess for recent antibiotic therapy and dietary intake.

9. Increase knowledge of HIV (the virus that causes AIDS).

 a. **Review universal precautions with staff.**

   b. Urge the client to use condoms during sexual intercourse and to avoid direct mouth contact with the penis, vagina, or rectum.

   c. Teach the client to avoid sexual practices that cut or tear the rectum, penis, or vagina.

   d. Caution the client to avoid sex with prostitutes and other high-risk persons.

   e. Teach a client who uses intravenous drugs to avoid contaminated needles or syringes.

10. Combat the client's sense of social isolation.

    a. Provide accurate information about disease transmission to allay fears or clear up misconceptions.

    b. Assess the client's normal patterns of communication.

    c. Observe for diminished interpersonal interactions, hospitality, or depression.

 d. **Encourage verbalization of feelings and concerns.**

    e. Collaborate with the client to identify available support systems and effective coping mechanisms.

    f. Provide care in an accepting, nonjudgmental manner.

    g. Provide diversional activities to relieve boredom.

11. Assess discharge needs.

    a. Assess home environment: adequacy of heating and cooling systems, availability of stove and refrigerator, stairs in house and their relationship to rooms used.

    b. Ask about finances: resources available to buy food, medications, and health insurance.

    c. Discuss support system: availability, reliability (family, friends, neighbors).

    d. Evaluate self-care: capability to care for self—prepare meals, bathe properly, administer medications, and ambulate with assistance.

12. Refer for social services, rehabilitation services, or home health care services as needed.

13. Provide client and family education.

    a. Name signs and symptoms of infection to watch for and report.

    b. Explain specifics of any drug therapy; use a medication calendar to describe clearly the drug, its dosage, and the time and length of therapy (for antibiotics).

    c. Define follow-up wound care; instruct on dressing changes and whether it is appropriate to shower.

    d. List activity limitations.

    e. Discuss stress-reduction measures.

   f. Encourage follow-up appointments with the physician.
   g. Talk about maintenance of proper nutrition.
   h. Point out the need to keep all immunizations up to date.

E. **Evaluation**

  1. The client displays no signs or symptoms of infection or inflammation.

  2. The client reports relief of pain; reduction of swelling is observed.

  3. The client maintains adequate nutritional intake.

  4. The client is afebrile.

  5. The client displays no signs of skin breakdown and maintains adequate circulation as evidenced by warm, pink extremities with palpable distal pulses.

  6. The client verbalizes a sense of being rested.

  7. The client's lungs are clear on auscultation.

  8. The client's arterial blood gas (ABG) values remain within normal ranges.

  9. The client regularly passes stools of normal color and consistency.

  10. The client maintains adequate hydration, as evidenced by normal blood urea nitrogen and hematocrit values, and elastic skin turgor and moist mucous membranes.

  11. The client verbalizes knowledge of prevention and transmission of HIV infection.

  12. The client verbalizes diminished sense of social isolation.

Bibliography

Bolander, V. R. (1994). *Sorensen and Luckmann's medical-surgical nursing: A psychophysiologic approach* (3rd ed.). Philadelphia: W. B. Saunders.

Cotran, R. S., Kumar, V., & Robbins, S. L. (1994). *Robbins pathologic basis of disease* (5th ed.). Philadelphia: W. B. Saunders.

Guyton, A. C. (1994). *Human physiology and mechanisms of disease* (5th ed.). Philadelphia: W. B. Saunders.

Paradiso, C. (Ed.). (1995). *Lippincott's review series: Pathophysiology.* Philadelphia: J. B. Lippincott.

Porth, C. M. (1994). *Pathophysiology: Concepts of altered health states* (4th ed.). Philadelphia: J. B. Lippincott.

Rosdahl, C. B. (1995). *Textbook of basic nursing* (6th ed.). Philadelphia: J. B. Lippincott.

Smeltzer, S. C., & Bare, B. G. (1996). *Brunner and Suddarth's textbook of medical-surgical nursing* (8th ed.). Philadelphia: Lippincott-Raven Publishers.

STUDY QUESTIONS

1. The part of the cell that is the control center and contains deoxyribonucleic acid (DNA) is called
   a. nucleus
   b. cytoplasm
   c. cell membrane
   d. protoplasm

2. Which of the following statements about the cell membrane is correct?
   a. It acts as a receptor for hormones.
   b. It extracts energy from nutrients and oxygen.
   c. It governs cell reproduction.
   d. It is involved in the synthesis of nonprotein substances.

3. Which of the following nursing diagnoses would most likely lead the nurse to believe that the client is experiencing a systemic response to cellular injury?
   a. Altered Body Temperature
   b. Impaired Skin Integrity: Actual
   c. Altered Oral Mucous Membrane
   d. Acute Pain

4. The most important factor in preventing the spread of a microorganism is
   a. using correct handwashing technique
   b. maintaining aseptic technique on indwelling catheter insertion
   c. wearing masks, gowns, and gloves when caring for AIDS clients
   d. cleaning blood spills with sodium hypochloride

5. A client is admitted with a hemoglobin level of 6.8, blood pressure 82/50 mmHg, pulse 136, and respirations 32 and shallow. The nurse would base the client's care on which of the following assumptions regarding the probable consequences of clinical status?
   a. vasodilation
   b. GI bleeding
   c. tissue hypoxia
   d. metabolic acidosis

6. Numerous factors can influence cellular repair. In planning care for a client with cellular injury, the nurse should consider that
   a. tissue with adequate blood supply (e.g., adipose tissue) may heal faster
   b. the presence of infection may slow the healing process
   c. nutritional needs remain unchanged for the well-nourished adult
   d. age is an insignificant factor in cellular repair

7. Appropriate nursing interventions for reducing pain due to cellular injury include
   a. administering antiinflammatory agents as prescribed
   b. elevating the injured area to decrease venous return to the heart
   c. keeping the skin clean and dry
   d. applying warm packs initially, followed by cool packs to reduce swelling

8. A client who has been admitted with fever of unknown origin complains of feeling weak and achy and reports anorexia. These symptoms are indicative of
   a. local signs of inflammation
   b. metaplasia
   c. psychosocial stress
   d. systemic signs of inflammation

9. A client who is admitted with bacterial pneumonia is febrile, diaphoretic, and short of breath. The medical history is significant for asthma. Based on these findings, the most important nursing intervention consideration would be to
   a. maintain adequate oxygenation
   b. prevent fluid volume excess
   c. reduce pain
   d. teach risk factors related to AIDS

10. Which of the following statements regarding stress and adaptation is true in relation to planning health promotion strategies?
    a. Health represents a pathologic adaptation to stress.

b. Illness represents an unsuccessful outcome to stress.
c. Sources of stress are always physiologic.
d. The inflammatory response occurs concurrently with the adaptive process.

11. Nursing interventions appropriate for maintaining normal bowel function include:
   a. assessing dietary intake
   b. providing bedrest and limiting physical activity
   c. having the client turn, cough, and do deep-breathing exercises
   d. decreasing fluid intake

12. An appropriate care plan for a hyperthermic client would include
   a. antiemetic administration
   b. axillary temperature measurement every 4 hours
   c. fluid restriction of 2000 mL/day
   d. reduction of room temperature

13. Which of the following terms is appropriate for signifying an increase in the number of cells in an organ or tissue?
   a. atrophy
   b. hypertrophy
   c. hyperplasia
   d. metaplasia

For additional questions, see
Lippincott's Self-Study Series Software
Available at your bookstore

ANSWER KEY

1. *Correct response: a*
   The control center for the cell is the nucleus, which contains deoxyribonucleic acid (DNA), comprising chromosomes.
   b. The cytoplasm which surrounds the nucleus is where the work of the cells takes place.
   c. The cell membrane is a semipermeable structure that surrounds the nucleus and cytoplasm.
   d. The cell is composed of protoplasm.
   Knowledge/Physiologic/Assessment

2. *Correct response: a*
   Cell membrane proteins attached to the lipid bilayer act as receptors for messages that regulate cellular activity.
   b. The mitochondria extract energy.
   c. The nucleus governs cell reproduction.
   d. The smooth endoplasmic reticulum is involved in synthesis of nonprotein substances.
   Knowledge/Physiologic/Assessment

3. *Correct response: a*
   Temperature elevation is caused by endogenous pyrogens released from neutrophils and macrophages.
   b, c, and d. These other diagnoses all represent local responses.
   Comprehension/Physiologic/ Analysis (Dx)

4. *Correct response: a*
   Handwashing remains the most effective procedure for controlling microorganisms and the incidence of nosocomial infections.
   b. Aseptic technique is essential with all indwelling lines, especially catheters.
   c. Masks, gowns, and gloves are necessary only when the likelihood of exposure to blood or body fluids is high.
   d. Spills of blood from clients with AIDS should be cleaned with sodium hypochloride.
   Application/Safe care/Implementation

5. *Correct response: c*
   Tissue hypoxia will result from the diminished oxygen-carrying capacity of the blood (hemoglobin), making the client susceptible to impaired skin integrity.
   a. Vasoconstriction, not vasodilation, would occur.
   b. GI bleeding would be a cause, not a consequence.
   d. Respiratory acidosis, not metabolic acidosis, would most likely occur.
   Analysis/Physiologic/Implementation

6. *Correct response: b*
   Infection impairs wound healing.
   a. Tissue of the head and hand have good blood supply; adipose tissue does not.
   c. Nutritional needs increase for all clients undergoing cellular repair.
   d. Elderly persons have a slower repair process because of diminished organ functioning and altered immunity.
   Application/Health promotion/Planning

7. *Correct response: a*
   Antiinflammatory agents will help reduce swelling and thus relieve pressure on nerve endings.
   b. Elevating the injured area would increase, not decrease, venous return to the heart.
   c. Maintaining clean, dry skin aids in preventing skin breakdown.
   d. Cool packs, not warm packs, should be used initially.
   Application/Safe care/Implementation

8. *Correct response: d*
   Fever, weakness, muscle aches, and anorexia represent systemic signs and symptoms of inflammation.
   a. Local signs and symptoms include redness, heat, swelling, and pain at the area of injury.
   b. Metaplasia is a type of pathologic adaptation in which one cell type is replaced by another.

c. Psychosocial stress may contribute to cellular injury, but no history of this is given.

Analysis/Physiologic/Assessment

9. **Correct response: a**

   Maintaining adequate oxygenation will reduce the risk of physiologic injury from cellular hypoxia—the leading cause of cell death.

   b. This client would be more likely to experience fluid volume deficit due to fever and diaphoresis.

   c. No information regarding pain is provided in this scenario.

   d. Teaching risk factors related to AIDS may be indicated later during hospitalization.

Application/Physiologic/Implementation

10. **Correct response: b**

    Health represents successful adaptation to stress.

    a. This is simply incorrect.

    c. Sources of stress may be both psychologic and physiologic.

    d. The inflammatory response occurs when the limits of adaptive capability are exceeded or when no adaptive response is possible.

Comprehension/Health promotion/ Planning

11. **Correct response: a**

    Assessing dietary intake may help determine if the client is prone to constipation or diarrhea.

b. This would be appropriate for promoting rest.

c. This would be appropriate for promoting gas exchange.

d. Fluid intake should be increased, not decreased.

Application/Safe care/Implementation

12. **Correct response: d**

    Reducing the room temperature may help decrease body temperature.

    a. Antipyretics—not antiemetics—are indicated to reduce fever.

    b. Oral or rectal temperature measurements are generally accepted as more accurate than axillary measurements.

    c. Fluids should be encouraged, not restricted, to compensate for insensible losses.

Application/Safe care/Planning

13. **Correct response: c**

    Hyperplasia is an increase in the number of cells in an organ or tissue, for example, breast changes in a pregnant female.

    a. Atrophy is a shrinking of the cell size through loss of cell substances.

    b. Hypertrophy is an increase in the cell size resulting in increased organ size.

    d. Metaplasia refers to a reversible change in which one adult cell type is replaced by another cell type.

Knowledge/Physiologic/Assessment

Fluid and Electrolytes

I. **Basic concepts**

   A. Composition

       1. **Fluid (water and electrolytes) accounts for about 60% of an adult's total body weight.**

      2. *Intracellular fluid* (ICF) constitutes about two thirds of this amount; *extracellular fluid* (ECF) accounts for the other one third.

   B. Electrolytes

      1. Potassium (K) and phosphate (PO_4) are the major electrolytes in ICF.

      2. Sodium (Na) and chloride (Cl) are the major electrolytes in ECF.

      3. Sodium level is the primary determinant of ECF concentration.

   C. Regulatory mechanisms

      1. Various mechanisms regulate fluid distribution between intracellular and extracellular compartments.

      2. *Osmosis* involves fluid shifting through membranes from an area of low solute concentration to an area of higher solute concentration in the attempt to achieve physiologic balance (homeostasis).

3. *Diffusion* involves fluid movement from an area of high solute concentration to one of lower solute concentration.

4. *Filtration* refers to movement of fluid out of solution in response, for example, to hydrostatic pressure of circulating blood (i.e., pressure of blood pushes fluids and electrolytes out of the vasculature and into the interstitial spaces).

5. *Active transport* is an energy-requiring process that transports ions across the cell membrane against a concentration gradient (e.g., the sodium–potassium pump).

D. **Sources of fluid loss (adults)**

1. Fluid loss constantly occurs as a normal result of body functions.

2. The *kidneys* normally produce a fluid output of 1 to 2 L daily.

3. From the *skin,* sensible losses (visible perspiration) normally range from 0 to 1000 mL/hour, depending on temperature. Insensible losses (water loss by evaporation) equal about 600 mL/day; these amounts increase with fever.

4. The *lungs* cause insensible loss (exhaled water vapor) of 300 to 400 mL/day, which increases with fever.

5. Losses from the *gastrointestinal* (GI) *tract* normally range from 100 to 200 mL/day.

E. **Homeostatic mechanisms**

1. Various organ systems and mechanisms interact to maintain homeostasis—optimal fluid and electrolyte balance.

2. The *kidneys*:
   a. Filter about 170 L of plasma daily
   b. Reabsorb HCO, secrete hydrogen ions in proximal and distal tubules, and produce ammonia (NH_3)
   c. Compensate for imbalances more slowly than the lungs; the kidneys may take up to several days to achieve balance

3. The *cardiovascular system* maintains adequate renal perfusion.

4. The *lungs* work to maintain acid–base balance by controlling carbon dioxide (CO_2) and H_2CO_3 excretion. PCO_2 (partial pressure of CO_2) is the most powerful respiratory stimulant, followed by pH, then PO_2 (partial pressure of oxygen).

5. *Buffers* are chemical systems that maintain body pH (acid–base balance) by inactivating or releasing hydrogen (H^+) ions. The primary buffer system involves bicarbonate–carbonic acid (HCO_3 to H_2CO_3). A HCO_3–H_2CO_3 ratio of 20:1 is necessary to maintain body pH; disruption of the ratio alters pH. Less important buffer systems are the phosphate buffer system (intracellular) and the protein buffer system.

6. The *pituitary gland* secretes antidiuretic hormone (ADH), which promotes water retention.
7. The *adrenal cortex* produces aldosterone, which causes sodium retention and potassium loss.
8. The *parathyroid glands* secrete parathyroid hormone, which regulates calcium and phosphate balance.
9. Normal laboratory values reflecting homeostasis include:
   a. pH: 7.35 to 7.45
   b. PO_2: 80 to 100 mmHg
   c. PCO_2: 35 to 45 mmHg
   d. HCO_3: 22 to 26 mEq/L

II. Fluid volume deficit (FVD)

A. **Description: excessive loss of water and electrolytes in equal proportion; vascular, cellular, or intracellular dehydration**
B. **Etiology**
   1. Inadequate fluid intake
   2. Increased output, for example, because of severe diarrhea, vomiting, or blood loss
   3. Massive third-space fluid shift, such as that which occurs with ascites due to liver dysfunction, pancreatitis, or burns
C. **Assessment findings**
   1. Common clinical manifestations include:
      a. Tented skin turgor
      b. Dry skin and mucous membranes
      c. Postural hypotension
      d. Increased heart rate
      e. Extreme thirst
      f. Change in mental status
      g. Renal shutdown and coma with severe FVD
   2. Laboratory findings may include:
      a. Urine specific gravity above 1.020
      b. Blood urea nitrogen (BUN) elevated disproportionately to serum creatinine
      c. Elevated hematocrit
D. **Nursing diagnoses**
   1. Fluid Volume Deficit
   2. Knowledge Deficit
E. **Planning and implementation**
   1. Monitor intake and output accurately.
   2. Monitor urine specific gravity.
   3. Weigh the client daily.
   4. Take vital signs every shift and as needed (p.r.n.).
   5. Monitor skin turgor.

      6.   Maintain adequate hydration through oral or IV fluid supplementation.

      7.   **Teach the client to change positions slowly to minimize postural hypotension.**

  F. **Evaluation**

      1.   The client exhibits adequate hydration, as evidenced by:

         a.   Elastic skin turgor

         b.   Moist mucous membranes

         c.   Absence of postural hypotension and tachycardia

      2.   The client's urine specific gravity, BUN, and hematocrit levels return to normal ranges.

III. **Fluid volume excess (FVE)**

  A. **Description: excessive retention of water and electrolytes in equal proportion; increased local or total body fluid volume**

  B. **Etiology**

      1.   Excessive fluid intake

      2.   Impaired ability to excrete fluid, such as in renal disease

      3.   Abnormal fluid retention, such as that which occurs in congestive heart failure or corticosteroid therapy

      4.   Excessive sodium intake (IV or oral)

  C. **Assessment findings**

      1.   Clinical manifestations may include:

         a.   Weight gain

         b.   Dependent edema (e.g., in feet, ankles, and sacrum)

         c.   Dyspnea and crackles (particularly in clients with a history of cardiac problems)

         d.   Change in mental status

      2.   Laboratory studies may reveal decreased BUN and hematocrit values.

  D. **Nursing diagnoses**

      1.   Fluid Volume Excess

      2.   Knowledge Deficit

  E. **Planning and implementation**

      1.   Monitor intake and output accurately.

      2.   Weigh the client daily.

      3.   Take vital signs every shift and p.r.n.

      4.   Assess for edema.

      5.   Assess lung sounds; if pulmonary edema occurs, elevate the head of the bed and have the client turn, cough, and deep breathe every 2 hours.

      6.   Teach the client the fundamentals of a sodium-restricted diet, as ordered.

      7.   Administer diuretics as prescribed.

      8.   Restrict sodium and water as ordered.

F. Evaluation

1. The client's weight decreases to preimbalance level.
2. The client's lungs are clear on auscultation.
3. The client exhibits minimal or no edema.
4. The client demonstrates compliance with the prescribed sodium-restricted diet.

IV. Hyponatremia (sodium deficiency)

A. Description: serum sodium level below 135 mEq/L resulting from excessive sodium loss or excessive water gain

B. Etiology

1. Fluid loss, such as from vomiting, diarrhea, fistulas, diaphoresis, diuretic therapy
2. Adrenal insufficiency
3. Syndrome of inappropriate antidiuretic hormone excretion (SIADH)
4. Excessive water gain from intake of sodium-deficient parenteral fluids or compulsive water drinking
5. Water pulled into cells because of decreased extracellular sodium level and increased cellular fluid concentration

C. Assessment findings

1. Clinical manifestations may include:
   a. Anorexia
   b. Muscle cramps
   c. Nausea
   d. Altered level of consciousness: lethargy, disorientation, headache, confusion, convulsions (with serum sodium level below 115 mEq/L)
2. Laboratory studies reveal:
   a. Serum sodium level below 135 mEq/L
   b. Urine sodium and specific gravity levels low if due to sodium loss; high if due to SIADH

D. Nursing diagnoses

1. Fluid Volume Excess
2. Risk for Injury
3. Knowledge Deficit
4. Altered Thought Processes

E. Planning and implementation

1. Monitor intake and output accurately.
2. Weigh the client daily.
3. Assess neurologic and GI status.
4. Administer sodium supplements as ordered.
5. Monitor for signs of fluid volume excess.
6. Infuse hypotonic solutions cautiously.
7. **Maintain seizure precautions.**

8. Restrict fluids, as ordered, if the client is normovolemic or hypervolemic.

F. **Evaluation**
1. The client displays adequate orientation to person, place, and time.
2. The client remains free of seizure activity.
3. The client maintains his or her normal body weight.
4. Serum sodium level returns to normal range.

V. Hypernatremia (sodium excess)

A. **Description: serum sodium level above 145 mEq/L due to a gain of sodium in excess of water or a loss of water in excess of sodium**

B. **Etiology**
1. Water loss, such as from:
   a. Diarrhea
   b. Fever
   c. Hyperventilation
   d. Diabetes insipidus
2. Inadequate water replacement, most commonly due to decreased intake in elderly, cognitively impaired, or comatose clients
3. Inability to swallow
4. Rarely, seawater ingestion or excessive oral or parenteral sodium intake
5. Water pulled from cells because of increased extracellular sodium level and decreased cellular fluid concentration

C. **Assessment findings**
1. Common clinical manifestations
   a. Thirst
   b. Dry skin and mucous membranes
   c. Elevated body temperature
   d. Lethargy and restlessness
2. Laboratory study results include:
   a. Serum sodium level above 145 mEq/L
   b. Elevated serum osmolality
   c. Elevated urine specific gravity

D. **Nursing diagnoses**
1. Risk for Altered Body Temperature
2. Risk for Fluid Volume Deficit
3. Risk for Injury
4. Altered Thought Processes

E. **Planning and implementation**
1. Monitor intake and output accurately.
2. Weigh the client daily.

n

3. Assess vital signs, skin turgor, and neurologic status.
4. **Protect the client from injury by:**
   a. **Repositioning frequently**
   b. **Securing all invasive lines**
   c. **Keeping bed side rails up**
   d. **Keeping bed brakes locked**
5. Encourage increased fluid intake as appropriate.
6. Infuse hypotonic solution as prescribed.

F. **Evaluation**
   1. The client exhibits adequate orientation to person, place, and time.
   2. The client remains free from injury.
   3. The client exhibits normal body temperature and elastic skin turgor.
   4. Serum sodium level returns to normal range.

VI. Hypokalemia (potassium deficiency)

A. **Description: serum potassium level below 3.5 mEq/L**
B. **Etiology**
   1. Inadequate dietary potassium intake
   2. Excessive loss due to:
      a. Treatments, such as carbenicillin, amphotericin B, diuretics, or steroid therapy; parenteral fluid therapy without potassium replacement; gastric suctioning; colostomy and ileostomy
      b. GI disorders, such as diarrhea, vomiting, or fistula
   3. Metabolic alkalosis
   4. Hyperaldosteronism
C. **Assessment findings**
   1. Common clinical manifestations include:
      a. Anorexia
      b. Fatigue
      c. Muscle weakness
      d. Paresthesia
   2. Laboratory and diagnostic test results typically include:
      a. Serum potassium level below 3.5 mEq/L
      b. ECG changes: flattened T wave, prominent U wave, depressed ST segment
D. **Nursing diagnoses**
   1. Risk for Injury
   2. Knowledge Deficit
   3. Altered Tissue Perfusion: Cardiopulmonary
E. **Planning and implementation**
   1. Monitor intake and output carefully.

    2. Infuse parenteral potassium supplement, as ordered; always dilute first, and monitor ECG during infusion.

    3. Teach the client to eat foods high in potassium, particularly if he or she is receiving steroid, diuretic, or digitalis therapy. Such foods include:

        a. Orange juice

        b. Bananas

        c. Cantaloupe

        d. Peaches

        e. Potatoes

        f. Dates

        g. Apricots

F. Evaluation

    1. The client exhibits a normal ECG pattern.

    2. The client demonstrates normal muscle strength and energy.

    3. The client verbalizes understanding of foods high in potassium.

    4. Serum potassium level returns to normal range.

VII. Hyperkalemia (potassium excess)

A. Description: serum potassium level above 5.5 mEq/L

B. Etiology

    1. "Pseudohyperkalemia" from hemolysis of blood sample

    2. Decreased renal excretion due to renal failure

    3. Hypoaldosteronism

    4. Acidosis

    5. Severe tissue trauma (e.g., burns, massive infection)

    6. Excessive intake of potassium supplement (rare)

C. Assessment findings

    1. Common clinical manifestations include:

        a. Muscle weakness, paresthesias, possibly paralysis

        b. Nausea

        c. Diarrhea

    2. Laboratory and diagnostic studies reveal:

        a. Serum potassium level above 5.5 mEq/L

        b. ECG changes: tall, narrow, symmetrically peaked T waves and short Q–T interval with serum potassium level between 5.5 and 7.8 mEq/L; shortened P–R interval, disappearing P wave, and widened QRS complex with continued rise in potassium level

D. Nursing diagnoses

    1. Knowledge Deficit

    2. Altered Tissue Perfusion: Cardiopulmonary

E. Planning and implementation

1. Evaluate all blood samples exhibiting potassium excess for hemolysis.
2. Teach clients at increased risk for hyperkalemia (such as those with renal failure) to avoid potassium-rich foods.
3. Monitor the ECG for abnormalities.
4. Prepare for and assist with aggressive therapy, as prescribed, which may include:
   a. Kayexalate
   b. Parenteral sodium bicarbonate
   c. Parenteral regular insulin and glucose
   d. Dialysis

F. Evaluation

1. The client exhibits normal ECG patterns.
2. The client verbalizes the importance of avoiding high-potassium foods.
3. Serum potassium level returns to normal range.

VIII. Hypocalcemia (calcium deficiency)

A. Description: serum calcium level below 8 mg/dL

B. Etiology

1. Primary or surgical hypoparathyroidism due to thyroidectomy
2. Pancreatitis
3. Inadequate vitamin D intake or synthesis
4. Renal failure
5. Drug therapy (e.g., aminoglycosides, corticosteroids, caffeine)
6. Insufficient calcium intake

C. Assessment findings

1. Clinical manifestations may include:
   a. Tetany (tingling in fingers and circumoral area; muscle spasms associated with pain in extremities and face)
   b. Positive Trousseau's sign (Fig. 4-1) and Chvostek's sign
   c. Seizures due to neuromuscular irritability
2. Laboratory and diagnostic studies may reveal:
   a. Serum calcium level above 8.5 mg/dL
   b. ECG changes: prolonged Q–T interval

D. Nursing diagnoses

1. Risk for Injury
2. Pain

E. Planning and implementation

1. **Institute and maintain seizure precautions.**
2. Administer parenteral calcium, as prescribed, taking precautions to prevent tissue infiltration, which can lead to tissue necrosis and sloughing.

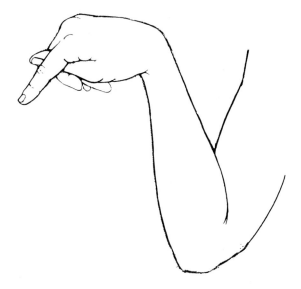

FIGURE 4-1.
In hypocalcemia, Trousseau's sign results after inflating a blood pressure
cuff to about 20 mmHg over systolic
pressure on the upper arm. As the
blood supply to the ulnar nerve is obstructed, carpopedal spasm develops,
usually within 2 to 5 minutes. (From
Smeltzer, S.C. & Bare, B.G. [1992].
*Brunner and Suddarth's textbook of
medical-surgical nursing* [7th ed.].
Philadelphia: J.B. Lippincott.)

3. Do not add calcium to parenteral solutions containing bicarbonate or phosphorus; this will cause a precipitate to form.
4. Administer calcium cautiously to a client receiving digitalis;
calcium potentiates the action of digitalis, increasing the risk
of cardiac arrest.
5. Maintain a relaxed, quiet environment, and promote adequate rest.

F. **Evaluation**
1. The client exhibits no tissue necrosis from IV calcium therapy.
2. The client reports reduced pain from muscle spasms.
3. The client exhibits no signs of seizure activity.
4. Serum calcium level returns to normal range.

IX. **Hypercalcemia (calcium excess)**
A. **Description: serum calcium level above 10.5 mg/dL**
B. **Etiology**
1. Excessive calcium administration or intake
2. Movement of calcium from bones to serum, as occurs in prolonged immobilization and malignant neoplastic diseases
3. Decreased renal excretion due to renal failure
4. Drug therapy with thiazide diuretics
5. Hyperparathyroidism
C. **Assessment findings**
1. Common clinical manifestations include:
a. Anorexia
b. Nausea and vomiting

    c.   Constipation

    d.   Altered level of consciousness: slurred speech, confusion, lethargy, coma

    e.   Polyuria, constipation

    f.   Possibly, renal calculi

  2.   Laboratory and diagnostic tests may reveal:

    a.   Serum calcium level above 10.5 mg/dL

    b.   ECG changes: shortened Q–T interval

D. **Nursing diagnoses**

  1.   Constipation

  2.   Risk for Injury

  3.   Knowledge Deficit

E. **Planning and implementation**

  1.   Provide client teaching on the causes and treatment of hypercalcemia, covering:

    a.   The importance of early ambulation to reduce calcium loss from bones during hospitalization

    b.   The need for daily weight-bearing activities

  2.   Encourage adequate fluid intake and dietary fiber intake.

  3.   **Take injury prevention measures, such as:**

    a.   **Keeping bed side rails up**

    b.   **Keeping bed brakes locked**

    c.   **Repositioning often**

    d.   **Securing all invasive lines**

  4.   Treat the underlying cause, as ordered; therapies may include:

    a.   Calcitonin for hyperparathyroidism

    b.   Mithramycin and corticosteroids for cancers

  5.   Administer parenteral saline solution, as prescribed, to dilute serum calcium and inhibit tubular reabsorption of calcium.

  6.   Administer parenteral phosphate, as prescribed, to enhance deposition of calcium.

F. **Evaluation**

  1.   The client remains injury-free.

  2.   The client demonstrates normal bowel elimination patterns.

  3.   The client verbalizes understanding of hypercalcemia and preventive measures.

  4.   Serum calcium level returns to normal range.

X. **Hypomagnesemia (magnesium deficiency)**

  A. **Description: serum magnesium level below 1.5 mEq/L**

  B. **Etiology**

    1.   Poor nutrition

    2.   Alcoholism

    3.   GI and renal losses without replacement

C. Assessment findings
1. Common clinical manifestations include:
   a. Positive Trousseau's and Chvostek's signs
   b. Tetany
   c. Facial twitching, jerking
   d. Tachycardia
   e. Hypotension
2. Symptoms typically do not occur until serum magnesium level drops below 1 mEq/L.
3. Laboratory and diagnostic tests reveal:
   a. Serum magnesium level below 1.5 mEq/L
   b. ECG changes: flattened T wave, prominent U wave, depressed ST segment

D. Nursing diagnoses
1. Risk for Injury
2. Knowledge Deficit
3. Pain
4. Altered Tissue Perfusion: Cardiopulmonary

E. Planning and implementation
1. Identify dietary sources of magnesium, including nuts, whole grains, cornmeal, spinach, bananas, and oranges; encourage increased intake of these foods.
2. Administer parenteral magnesium replacement therapy as prescribed.
3. **Monitor for signs of magnesium toxicity, including:**
   a. **Hot, flushed skin**
   b. **Diaphoresis**
   c. **Anxiety or lethargy**
   d. **Hypotension**
4. **Institute and maintain seizure precautions.**
5. Monitor ECG and pulse for abnormalities.

F. Evaluation
1. The client remains injury-free.
2. The client displays normal cardiac rate and rhythm.
3. The client verbalizes knowledge of magnesium-rich foods.
4. Serum magnesium level returns to normal range.

XI. Hypermagnesemia (magnesium excess)
A. Description: serum magnesium level above 2.5 mEq/L
B. Etiology
1. Renal failure
2. Overuse of magnesium-containing antacids
3. Excessive magnesium administration
4. Overuse of enemas or laxatives containing magnesium
5. Severe dehydration, such as occurs in diabetic ketoacidosis

C. **Assessment findings**
   1. Clinical manifestations may include:
      a. Hot, flushed skin
      b. Diaphoresis
      c. Hypotension
      d. Lethargy, drowsiness, absent deep tendon reflexes with increasing magnesium level
      e. Possible progression to coma and cardiac arrest
   2. Laboratory studies reveal serum magnesium level above 2.5 mEq/L.

D. **Nursing diagnoses**
   1. Risk for Injury
   2. Knowledge Deficit
   3. Altered Tissue Perfusion: Cardiopulmonary

E. **Planning and implementation**
   1. Teach the client about the adverse effects associated with overuse of magnesium-containing antacids and cathartics.
   2. Instruct the client to read all over-the-counter drug labels carefully for magnesium content.
   3. **Monitor cardiovascular status closely.**
   4. Institute safety precautions, such as:
      a. Keeping bed side rails up
      b. Keeping bed brakes locked
      c. Repositioning often

F. **Evaluation**
   1. The client verbalizes understanding of the adverse effects associated with magnesium overdose.
   2. The client remains injury-free.
   3. The client exhibits normal cardiac rate and rhythm.
   4. Serum magnesium level returns to normal range.

XII. **Metabolic acidosis**

A. Description: an acid–base imbalance resulting from excessive absorption or retention of acid or excessive excretion of bicarbonate (HCO_3)

B. **Etiology**
   1. Ketoacidosis
   2. Lactic acidosis
   3. Prolonged fasting
   4. Salicylic poisoning
   5. Oliguric renal disease
   6. Abnormal HCO_3 losses, which can occur in loss of fluid from the lower GI tract from surgery, drains, or severe diarrhea

C. **Assessment findings**
   1. Common clinical manifestations include:

   a. Headache
   b. Drowsiness, confusion
   c. Weakness
   d. Increased respiratory rate and depth
  2. Laboratory and diagnostic studies typically reveal:
   a. Abnormal arterial blood gas (ABG) values: pH below 7.35 and HCO_3 below 22 mEq/L
   b. Diminished cardiac output with pH below 7
   c. Possible hyperkalemia

D. **Nursing diagnoses**
  1. Risk for Injury
  2. Altered Tissue Perfusion: Cardiopulmonary

E. **Planning and implementation**
  1. Monitor cardiovascular status closely, noting:
   a. Blood pressure
   b. Pulse rate and rhythm
   c. Capillary refill
   d. Warmth and color of extremities

  2. **Institute safety precautions, such as:**
   a. **Keeping bed side rails up**
   b. **Keeping bed brakes locked**
   c. **Securing all invasive lines properly**
  3. When appropriate, administer sodium bicarbonate.

F. **Evaluation**
  1. The client remains injury-free.
  2. The client exhibits adequate tissue perfusion, as evidenced by warm, dry, and normal-colored skin.
  3. Vital signs remain within normal ranges.
  4. ABG values return to normal ranges.

XIII. Metabolic alkalosis

A. **Description: an acid–base imbalance characterized by excessive loss of acid or excessive gain of HCO_3**

B. **Etiology**
  1. Loss of hydrogen and chloride ions due to prolonged vomiting or gastric suctioning (most common cause)
  2. Excessive intake of alkali, as in antacids or baking soda
  3. Any condition that causes hyperventilation

C. **Assessment findings**
  1. Clinical manifestations may include:
   a. Belligerence, confusion
   b. Tetany
   c. Slow, shallow respirations; possibly apnea
  2. Laboratory study results include:
   a. ABGs: pH above 7.45 and HCO_3 above 26 mEq/L

b.   Hypokalemia
D.   Nursing diagnoses
1.   Ineffective Breathing Pattern
2.   Risk for Injury
E.   Planning and implementation
1.   **Institute safety precautions, such as:**
   a.   **Keeping bed side rails up**
   b.   **Keeping bed brakes locked**
   c.   **Securing all invasive lines properly**
2.   Monitor respiratory rate and pattern, lung sounds, skin color, and mental status.
3.   Provide treatment to correct the underlying cause as ordered.
4.   Promote adequate hydration.
5.   Correct electrolyte deficits, particularly of potassium and sodium, as ordered.
F.   Evaluation
1.   The client remains injury-free.
2.   The client's lungs are clear on auscultation.
3.   Respiratory rate and pattern are within normal ranges.
4.   ABG values return to normal ranges.

XIV.   Respiratory acidosis
A.   Description: an acid–base imbalance characterized by increased arterial PCO_2 and decreased blood pH
B.   Etiology
1.   Chronic obstructive respiratory disorders, such as bronchial asthma and emphysema
2.   Acute disorders such as chest wall trauma, pulmonary edema, atelectasis, pneumothorax, drug overdoses, pneumonia, and Guillain-Barré syndrome
3.   Any condition that results in hypoventilation
C.   Assessment findings
1.   Clinical manifestations may include:
   a.   Dyspnea, wheezing, tachypnea
   b.   Tachycardia
   c.   Disorientation
2.   Laboratory studies reveal ABG abnormalities: pH below 7.35 and PCO_2 above 42 mmHg.
D.   Nursing diagnoses
1.   Activity Intolerance
2.   Ineffective Breathing Pattern
3.   Altered Tissue Perfusion: Cardiopulmonary
E.   Planning and implementation
1.   Monitor ABG values.

2. Administer low-flow oxygen therapy to clients with chronic PCO_2 above 50 mmHg (clients who have chronic obstructive pulmonary disease and who have hypoxic stimulus for breathing); assess for adequacy of delivery.

3. Position the client in semi-Fowler's or another comfortable position to ease the work of breathing.

4. Improve ventilation with bronchodilators; postural drainage; antibiotic therapy to treat infection; regular coughing, turning, and deep breathing; and mechanical ventilation as appropriate.

5. Maintain a quiet, relaxing environment; cluster activities to allow for periods of uninterrupted rest.

6. Keep needed items within the client's reach.

7. **Monitor cardiovascular status, noting:**
   a. **Blood pressure**
   b. **Pulse rate and rhythm**
   c. **Capillary refill**
   d. **Warmth and color of extremities**

8. Maintain fluid and electrolyte balance.

9. Intervene to correct the underlying cause.

F. Evaluation
   1. The client displays normal respiratory rate and pattern.
   2. The client exhibits adequate tissue perfusion, as evidenced by stable vital signs and warm, dry, and normal-colored skin.
   3. The client reports no dyspnea on activity.
   4. ABG values return to normal ranges.

XV. **Respiratory alkalosis**
   A. **Description: an acid–base imbalance characterized by decreased arterial PCO_2 and increased blood pH**
   B. **Etiology**
      1. Most commonly, hyperventilation due to anxiety, hypoxia, improper mechanical ventilation
      2. Fever
      3. Salicylate poisoning
   C. **Assessment findings**
      1. Common clinical manifestations include:
         a. Lightheadedness
         b. Inability to concentrate
         c. Convulsions
         d. Positive Chvostek's sign
         e. Muscle twitching
      2. Laboratory studies reveal ABG abnormalities: pH above 7.45 and PCO_2 below 38 mmHg.

D. **Nursing diagnoses**
  1. Ineffective Breathing Pattern
  2. Risk for Injury
E. **Planning and implementation**
  1. Monitor ABG values and respiratory rate and pattern.
  2. **Institute and maintain seizure precautions as necessary.**
  3. Assess sources of anxiety and intervene to help reduce anxiety.
  4. Encourage slow, deep breathing; instruct the client to breathe into and out of a paper bag, if necessary, to reverse hyperventilation.
  5. Assist the client with activities as necessary.
F. **Evaluation**
  1. The client remains injury-free.
  2. The client demonstrates normal respiratory rate and pattern.
  3. ABG values return to normal ranges.

Bibliography

Bolander, V. B. (1994). *Sorensen and Luckmann's basic nursing: A psychophysiologic approach* (3rd ed.). Philadelphia: W. B. Saunders.

Cotran, R. S., Kumar, V., & Robbins, S. L. (1992). *Robbins pathologic basis of disease* (5th ed.). Philadelphia: W. B. Saunders.

Gordon, M. (1995). *Manual of nursing diagnosis 1995–1996.* St. Louis: C. V. Mosby

Guyton, A. C. (1992). *Human physiology and mechanisms of disease* (5th ed.). Philadelphia: W. B. Saunders.

North American Nursing Diagnosis Association. (1994). *NANDA nursing diagnosis: Definitions and classification 1995–1996.* Philadelphia: NANDA.

Porth, C. (1994). *Pathophysiology: Concepts of altered health states* (4th ed.). Philadelphia: J. B. Lippincott.

Smeltzer, S. C., & Bare, B. G. (1996). *Brunner and Suddarth's textbook of medical-surgical nursing* (8th ed.). Philadelphia: Lippincott-Raven Publishers.

STUDY QUESTIONS

1. A client who is admitted with seizure activity has electrolyte values as follows: Na, 115 mEq/L; K, 3.0 mEq/L; Ca, 8.0 mg/dL; and Mg, 1.0 mEq/L. Which imbalances must be controlled to reduce seizure activity?
   a. K and Ca
   b. Na and Ca
   c. Na and K
   d. Mg and K

2. A client is admitted with altered level of consciousness. Laboratory results show pH, 7.28; PCO_2, 20 mmHg; PO_2, 65 mmHg; and HCO_3, 18 mEq/L. The most appropriate nursing diagnosis for this client likely would be
   a. Pain
   b. Fluid Volume Excess
   c. Ineffective Breathing Pattern
   d. Ineffective Thermoregulation

3. Laboratory data on a client show serum Na, 128 mEq/L and K, 3.0 mEq/L. The nurse would evaluate this client's progress based on resolution of which of the following complications?
   a. The client exhibits decreased diuresis.
   b. The client's urine output increases to normal level.
   c. The client demonstrates reduced GI fluid loss.
   d. The client exhibits resolution of diabetic ketoacidosis.

4. Which of the following homeostatic mechanisms help regulate fluid, electrolyte, and acid–base balance?
   a. cardiovascular system
   b. pituitary gland
   c. chemical buffers
   d. renal system

5. A client has a history of COPD; laboratory tests reveal the following ABG values: PO_2, 55 mmHg and PCO_2, 60 mmHg. When attempting to improve the client's blood gas values through improved ventilation and oxygen therapy, the nurse should understand that this client's primary stimulus for breathing is
   a. high PCO_2
   b. low PO_2
   c. normal pH
   d. low PCO_2

6. Evaluation of successful resolution of a fluid volume deficit may be demonstrated by which of the following?
   a. The client demonstrates adequate hydration by an absence of postural hypotension and tachycardia.
   b. The client adheres to prescribed dietary sodium restrictions.
   c. The client maintains weight loss.
   d. The client maintains a serum sodium level above 145 mEq/L.

7. When planning care for a client with hypocalcemia, the nurse's priority consideration should be
   a. the effects of hypoirritability, such as coma
   b. the effects of hyperirritability, such as tetany
   c. the effects of bedrest on calcium levels
   d. the effects of certain medications (e.g., antacids and cathartics)

8. When administering an intravenous electrolyte solution, the nurse should take which of the following precautions?
   a. Infuse hypertonic solutions rapidly.
   b. Mix no more than 80 mEq of potassium per liter of fluid.
   c. Prevent infiltration of calcium, which will cause tissue necrosis and sloughing.
   d. As appropriate, reevaluate the client's digitalis dosage; he or she may need an increased dosage since IV calcium diminishes digitalis' action.

9. Teaching about the need to avoid foods high in potassium would be most important for which client?
   a. a client receiving diuretic therapy

b. a client with an ileostomy

c. a client with metabolic alkalosis

d. a client with renal disease

10. What do the following ABG values—pH, 7.38; PO_2, 78 mmHg; PCO_2, 36 mmHg; HCO_3, 24 mEq/L—indicate?

a. metabolic alkalosis

b. homeostasis

c. respiratory acidosis

d. respiratory alkalosis

11. The major electrolytes in the extracellular fluid are

a. potassium and chloride

b. potassium and phosphate

c. sodium and chloride

d. sodium and phosphate

12. Which physiologic mechanism best describes the function of the sodium–potassium pump?

a. active transport

b. diffusion

c. filtration

d. osmosis

13. Laboratory tests reveal the following electrolyte values for the client: Na, 135 mEq/L; Ca, 8.5 mg/dL; Cl, 102 mEq/L; K, 2.0 mEq/L. Which of these values should the nurse report to the physician because of its potential risk to the client?

a. Ca

b. K

c. Na

d. Cl

14. A client receiving furosemide (Lasix) and digitalis requires careful observation and care. In planning care for this client, the nurse should be alert for one of the following electrolyte imbalances, requiring nursing intervention. Which one?

a. hyperkalemia

b. hypernatremia

c. hypokalemia

d. hypomagnesemia

For additional questions, see
Lippincott's Self-Study Series Software
Available at your bookstore

ANSWER KEY

1. **Correct response: b**
   Hyponatremia, hypomagnesemia, and hypocalcemia all may result in neuro-muscular irritability with seizure activity.
   a, c, and d. Hypokalemia commonly produces arrhythmias, weakness, and anorexia but is not associated with seizure activity.
   Application/Health promotion/Implementation

2. **Correct response: c**
   A pH below 7.35 indicates acidosis. Alteration in PCO_2 points to the regulatory mechanism of acid–base balance—the lungs. Decreased HCO_3 supports metabolic acidosis; decreased PCO_2 supports attempts to compensate. Kussmaul's respirations would be a classic response to metabolic acidosis.
   a, b, and d. These diagnoses would not be expected with metabolic acidosis.
   Application/Physiologic/Analysis (Dx)

3. **Correct response: c**
   Decreased Na and K levels can result from GI fluid loss, as occurs with diarrhea and vomiting. This can lead to cardiac dysrhythmias.
   a and b. Increased fluid output would increase serum Na level.
   d. Decreased renal excretion and acidosis would increase serum K level.
   Analysis/Physiologic/Evaluation

4. **Correct response: d**
   Homeostatic regulators common to fluid, electrolyte, and acid–base balance are the kidneys and lungs.
   a and b. Cardiovascular and pituitary mechanisms are involved in fluid and electrolyte balance only.
   c. Chemical buffers are specific to acid–base balance.
   Application/Physiologic/Assessment

5. **Correct response: b**
   Chronically elevated PCO_2 (above 50 mmHg) is associated with inadequate response of the respiratory center to plasma CO_2. The major stimulus to breathing then becomes hypoxia (low PO_2).
   a, c, and d. These blood gas parameters would not be primary stimuli for breathing in this client.
   Analysis/Safe care/Implementation

6. **Correct response: a**
   This client would exhibit signs of adequate hydration such as stable blood pressure and pulse.
   b and c. Sodium restrictions would apply if the client exhibited fluid volume excess, as would weight loss.
   d. Serum sodium level above 145 mEq/L would indicate hypernatremia.
   Analysis/Health promotion/Evaluation

7. **Correct response: b**
   Hyperirritability, such as tetany, is associated with hypocalcemia.
   a. In contrast, hypercalcemia may result in mental status changes, such as lethargy and coma.
   c. Prolonged bedrest is associated with calcium loss from bones in hypercalcemia.
   d. Antacid and cathartic use may potentiate hypermagnesemia.
   Comprehension/Safe care/Planning

8. **Correct response: c**
   Preventing tissue infiltration is necessary to avoid skin damage.
   a. Hypertonic solutions should be infused cautiously.
   b. Potassium should be mixed at a concentration not exceeding 60 mEq/L.
   d. Calcium (particularly intravenous) potentiates the action of digitalis.
   Application/Safe care/Implementation

9. *Correct response: d*

Clients with renal disease are predisposed to hyperkalemia and thus should avoid foods high in potassium.

a, b, and c. Clients receiving diuretics, with ileostomies, or with metabolic alkalosis all may be hypokalemic and thus should be encouraged to eat foods high in potassium.

Analysis/Health promotion/Planning

10. *Correct response: b*

These ABG values are within normal limits.

a, c, and d. These ABG values indicate none of these acid–base disturbances.

Analysis/Physiologic/Evaluation

11. *Correct response: c*

Sodium and chloride are the major electrolytes in the extracellular fluid.

Knowledge/Physiologic/Assessment

12. *Correct response: a*

Active transport is a process requiring energy to transport ions against a concentration gradient, as is needed in the sodium–potassium pump.

b, c, and d. Diffusion, filtration, and osmosis are other regulatory mechanisms involved in fluid and electrolyte balance.

Knowledge/Physiologic/Assessment

13. *Correct response: b*

Normal serum potassium level ranges between 3.5 and 5.5 mEq/L.

a, c, and d. These Na, Ca, and Cl levels are within normal ranges.

Comprehension/Safe care/
Implementation

14. *Correct response: c*

Diuretics such as furosemide may deplete serum potassium. Additionally, the action of digitalis may be potentiated by hypokalemia.

a. These drugs are not associated with hyperkalemia.

b. Diuretic therapy could cause hyponatremia, not hypernatremia.

d. Hypomagnesemia generally is associated with poor nutrition, alcoholism, and excessive GI or renal losses.

Comprehension/Health promotion/
Planning

Pain

I. Anatomy and physiology of pain

  A. Peripheral nervous system

    1. The peripheral nervous system, including spinal and cranial nerves, carries pain impulses to and from the central nervous system (CNS).

      a. Afferent nerve fibers carry impulses *to* the CNS.

      b. Efferent nerve fibers carry impulses *from* the CNS.

    2. Nerve receptors on the skin surface specific for pain are known as nociceptors.

    3. Various types of afferent nerve fibers conduct impulses from the nociceptors to the spinal cord:

      a. A-alpha, A-beta, and A-gamma fibers (myelinated) transmit touch, pressure, heat, cold, and movement impulses at speeds of up to 120 m/sec.

      b. A-delta fibers (myelinated) transmit sharp, piercing pain impulses at 30 to 60 m/sec.

      c. Type C fibers (unmyelinated) transmit aching and burning pain at 0.5 to 2 m/sec and account for more than two thirds of all fibers in the peripheral nervous system.

  B. Autonomic nervous system

    1. The autonomic nervous system regulates involuntary vital functions. It comprises sympathetic and parasympathetic divisions.

2. This system also contains two types of neurotransmitters, which are chemicals that modify or enable transmission of nerve impulses between synapses.
3. Cholinergic neurotransmitters involve acetylcholine.
4. Adrenergic neurotransmitters include:
   a. Epinephrine
   b. Norepinephrine
   c. Dopamine
   d. Serotonin
5. Sympathetic nervous system functions include:
   a. Fight, flight, or freeze response to alarm or stress (e.g., pain)
   b. Whole person response, by which the body mobilizes defenses in response to stress
   c. Control of the adrenal medullae, sweat glands, blood vessels, and piloerector muscles in hair
6. Parasympathetic nervous system functions include:
   a. Exhaustion or shock response with intense or prolonged stress (pain); triggered when sympathetic system no longer functions
   b. Specific organ responses
   c. Control of many body functions, such as digestion and elimination

C. Central nervous system
1. The CNS comprises the spinal cord and the brain.
2. The spinal cord transmits painful stimuli to the brain and motor responses and pain perception to the periphery.
3. The brain processes and interprets transmitted pain impulses.
4. Spinal cord pathways (nerve tracts) consist of:
   a. Afferent tracts to the brain
   b. Efferent tracts from the brain
5. In the substantia gelatinosa (SG), located in lamina II of the spinal cord's dorsal horn, fibers carrying information about pain from the periphery converge with large fibers and form connections (synapses) with T cells and fibers from the brain that carry inhibitory pain information.
6. The midbrain contains many centers for control, association, and relay of impulses, including:
   a. Reticular formation
   b. Medulla
   c. Hypothalamus: center for brain opiates
   d. Thalamus: relay station and center for perception of pain
   e. Limbic system: center for emotion, responses to environment

7. In the sensory cortex, tactile sensory impulses from the periphery are interpreted and understood.
8. The motor cortex initiates motor responses to data reaching the sensory cortex.
9. The frontal lobes contain areas for:
   a. Attention (an essential component of the pain experience)
   b. Memory
   c. Cognition
   d. Emotion
   e. Decision making

D. Physiology of pain
1. Various models and theories of pain transmission and perception have been proposed.
2. Gate control model
   a. Nerve fibers carry touch and pain impulses from receptors on the skin to the spinal cord.
   b. Nerve cells in the SG of the spinal cord receive these touch and pain impulses.
   c. Impulses then proceed through transmission cells (T cells) to the brain.
   d. Increased input over large fibers (A-alpha, A-beta, and A-gamma) inhibits some pain impulses over smaller fibers (A-delta and Type C fibers); thus, fewer pain impulses reach T cells for transmission to the brain.
   e. Decreased input over large fibers allows more pain impulses to reach T cells.
   f. Fibers from the brain send inhibiting information to the SG, which serves as a gate for control of pain.
3. Central control theory of pain
   a. Some neuropeptides (e.g., substance P) present in the SG seem to be pain-specific neurotransmitters that facilitate pain transmission.
   b. Endogenous molecular neuropeptides called brain opiates (endorphins, enkephalins, and others) are opium-like compounds that have profound analgesic properties.
   c. Specific neuroreceptors bind with morphine and brain opiates.
   d. Certain events or situations trigger the release of brain opiates (e.g., cutaneous stimulation such as massage, electrical stimulation, pain itself, tissue injury, placebos, acupuncture, transcutaneous electric nerve stimulation [TENS]).
4. *Note:* The gate control model and the central control theory overlap somewhat in current thought; however, both are useful.

    5. Specificity theory

        a. This theory posits that pain originates in specific pain receptors, not in free nerve endings.

        b. This theory does not explain pain modulation by variables such as social and cultural factors.

        c. It also does not account for pain syndromes such as causalgia and phantom pain.

    6. Pattern theory

        a. This theory has been proposed because of the inadequacies of the specificity theory.

        b. However, it does not explain psychologic factors related to pain.

    7. Psychologic theories

        a. In many cases, pain results from emotion, hostility, guilt, or depression.

        b. Persons with pain-prone personalities use pain as a means to communicate.

        c. According to the psychogenic theory, pain arises from a perceived threat to self.

II. Overview of pain

A. Description

    1. Features of the pain experience have various facets.

        a. **Pain is subjective and personal; it exists wherever and whenever a client says it does.**

        b. Physiologic pain may sometimes broaden to encompass emotional hurt.

        c. Pain is a symptom, not a disease entity.

        d. Pain is a valuable diagnostic indicator; it usually indicates tissue damage or pathology.

        e. Pain is usually reported as severe discomfort or an uncomfortable sensation.

    2. Components of pain include:

        a. Stimulus, which may be mechanical, chemical, thermal, or mental

        b. Sensation of hurt, which relies on intact reception, transmission, perception, and interpretation

        c. Reaction, which may involve musculoskeletal, autonomic, and psychologic responses

    3. An intact nervous system is essential to the sensation of and reaction to pain.

    4. Phases of the pain experience include:

        a. Anticipation of pain: Fear and anxiety affect a person's response to sensation and typically intensify the perception of pain.

      b.   Sensation of pain: Affected by how anticipation was managed; pain increases anxiety, which in turn increases pain.

      c.   Aftermath of pain: The most neglected phase; response may indicate fear, embarrassment, or guilt, all of which can affect future experiences with pain.

5.   Pain can have certain beneficial effects, primarily as a warning sign of injury and signal of the need for treatment.

6.   Detrimental effects of pain

      a.   Poses a threat to basic needs: interferes with meeting food, fluid, and sleep needs; affects elimination; interferes with breathing and meeting oxygen needs; limits mobility and leads to impaired skin integrity and altered ability for self-care

      b.   Poses a threat to higher-level needs: interferes with relationships with significant others, communication, sexuality, social involvement, job performance; causes spiritual distress and may even lead to violence

      c.   Delays rehabilitation: Pain itself may become the disability.

B.   **Types of pain**

   1.   *Acute pain* can be described as:

      a.   Rapid in onset

      b.   Usually temporary, lasting no more than 6 months

      c.   Subsiding spontaneously, with or without treatment

   2.   Characteristics of *chronic pain* include:

      a.   Gradual onset

      b.   Lengthy duration, more than 6 months

      c.   Recurrent periodically

      d.   Without a useful purpose

      e.   Potential for becoming a major complication

   3.   *Cutaneous and superficial pain* involves:

      a.   Abrupt onset

      b.   Sharp, stinging quality

   4.   *Deep pain* is marked by:

      a.   Somatic pain from organs in any body cavity

      b.   Slower onset

      c.   Burning quality

      d.   Diffusion and radiation

      e.   Possibly causing nausea and vomiting

   5.   *Referred pain* is pain at one site perceived in another; referred pain follows dermatome and nerve root patterns.

   6.   *Phantom pain* may follow amputation or mastectomy; the client feels pain as if it were in the absent part.

   7.   *Intractable pain* refers to moderate to severe pain that cannot be relieved by any known treatment.

C. Etiology of pain

1. **Pain commonly results from an injury or disease process; other physiologic factors may contribute. Common causes include:**
   a. **Musculoskeletal disorder caused by spasm, rupture, ischemia, or stretching**
   b. **Visceral disorders**
   c. **Cancer**
   d. **Vascular disorders (caused by cold, pulling, displacement, or distention)**
   e. **Inflammation**
   f. **Contagious disease**
   g. **Trauma (surgical or accidental)**
   h. **Diagnostic tests (e.g., biopsy, venipuncture, invasive scanning)**
   i. **Unmet basic needs (e.g., flatus following abdominal surgery)**
   j. **Necessary nursing interventions (e.g., ambulation or coughing after surgery)**
   k. **Pregnancy, labor, and delivery**
   l. **Chemical irritants (e.g., release of histamine, bradykinin, prostaglandins, and leukokinins)**
   m. **Allergic responses**
   n. **Neuralgia, such as that which follows herpes zoster due to scarring and degenerative changes in nerves**
   o. **Causalgia, such as that which follows peripheral nerve injury**
2. **Pain also may arise from or be augmented by psychologic or emotional factors. Stress or emotion may produce observable physiologic changes (e.g., chronic excessive muscle contractions).**
3. Psychologic factors that can cause a person to interpret pain as more severe or less severe include:
   a. Isolation
   b. Anxiety
   c. Fear
   d. Anticipation of pain
4. A person's past experiences with pain influence the meaning he or she attaches to the pain experience and affect his or her expectations of the health care team.
5. Social factors that can affect pain perception include:
   a. Group status
   b. State of involvement at time of pain episode (e.g., an injury sustained during a sporting event may not be perceived as significant until after the event is over)

     c.   Role changes in family and social groups

6.   Economic factors that can contribute to pain perception include:
   a.   Threat to job or work role
   b.   Cost of treatment
   c.   Cost of caregiver or care for family

7.   Cultural factors influencing pain perception may include:
   a.   Whether the person's culture encourages or discourages expression of pain
   b.   Whether or not the culture teaches that suffering can serve some higher purpose (such as spiritual cleansing or a test of faith)
   c.   The culture's view of the role of the health care system and of health care providers

D.   Responses to pain

1.   Sympathetic nervous system responses occur with pain of low to moderate intensity or with severe superficial pain of short duration; these responses may include:
   a.   Skin pallor, coldness, clamminess
   b.   Altered vital signs (i.e., elevated blood pressure, pulse rate, and respiratory rate)
   c.   Diaphoresis
   d.   Dilated pupils

2.   Parasympathetic nervous system responses occur with pain of severe intensity and long duration or deep pain; these may include:
   a.   Skin pallor
   b.   Altered vital signs, i.e., decreased blood pressure and pulse rate
   c.   Nausea and vomiting
   d.   Weakness, fainting, prostration
   e.   Possible loss of consciousness

3.   Behavioral and musculoskeletal responses include:
   a.   Reports of pain
   b.   Postures to splint, hold, or protect painful areas
   c.   Muscle spasms
   d.   Skeletal muscle rigidity
   e.   Reflex abnormalities
   f.   Grimacing, clenching of jaws or fists
   g.   Rapid blinking, squinting eyes, or darting glance
   h.   Drawn facial expression, twitching facial muscles
   i.   Moaning, sighing, crying
   j.   Restlessness
   k.   Immobility, becoming quiet and withdrawn when touched
   l.   Anorexia, nausea, and vomiting

4. Psychologic responses may include:
   a. Fear
   b. Anxiety
   c. Anger or irritation
   d. Depression
   e. Inability to concentrate
   f. Desire for extra attention from others
5. Some persons demonstrate atypical response patterns to pain; variations in adaptation depend on such factors as:
   a. Personal perception of appropriate behavior
   b. Ability for self-distraction
   c. Attempts to adjust to prolonged pain

E. **Common pain medications**

1. *Narcotic analgesics* (opiates) which depress the CNS and inhibit pain impulses
   a. Examples: morphine (Duramorph), codeine (Paveral), meperidine (Demerol), pentazocine (Talwin), oxycodone (Roxicodone), propoxyphene (Darvon)
   b. Selected nursing considerations

   m ▸ **Avoid overdosing, which can lead to tolerance and dependence.**
   ▸ **Monitor respiratory function.**

2. *Nonnarcotic analgesics,* which act by a peripheral mechanism that blocks the generation of pain impulses
   a. Examples: acetaminophen (Tylenol); acetylsalicylic acid (aspirin); nonsteroidal analgesic drugs (NSAIDs), such as salicylates (Dolobid), ibuprofen (Advil, Motrin), indomethacin (Indocin), naproxen (Naprosyn, Aleve), ketorolac (Toradol)
   b. Selected nursing considerations

   m ▸ **Administer with food to minimize gastric upset.**
   ▸ **Inform client that medication may have anticoagulant effect.**

3. *Skeletal muscle relaxants,* which relieve pain-producing muscle spasm and spasticity
   a. Examples: benzodiazepine (T-Quil), cyclobenzaprine (Flexeril), methocarbamol (Marbaxin), dantrolene (Dantrium)
   b. Selected nursing considerations

   m ▸ **Caution client that alcohol and other drugs, such as antihistamines, potentiate the effect of muscle relaxants.**

4. *Antiinfective agents,* which reduce discomfort, fever, swelling, and inflammation associated with infection.

a. Examples: penicillins, such as penicillin G; cephalosporins, such as cefaclor (Ceclor); sulfonamides, such as sulfisoxazole (Gantrisin); tetracyclines (Tetracyn); aminoglycosides, such as streptomycin; urinary tract antiseptics
b. Selected nursing considerations

𝕟 ▸ **Check client history for drug allergies before administering.**

5. *Tranquilizers,* which decrease stress and anxiety, thereby reducing interpretation of pain
   a. Examples: hydroxyzine (Vistaril), diazepam (Valium)
   b. Selected nursing considerations

𝕟 ▸ **Caution client that alcohol and other drugs, such as antihistamines, potentiate the effect of tranquilizers.**

6. *For cardiac pain* (e.g., angina), sublingual nitroglycerin (Nitrobid), a fast-acting nitrate, usually is prescribed. The client should take medication exactly as directed and should move cautiously to minimize effects of possible orthostatic hypotension.

𝕟 F. **Special considerations**
   1. **After assessing pain (nature, location, and type), rule out complications: Make sure that the pain relates to the client's identified condition and is not a sign of developing complications. For example, a client is expected to have pain soon after abdominal or hip surgery. However, the nurse needs to make sure that the client's pain results from the surgery, not from a complication such as hemorrhage. In such a case the nurse should:**
      a. **Assess the surgical dressing.**
      b. **Assess bowel sounds (or neurovascular status of both legs in the case of hip surgery).**
      c. **Assess vital signs, such as blood pressure and pulse rate.**
   2. **Take action and intervene (see Section IIIC) as follows:**
      a. **If the assessment data are within normal limits for the client's condition, administer appropriate medication as prescribed.**
      b. **If the assessment data are abnormal for the client's condition, assess further. If indicated, notify the physician or perform appropriate activities, such as repositioning, ambulation, or distraction.**
   3. **Assess risk for injury and institute safety measures after administering pain medications that may cause drowsiness,**

impaired judgment, memory loss, or disorientation (e.g., raise the bed side rails, lower the bed, place call signal in position for easy use).

4. Evaluate effectiveness of medication interventions 30 minutes after administration (e.g., use a 10-point scale to measure and compare the client's comfort/discomfort level before and after medication).

5. Document pain, related nursing interventions, and the client's responses.

III. Nursing care of a client in pain

A. Assessment

 1. Always believe the client's account and rating of pain. Keep in mind that pain assessment depends mainly on subjective data; objective signs must be confirmed by the client, except in certain cases when physiologic changes are obvious.

2. Ask the client about the nature of the pain, including:
   a. Description (e.g., piercing, aching, shooting, burning, stinging, constant, intermittent, sharp, dull)
   b. Onset or time of occurrence: when it began, how often it occurs, what time of day it occurs
   c. Duration: how long it lasts, whether it is constant or intermittent
   d. Location: have the client describe or point to the area or areas (*Note:* When documenting, use the client's words and give the correct anatomic terms.)
   e. Intensity or severity: mild, moderate, severe, excruciating; have the client rate the severity of pain on a scale of 1 to 10, with 1 representing the least pain and 10 the most severe pain; or use a color scale, with green representing the least pain and red the most severe
   f. Apparent or suspected cause
   g. Meaning of the pain to the client
   h. Apparent or suspected precipitating, aggravating, or alleviating factors

3. Listen carefully to how the client describes the pain and evaluate implied messages about pain.

4. Using all of your senses, observe:
   a. Nonverbal behavior
   b. The painful body part or area
   c. Unusual odors
   d. Position or posture
   e. Environment
   f. Relationships, if others are present

5. Palpate painful areas for:
   a. Heat

   b. Swelling

   c. Masses

  6. Assess vital signs.

B. **Nursing diagnoses**

  1. Pain

  2. Chronic Pain

  3. Associated nursing diagnoses reflecting aggravating factors or consequences of pain; for example:

   a. Activity Intolerance

   b. Ineffective Airway Clearance

   c. Anxiety

   d. Constipation

   e. Fear

   f. Fluid Volume Deficit

   g. Risk for Injury

   h. Knowledge Deficit

   i. Impaired Physical Mobility

   j. Altered Nutrition: Less than body requirements

   k. Powerlessness

   l. Altered Role Performance

   m. Self Care Deficit

   n. Sleep Pattern Disturbance

   o. Urinary Retention

C. **Planning and implementation**

  1. Intervene to alter the source or progress of pain:

   a. Prepare the client for surgery or other treatment, such as radiation, if scheduled, to remove or reduce the cause of pain (e.g., tumor or infection).

   b. Explain simply how treatment will work to control pain.

   c. Explain alternative therapies, for example, hypnosis, if the client or physician desires. (*Note:* Why hypnosis is effective for some clients remains unclear; it may stimulate brain opiates or produce a purely psychologic effect.)

   d. Administer medication for pain as prescribed.

   e. As prescribed, administer medication for other problems causing pain (e.g., infection, postsurgical flatus).

   f. Relieve or prevent factors that aggravate pain (e.g., coughing, vomiting, diarrhea, constipation, bladder fullness, infection).

   g. Reduce or remove noxious stimuli (e.g., cast, elastic bandage, or weight; foreign body in eye; wrinkles in sheets; unsupported heavy bedding; excessive noise; excessively hot or cold environment; glaring lights).

   h. As prescribed, provide nonpharmacologic pain relief interventions, such as cutaneous stimulation, backrubs, biofeedback, acupuncture, transcutaneous electrical stimulation (TENS), dorsal column stimulation, counter irritation, and contralateral stimulation.

i. Encourage noninvasive pain management techniques such as guided imagery and relaxation.

j. Provide heat and cold application or menthol rubs as prescribed; these methods may relieve swelling and may produce anesthesia.

k. Note any age-related effects on the client's response to pain and medication administration, and adjust interventions accordingly.

l. Refer the client to a pain center or pain clinic, as recommended, for special treatment of pain that does not respond to therapy.

m. Encourage activity or perform passive range-of-motion exercises. Mild activity or assisted activity, although painful, helps relieve stiffness of arthritic joints and sore muscles, thus eventually reducing pain; activity may also increase endorphins.

n. Ensure proper body alignment and reposition regularly; although movement may hurt, repositioning and proper alignment relieves muscle strain and joint stiffness and helps relieve pain.

o. Provide distraction (e.g., with music, TV, radio, reading) to reduce focus on pain and increase other impulses, which may help block pain impulses.

p. Use behavior modification techniques as appropriate.

q. Involve family members to help them understand pain control and the client's response, and to enhance their ability to provide comfort and emotional support.

r. Involve other disciplines (e.g., clergy, social worker, counselor, occupational therapist) as necessary.

s. When performing painful procedures, work gently, swiftly, and skillfully to minimize the amount of pain generated and the time required.

t. Provide adequate rest for the client or the painful body part.

2. Intervene to alter psychosocial, economic, and cultural factors influencing pain:

a. Explain all interventions, treatments, or symptoms that may frighten or worry the client; anxiety or fear increase a client's perception of the severity of pain.

b. Discuss with the client what the pain means to him or her to help decrease the client's concerns about the cause of pain (e.g., cancer or incurable disease).

    c. Stay with the client during pain episodes, and convey your empathy and concern; this can help decrease stress and anxiety and ease feelings of isolation and loneliness.

    d. Establish a trusting relationship with the client by keeping your promises and providing excellent physical care.

    e. Promote the client's sense of control and participation in pain control by allowing him or her to make choices regarding therapy, as appropriate, and (if applicable) by using client-controlled analgesia (PCA).

    f. When talking with the client, avoid words like "complain," "attack," and "victim," which imply helplessness and criticism and may interfere with pain control; instead, use neutral or positive terms such as "explain," "episode," and "experience."

    g. As prescribed, administer medication to reduce stress and anxiety that may contribute to pain.

    h. Discuss with the client the painful experience both before and after episodes to help decrease any fear or shame associated with perceived inability to cope with pain appropriately.

    i. Discuss the client's previous experiences with pain, including how it was managed and how the client wants to manage current pain.

    j. Discuss situational factors that may influence pain (e.g., loss of job, recent divorce, death in family, serious illness); this may help decrease anxiety and reassure the client that others are there to help, which can combat feelings of isolation and loneliness.

    k. As necessary, refer the client to psychologic counseling, occupational therapy, and other resources to help deal with psychosocial problems.

    l. Teach the client what he or she needs to learn to meet any knowledge deficit related to pain or treatment.

D. Evaluation

    1. The client reports reduced pain after pain-relief interventions.

    2. The client displays a change in various responses to pain, for example:

        a. Sympathetic nervous system responses

        b. Parasympathetic nervous system responses

        c. Behavioral and musculoskeletal responses: verbal and nonverbal

        d. Psychologic responses

Bibliography

Carpenito, L. J. (1995). *Nursing diagnosis: Application to clinical practice* (6th ed.). Philadelphia: J. B. Lippincott.

Guyton, A. C. (1991). *Textbook of medical physiology.* Philadelphia: W. B. Saunders.

Karch, A. (1995). *1996 Lippincott's nursing drug guide.* Philadelphia: J. B. Lippincott.

Melzack, R. (1983). *Pain measurement and assessment.* New York: Raven Press.

Nettina, S. (1996). *The Lippincott manual of nursing practice* (6th ed.). Philadelphia: Lippincott-Raven Publishers.

Smeltzer, S. C., & Bare, B. G. (1996). *Brunner and Suddarth's textbook of medical-surgical nursing* (8th ed.). Philadelphia: Lippincott-Raven Publishers.

STUDY QUESTIONS

1. A client who had abdominal surgery 3 days ago complains of sharp, throbbing abdominal pain that ranks "8" on a scale of 1 (no pain) to 10 (worst pain). The nurse's first action should be to
   a. medicate the client with pain medication as needed
   b. assess the client to rule out possible pain-causing complications secondary to surgery
   c. check the nurse's notes to determine when pain medication was last administered
   d. explain to the client that the pain should not be this severe 3 days postoperatively

2. Assessment of a client with postoperative abdominal pain discloses no urine output for 12 hours, with an IV fluid intake of 1000 mL and a distended lower abdomen. Which of the following nursing diagnoses would be made 1 hour after analgesic administration?
   a. Pain related to abdominal surgery
   b. Fear related to urinary catheterization
   c. Pain related to pressure of a full bladder
   d. Anxiety related to past experiences with pain

3. Which of the following interventions should the nurse plan for a client with arthritis who remains in bed too long because "It hurts to get started?"
   a. Tell the client to absolutely limit movement of inflamed joints.
   b. Teach significant others to lift the client into a wheelchair.
   c. Teach the client the proper way of massaging inflamed joints.
   d. Administer aspirin, and tell the client to gently perform range-of-motion exercises before rising.

4. A 20-year-old victim of a motorcycle accident has a fractured right femur and spinal cord injuries. The client cannot move either leg. Skeletal traction is ap- plied to the injured leg. The nurse notes an elevated blood pressure and redness around the pain site, although the client does not complain of pain. Which of the following nursing diagnoses would be the most likely explanation for the client's failure to report pain to the nurse?
   a. Ineffective Individual Coping
   b. Sensory/Perceptual Alterations: Tactile
   c. Unilateral Neglect
   d. Knowledge Deficit

5. A 10-year-old boy falls off his bicycle, grabs his wrist, and cries, "Oh, my wrist. Help. The pain is so sharp, I think I broke it." Based on these data, the pain the boy is experiencing is caused by impulses traveling from receptors to the spinal cord along which type of nerve fibers?
   a. A-alpha
   b. Type C
   c. A-gamma
   d. A-delta

6. A client arrives in the emergency room complaining of severe leg pain which occurred after the client fell out of a tree. Nursing assessment reveals parasympathetic nervous system responses to pain. Which of the following outcomes would indicate resolution of these responses?
   a. a rise in blood pressure and pulse rate within normal range
   b. decreased blood pressure and pulse rate within normal range
   c. reduced skeletal muscle rigidity
   d. reduced diaphoresis

7. Of the various theories of pain, which provides the information most useful to the nurse in planning pain reduction interventions?
   a. central control theory
   b. gate control theory
   c. specificity theory
   d. pattern theory

8. One day after open reduction and inter-

nal fixation (ORIF) of the left hip, which of the following data would the nurse report to the physician instead of administering pain medication?
a. left hip dressing dry and intact
b. BP, 114/78; pulse rate, 82
c. left leg in functional anatomic position
d. left foot cold to touch; no palpable pedal pulse

9. A client who has sustained burns over most of the trunk and arms dreads physical therapy and resists activity. The client reports difficulty sleeping due to pain and fatigue after treatments. Based on this information, the priority nursing diagnosis would be
a. Activity Intolerance related to pain secondary to burns
b. Altered Nutrition: Less than body requirements related to pain secondary to burns
c. Sleep Pattern Disturbance related to pain secondary to burns
d. Pain related to burns

10. Six months after sustaining severe burn injuries, a client expresses concern about possible loss of abilities needed for job performance and about physical disfigurement. The nurse can best intervene for this kind of pain by
a. referring the client for counseling and occupational therapy
b. staying with the client as much as possible and building trust
c. providing cutaneous stimulation and pharmacologic therapy
d. providing distraction and guided imagery

11. The client who has chronic pain, loss of self-esteem, no job, and bodily disfigurement secondary to severe burns over the trunk and arms is admitted to a pain center. Evaluation criteria for the client's successful rehabilitation should include which of the following?
a. The client has no aftermath phase of the pain experience.
b. The client experiences decreased frequency of acute pain episodes.

c. The client continues normal growth and development with support systems intact.
d. The client develops increased tolerance for severe pain in the future.

12. Which of the following statements regarding pain is correct?
a. Intractable pain may be relieved by treatment.
b. Pain is an objective sign of a more serious problem.
c. Psychologic factors rarely contribute to a client's pain perception.
d. Pain sensation is affected by a client's anticipation of pain.

13. A 5-year-old boy received a small paper cut on his finger. His mother let him wash it and apply a small amount of antibacterial ointment and a bandage. She then let him watch TV and eat an apple. Her interventions for pain are examples of
a. providing pharmacologic therapy
b. providing control and distraction
c. altering Billy's environment
d. providing cutaneous stimulation

14. Which of the following represents the best rationale for using noninvasive and nonpharmacologic pain control measures in conjunction with other measures?
a. These measures are more effective than analgesics.
b. These measures decrease input to large fibers, reducing transmission of pain impulses to the CNS.
c. These measures help potentiate the effects of analgesics.
d. These measures help block transmission of impulses from Type C fibers.

15. In evaluating a client's adaptation to pain, which of the following behaviors would indicate appropriate adaptation?
a. The client can distract himself or herself during pain episodes.
b. The client denies pain.
c. The client reports no need for family support.
d. The client reports pain reduction with decreased activity.

ANSWER KEY

1. **Correct response: b**
   The nurse must rule out complications. The physician ordered the pain medication for routine postoperative pain that is expected after abdominal surgery, not for a complication such as hemorrhage, infection, or dehiscence.
   a. The nurse should never administer pain medication without assessing the client.
   c. This is appropriate, but it is not the first action.
   d. Always believe the client. Pain is subjective and each person has his or her own level of pain tolerance.

   Application/Physiologic/Planning

2. **Correct response: c**
   Data reveal that the client's bladder is probably full and causing pressure.
   a. Pain related to surgery should have been relieved by the analgesic.
   b and d. There are no data to support a diagnosis of fear or anxiety.

   Comprehension/Physiologic/
   Analysis (Dx)

3. **Correct response: d**
   Aspirin raises the pain threshold; although range-of-motion will hurt, mild exercise will relieve pain on rising.
   a. Limitation of motion will increase pain.
   b. Lifting the client into a wheelchair will not increase mobility.
   c. Massaging will increase inflammation.

   Application/Health promotion/Planning

4. **Correct response: b**
   An intact nervous system is essential for a client to experience or respond to pain. Even though evidence indicates that the client should be experiencing pain, pain impulse transmission apparently is impaired because of the spinal cord injury.
   a and d. No evidence indicates that either knowledge deficit or poor coping would interfere with reporting the pain.
   c. Unilateral neglect would result from cerebral dysfunction leading to loss of recognition of one side of the body.

   Analysis/Safe care/Analysis (Dx)

5. **Correct response: d**
   Only A-delta fibers transmit sharp, piercing pain.
   a and c. A-alpha and A-gamma fibers transmit touch, pressure, heat, cold, and movement impulses.
   b. C fibers transmit aching and burning pain.

   Application/Physiologic/Assessment

6. **Correct response: a**
   Blood pressure and pulse rate decrease with parasympathetic involvement.
   b. Blood pressure and pulse rate increase with sympathetic involvement.
   c. Skeletal muscle rigidity is a musculoskeletal response.
   d. Diaphoresis indicates sympathetic involvement.

   Analysis/Physiologic/Evaluation

7. **Correct response: a**
   No one theory explains all the factors underlying the pain experience, but the central control theory discusses brain opiates with analgesic properties and how their release can be affected by actions initiated by the client and caregivers.
   b, c, and d. These theories do not address pain control in the depth included in the central control theory.

   Knowledge/Health promotion/Planning

8. **Correct response: d**
   These data represent abnormal findings on neurovascular assessment of the left leg which require immediate medical intervention.
   a, b, and c. All of these data are nor-

mal and would not require medical intervention.
Analysis/Physiologic/Evaluation

9. Correct response: d
Pain is the cause of the other diagnoses; they could be resolved if pain could be prevented.
  a, b, and c. These diagnoses are all secondary to the primary diagnosis of pain.
Application/Physiologic/Analysis (Dx)

10. Correct response: a
The client needs professional help to get on with life and handle the limitations imposed by the current problems.
  b, c, and d. These interventions would have been more appropriate in earlier stages of postburn injury, when physical pain was most severe and fewer psychologic factors needed to be addressed.
Analysis/Health promotion/ Implementation

11. Correct response: c
Even though the client may experience an aftermath phase, progress is still possible as is effective rehabilitation.
  a. Aftermath may occur but need not interfere with rehabilitation.
  b. Acute pain would not be expected at this stage of recovery.
  d. Conditioning likely will produce less pain tolerance.
Analysis/Health promotion/Evaluation

12. Correct response: d
Phases of the pain experience include the anticipation of pain. Fear and anxiety affect a person's response to sensation.
  a. Intractable pain is moderate to severe pain that cannot be relieved by any known treatment.
  b. Pain is a subjective sensation than cannot be quantified by anyone except the person experiencing it.

  c. Psychologic factors contribute to a client's pain perception. In many cases, pain results from emotions, such as hostility, guilt, or depression.
Comprehension/Self-care/Planning

13. Correct response: b
Involving the child in care and providing distraction took his mind off the pain.
  a. Pharmacologic agents for pain—analgesics—were not used.
  c. The home environment was not changed.
  d. Cutaneous stimulation was not provided.
Application/Physiologic/Implementation

14. Correct response: c
Noninvasive measures may result in release of endogenous molecular neuropeptides with analgesic properties.
  a. No evidence indicates that noninvasive and nonpharmacologic measures are more effective than analgesics in relieving pain.
  b. Decreased input over large fibers allows more pain impulses to reach the CNS.
  d. This is simply incorrect.
Application/Safe care/Implementation

15. Correct response: a
Distraction is an appropriate method of reducing pain.
  b. Not reporting experienced pain is an inappropriate response.
  c. Exclusion of family members and other sources of support represents a maladaptive response.
  d. Range-of-motion exercises and at least mild activity can help reduce pain and are important to prevent complications of immobility.
Application/Physiologic/Evaluation

Respiratory Disorders

I. Respiratory system

A. Structures

 1. The *upper airways* consist of the nose and sinuses, pharynx, epiglottis, and larynx; all are lined with mucus-
secreting cells and cilia. The uppermost structures contain olfactory sensors.

2. The *lower airways* consist of the trachea, right and left
mainstem bronchi, segmental bronchi, terminal bronchioles, and alveoli.

3. The *lungs* are situated in the thoracic cavity on either side of
heart, bounded by the clavicles, ribs, vertebrae, and diaphragm.

 **4. The right lung contains three lobes; the left lung, two
lobes.**

5. The lungs' primary lobules contain millions of alveolar sacs.

6. Blood supply to the lungs is provided by the pulmonary and
bronchial arteries.

7. Neurologic control of ventilation is governed by the *medulla
oblongata,* which contains both inspiratory and expiratory
centers and controls the rate and depth of respiration to meet
the body's metabolic needs.

8. Parietal and visceral pleura surround the lungs; these two layers are separated by the intrapleural space.

9. The *diaphragm,* a dome-shaped muscle separating the thoracic and abdominal cavities, is innervated by the phrenic
nerve (a branch of the vagus nerve).

B. Function

 1. Upper airway functions include:
   a. **Conduct air to lower airways**
   b. **Protect lungs from foreign matter**
   c. **Warm, filter, and humidify inspired air**

2. The bronchi conduct air to the alveoli.

3. Cilia and mucus help clear particulate matter from inspired air.
4. The alveoli receive air and exchange oxygen (O_2) and carbon dioxide (CO_2) across the alveolar membrane to the pulmonary capillaries.
5. The lungs are the organs of ventilation which involves:
    a. The cyclic process of inspiration and expiration
    b. Pulmonary inflation and deflation, causing O_2 and CO_2 gas exchange at the pulmonary capillary–alveolar interface in the lung parenchyma
6. The lungs provide the body's primary mechanism for altering CO_2 as a buffer to maintain acid–base balance.
7. Diffusion of gases occurs across the alveolar membrane according to pressure gradients from areas of high to low concentration.
8. The pressure gradient of O_2 is greater in the lung than in the pulmonary capillaries, causing O_2 to diffuse across the alveolar membrane into the pulmonary capillaries.
9. The pressure gradient of CO_2 is lower in the lung than in the pulmonary capillaries, causing CO_2 to diffuse from the pulmonary blood vessels to the lungs.
10. In normal anatomic shunting, a small amount of blood from bronchial, pleural, and coronary circulation bypasses pulmonary circulation and therefore is not oxygenated.
11. In abnormal physiologic shunting, a large amount of unoxygenated venous blood mixes with oxygenated blood in the left heart chambers as a result of adequate pulmonary perfusion with inadequate or absent alveolar ventilation.
12. Inspired air has a high O_2 concentration (O_2 = 158 mmHg); expired air, a high CO_2 concentration (CO_2 = 46 mmHg).
13. Negative pressure created by the intrapleural space helps effect elastic recoil of lungs.
14. The major muscle of respiration, the diaphragm assists breathing by rising on expiration and lowering on inspiration.

II. Overview of respiratory disorders
A. Assessment
1. Nursing health history should focus on risk factors for respiratory dysfunction, including:
    a. Personal or family history of lung disease
    b. **Smoking (the most significant contributing factor in lung disease)**
    c. Occupational or avocational exposure to allergens or environmental pollutants
    d. Age-related changes in lung capacity and respiratory function

    e.   History of upper respiratory infection

    f.   Postoperative changes resulting in diminished respiratory excursion

2.   Inspection involves:

    a.   General appearance: body size, age, skin quality and color, posture

    b.   Configuration and movement of the thorax during respiration

    c.   Characteristics of respiration: rate, rhythm, depth, and muscles used for breathing (*Note:* The normal resting adult breathes at 12–20 breaths per minute.)

    d.   Presence of cough, nature and character of sputum (clear, purulent, bloody, tenacious)

    e.   Clubbing of fingers: angle of nailbed greater than 160 degrees, distal phalangeal depth greater than interphalangeal depth; softening of nailbeds

3.   Palpation of the chest is done to:

    a.   Detect painful areas or masses on the chest surface

    b.   Evaluate chest excursion and the presence or absence of fremitus (vibration)

4.   Chest percussion elicits sound to evaluate underlying tissues.

    a.   Resonant sound: indicates air-filled lung (normal)

    b.   Dull or flat sound: suggests presence of firm mass (usually abnormal)

5.   Auscultation involves listening to air movement in lungs to detect normal or adventitious breath sounds, including:

    a.   Vesicular sounds: low-pitched rustling sound heard over most of lung field, most prominently on inspiration; indicative of normal, clear lungs

    b.   Bronchial sounds: high-pitched tubular sound with slight pause between inspiration and expiration; normal over large airways

    c.   Bronchovesicular sounds: combination of vesicular and bronchial sounds, normally heard anteriorly to the right or left of the sternum and posteriorly between the scapulae; inspiration and expiration equal

    d.   Adventitious breath sounds: crackles (fine to coarse), wheezes (sibilant, sonorous), pleural friction rub

6.   During assessment, the nurse should be alert for cardinal signs and symptoms of respiratory dysfunction, including:

    a.   Dyspnea (labored breathing)

    b.   Orthopnea (difficulty breathing in all positions except upright)

    c.   **Cough: may be hacking, brassy, wheezing, productive, or nonproductive**

    d.   **Increased sputum production; purulent (yellow or green), rusty, bloody, or mucoid sputum**

    e.   **Chest pain**

    f.   **Wheezing, crackles**

    g.   **Clubbing of fingers**

    h.   **Hemoptysis**

    i.   **Cyanosis (buccal, peripheral)**

B.   **Laboratory studies and diagnostic tests**

   1.   Radiographic and scanning studies, done to visualize respiratory system structures, include:

    a.   Chest radiography

    b.   Chest tomography

    c.   Lung scan

    d.   Computed tomography (CT) scan

    e.   Positron-emission tomography scan

    f.   Fluoroscopy

    g.   Barium swallow

   2.   Endoscopic studies, invasive techniques performed to visualize pulmonary structures and obtain tissue specimens, include:

    a.   Bronchoscopy

    b.   Esophagoscopy

    c.   Mediastinoscopy

   3.   Thoracentesis involves needle aspiration of pleural fluid for diagnostic and therapeutic purposes.

   4.   Needle biopsy is an invasive technique involving entering the lung or pleura to obtain tissue for analysis.

   5.   Spirometry (pulmonary function testing) is a noninvasive technique used to determine lung volumes, ventilatory function, airway resistance, and distribution of gases.

   6.   Sputum culture determines the presence of pathogenic organisms.

   7.   Arterial blood gas (ABG) studies determine O_2 and CO_2 content and evaluate the body's acid–base balance (Tables 6-1 and 6-2).

C.   **Psychosocial implications**

   1.   A client with respiratory dysfunction may experience coping difficulties related to:

    a.   Progressive nature of disease

    b.   Chronicity of disease

    c.   Diminished respiratory function

    d.   Fear of dying

TABLE 6-1.
Normal Arterial Blood Gas Values at Sea Level

PARAMETER	NORMAL RANGE
pH (hydrogen ion concentration)	7.35 to 7.45
PaO_2 (partial pressure of oxygen)	80 to 100 mmHg
$PaCO_2$ (partial pressure of carbon dioxide)	35 to 45 mmHg
HCO_3	22 to 26 mEq/L
BE (base excess)	−2 to +2 mEq/L
SaO_2 (saturation of hemoglobin)	>95%

2. The client also may develop self-concept concerns due to:
   a. Role changes involving increased dependence
   b. Body image changes with the use of breathing apparatus
3. Lifestyle concerns related to respiratory dysfunction may include potential changes in:
   a. Activity tolerance
   b. Physical mobility
   c. Work performance, with potential for job loss
   d. Self-care ability
4. The chronically ill client may develop concerns about social interaction, leading to feelings of:
   a. Isolation and loneliness
   b. Depression
   c. Hopelessness
D. **Medications used to treat respiratory problems (additional medications may be included with specific diseases)**
   1. *Adrenergics* (also called sympathomimetics), which dilate bronchial smooth muscles to relieve bronchospasm
      a. Examples: isoetharine (Bronkosol), metaproterenol (Alupent), albuterol (Ventolin), terbutaline (Brethine),

TABLE 6-2.
Blood Gas Changes in Acid–Base Disorders

DISORDER	BLOOD GAS CHANGES
Respiratory acidosis	↓ pH, ↑ $PaCO_2$
Respiratory alkalosis	↑ pH, ↓ $PaCO_2$
Metabolic acidosis	↓ pH, ↓ HCO_3, ↓ BE
Metabolic alkalosis	↑ pH, ↑ HCO_3, ↑ BE

epinephrine (Bronkaid), isoproterenol (Isuprel), ephedrine (Adrenalin, Primatene)

b. Selected nursing considerations

- ▶ Instruct client to inhale twice as follows: inhale once, wait 1 minute, and inhale once more.
- ▶ Monitor vital signs closely.
- ▶ Instruct client that nervousness, anxiety, or insomnia will occur.

2. *Xanthine derivatives,* which relax bronchial smooth muscle, in asthma

a. Examples: aminophylline (Phyllocontin), theophylline (Theo-Dur), ephedrine (Adrenalin, Primatene)

b. Selected nursing considerations

- ▶ **Monitor serum level of theophylline (normal level, 10–20 mcg/mL).**
- ▶ **Provide medication at regular intervals.**
- ▶ **Instruct client to notify physician of irritability, restlessness, headache, insomnia, dizziness.**

3. *Corticosteroids* (oral or inhalable), which are used in severe immune or inflammatory responses

a. Examples: oral—hydrocortisone, methylprednisolone, dexamethasone, prednisone; inhalable—beclomethasone

b. Selected nursing considerations

- ▶ **Instruct client to take medication exactly as directed and to taper discontinuation of drug rather than stop abruptly, which could cause serious withdrawal symptoms leading to adrenal insufficiency, shock, and death.**
- ▶ **Forewarn client that drug may cause reportable Cushingoid effects (weight gain, moon face, buffalo hump, and hirsutism) and may mask signs and symptoms of infection.**

4. *Cromolyn sodium,* which has bronchodilating effect

a. Example: Intal

b. Selected nursing considerations

- ▶ **Teach client to insert capsule in nebulizer device, exhale completely, place mouthpiece between lips, inhale deeply and hold breath for 10 seconds, and then exhale.**

5. *Mucolytic, expectorant, and antitussive agents,* which facilitate sputum expectoration, are indicated primarily for clients with cystic fibrosis or other disorders characterized by thick, resistant secretions; acetylcysteine (Mucomyst), guaifenesin (Robitussin), and potassium iodide (SSKI) are commonly used.

III. Pneumonia

A. Description

1. Pneumonia is an inflammatory process involving the respiratory bronchioles, alveolar space and walls, and lobes, caused primarily by specific organisms (bacteria, viruses, fungi, parasites, mycoplasma, or chemical irritants).
2. It can be broadly classified as bacterial or nonbacterial.

B. Etiology and incidence

1. Causative organisms in bacterial pneumonia include:
   a. *Streptococcus pneumoniae* (hemolytic type A) accounts for 90% of cases.
   b. *Staphylococcus aureus*
   c. *Haemophilus influenzae* (type B)
   d. *Klebsiella pneumoniae, Pseudomonas aeruginosa, Escherichia coli, Enterobacter,* and other gram-negative enteric bacilli
2. Causes of nonbacterial pneumonia include:
   a. *Mycoplasma pneumoniae*
   b. Influenza viruses, parainfluenza viruses, and other viral infections
   c. *Pneumocystis carinii*
   d. *Aspergillus fumigatus*
3. Pneumonia is the most common cause of death from infectious disease in North America.

C. Pathophysiology and management

1. The infecting organisms trigger inflammation of the airways.
2. Inflammatory exudate fills the alveolar air spaces, producing lung consolidation.
3. Impaired gas exchange in the alveoli leads to varying degrees of hypoxia, depending on the amount of lung tissue affected.
4. Management involves lifestyle changes and medication use.

D. Assessment findings

1. Common clinical manifestations include:
   a. Dullness on percussion of chest with consolidation
   b. Bronchial breath sounds auscultated over consolidated lung fields
   c. Fever: sudden onset over 100°F
   d. Shaking chills (with bacterial pneumonia)
   e. Chest pain
   f. Dyspnea
   g. Hacking cough
   h. Anxiety and confusion
2. Laboratory and diagnostic studies may reveal:

a. Density changes, primarily in lower lung fields, seen on chest radiograph
b. Sputum culture and sensitivity positive for specific causative organism
c. Elevated white blood cell (WBC) count; depressed in pneumonia of mycoplasmal or viral origin

E. Nursing diagnoses
1. Risk for Altered Body Temperature
2. Ineffective Breathing Pattern
3. Fluid Volume Deficit
4. Impaired Gas Exchange
5. Pain
6. Knowledge Deficit

F. Planning and implementation
1. Encourage adequate fluid intake with IV fluid administration and oral hydration as appropriate (2 to 3 L/day).
2. Humidify inspired air.
3. Encourage effective coughing.
4. Encourage the client to rest and remain in comfortable position (e.g., semi-Fowler's) and to avoid overexertion that may exacerbate symptoms.
5. Analyze ABG values to determine the need for oxygen and to evaluate the client's response to oxygen therapy.
6. Relieve pain with analgesics, as prescribed, and monitor for signs of respiratory depression.
7. **Assess for allergies, especially drug allergies, for example to antibiotics.**
8. Administer antibiotics, as prescribed, specific for the causative organism which may include penicillin, erythromycin, nafcillin, gentamycin, tobramycin, and tetracycline.
9. Administer mucolytics or expectorants as prescribed (see Section II.D).
10. Provide client and family teaching, covering:
    a. Disease process, cause, treatments (including medications), expected response
    b. Deep breathing and coughing techniques
    c. The importance of thorough handwashing to help prevent infection transmission
    d. The importance of nutrition; rest; avoiding fatigue, overexertion, alcohol, tobacco, and secondhand smoke
    e. The importance of follow-up medical visit for a chest x-ray and for influenza immunizations at prescribed times

G. **Evaluation**
1. The client demonstrates response to therapy within 48 hours if no complications occur.
2. The client demonstrates improved respiratory function and ABG values within normal ranges.
3. The client exhibits diminished cough and sputum production.
4. The client demonstrates resolution of disease process on radiograph.

IV. Chronic obstructive pulmonary disease (COPD)

A. **Description: COPD is a group of disorders associated with persistent or recurrent obstruction of airflow; includes chronic bronchitis, emphysema, and asthma, often with overlap of these disorders**

B. **Etiology and incidence**
1. Major causes of and contributing factors to chronic bronchitis and emphysema which are irreversible include:
   a. Smoking
   b. Air pollution
   c. Occupational exposure to respiratory irritants
   d. Allergies
   e. Autoimmunity
   f. Infection
   g. Genetic predisposition
   h. Aging
2. Asthma is a reversible diffuse airway obstruction. It may be extrinsic or intrinsic; possible causes include:
   a. Extrinsic: external agents or specific allergens (e.g., dust, foods, mold spores, insecticides)
   b. Intrinsic: upper respiratory infection, exercise, emotional stress, cold, or other nonspecific factors
3. The most common chronic lung disease, COPD affects an estimated 17 million persons in the United States; incidence is rising.

C. **Pathophysiology and management**
1. Basic pathologic changes in COPD include:
   a. Hypertrophy and hypersecretion in goblet cells and bronchial mucus glands leading to increased sputum secretion, bronchial congestion, narrowing of bronchioles, and small bronchi (chronic bronchitis)
   b. Increased size of air spaces; loss of elastic recoil of lung due to hyperinflation of distal airways; destruction of alveolar walls; and diffuse airway narrowing causing resistance to airflow due to loss of supporting structure and bronchospasm (emphysema)

     c.   Narrowing of the bronchial airways (asthma)
2. These conditions frequently overlap; most commonly, bronchitis and emphysema occur together.
3. These changes disrupt airway dynamics, resulting in obstruction of airflow into or out of the lungs.

D. Assessment findings

1. Health history findings, clinical manifestations, and laboratory and diagnostic study results in *chronic bronchitis* may include:
    a. Recurrent acute respiratory infections
    b. Persistent cough
    c. Persistent sputum production
    d. Slow development, typically over several years
    e. History of smoking, air pollution, occupational exposure
    f. Pulmonary function studies: decreased forced expiratory volume (FEV), decreased forced vital capacity (FVC), increased residual volume (RV)
    g. Chest radiograph: flattened diaphragm
    h. ABG values during acute phase: significantly increased $PaCO_2$, decreased PaO_2
    i. Sputum culture: secondary bacterial infection with gram-negative or gram-positive organisms, such as *Diplococcus pneumoniae* and *Haemophilus influenzae*

2. Common assessment findings in *emphysema* include:
    a. History of chronic bronchitis
    b. Slow onset of symptoms (typically over several years)
    c. Progressive dyspnea, initially only on exertion and later also at rest
    d. Progressive cough and increased sputum production, especially during bouts of infection
    e. Anorexia with weight loss
    f. Profound weakness
    g. Pulmonary function studies: decreased FEV, decreased FVC, increased RV
    h. Chest radiograph: flattened diaphragm, decreased vascular markings with hyperradiolucence, increased anteroposterior (AP) diameter ("barrel chest")
    i. ABGs: increased $PaCO_2$, decreased PaO_2
    j. Clubbing of fingers

3. Assessment findings in *asthma* typically include:
    a. Chest tightness
    b. Cough
    c. Wheezing

      d.   Expiration more strenuous and prolonged than inspiration

      e.   Use of accessory muscles of respiration

      f.   Hypoxia with cyanosis, weak pulse, diaphoresis

      g.   Can occur alone without triad of bronchitis, emphysema, and asthma; usually associated with allergy

      h.   Commonly triggered by emotional stress, exercise, change in weather, exposure to allergen

      i.   Pulmonary function studies during acute episode: markedly decreased FEV, increased RV, increased TLC, decreased peak flow (PEFR) that improve after treatment

E. Nursing diagnoses

    1.   Activity Intolerance

    2.   Anxiety

    3.   Ineffective Breathing Pattern

    4.   Impaired Verbal Communication

    5.   Fatigue

    6.   Impaired Gas Exchange

    7.   Impaired Home Maintenance Management

    8.   Altered Nutrition: Less than body requirements

    9.   Pain

  10.   Chronic Pain

  11.   Altered Tissue Perfusion: Peripheral

F. Planning and implementation

    1.   For a client with bronchitis or emphysema:

      a.   Eliminate or minimize exposure to all pulmonary irritants.

      b.   Clear airways with postural drainage, clapping or vibrating and suctioning as appropriate.

      c.   Encourage the client to perform graded physical exercise, deep breathing and coughing, and relaxation techniques.

      d.   Administer low-flow O_2 to help prevent hypoxia due to loss of respiratory drive (2 to 4 L according to ABG values).

      e.   Avoid narcotics, sedatives, and tranquilizers, which can further depress respirations.

      f.   Encourage rest. Have client remain in a comfortable position (e.g., semi-Fowler's) and avoid overexertion that may exacerbate symptoms.

      g.   Assess for drug allergies, especially to antibiotics before administering as prescribed for the causative organism (*Streptococcus pneumonise* and *Haemophilus influenzae* are the most common).

  h. Also as prescribed, administer bronchodilators, mucolytic agents, and corticosteroids (see Section II.D).

  i. Provide client and family teaching, covering disease process and treatments; breathing retraining exercises; energy conservation; use of inhalers and nebulizers; medication administration and the importance of compliance; prevention of complications and infections by receiving influenza immunizations and taking medications as prescribed.

 2. For a client with asthma:

  a. Identify and eliminate or minimize exposure to pulmonary irritants.

  b. As prescribed, administer bronchodilators and corticosteroids as for a client with bronchitis or emphysema (see Section II.D).

  c. As prescribed, encourage use of cromolyn sodium as a prophylactic treatment; not for acute attacks (see Section II.D).

  d. Encourage the client to perform graded physical, breathing, and relaxation exercises with acute attacks.

  e. Provide client and family teaching, covering disease process and triggering factors; breathing retraining exercises; energy conservation; medication administration, including indications, expected responses, potential side effects, importance of compliance, and use of inhaler or nebulizer; importance of receiving influenza immunization as prescribed; and prevention of complications and infection.

G. Evaluation

 1. The client displays improved ABG values with compensation.

 2. The client exhibits improved pulmonary function studies with compensation.

 3. The client demonstrates resolution of acute processes.

 4. The client reports eased breathing effort.

 5. The client produces sputum that is more liquid and controlled by coughing.

 6. The client reports and exhibits reduced anxiety.

 7. The client reports symptom improvement with use of work modification strategies.

 8. The client verbalizes an understanding of administration and purpose of prescribed medications.

 9. The client verbalizes an understanding of the disease process and measures to prevent complications, including infection.

 10. The client incorporates health maintenance behaviors into his or her lifestyle.

V. Occupational lung disease (pneumoconioses)

A. Description

1. Commonly producing no signs or symptoms in early stages, occupational lung disorders result from exposure in the workplace to organic or inorganic dusts and noxious gases.

2. The most common types include silicosis, asbestosis, and coal workers' pneumoconiosis (CWP, "black lung").

B. Etiology and incidence

1. Silicosis results from inhaling silica dust in such occupations as mineral mining, stone cutting, quarrying, abrasives manufacturing, and ceramic and pottery work.

2. Asbestosis results from inhaling asbestos dust and particles in occupations related to manufacture, handling, and removal of asbestos-containing materials. (*Note:* There are more than 4000 known uses of asbestos fiber.)

3. CWP results from accumulation of coal dust in the lungs, most commonly from coal mining.

C. Pathophysiology and management

1. The effects of inhaling dusts, particles, or gases depend on the substance's composition, its antigenic or irritating properties, the amount inhaled, duration of exposure, and the person's overall health status.

2. Chronic inhalation of silica particles produces nodular lesions throughout the lungs. These lesions become fibrotic, enlarge, and fuse, resulting in obstructive and restrictive lung changes.

3. In asbestosis, inhaled asbestos fibers enter the alveoli which eventually become obliterated by fibrous tissue surrounding the particles. Progressive pleural fibrosis and plaque formation lead to restrictive lung disease, diminished lung volume, impaired gas exchange, hypoxemia, and eventually, cor pulmonale. Asbestosis also is associated with bronchogenic cancer.

4. In CWP, inhaled coal dust is deposited in the alveoli and bronchioles. Eventually, the alveoli and bronchioles become clogged with dust, macrophages, and fibroblasts, leading to the formation of coal macules, the primary lesion of CWP. As these macules enlarge, bronchiolar dilation and emphysema result.

5. Management involves treatment to improve oxygenation and activity tolerance, and measures to avoid infection, disease progression, and other complications.

D. Assessment findings

1. Common clinical manifestations include:

      a. Chronic cough, often nonproductive in silicosis and asbestosis but producing black fluid in CWP

      b. Progressive dyspnea

      c. Susceptibility to recurrent upper respiratory infections

      d. Impaired diaphragmatic excursion

      e. Diminished breath sounds with decreased chest expansion

      f. Tachypnea

      g. Clubbing of fingers and toes

  2. Chest radiograph findings typically include:

      a. Silicosis: nodular formation to massive fibrosis and densities in lung fields as disease progresses

      b. Asbestosis: interstitial density in lower lung fields

      c. CWP: nodular densities in upper lung fields

  3. Pulmonary function tests commonly reveal decreased FVC, FEV, TLC, and diffusing capacity of CO_2 as the disease progresses.

  4. ABG values demonstrate decreasing PaO_2 and increasing $PaCO_2$ with disease progression.

E. Nursing diagnoses

  1. Activity Intolerance

  2. Anxiety

  3. Impaired Verbal Communication

  4. Fatigue

  5. Altered Health Maintenance

  6. Health Seeking Behaviors

  7. Impaired Home Maintenance Management

  8. Pain

  9. Altered Tissue Perfusion: Peripheral

F. Planning and implementation

  1. For a client experiencing acute symptoms:

      a. Maintain a patent airway by suctioning or endotracheal intubation.

      b. Provide adequate oxygenation.

      c. Maintain cardiac output.

      d. Initiate mechanical ventilation if respiratory failure occurs.

  2. Interventions for chronic disease include:

      a. Maintain bronchial hygiene.

      b. As prescribed, administer broad-spectrum antibiotics as a prophylactic treatment against lung infections.

      c. See Section IV.F for additional interventions.

G. Evaluation (see Section IV.G)

VI. **Acute respiratory failure (ARF)**

   A. Description: the condition resulting when the exchange of O_2 for CO_2 in the normal lungs cannot match the rate of O_2 consumption and CO_2 production in body cells

   B. Etiology and incidence: possible causes of ARF include:

   1. Airway obstruction
   2. Restrictive lung disease
   3. Central nervous system disorder, such as head trauma or cerebrovascular accident
   4. Drug overdose
   5. Anesthesia and surgical procedures

   C. Pathophysiology and management

   1. ARF occurs whenever O_2 and CO_2 exchange in normal lungs fails to fulfill oxygen needs of body causing alveolar hypoventilation.
   2. Effects include hypoxia (PaO_2 < 60 mmHg) with or without hypercapnia ($PaCO_2$ > 50 mmHg).

   D. Assessment findings

   1. Clinical manifestations of ARF may include:
      a. Dyspnea
      b. Tachypnea
      c. Tachycardia
      d. Headache
      e. Cyanosis
      f. Anxiety, confusion, restlessness
      g. Decreased or absent breath sounds
      h. Adventitious breath sounds: crackles, wheezing
   2. Laboratory and diagnostic studies may reveal:
      a. ABGs: PaO_2 < 60 mmHg; $PaCO_2$ > 50 mmHg; pH < 7.35
      b. ECG: cardiac arrhythmias
      c. Chest radiograph: various lung field changes depending on causative factors
   3. Evaluation of the precipitating event is important in differentiating ARF from acute lung damage (e.g., adult respiratory distress syndrome [ARDS]) and chronic respiratory conditions with acute changes (e.g., COPD).

   E. Nursing diagnoses

   1. Activity Intolerance
   2. Ineffective Airway Clearance
   3. Anxiety
   4. Ineffective Breathing Pattern
   5. Decreased Cardiac Output
   6. Impaired Verbal Communication

   7. Ineffective Individual Coping
   8. Fluid Volume Excess
   9. Impaired Gas Exchange
 F. **Planning and implementation**
   1. Restore and maintain a patent airway by suctioning or performing endotracheal intubation as ordered.
   2. Administer oxygen therapy to maintain adequate alveolar ventilation.
   3. Institute mechanical ventilation if the client's condition deteriorates.
   4. Maintain effective tracheobronchial hygiene.
   5. Monitor cardiac status.
   6. Monitor ABG values.
 G. **Evaluation**
   1. The client maintains ABG values within preillness ranges.
   2. The client demonstrates restoration of adequate pulmonary function.
   3. The client exhibits and reports reduced anxiety and confusion.

VII. Pulmonary embolism
 A. **Description: obstruction of one or more pulmonary arteries by a thrombus or thrombi, originating somewhere in the venous system or in the right side of the heart**
 B. **Etiology and incidence**
   1. Thrombus formation may result from:
      a. Venous stasis, as may result from prolonged immobilization, sitting, or standing
      b. Vessel wall injury
      c. Hypercoagulability of the blood
   2. **Predisposing factors to pulmonary embolism include:**
      a. **Prolonged immobility**
      b. **Chronic lung disease**
      c. **Congestive heart failure**
      d. **Thrombophlebitis**
      e. **Hematologic disorders**
      f. **Lower extremity fractures or surgery**
      g. **Pregnancy or oral contraceptive use**
   3. Pulmonary embolism affects an estimated 6 million adult Americans yearly, resulting in about 100,000 deaths.
 C. **Pathophysiology and management**
   1. Thrombus formation may occur in the deep veins of the legs (most common site); pelvic, renal, or hepatic veins; right heart; and upper extremities.

2. A dislodged thrombus may travel to the pulmonary arterial bed, where obstruction leads to:
    a. Altered ventilation–perfusion ratio
    b. Increase in alveolar dead space
3. The area of obstruction continues to ventilate but receives little or no blood supply, resulting in:
    a. Decreased pulmonary vascular blood pressure
    b. Increased pulmonary artery pressure
4. Unrelieved obstruction may result in right ventricular heart failure and shock; total occlusion of the main pulmonary artery is rapidly fatal.

D. Assessment findings
1. Clinical manifestations commonly include:
    a. Chest pain: may be sudden, sharp or mild, substernal or pleuritic, depending on the site and extent of obstruction
    b. Tachycardia
    c. Dyspnea
    d. Anxiety and restlessness
    e. Decreased breath sounds on auscultation, usually with plural friction rub
    f. Signs of circulatory collapse (weak, rapid pulse; hypotension)
2. Laboratory and diagnostic studies may reveal:
    a. ABGs: PaO_2 < 60 mmHg, indicating hypoxemia
    b. Elevated LDH, bilirubin, and fibrin split products
    c. Deficient perfusion and ventilation lung scans
    d. Pulmonary angiogram (most specific for diagnosis): intraarterial filling defect, obstruction of pulmonary artery branch

E. Nursing diagnoses
1. Activity Intolerance
2. Anxiety
3. Impaired Verbal Communication
4. Impaired Gas Exchange
5. Pain

F. Planning and implementation
1. Administer prescribed medications, which may include:
    a. Anticoagulants: initial therapy includes IV heparin followed by warfarin
    b. Thrombolytics (urokinase, streptokinase, or t-PA)
2. Monitor activated partial thromboplastin time (APTT) when administering heparin. The goal of heparin therapy is an APTT that is 1.5 to 2 times the normal value of 30 to 40 seconds; the antidote for heparin overdose is protamine sulfate.

3. Monitor prothrombin time (PT) when administering warfarin sodium (Coumadin). The goal of anticoagulant therapy is a PT 1.5 to 2.5 times the normal value of 12 seconds; the antidote for Coumadin overdose is vitamin K (Aquamephyton).

4. **Monitor for bleeding; common locations are gastrointestinal tract, urinary tract, mucosal surfaces such as gums, nasal passages.**

5. Administer pain medication as prescribed to relieve chest pain.

6. Correct hypoxemia with oxygen therapy, as necessary.

7. Help reduce venous stasis in legs by applying antiembolism stockings.

8. Provide client teaching covering:
   a. Leg exercises to maintain peripheral circulation
   b. Correct use of anticoagulant therapy and monitoring for bleeding
   c. Safety measures to avoid bleeding, such as using an electric razor and a soft toothbrush, wearing shoes at all times, wearing gloves when working in the garden, and being careful with sharp objects
   d. Measures to take if bleeding occurs, such as applying direct pressure to the wound; if bleeding does not stop in 5 minutes, getting medical assistance

G. **Evaluation**
   1. The client maintains gas exchange at preemboli level.
   2. The client maintains normal vital signs, including temperature.
   3. The client demonstrates return of breath sounds to normal, with no evidence of pleural friction rub.
   4. The client demonstrates compliance with prescribed anticoagulant therapy to prevent recurrence of thrombi.

VII. Lung cancer

A. **Description**
   1. Lung cancer refers to a malignant tumor arising within the wall or epithelial lining of the bronchus or resulting from metastatic spread of cancer arising elsewhere in the body.
   2. Types include:
      a. Squamous cell (epidermoid): the most common type
      b. Adenocarcinoma
      c. Small cell undifferentiated (oat cell)
      d. Large cell undifferentiated

B. **Etiology and incidence**
   1. Predisposing factors to lung cancer include:
      a. Smoking (Lung cancer is 10 times more prevalent in smokers than nonsmokers.)

       b.   Occupational exposure to carcinogenic substances, such as asbestos, arsenic, chromium, nickel, radioactive substances, coal dust, and iron oxides

       c.   Family history of lung cancer

  2.   The most common cause of cancer death in men, lung cancer, has a 5-year survival rate of only 13%.

C. **Pathophysiology and management**

  1.   Squamous cell carcinomas arise most often in the upper lobes, usually in the main stem lobar segmental bronchi. They grow relatively slowly and tend to metastasize late in their course.

  2.   Adenocarcinomas tend to arise in more peripheral lung areas and grow even more slowly than squamous cell carcinomas. They metastasize relatively early in their course.

  3.   Small cell carcinomas arise more peripherally than squamous cell carcinomas and grow rapidly. Metastasis commonly is well established by the time of diagnosis.

  4.   Large cell carcinomas arise more centrally than small cell carcinomas and tend to metastasize early in their course.

  5.   Regardless of cell type, lung cancer produces some combination of pulmonary effects (principally, disturbance in ventilation and perfusion of lung fields invaded by the tumor), systemic effects, and effects of metastatic spread.

  6.   Choice of treatment modalities depends on disease stage, tumor type, and the client's condition, and may include:

       a.   Surgical resection of the tumor or lung tissue

       b.   Radiation therapy

       c.   Chemotherapy

       d.   Immunotherapy

D. **Assessment findings**

  1.   Symptoms usually occur relatively late and are related to tumor size and location.

  2.   Common clinical manifestations include:

       a.   Change in nature of normal cough

       b.   Hemoptysis

       c.   Dyspnea

       d.   Hoarseness and wheezing

       e.   Chest pain

       f.   Weight loss and fatigue

  3.   Test results may reveal:

       a.   Radiograph: chest mass

       b.   Sputum studies: malignant cells

       c.   Bronchoscopy specimen: positive for malignant cells

       d.   CT lung scan: positive

       e.   Pulmonary function studies: decreased pulmonary reserve

E. **Nursing diagnoses**
   1. Activity Intolerance
   2. Anxiety
   3. Ineffective Individual Coping
   4. Altered Health Maintenance
   5. Impaired Home Maintenance Management
   6. Altered Nutrition: Less than body requirements
   7. Pain
F. **Planning and implementation (*Note:* See Chapter 21, Cancer Nursing, for more detailed nursing interventions applicable to all types of cancer.)**
   1. Prepare the client for planned tests and treatments.
   2. Maintain adequate nutritional status.
   3. Control pain with prescribed analgesics or other measures.
   4. Provide emotional support to the client and family; address concerns and uncertainty that contribute to anxiety and depression.
G. **Evaluation**
   1. The client reports relief or control of dyspnea and chest discomfort.
   2. The client demonstrates improved nutritional status.
   3. The client reports reduced anxiety and depression.
   4. The client and family members report acceptance of the diagnosis and make realistic plans.

IX. Chest trauma
   A. **Description**
      1. Injury to the chest wall or lungs can interfere with inspiration, gas exchange, or expiration.
      2. Types include:
         a. Hemothorax: blood in the pleural space
         b. Pneumothorax: air in the pleural space
         c. Open pneumothorax: sucking wound of the chest
   B. **Etiology and incidence**
      1. Hemothorax results from penetrating or blunt chest injury.
      2. Pneumothorax can result from disease or injury, most commonly from laceration of the lung parenchyma, tracheobronchial tree, or esophagus.
      3. Open pneumothorax most commonly results from penetrating chest injury.
   C. **Pathophysiology and management**
      1. In hemothorax, blood in the pleural cavity compresses the lungs and can produce blood loss resulting in shock.
      2. In tension pneumothorax—considered a medical emergency—pressure in the pleural space compromises ventilation

and can lead to lung collapse, decreased ventilation in the other lung, and decreased venous return to the heart, known as a mediastinal shift.

3. Open pneumothorax, an acutely life-threatening condition, involves an opening in the chest wall large enough to allow air passage into and out of the chest cavity with each attempted respiration; the rush of air produces a characteristic "sucking" sound. Tidal volume diminishes, and ventilation is compromised.

D. Assessment findings

1. Clinical manifestations may include:
   a. Dyspnea
   b. Tachypnea
   c. Pain on breathing
   d. Rapid development of cyanosis
   e. Asymmetric chest movement
   f. Hypotension progressing to shock (hemothorax)
2. ECG may reveal cardiac arrhythmias

E. Nursing diagnoses

1. Ineffective Airway Clearance
2. Ineffective Breathing Pattern
3. Decreased Cardiac Output
4. Impaired Verbal Communication
5. Fluid Volume Deficit
6. Impaired Gas Exchange

F. Planning and implementation

1. Establish and maintain a patent airway by suctioning and endotracheal intubation as appropriate.
2. Administer oxygen to correct hypoxemia as necessary.
3. Control hemorrhage; treat damage to chest and other injured structures.
4. Stabilize the chest wall if necessary.
5. As ordered, assist with insertion of chest tube, and maintain closed drainage system (Fig. 6-1).
6. Provide emotional support to reduce anxiety and fear.
7. Prepare the client for surgery if appropriate, based on the nature of the injury.

G. Evaluation

1. The client displays normal cardiopulmonary function.
2. The client exhibits healing of penetrating chest wound without infection.
3. The client demonstrates resolution of arrhythmias.
4. Vital signs remain in normal ranges.
5. The client's lungs are clear on auscultation.

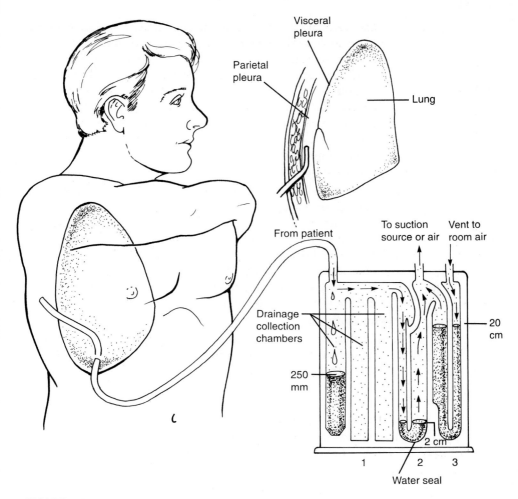

FIGURE 6-1.
Common chest tube and drainage-suction system used in patients with pulmonary injury, such as hemothorax or pneumothorax. The Pleur-Evac system (shown) works much like the traditional bottle-suction systems.

X. Adult respiratory distress syndrome (ARDS)

A. Description: a clinical syndrome characterized by pulmonary edema and progressive decrease in arterial oxygen content; occurs after a serious illness or injury and accumulation of lung fluids, also known as noncardiogenic pulmonary edema

B. Etiology and incidence

 1. ARDS is *always* secondary to another injury or illness. Numerous factors are associated with the development of ARDS and include any direct injury to the lungs or indirect insult to the body.

2. Causes may include aspiration; drug overdose; prolonged inhalation of high concentrations of oxygen, smoke, or corrosive substances; shock (any cause); trauma (e.g., pulmonary contusion, multiple fractures, head injury); and systemic infection.

3. ARDS has been associated with a mortality rate as high as 50% to 60%. Early diagnosis and prompt treatment increase survival rate.

C. **Pathophysiology and management**

1. Injury to the alveolar capillary membrane results in leakage of blood and fluid into the alveolar interstitial spaces and alteration in the capillary bed.

2. The fluid in the alveoli impairs gas exchange and causes extensive shunting of blood in the lungs. This leads to a ventilation–perfusion imbalance which in turn leads to noncardiogenic pulmonary edema.

3. Early diagnosis and treatment is crucial for recovery and may involve ventilatory support, medication, and supportive care.

D. **Assessment findings**

1. Clinical manifestations usually occur 12 to 48 hours after a serious injury or illness and include:

   a. Anxiety
   b. Decreased level of consciousness
   c. Dyspnea
   d. Tachypnea
   e. Auscultated crackles
   f. Decreased functional residual capacity
   g. Hypocapnia
   h. Severe hypoxia
   i. Marked buccal peripheral cyanosis

2. Laboratory and diagnostic studies may reveal:

   a. Chest x-ray: bilateral pulmonary infiltrates

   b. **ABG analysis: decreased PaO_2 (below 60 mmHG) despite administration of oxygen at a high flow rate (10 L/min)**

E. **Nursing diagnoses**

1. Impaired Gas Exchange
2. Ineffective Breathing Pattern
3. Fluid Volume Excess
4. Anxiety
5. Decreased Cardiac Output
6. Ineffective Individual Coping

F. **Planning and implementation**

1. Assist with endotracheal intubation and mechanical ventilation; as prescribed, institute positive end-expiratory pressure (PEEP) to keep alveoli distended, stretch stiff lungs, and increase oxygen–carbon dioxide diffusion.

2. Administer corticosteroids, as prescribed, to decrease inflammation surrounding the alveoli and to stabilize the capillary membranes. Keep in mind that this therapy remains controversial because of the belief that corticosteroid use may precipitate superinfection and further impair pulmonary function (see Section II.O).

3. Encourage semi-Fowler's or high-Fowler's position.

4. Assess client for signs and symptoms of fluid volume overload including peripheral edema and jugular vein distention.

5. Provide adequate nutritional support that is not high in carbohydrates, which metabolize to form excess CO_2. The diet should include 35 to 45 kcal/kg a day to meet normal requirements, with enteral or parental feeding support if necessary.

6. Reassure client, explain all procedures, and remain calm to reduce client's anxiety and thereby decrease oxygen need.

7. Monitor ABG levels.

8. Maintain effective tracheobronchial hygiene.

9. Monitor hemodynamic status.

G. Evaluation

1. The client maintains ABG values within preillness ranges.

2. The client demonstrates restoration of adequate pulmonary function.

3. The client recovers from the precipitating cause of ARDS.

XI. **Thoracic surgery (thoracotomy)**

A. Description

1. Surgical intervention is viewed as deliberate trauma to the chest to correct an underlying problem (e.g., tumor resection, organ repair, transplant).

2. Surgery disrupts the negative pressure of the chest, requiring controlled ventilation throughout the procedure to maintain ventilation and pulmonary circulation.

B. Assessment

1. Evaluate the client's preoperative status (see Chapter 24 for information on general preoperative and postoperative nursing assessment).

   a. Physiologic condition, particularly cardiovascular and respiratory status

   b. Coping abilities

2. Assess the client's and family's teaching needs related, for example, to postoperative measures, such as deep breathing,

coughing, and incentive spirometry to improve alveolar ventilation and respiratory function.

C. **Nursing diagnoses**
1. Ineffective Breathing Pattern
2. Risk for Disuse Syndrome
3. Impaired Gas Exchange
4. Risk for Infection
5. Impaired Physical Mobility
6. Pain
7. Risk for Impaired Skin Integrity

D. **Planning and implementation**
1. Preoperative
   a. Prepare the client for scheduled diagnostic and laboratory tests, such as chest radiography, pulmonary function studies, lung scan, ECG, hematologic studies, and ABG analysis and other blood tests.
   b. See Chapter 24 for general preoperative and postoperative nursing interventions.
   c. Provide explanations, reassurance, and support for the planned surgical procedure.
   d. Describe what the client can expect to see, hear, and feel before and after surgery. Also describe nursing care that will be provided.
2. Postoperative
   a. Maintain effective gas exchange by suctioning or mechanical ventilation as appropriate.
   b. Encourage the client to perform incentive spirometry to aid reinflation of the affected lung.
   c. Monitor chest tube function, and evaluate the amount and nature of drainage.
   d. Assess for pain related to surgical incision and presence of chest tubes. Help relieve pain by:

   ► Instructing the client to splint the incision when coughing
   ► Maintaining the client in Fowler's position
   ► Administering analgesics as ordered (in moderation to avoid respiratory depression)

   e. Maintain fluid therapy and blood replacement as ordered.
   f. Monitor ABG values for hypoxia or hypercapnia.
   g. Monitor vital signs.
   h. Assess for signs and symptoms of complications, such as hemorrhage, respiratory failure, wound infection, and cardiac abnormalities.

E.   Evaluation
1.   The client maintains effective respiration without assistance.
2.   The client reports pain control or relief.
3.   The client demonstrates restoration of chest and arm mobility.
4.   The client's ABG values remain within normal ranges.

Bibliography

Bolander, V.C. (1994). *Sorensen and Luckmann's medical-surgical nursing: A psychophysiologic approach* (3rd ed.). Philadelphia: W. B. Saunders.

Carpenito, L. J. (1992). *Nursing diagnosis: Application to clinical practice* (3rd ed.). Philadelphia: J. B. Lippincott.

Clark, J., Queener, S., & Karb, V. (1993). *Pharmacological basis of nursing practice* (4th ed.). St. Louis: C. V. Mosby.

Nettina, S. (1996). *The Lippincott manual of nursing practice* (6th ed.). Philadelphia: Lippincott-Raven Publishers.

Smeltzer, S. C., & Bare, B. G. (1996). *Brunner and Suddarth's textbook of medical-surgical nursing* (8th ed.). Philadelphia: Lippincott-Raven Publishers.

Springhouse Corporation. (1992). *Nursing student's guide to drugs*. Spring House, PA: Springhouse Corp.

STUDY QUESTIONS

1. An accountant complains of shortness of breath and tightness in the chest after a short run. The client denies sore throat, fever, or productive cough but admits to having had a cold last week. Based on these data the nurse would surmise the symptoms are related to
   a. asthma
   b. pneumoconioses
   c. bronchitis
   d. pneumonia

2. In addition to fever, hacking cough, and general complaints of malaise, additional assessment data the nurse would expect to uncover in a client with pneumonia would include:
   a. conjunctivitis and nasal swelling
   b. tonsillar exudate and pain on swallowing
   c. bronchial breath sounds over lung field with consolidation
   d. productive cough with excess mucus

3. A client diagnosed with pulmonary embolism is being discharged. The nursing diagnosis of knowledge deficit would be based on the client's need to know which of the following self-care measures?
   a. Reduce walking to only necessary activities around the house.
   b. Maintain peripheral circulation with leg exercises.
   c. Soak feet nightly in warm water to increase circulation.
   d. Avoid bending to pick up objects.

4. The long-term goal in the nursing care of a client diagnosed with COPD would be to
   a. Decrease activity to conserve functional lung tissue.
   b. Increase the frequency of postural drainage to every 2 hours while awake.
   c. Increase the residual volume.
   d. Improve and maintain pulmonary ventilation and gas exchange.

5. The primary nursing intervention most commonly required in caring for a client who has COPD and who is in acute respiratory failure is
   a. Establish initial stage of activity.
   b. Discourage client from sitting in Fowler's position, which increases the work of the heart.
   c. Remove bronchial secretions, and manage oxygen therapy.
   d. Plan with family for home care.

6. The nursing care for the client with COPD should include assisting the client to develop ways to cope with chronic obstructive pulmonary disease by
   a. encouraging the family to take increased responsibility for the client's care
   b. discouraging the client from performing activities of daily living if they promote fatigue
   c. teaching the client relaxation techniques and breathing retraining exercises
   d. protecting the client from knowing the prognosis of the disease

7. A nursing diagnosis appropriate for the client with pneumonia would include which of the following?
   a. Fluid Volume Deficit related to vomiting and diarrhea
   b. Pain related to chest pain radiating to the left shoulder and arm
   c. Hyperthermia related to sudden onset of chills with a rising fever and chest pain
   d. Ineffective Breathing Pattern related to slow, shallow respiration

8. A client hospitalized for acute bacterial pneumonia is now recovering after a course of therapy with penicillin G. In evaluating the effect of care, the nurse should expect which of the following outcomes?
   a. The client displays PaO_2 of 85 mmHg or above.
   b. The client displays $PaCO_2$ of 80 mmHg or above.

c. The client demonstrates decreased breath sounds.

d. The client demonstrates signs of restlessness and confusion.

9. The postoperative nursing care for the client who has just undergone chest surgery for a right lower lobectomy would include which of the following?
   a. Encourage coughing to mobilize secretions.
   b. Ensure that the thoracotomy tube is attached to open chest drainage.
   c. Restrict IV fluids for 24 hours.
   d. Prevent coughing to ensure incision integrity.

10. A potential complication of tracheobronchial suctioning is lobar collapse. This can be avoided by
    a. using a large catheter the same diameter as the trachea
    b. applying suction at high pressure to accomplish the procedure as quickly as possible
    c. applying suction continuously for 30 seconds or more
    d. using a catheter that is narrow enough not to occlude the airway during application of suction

11. The client diagnosed with respiratory insufficiency resulting from longstanding restrictive lung disease should be advised to prevent or control respiratory infections by
    a. taking penicillin prophylactically for life
    b. smoking low-tar cigarettes
    c. taking influenza injections and broad-spectrum antibiotics as prescribed
    d. having periodic blood studies to monitor PO_2

12. The neurologic control of ventilation rests in several areas of the nervous system. The primary control of inspiration and expiration occurs in the
    a. baroreceptors
    b. medulla oblongata
    c. alveoli
    d. pons

13. The nurse would suspect adult respiratory distress syndrome (ARDS) in the client diagnosed with hypovolemic shock secondary to multiple trauma when the client exhibits which of the following?
    a. PaO_2 of 62 mmHg after 2 hours of oxygen administered at a rate of 10 L/min by nasal cannula
    b. Increased breath sounds with increased chest expansion
    c. $PaCO_2$ of 65 mmHg with a PaO_2 of 85 mmHg
    d. Greenish tenacious sputum and tachypnea

14. Nursing assessment findings in a client with a right-sided pneumothorax would include
    a. bradypnea and bronchovesicular breath sounds
    b. chronic cough and sudden onset of chills
    c. rust-colored sputum and increased temperature
    d. dyspnea and asymmetrical chest expansion

15. Nursing care of the client with ARDS would include
    a. keeping the client in prone position
    b. assessing the client for fluid volume deficit
    c. monitoring ABG levels and cardiac status
    d. administering oxygen at a rate of 4 L/min by nasal cannula

16. The client with a pulmonary embolism is receiving anticoagulation therapy with warfarin (Coumadin). Before administering the next dose, the nurse evaluates the client's current lab values which are PT 25/PTT 39. Based on these values the nurse would
    a. give the prescribed dose
    b. prepare to administer protamine sulfate
    c. withhold the dose and notify the physician
    d. prepare to administer vitamin K (Aquamephyton)

ANSWER KEY

1. **Correct response: a**
   The reported symptoms and lack of symptoms are characteristic of asthma. The previous viral infection may have made the client more prone to bronchial spasms in response to exercise or cold temperatures.
   b. The client's occupation as an accountant would decrease the likelihood of pneumoconioses.
   c and d. The client's lack of productive cough or fever would decrease the probability of either bronchitis or pneumonia.
   Application/Physiologic/Assessment

2. **Correct response: c**
   Bronchial breath sounds are commonly found over lung fields with infiltration and consolidation in pneumonia.
   a. Eye and nose symptoms are not typical in pneumonia.
   b. Tonsillar exudate and pain on swallowing are cardinal symptoms of streptococcal sore throat caused by infection of the pharynx.
   d. Cough associated with pneumonia is typically hacking and nonproductive.
   Application/Physiologic/Assessment

3. **Correct response: b**
   Leg exercises are important in reducing the risk of further thrombus development.
   a. Reduction of walking is contraindicated.
   c. Soaking the feet is not necessary to increase circulation and is inappropriate, especially in an older person, because of its drying effect on skin.
   d. No physiologic contraindication to bending is associated with this medical diagnosis.
   Analysis/Health promotion/
   Analysis (Dx)

4. **Correct response: d**
   The underlying pathology of COPD affects the lungs' ability to ventilate and exchange O_2 and CO_2. Ventilation and gas exchange are directly dependent on each other. An effective relationship between the two parameters is absolutely necessary for effective physiologic and mental functioning.
   a. Decreasing activity level will not conserve functional lung tissue. Rather, treatment should aim to increase activity while implementing work modification techniques.
   b. Postural drainage performed every 2 hours would be unnecessary since no evidence links the client's problem to retained secretions.
   c. The goal would be to decrease rather than increase residual volume, which usually is high in COPD.
   Application/Health promotion/
   Implementation

5. **Correct response: c**
   Acute respiratory failure results from inadequate gas exchange in the lungs. Increasing the availability of oxygen and assisting with secretion removal will improve ventilation.
   a. A client experiencing acute respiratory failure should usually not be started on an activity program: conservation of energy is critical at this stage.
   b. The client most likely will find that semi-Fowler's or Fowler's position facilitates breathing.
   d. Planning for home care is important—but not at this stage; the client's level of self-care deficit is unknown at this point.
   Knowledge/Safe care/Implementation

6. **Correct response: c**
   Relaxation techniques and breathing retraining will help a client with COPD maximize energy supplies and effectively use available oxygen.
   a and b. A COPD client should be encouraged to be as independent as

possible within physiologic capabilities; total care encourages deterioration.

d. Knowledge of the disease process may help the client better understand how to make the most of his or her life.

Application/Psychosocial/Implementation

7. **Correct response: c**
Chills, fever, and pain result from inflammation of the terminal airways and alveoli caused by bacterial, viral, or fungal infection.
a, b, and d. These signs and symptoms are not associated with pneumonia.

Comprehension/Physiologic/ Analysis (Dx)

8. **Correct response: a**
As lung infection progresses, ventilation is interrupted. PO_2 usually decreases, and a degree of respiratory insufficiency occurs. As the infection subsides and lung function returns, PO_2 typically rises between 85 and 100 mmHg.
b. PCO_2 of 80 mmHg indicates respiratory failure.
c. Decreased breath sounds is an abnormal manifestation.
d. Restlessness and confusion would indicate hypoxia rather than improvement.

Analysis/Physiologic/Evaluation

9. **Correct response: a**
The client should be encouraged to cough to raise and expectorate sputum. Splinting the incision during coughing is recommended to minimize discomfort.
b. Thoracotomy tubes are always attached to closed, sealed drainage to reexpand lung tissue and prevent pneumothorax.
c. IV fluid infusion is indicated following surgery because the client will not be able to tolerate oral fluids for a time. Restricting fluids would encourage dehydration.

d. Coughing is indicated to mobilize secretions.

Analysis/Safe care/Planning

10. **Correct response: d**
Suctioning may produce lobar collapse if the suction catheter diameter is too large for the size of the airway. Lobar collapse occurs when air cannot enter the lung from around the catheter while suction is applied.
a. This catheter is too large in diameter.
b and c. Performing intermittent suctioning for no more than 8 seconds at a time and using low pressure reduce the risk of trauma or hypoxia.

Application/Safe care/Planning

11. **Correct response: c**
Broad-spectrum antibiotics are indicated under medical supervision as a prophylactic treatment against lung infections, particularly during winter months. Influenza injections are regularly recommended for clients with chronic chest problems.
a. Penicillin is not a broad-spectrum antibiotic.
b. Clients with lung disease should not smoke any substance in any form.
d. PO_2 studies are indicated only if exacerbation occurs.

Comprehension/Health promotion/ Planning

12. **Correct response: b**
The rhythmicity of breathing is controlled by respiratory centers located in the medulla oblongata of the brain. These inspiratory and expiratory centers control the rate and depth of respiration to meet the body's metabolic demands.
a. Located in the aortic arch and carotid bodies, baroreceptors respond to increase and decrease in arterial blood pressure and cause reflex hypoventilation and hyperventilation.
c. The alveoli contain stretch receptors

that mediate overdistention of the lung.

    d. The pons houses the pneumotaxic center, which is thought to stimulate the expiratory medullary center.

Comprehension/Physiologic/Assessment

13. ***Correct response: a***

One of the cardinal signs of ARDS is low $PaCO_2$ after administration of a high concentration of oxygen. The oxygen cannot cross the alveoli because of the fluid in the interstitial space.

    b. Crackles would be heard throughout the lungs.

    c. The $PaCO_2$ (normal 35–45 mmHg) is not immediately increased because carbon dioxide can diffuse across the alveoli more easily than can oxygen. PaO_2 of 85 mmHg is within normal limits.

    d. Greenish, tenacious sputum is indicative of pneumonia, not of ARDS.

Application/Physiologic/Assessment

14. ***Correct response: d***

The client with a pneumothorax would have dyspnea secondary to decreased lung expansion. The breathing pattern would be asymmetrical secondary to the air in pleural space.

    a. The client would have tachypnea and decreased breath sounds over the pneumothorax. Bronchovesicular breath sounds are normal.

    b and c. These signs and symptoms would not be indicative of pneumothorax but would be indicative of pneumonia of COPD.

Application/Physiologic/Assessment

15. ***Correct response: c***

Monitoring ABG values is of paramount importance in diagnosing as well as evaluating effectiveness of treatment. Decreased PaO_2 despite a high oxygen concentration is a cardinal sign. A rising level of PaO_2 reflects progress.

    a. The client would need to be in semi-Fowler's or high-Fowler's position to ease breathing.

    b. The nurse would need to assess for fluid volume overload secondary to noncardiogenic pulmonary edema.

    d. Low flow oxygen administration is indicated in COPD; high flow oxygen administration is indicated in ARDS.

Application/Physiologic/Implementation

16. ***Correct response: a***

Anticoagulant therapy with warfarin (Coumadin) requires monitoring the client's PT. Normal PT is 12 seconds. A therapeutic level of Coumadin is 1.5 to 2.5 times the normal 12 seconds (between 18 and 30 sec). The client's PT is 25; therefore, the nurse would administer the dose.

    b. Protamine sulfate is the antidote for heparin overdose.

    c. There is no need to withhold the dose since the PT/PTT indicates that the drug is at a therapeutic level.

    d. Vitamin K (Aquamephyton) is the antidote for warfarin overdosage but the data reflect that the drug is within a normal therapeutic level.

Comprehension/Safe care/Planning

Cardiovascular Disorders

I. Cardiovascular system

A. Structures

1. A hollow, muscular organ, the heart lies in the mediastinum (the space between the two lungs) and rests on the diaphragm.

2. The heart is encased in the *pericardium,* a thin, membranous sac that has two layers: a *visceral* layer in contact with the heart and an outer *parietal* layer.

3. The space between the pericardial layers contains 20 to 30 mL of serous fluid, which protects the heart from trauma and friction.

4. The heart wall, specialized muscle tissue, consists of three tissue layers:

    a. *Epicardium,* the thin, serous outer layer

    b. *Myocardium,* the thick, muscular middle layer

    c. *Endocardium,* the smooth inner layer that comes in contact with blood

5. A membranous muscular *septum* divides the heart into two distinct sides, each containing two chambers: an atrium and a ventricle (Fig. 7-1).

6. The *right atrium,* a low-pressure chamber, receives systemic venous blood via the superior vena cava, inferior vena cava, and coronary sinus.

7. The *right ventricle,* another low-pressure chamber, receives blood from the right atrium through the tricuspid valve during ventricular diastole, then ejects deoxygenated blood via the pulmonic valve through the pulmonary artery and into pulmonary circulation during ventricular systole.

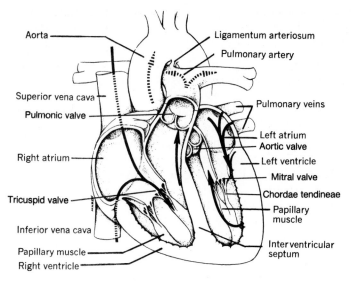

FIGURE 7-1.
Structure of the heart and course of blood flow (arrows) through the chambers. (From Chaffee, E.E. & Greisheimer, E.M. *Basic physiology and anatomy*. Philadelphia: J.B. Lippincott.)

8. The *left atrium,* a low-pressure chamber, receives oxygenated blood returning to the heart from the lung via four pulmonary veins.
9. The *left ventricle,* a high-pressure chamber, receives blood from the left atrium through the mitral valve during ventricular diastole and ejects oxygenated blood via the aortic valve through the aorta and into systemic circulation during ventricular systole.
10. Valves connect the chambers and outflow tracts; types include atrioventricular and semilunar valves (see Fig. 7-1).
11. *Atrioventricular* (AV) *valves,* separating the atria from the ventricles, include:
    a. The *tricuspid valve* (so called because it contains three cusps, or leaflets) between the right atrium and ventricle
    b. The *mitral valve* (or bicuspid valve, with two cusps) between the left atrium and ventricle
12. Situated between each ventricle and its corresponding artery, *semilunar valves* (each containing three cusps) include:
    a. The *pulmonic valve* between the right ventricle and pulmonary artery
    b. The *aortic valve* between the left ventricle and aorta
13. *Papillary muscles,* muscle bundles on the ventricular walls, and *chordae tendineae,* fibrous bands extending from the papillary muscles to the valve cusps, keep the valves closed during

systole, maintaining unidirectional blood flow through the AV valves and preventing backflow of blood.

14. The *cardiac conduction system* consists of specialized cardiac cells that either initiate or propagate electrical impulses throughout the myocardium as a precursor to cardiac muscle contraction (Fig. 7-2).

15. Located at the junction of the right atrium and the superior vena cava, the *sinoatrial (SA) node* functions as the pacemaker for the myocardium, initiating rhythmic electrical impulses at an intrinsic rate of 60 to 100 impulses per minute.

16. The *AV node,* located in the right atrial wall near the tricuspid valve, receives impulses from the SA node and relays them to the ventricles.

17. These impulses travel through a bundle of specialized muscle fibers in the myocardial septum—the *bundle of His*—that divides into right and left branches:
    a. The *right bundle branch* (RBB), which conducts impulses down the right side of the septum
    b. The *left bundle branch* (LBB), which divides again into right and left fascicles that fan out into the left ventricular muscle

18. The RBB and LBB terminate in the *Purkinje fibers,* which propagate electrical impulses into the endocardium and on to the myocardium.

19. The *coronary arteries* supply the heart with blood from branches that originate in either the right or left sinus of Valsalva of the aortic valve cusps.

20. The *right coronary artery* supplies blood to the right heart

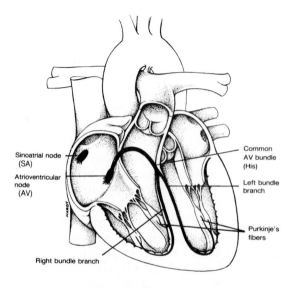

Sinoatrial node (SA)

Atrioventricular node (AV)

Right bundle branch

Common AV bundle (His)

Left bundle branch

Purkinje's fibers

FIGURE 7-2.
Cardiac conduction system and landmarks, beginning with the sinoatrial node and progressing along the atrioventricular node, the common atrioventricular bundle (the bundle of His) and its branches. (From Chaffee, E.E. & Greisheimer, E.M. *Basic physiology and anatomy.* Philadelphia: J.B. Lippincott.)

wall. The *left main coronary artery,* which divides into two branches—the left anterior descending (LAD) coronary artery and the circumflex artery—supplies most of the blood to the left heart wall.

B. **Function**

1. The heart has electrophysiologic, mechanical, and neurologic properties that coordinate to produce effective myocardial contraction and pumping of blood.
2. Each complete heartbeat, or *cardiac cycle,* consists of two phases in response to electrical stimulation:
   a. *Systole,* the contraction phase
   b. *Diastole,* the relaxation (filling) phase
3. Systole is triggered by *depolarization* of cardiac muscle cells, which involves a transient change in sodium and potassium ion concentration inside and outside the cell.
4. Immediately after depolarization is completed, the process reverses itself, resulting in *repolarization* and a return to the resting state, or diastole.

5. **Heart sounds result from vibrations caused by valve closure and ventricular filling; they include:**
   a. **The *first heart sound* (S1), associated with tricuspid and mitral valve closure**
   b. **The *second heart sound* (S2), associated with aortic and pulmonic valve closure**
   c. **The *physiologic third heart sound* (S3), often normal in persons under age 30 but pathologic in older persons (known as *ventricular gallop*), occurring during the rapid ventricular filling stage of diastole**
   d. **The *fourth heart sound* (S4), or atrial gallop, linked to resistance to ventricular filling, as in hypertrophy or injury of the ventricular wall**
6. **Cardiac output (CO) is defined as the volume of blood ejected by each ventricle in 1 minute; CO = SV (stroke volume) × HR (heart rate).**
7. Several factors influence CO indirectly by affecting SV, including:
   a. *Preload,* the end-diastolic filling volume of the ventricle; increased by increased returning volume to ventricle
   b. *Afterload,* the resistance to left ventricular ejection; increased by increased systemic arterial pressure
8. Various neurologic factors regulate heart function, including:
   a. Sympathetic nervous system stimulation, with release of norepinephrine, which results in arteriolar vasoconstriction, increased heart rate, and a positive inotropic effect

b. Parasympathetic nervous system stimulation, with release of acetylcholine, resulting in decreased heart rate and slowed AV conduction

c. Response of chemoreceptors located in carotid and aortic bodies to decrease in O_2 and increase in CO_2, leading to increased heart rate

d. Response of baroreceptors located in the aortic arch, carotid sinus, vena cava, pulmonary arteries, and atria to blood pressure changes; either decrease or increase heart rate, resulting in blood pressure changes

II. Overview of cardiovascular disorders

A. Assessment

1. During the health history, the nurse should elicit a description of symptoms, including onset, course, duration, location, and precipitating and alleviating factors; significant symptoms in cardiovascular dysfunction include:

   a. Pain: character, quality, radiation, associated symptoms; may be an indicator of myocardial ischemia

   b. Palpitations, characterized by rapid irregular or pounding heart beat; may be associated with arrhythmias or ischemia

   c. Intermittent claudication, characterized by extremity pain with exercise; indicative of peripheral vascular disease

   d. Dyspnea, characterized by difficult breathing or shortness of breath with activity (dyspnea on exertion), in the supine position (orthopnea), or sudden onset at night (paroxysmal nocturnal dyspnea); commonly associated with compromised cardiac function

   e. Fatigue with or without activity; may be associated with decreased cardiac output (CO)

   f. Syncope with or without dizziness; can result from sudden decrease in CO

   g. Diaphoresis with associated clamminess and cyanosis; reflects decreased CO and poor peripheral perfusion

   h. Edema or weight gain (>3 lb in 24 hours); may indicate heart failure

2. The nurse also should explore the client's health history for risk factors associated with cardiovascular disease, including:

   a. Positive family history for cardiovascular disease

   b. Age (incidence increases after age 40)

   c. Sex (mortality from cardiovascular disease is greater in men than in women; difference decreases after menopause)

   d. Race (mortality is greater in nonwhites than in whites)

     e.   Smoking (the risk of cardiovascular disease is 2 to 4 times greater in cigarette smokers than in nonsmokers)

     f.   Hypertension, particularly elevated systolic pressure

     g.   Hyperlipidemia (the ratio of high-density lipoproteins [HDL] to low-density lipoproteins [LDL] is the best predictor)

     h.   Obesity, which contributes to the severity of other risk factors

     i.   Physical inactivity (sedentary lifestyle)

     j.   Diabetes (uncontrolled elevated blood glucose level increases risk)

     k.   Stress, which may contribute to developing coronary artery disease (CAD)

     l.   Use of oral contraceptives

3.   Physical assessment should include the following:

     a.   Assess the client's general appearance for signs of distress, anxiety, and altered level of consciousness.

     b.   Assess vital signs, particularly pulse, blood pressure, and respirations.

     c.   Assess peripheral pulses.

     d.   Inspect the lips, earlobes, and buccal mucosa for central cyanosis, reflecting hypoxia.

     e.   Inspect and palpate the carotid arteries.

     f.   Assess jugular venous pressure, and observe for venous distention.

     g.   Inspect and palpate the precordium to locate the point of maximal impulse (PMI) or the apical impulse.

     h.   Systematically auscultate the heart for normal and abnormal heart sounds, murmurs, and friction rub, covering four main areas: aortic area, pulmonary area, mitral area, and tricuspid area.

     i.   Perform a respiratory assessment (see Chapter 6, Section II.A). Findings pointing to cardiovascular problems may include cough (possibly reflecting pulmonary congestion); rales, crackles, or wheezing (reflecting airway narrowing, atelectasis, or left ventricular failure); hemoptysis (possibly pointing to acute pulmonary edema); Cheyne-Stokes respiration (possibly associated with severe left ventricular failure).

     j.   Perform an abdominal assessment (see Chapter 9, Section II.A) noting particularly liver enlargement and ascites (indicating decreased venous return secondary to right ventricular failure); bladder distention (possibly pointing to decreased cardiac output); and bruits just above the umbilicus (may reflect abdominal aortic obstruction or aneurysm).

B. **Laboratory studies and diagnostic tests**
1. Important laboratory studies in cardiovascular evaluation include:
   a. Leukocyte count
   b. Lipid profile: cholesterol (LDL and HDL), triglycerides
   c. Cardiac enzymes: lactic dehydrogenase (LDH), creatinine phosphokinase (CPK), and their isoenzymes
   d. Blood coagulation: prothrombin time (PT), partial thromboplastin time (PTT)
2. Noninvasive diagnostic studies include:
   a. Chest radiograph, to determine heart size and silhouette and visualize the pulmonary system
   b. Electrocardiography (ECG), to evaluate the heart's electrical activity
   c. Ambulatory ECG, to allow 24-hour continuous measurement of the heart's electrical activity
   d. Exercise ECG (graded exercise test), to evaluate electrical activity during physical stress
   e. Vectorcardiography, which provides a graphic representation of the direction and magnitude of the heart's electrical activity
   f. Echocardiography, which yields information about cardiac structures (especially valvular) and function
   g. Radionuclide testing, which evaluates ventricular function and myocardial blood flow and detects areas of myocardial damage
3. Invasive diagnostic studies include:
   a. Cardiac catheterization, which enables measurement of chamber pressures and oxygen saturation
   b. Arteriography, done to visualize coronary arteries with injections of radiopaque contrast media
   c. Ventriculography, to visualize ventricles with injection of radiopaque contrast media
   d. Central venous pressure (CVP), which reflects filling pressure of the right ventricle and helps assess cardiac function and intravascular volume status
   e. Pulmonary artery pressure (PAP) and pulmonary artery wedge pressure (PAWP), which measure left heart pressures
   f. Arterial line, which allows continuous monitoring of peripheral arterial pressures

C. **Psychosocial implications**
1. A client with cardiovascular dysfunction commonly experiences problems in coping with the disease process, related to such factors as:

       a.   Sense of loss of control

       b.   Perception of the heart as a center of emotion and personality

       c.   Uncertain prognosis

       d.   Fear of rejection and isolation

       e.   Fear of dying

2.   The client also may experience self-concept changes related to fear of:

       a.   Sexual dysfunction

       b.   Role change toward increased dependence

       c.   Body image changes if surgery or an adjunctive device (such as a pacemaker) is needed

3.   The client may have concerns associated with changes in lifestyle due to alterations in:

       a.   Physical activity

       b.   Work performance, with potential for job loss

D. **Medications used to treat cardiovascular disorders (additional medications may be included with specific diseases)**

    1.   *Antiarrhythmics,* which reduce or prevent cardiac arrhythmias by directly depressing the excitability of cardiac tissue

       a.   Examples: amiodarone (Cordarone), bretylium (Bretylol), disopyramide (Norpace), lidocaine (Xylocaine), procainamide (Pronestyl), quinidine (Cardioquin), propranolol (Inderal)

       b.   Selected nursing considerations

       m ▸ **Take apical pulse rate before administering drug. Notify physician if rate falls below 60. Teach client to take pulse.**

    2.   *Anticoagulants,* which disrupt the coagulation pathways and prevent platelet aggregations, thereby preventing deep vein thrombosis or pulmonary emboli

       a.   Examples: heparin, warfarin sodium (Coumadin)

       b.   Selected nursing considerations

       m ▸ **In clients receiving heparin, monitor activated partial thromboplastin time (APTT) which should be 1.5 to 2 times the normal value of 30 to 40 sec.**

           ▸ **In clients receiving warfarin, monitor prothrombin time (PT) which should be 1.5 to 2.5 times the normal value of 12 sec.**

           ▸ **Instruct client to report any prolonged or unexplained bleeding.**

    3.   *Antilipemics,* which lower serum cholesterol level by binding bile salts in the bowel and forming an insoluble complex that is excreted in the stool

a. Examples: cholestyramine (Questran), clofibrate (Atromid-S), colestipol (Colestid), probucol (Lorelco)
b. Selected nursing considerations

m ▸ **Mix medication with 60 mL water or fruit juice to mask the unpleasant flavor.**
▸ **Instruct client to increase fluid intake to prevent constipation.**

4. *Beta-adrenergic blockers,* which decrease the heart rate and the force of contraction and reduce vasoconstriction by antagonizing beta receptors in the myocardium and vasculature; used in stable or unstable angina, arrhythmias, and hypertension in coronary artery disease (CAD)
a. Examples: atenolol (Tenormin), metoprolol (Lopressor), nadolol (Corgard), propranolol (Inderal)
b. Selected nursing considerations

m ▸ **Monitor blood pressure frequently.**
▸ **Hold drug if apical pulse rate falls below 60.**

5. *Calcium-channel blockers,* which inhibit calcium ions from crossing myocardial and vascular smooth muscle and thereby produce vasodilation and decreased myocardial contractility
a. Examples: diltiazem (Cardiazem), nifedipine (Procardia), verapamil
b. Selected nursing considerations

m ▸ **Do not administer when client's blood pressure is lower than 90/60 and apical pulse is less than 60.**
▸ **Monitor intake and output and daily weight.**

6. *Cardiac glycosides,* which increase the force of myocardial contractions and slow heart rate and conduction through the AV node and bundle of His, are used to treat CHF and atrial arrhythmias
a. Examples: digoxin, digitoxin
b. Selected nursing considerations

m ▸ **Do not administer when client's apical pulse rate is lower than 60.**
▸ **Monitor frequently for life-threatening arrhythmias.**

7. *Nitrates,* which reduce myocardial oxygen demand by promoting vasodilation and by increasing oxygen supply to myocardial tissue; used to treat angina and coronary artery spasm
a. Examples: isosorbide dinitrate, nitroglycerin
b. Selected nursing considerations

m ▸ **Inform client that a headache is a common side effect.**

8. *Thrombolytic agents,* which dissolve thrombi or emboli, especially in cases of acute disorders
   a. Examples: alteplase (t-PA), streptokinase, urokinase
   b. Selected nursing considerations

   > ► **Administer intravenously as prescribed.**
   > ► **Monitor for internal bleeding every 15 minutes to 30 minutes for the first 8 hours and then every 4 hours throughout therapy.**

III. Arrhythmias

A. Overview

1. Arrhythmia (or dysrhythmia) refers to any cardiac rhythm deviating from normal sinus rhythm.
2. Normal sinus rhythm has the following characteristics:
   a. Rate: 60 to 100 beats per minute
   b. P waves: preceding each QRS complex
   c. P–R interval: 0.12 to 0.20 seconds
   d. QRS complex: 0.04 to 0.1 seconds
   e. Conduction: forward and cyclically through the conduction system
   f. Rhythm: regular with no abnormal delay
3. Arrhythmias result from altered impulse formation, altered impulse conduction, or both.
4. Symptomatology varies from asymptomatic to death.
5. Treatment of choice varies depending on type and severity.

B. Sinus tachycardia

1. Description: heart rate greater than 100 beats per minute; originates in the sinus node
2. Characteristics
   a. Rate: 100 to 180 beats per minute
   b. P waves: precede each QRS complex
   c. P–R interval: normal
   d. QRS complex: normal
   e. Conduction: normal
   f. Rhythm: regular
3. Causes include exercise, anxiety, fever, drugs, anemia, heart failure, hypovolemia, shock.
4. Clinical manifestations
   a. Usually asymptomatic
   b. Occasionally palpitations
   c. Hypotension, angina with cardiovascular disease
5. Treatment is directed at the primary cause, which usually is not cardiac related.

C. **Sinus bradycardia**

1. Description: heart rate less than 60 beats per minute; originates in the sinus node
2. Characteristics
   a. Rate: less than 60 beats per minute
   b. P waves: precede each QRS complex
   c. P–R interval: normal
   d. QRS complex: normal
   e. Conduction: normal
   f. Rhythm: regular
3. Causes include drugs, vagal stimulation, hypoendocrine states, anorexia, hypothermia or sinus node involvement in myocardial infarction; may be normal in athletes.
4. Clinical manifestations
   a. Often asymptomatic
   b. Fatigue
   c. Lightheadedness
   d. Syncope
5. Treatment is aimed at maintaining adequate CO through treating the underlying cause and administering atropine, which antagonizes the ability of acetylcholine to act on the sinoatrial node to slow heart rate, or using a pacemaker if necessary.

D. **PAT or PSVT**

1. Description: Paroxysmal atrial tachycardia (PAT) or paroxysmal supraventricular tachycardia (PSVT)—abrupt onset and cessation of rapid heartbeat (palpitations); originates in the atria
2. Characteristics
   a. Rate: 150 to 250 beats per minute
   b. P waves: ectopic, may be found in preceding T waves
   c. P–R interval: shortened, 0.12 second
   d. QRS complex: normal, may be distorted due to aberrancy
   e. Conduction: normal
   f. Rhythm: regular
3. Causes include emotions, drugs, alcohol, smoking, hormones; usually not associated with heart disease.
4. Clinical manifestations
   a. Palpitations
   b. Lightheadedness
   c. Dyspnea
   d. Anginal pain
5. Treatment depends on the client's overall clinical situation and how well he or she tolerates the arrhythmia; treatment

aims at decreasing heart rate and eliminating the underlying cause and may include:

    a.   Carotid sinus pressure or any vagal maneuver

    b.   Medication with digitalis, verapamil, propranolol, and/ or quinidine (see Section II.D)

     c.   **Medication with adenosine which inhibits SA and AV nodal impulse conduction and which clears the bloodstream in less than 1 minute; stay with the client after administering adenosine because the drug can cause severe hypotension.**

    d.   Cardioversion

E. Atrial fibrillation

  1. Description: disorganized and uncoordinated twitching of atrial musculature due to overrapid production of atrial impulses

  2. Characteristics

    a.   Rate: atrial rate, 350 to 600 beats per minute; ventricular response rate, 120 to 200 beats per minute

    b.   P wave: none discernible, irregular baseline

    c.   P–R interval: not measurable

    d.   QRS complex: normal

    e.   Conduction: normal through ventricle, irregular through AV junction because of overwhelming number of impulses from atria

    f.   Rhythm: irregularly irregular, usually rapid unless controlled

  3. Causes include atherosclerosis, rheumatic mitral valve stenosis, congestive heart failure, congenital, chronic obstructive pulmonary disease, thyrotoxicosis.

  4. Clinical manifestations

    a.   Asymptomatic

    b.   Palpitations

    c.   Dyspnea

    d.   Pulmonary edema

    e.   Signs of cerebrovascular insufficiency

  5. Treatment is directed at decreasing ventricular response, decreasing atrial irritability, and eliminating the cause and may include:

    a.   Medication with a cardiac glycoside, calcium-channel blocker, or antiarrhythmic agent (see Section II.D)

    b.   Cardioversion

F. AV blocks

  1. Description: conduction defect within the atrioventricular (AV) junction that impairs conduction of atrial impulses to ventricular pathways; three types exist: first degree, second degree, and third degree

2. Characteristics
   a. Rate: first degree—usually 60 to 100 beats per minute or the inherent ventricular rate; second degree—slowed, atrial rate 2 to 4 times faster than the ventricular rate; third degree—slowed, 40 to 60 beats per minute or the inherent ventricular rate
   b. P wave: normal and present in each type of block
   c. P–R intervals: first degree—prolonged, 0.20 second; second degree—may be progressively lengthening, as in Type I (Mobitz I or Wenckebach) or fixed, as in Type II (Mobitz II); third degree—no relationship between P waves and QRS complexes; cannot be measured
   d. QRS complex: first and second degrees—usually normal; third degree—widened (0.10 second) if originating from ventricles, or normal duration if originating from the AV junction below the block
   e. Conduction: first degree—delayed in AV junction; second degree—impulses not regularly conducted through the AV junction; third degree—all sinus impulses blocked, conduction through ventricles abnormal
   f. Rhythm: regular
3. Causes include congenital and atherosclerotic heart disease (most common), certain drugs (digitalis, vagotonic agents, sympatholytic agents, beta-adrenergic blockers), hypokalemia
4. Clinical manifestations
   a. First degree: asymptomatic
   b. Second degree: vertigo, weakness, irregular pulse
   c. Third degree: hypotension, angina, heart failure
5. Treatment
   a. First degree: no treatment necessary; may need to discontinue causative drug
   b. Second degree: increase heart rate with atropine (which antagonizes the ability of acetylcholine to act on the SA node to slow heart rate); may need a pacemaker with certain types of myocardial infarction
   c. Third degree: support of ventricular escape rhythm by using atropine (which antagonizes the ability of acetylcholine to act on the SA node to slow heart rate); isoproterenol (a beta agonist and vasodilator that reduces diastolic blood pressure and peripheral resistance)
   d. Pacemaker insertion: provide repetitive electrical stimuli to the heart muscle to control the heart rate

G. **Premature ventricular contractions**

1. Description: early or premature ventricular contractions (PVCs) due to increased automaticity of ventricular muscle cells; usually not considered harmful but are of concern if more than six occur in 1 minute, if they occur in pairs or triplets, if they are multifocal, or if they occur on or near a T wave

2. Characteristics
   a. Rate: of underlying rhythm, usually 60 to 100 beats per minute
   b. P wave: of underlying rhythm, normal; of premature beat, no P wave
   c. P–R interval: of underlying rhythm, normal; of premature beat, no P–R interval
   d. QRS complex: of underlying rhythm, normal; of premature beat, wide and bizarre (>0.10 second); may have one focus or variety of foci, resulting in many different configurations (multifocal)
   e. Conduction: retrograde through conduction system
   f. Rhythm: usually irregular when premature beat occurs; may be in a regular pattern, as in bigeminy

3. Causes include factors linked to irritability of ventricular muscle cells, including normal variance, exercise, increased catecholamines, electrolyte imbalance, digitalis toxicity, and hypoxia and myocardial damage.

4. Clinical manifestations
   a. Asymptomatic
   b. Palpitations
   c. Weakness
   d. Lightheadedness

5. Treatment is indicated if the client has underlying disease because PVCs may precipitate ventricular tachycardia or fibrillation. Antiarrhythmic drugs, which slow depolarization thereby reducing cardiac contractile force and normalizing cardiac electrical stimulation, may be used. Lidocaine IV is the drug of choice. If lidocaine is not successful, procainamide IV or bretylium IV may be tried. Other antiarrhythmic agents include amiodarone and disopyramide phosphate (see Section II.D).

H. **Ventricular tachycardia (VT)**

1. Description: three or more consecutive PVCs; considered a medical emergency since cardiac output cannot be maintained because of decreased diastolic filling

2. Characteristics
   a. Rate: 100 to 250 beats per minute

   b.   P wave: blurred in QRS, but QRS complexes have no association with P waves
   c.   P–R interval: none
   d.   QRS complex: wide, bizarre, T waves in opposite direction
   e.   Conduction: abnormal through ventricular tissue
   f.   Rhythm: usually regular
3.   Causes linked to irritability of ventricular muscle (see Section III.G.3)
4.   Clinical manifestations
   a.   Lightheadedness
   b.   Weakness
   c.   Dyspnea
   d.   Unconsciousness
5.   Treatment
   a.   If the client is conscious, lidocaine IV; if lidocaine is not successful, procainamide or bretylium (see Section III.G.5)
   b.   If the client is conscious or if lidocaine is unsuccessful, cardioversion
   c.   If rhythm deteriorates to ventricular fibrillation, or if the client is pulseless, defibrillation and cardiopulmonary resuscitation (CPR)

I.   **Ventricular fibrillation**
   1.   Description: rapid, ineffective quivering of ventricles that may be rapidly fatal
   2.   Characteristics
      a.   Rate: rapid, uncoordinated, ineffective motions
      b.   P wave: not seen
      c.   P–R interval: not seen
      d.   QRS complex: seen as undulation with no specific pattern
      e.   Conduction: no organized conduction, many foci firing at once
      f.   Rhythm: irregular without pattern
   3.   Cause is most commonly myocardial ischemia or infarction; also may result from untreated VT, electrolyte imbalances (hypokalemia and hypercalcemia), digitalis or quinidine toxicity, or hypothermia.
   4.   Clinical manifestations
      a.   Loss of consciousness
      b.   Pulselessness
      c.   Loss of blood pressure
      d.   Cessation of respirations
      e.   Possible seizures
      f.   Sudden death

      5.   Treatment involves defibrillation, CPR, and drugs such as lidocaine, bretylium, or procainamide (see Section III. G. 5).

IV. **Coronary artery disease (coronary atherosclerosis)**

   A.   Description: results from focal narrowing of large and medium-sized coronary arteries due to intimal plaque formation; the most common cardiac disorder in the United States

   B.   Etiology and incidence

      1.   Causes vary and may involve a combination of factors such as genetic predisposition, metabolic disturbances, arterial hypertension, and altered platelet function that predisposes the vessel to plaque formation.

      2.   Risk factors for coronary atherosclerosis include:

         a.   Advanced age

         b.   Male or postmenopausal female

         c.   Hyperlipidemia

         d.   Smoking

         e.   Hypertension

         f.   Diabetes mellitus

         g.   Obesity

         h.   Sedentary lifestyle

         i.   Family history

         j.   Chronic stress

         k.   Oral contraceptive use

      3.   Incidence increases progressively with age.

   C.   Pathophysiology and management

      1.   Atherosclerosis begins with formation of fatty, fibrous plaques on the intima of coronary arteries.

      2.   These plaques narrow the arterial lumen, reducing the volume of blood that can flow through the artery to the heart.

      3.   Reduced coronary blood flow leads to myocardial ischemia and varying degrees of cell damage.

      4.   Plaque formation also predisposes the vessel to thrombus formation and subsequent embolism.

      5.   Treatment modalities include thrombolytic agents, angioplasty, and bypass surgery.

   D.   Assessment findings

      1.   Common clinical manifestations include:

         a.   Chest pain (angina), the most characteristic symptom, marked by mild to severe retrosternal pain typically described as burning or squeezing that may radiate to the arm, jaw, neck, or shoulder; usually precipitated by exertion, cold, heavy meal, smoking, or excitement (or may occur at rest because of vasospasm), and relieved by rest and nitrates

         b.   Nausea and vomiting

        c.   Dizziness, syncope

        d.   Diaphoresis; cool, clammy skin

        e.   Apprehension, a sense of impending doom

    2.   The client's ECG may appear normal when pain-free and may show ischemic changes (ST depression, T-wave inversion) during angina episodes or exercise.

E.   Nursing diagnoses

    1.   Activity Intolerance

    2.   Altered Family Processes

    3.   Fear

    4.   Knowledge Deficit

    5.   Pain

F.   Planning and implementation

    1.   Reduce activity to a point at which pain does not occur.

    2.   Assess blood pressure and pulse rate during anginal episodes.

    3.   Monitor ECG during anginal episodes.

    4.   Support and reassure the client during anginal episodes.

    5.   Administer oxygen therapy as prescribed.

    6.   Administer nitrates as prescribed (see Section II.D).

    7.   **Administer analgesics as prescribed. The drug of choice is usually morphine IV. Keep in mind that IM medications may falsely elevate cardiac enzymes.**

    8.   Prepare client for possible treatment, such as:

        a.   Thrombolytic therapy, for example with alteplase (t-PA), to dissolve thrombi or emboli (see Section II.D)

        b.   Angioplasty, which compresses the blockage (atheroma) into the intimal lining of the artery, thereby increasing blood flow through the artery

        c.   Coronary artery bypass grafting (CABG), which uses a blood vessel from the body to bypass the occluded vessel, thereby increasing blood flow to the myocardium

    9.   Provide client and family teaching, covering:

        a.   Basic pathophysiology of coronary atherosclerosis, its effects, and treatments

        b.   Recognition and avoidance of events precipitating angina

        c.   Name, purpose, effects, dosage, and side effects of the client's medications, for example, calcium-channel blockers, nitrates, beta-adrenergic blockers, and antilipemics (see Section II.D)

        d.   Lifestyle modifications to reduce risk factors

        e.   Signs and symptoms to report promptly

        f.   Appropriate action to take when pain occurs

        g.   Cardiopulmonary resuscitation (CPR) techniques

G. Evaluation
   1. The client verbalizes factors and events that precipitate pain.
   2. The client reports no pain during normal activities.
   3. The client reports relief of anginal pain with nitrate administration.
   4. The client displays decreased anxiety.
   5. The client and family members or significant others verbalize understanding of the disease process, its effects, and prescribed treatment.

V. Myocardial infarction (MI)
   A. Description: destruction of myocardial tissue in regions of the heart abruptly deprived of adequate blood supply due to reduced coronary blood flow
   B. Etiology and incidence
   1. Causes of myocardial infarction (MI) include:
      a. Coronary artery narrowing due to atherosclerosis, coronary artery spasm, or complete arterial occlusion by embolism or thrombus
      b. Decreased coronary blood flow due to hemorrhage or shock, causing a profound imbalance between myocardial oxygen supply and demand
   2. In the United States, well over 1 million cases of MI are reported annually. Incidence is far greater in men than in women.
   C. Pathophysiology and management
   1. In MI, inadequate coronary blood flow rapidly results in myocardial ischemia in the affected area. The location and extent of the infarct determine the effects on cardiac function.
   2. Ischemia depresses cardiac function and triggers autonomic nervous system responses that exacerbate the imbalance between myocardial oxygen supply and demand.
   3. Persistent ischemia results in tissue necrosis and scar tissue formation, with permanent loss of myocardial contractility in the affected area.
   4. Cardiogenic shock may develop due to inadequate cardiac output secondary to decreased myocardial contractility and pumping capacity.
   5. Treatment consists of medications, lifestyle modifications, and, possibly, angioplasty or bypass grafting.
   D. Assessment findings
   1. Common clinical manifestations include:
      a. Chest pain (typically persistent and crushing; located substernally with radiation to the arm, neck, jaw, or

back and unrelieved by rest or nitrates); a so-called silent MI may produce no pain

   b. Diaphoresis and cool, clammy, pale skin

   c. Nausea and vomiting

   d. Dyspnea with or without crackles

   e. Palpitations or syncope

   f. Restlessness and anxiety, feeling of impending doom

   g. Tachycardia or bradycardia

   h. Decreased blood pressure

   i. Heart sounds: S4, possibly a systolic murmur

2. Laboratory studies may reveal:

   a. ECG changes: ST segment and T-wave changes, Q waves; location of changes on the monitoring strip depends on the location of the infarct in the heart

   b. Serum enzyme elevations: CPK and CPK-MB, LDH

   c. Elevated WBC count

E. Nursing diagnoses

1. Anxiety

2. Decreased Cardiac Output

3. Impaired Gas Exchange

4. Pain

F. Planning and implementation

1. Monitor the electrocardiogram (ECG) to assess continually heart rate, rhythm, and conduction.

2. Monitor vital signs: temperature, blood pressure, pulse and respiratory rates; monitor cardiac enzymes.

3. As prescribed, administer nitrates to reduce oxygen demand and increase supply (see Section II.D).

4. Administer analgesics as prescribed. Drug of choice is usually morphine IV; IM medications may falsely elevate cardiac enzyme levels.

5. Prepare client for possible treatment

   a. t-PA therapy (thrombolytic agents used in acute management of thrombus formation and to dissolve thrombi or emboli in acute myocardial infarction; see Section II.D)

   b. angioplasty, which opens the arterial passage by compressing the blockage

   c. CABG, which increases myocardial blood flow by using another vessel to bypass the occlusion

6. Establish a patent IV line to enable rapid medication and fluid administration if needed.

7. Maintain the client on bedrest in semi-Fowler's position.

8. Administer oxygen therapy as prescribed.

9. Monitor hemodynamic parameters as necessary.

10. Carefully record urine intake and output.
11. Reassure the client, and explain procedures as the situation warrants.
12. Provide a quiet, restful environment to the extent possible.
13. Assess heart and lung sounds regularly.
14. Institute a liquid diet; advance to a low-sodium, solid diet as tolerated.
15. Administer stool softeners, as ordered, to prevent the client from straining on defecation.
16. Initiate client and family teaching covering:
    a. Basic pathophysiology of MI, its effects, and treatment
    b. Necessary lifestyle modifications (e.g., diet) to reduce risk factors for another MI
    c. Exercise program to begin during hospitalization and continue after discharge
    d. Signs and symptoms of further heart damage to watch for and report
    e. Protocol to follow in the event of recurrence of chest pain or other symptoms of MI
    f. Resumption of sexual activity
    g. Proper use of medications: their name, purpose, effects, dosage, and side effects; common medications for MI include calcium-channel blockers; nitrates; beta-adrenergic blockers, such as propranolol; and antilipemics (see Section II.D).

G. **Evaluation**
1. The client demonstrates stable cardiac rhythm, vital signs, and hemodynamic parameters.
2. The client reports no pain during normal activities.
3. The client enters a cardiac rehabilitation or exercise program.
4. The client exhibits decreased anxiety.
5. The client and family members or significant others verbalize an understanding of the disease process, its effects, and treatment.

VI. Congestive heart failure (CHF)
A. **Description**
1. Congestive heart failure (CHF) is a syndrome of pulmonary or systemic circulatory congestion due to decreased myocardial contractility, resulting in inadequate cardiac output to meet oxygen requirements of tissues.
2. CHF may be classified as:
    a. Left sided (or left ventricular)
    b. Right sided (or right ventricular)
    c. Biventricular

B. **Etiology and incidence**

1. The primary causes of CHF are disorders producing decreased myocardial contractility (e.g., MI, valvular heart disease, hypertension, cardiomyopathy).
2. Other possible causes include:
   a. Conditions increasing afterload (e.g., acute systemic hypertension)
   b. Conditions causing abnormalities in preload (e.g., severe renal failure, constrictive pericarditis)
3. Incidence increases with aging.

C. **Pathophysiology and management**

1. Left-sided CHF
   a. Congestion occurs primarily in the lungs from backup of blood into pulmonary veins and capillaries due to left ventricular pump failure.
   b. As blood backs up into the pulmonary bed, increased hydrostatic pressure causes fluid accumulation in the lungs.
   c. Blood flow is consequently decreased to the brain, kidneys, and other tissues.
2. Right-sided CHF
   a. Congestion in systemic circulation results from right ventricular pump failure.
   b. As blood backs up into systemic circulation, increased hydrostatic pressure produces peripheral and dependent pitting edema.
   c. Venous congestion in the kidneys, liver, and GI tract also develops.
3. Treatment is mainly pharmacologic.

D. **Assessment findings**

1. Clinical manifestations of left-sided CHF may include:
   a. Dyspnea on exertion, nocturnal dyspnea, orthopnea
   b. Moist crackles on lung auscultation
   c. Tachycardia with S3 heart sound
   d. Easy fatigability
   e. Insomnia and restlessness
2. Right-sided CHF may be marked by:
   a. Dependent pitting edema
   b. Weight gain
   c. Nausea, anorexia
   d. Distended neck veins
   e. Liver congestion (hepatomegaly), ascites, weakness
3. Laboratory and diagnostic test results in CHF commonly include:

a. Cardiomegaly and vascular congestion of lung fields on chest radiograph
b. ECG findings consistent with hypertrophy or myocardial damage
c. Arterial blood gas values: decreased PaO_2, increased $PaCO_2$
d. Hemodynamic changes: elevated pulmonary artery and capillary wedge pressures (left-sided CHF), elevated central venous pressure (right-sided CHF)

E. Nursing diagnoses
1. Activity Intolerance
2. Decreased Cardiac Output
3. Fear
4. Impaired Gas Exchange
5. Knowledge Deficit
6. Sleep Pattern Disturbance
7. Altered Tissue Perfusion: Cardiopulmonary

F. Planning and implementation
1. Promote measures to provide rest for the heart; for example:
    a. Maintain bedrest with limited activity.
    b. Ensure a quiet, relaxed environment.
    c. Cluster necessary nursing care to minimize disruptions.
2. Maintain adequate ventilation:
    a. Monitor respiratory status.
    b. Administer oxygen therapy as prescribed.
    c. Position the client in semi- or high-Fowler's position.
    d. Monitor ABG values as prescribed.
3. Maintain adequate circulation:
    a. Monitor hemodynamic parameters and heart rate and rhythm.

    b. **As prescribed, administer digoxin, which strengthens myocardial contractions, reduces the heart rate, and slows conduction through the AV node and the bundle of His. If apical pulse rate falls below 60, monitor digoxin level. If digoxin level exceeds 2 ng/mL (the toxicity level), withhold the drug and notify the physician. Notify the physician of persistent nausea or vomiting or such visual effects as a yellow haze over objects.**

    c. **Monitor intake, output, and potassium level when administering diuretics, such as thiazide, loop, or potassium-sparing diuretics. These agents increase urine output which leads to decreased blood volume, which in turn decreases the workload of the heart.**

4. Weigh the client daily. Notify physician if client gains 3 lb or more a day—a sign of fluid retention.
5. Assess for peripheral and dependent edema.
6. Keep accurate intake and output records.
7. Provide a low-sodium diet as prescribed.
8. Monitor serum electrolyte levels daily.
9. Instruct the client in or assist in performing range-of-motion exercises, and apply antiembolism stockings to prevent deep vein thrombosis.
10. Provide client and family teaching, covering:
    a. Basic pathophysiology of CHF, its effects, and prescribed treatment
    b. Dietary guidelines, including low-sodium foods and, if applicable, high-potassium foods to replace potassium lost through diuretic therapy
    c. Proper use of medications including purpose, action, dosage, and side effects, for example:

    𝑛 ► **Explain the purpose of cardiac glycosides, such as digoxin and digitoxin. Demonstrate how to take the radial pulse. Caution the client not to take the medication if his or her pulse rate is lower than 60 (signifying toxicity) and to notify the physician of persistent nausea or vomiting or of vision problems such as seeing objects through a yellow haze.**
    ► **Explain that diuretics, such as furosemide (Lasix), will decrease blood volume and, therefore, decrease the workload of the heart. Teach the client to recognize signs and symptoms of fluid volume deficit or overload.**

    d. Signs and symptoms of complications to watch for and report
    e. The need for regular follow-up examinations
    f. The importance of getting adequate rest and avoiding fatigue

G. Evaluation
1. The client demonstrates stable cardiac rhythm, vital signs, hemodynamic parameters, and urinary output.
2. The client limits activities to a level that permits the heart to rest.
3. The client exhibits weight loss, indicating reduced fluid overload.
4. The client displays decreased anxiety.
5. The client and family members or significant others verbalize an understanding of the disease process, its effects, and treatment.

VII. Acute pulmonary edema

A. Description: rapid fluid accumulation in the extravascular (alveoli and interstitial) lung spaces; considered a medical emergency

B. Etiology and incidence

1. Major causes of acute pulmonary edema include:
    a. Left ventricular CHF (most common cause), MI, or other cardiac disorders
    b. Circulatory overload from infusions or transfusions
    c. Lung injury (e.g., smoke inhalation, pulmonary embolism)
    d. Drug hypersensitivity, allergy, poisoning, narcotic overdose
    e. Central nervous system damage (e.g., cerebrovascular accident, head trauma)
    f. Pulmonary infections (e.g., viral, bacterial, or parasitic pneumonia)
2. Acute pulmonary edema also may develop after certain procedures and treatments (e.g., cardioversion, coronary artery bypass grafting, postanesthesia).

C. Pathophysiology and management

1. Engorged with blood, the pulmonary capillaries eventually cannot hold their contents, and fluid leaks into adjacent alveoli or interstitial spaces.
2. Fluid accumulation causes the lungs to stiffen and impairs normal expansion, resulting in severe hypoxia.

D. Assessment findings

1. Signs and symptoms of acute pulmonary edema include:
    a. Dyspnea and cough producing copious blood-tinged, frothy sputum
    b. Crackles and wheezes heard throughout the lung fields on auscultation
    c. Tachycardia, other arrhythmias
    d. Cyanotic, cold, clammy, diaphoretic skin
    e. Restlessness, anxiety
    f. Jugular venous distension
2. Laboratory and diagnostic test findings may reveal:
    a. Vascular congestion of lung fields ("butterfly" appearance) on chest radiograph
    b. Hemodynamic changes: elevated central venous, pulmonary artery, and capillary wedge pressures
    c. ABG alterations: decreased PaO_2, increased $PaCO_2$

E. Nursing diagnoses

1. Activity Intolerance

    2. Decreased Cardiac Output

    3. Fear

    4. Impaired Gas Exchange

    5. Knowledge Deficit

    6. Sleep Pattern Disturbance

    7. Altered Tissue Perfusion: Cardiopulmonary

F. **Planning and implementation**

    1. Position the client upright to decrease venous return and allow maximum lung expansion.

    2. Administer oxygen therapy, as ordered (usually 40% to 60% concentration via face mask).

    3. Monitor ventilation; assist with intubation or other measures as necessary.

    4. Administer morphine IV, as ordered, to decrease peripheral resistance and venous capacitance; monitor for respiratory depression.

    5. As prescribed, administer cardiac glycosides and diuretics (see Section VI.F.3).

𝕟   **7.** **Administer aminophylline to relieve bronchospasm, promote diuresis, and increase cardiac output. Monitor aminophylline level. The therapeutic level ranges between 10 and 20 μg/mL.**

    8. Monitor vital signs and hemodynamic parameters, assessing respiratory and cardiovascular status at least hourly.

    9. Apply rotating tourniquets to decrease venous return if necessary.

  10. Provide reassurance and support to the client and family members or significant others.

  11. Assess renal status through output and electrolyte monitoring.

  12. Provide client and family teaching, covering:

    a. Importance of daily weight measurement and intake and output monitoring to determine the need for further diuresis

    b. Plan for rest periods, gradually increasing daily activity

    c. Dietary guidelines, including foods low in sodium and high in potassium to replace that lost from diuretic therapy

    d. Proper use of medications: purpose, action, dosage, and side effects (see Section VI.F.10.C).

G. **Evaluation**

    1. The client demonstrates stable cardiac rhythm, vital signs, hemodynamic parameters, and urine output.

2. The client limits activities to a level that allows the heart to rest.
3. The client exhibits weight loss, indicating reduced fluid overload.
4. The client displays decreased anxiety.
5. The client and family members or significant others verbalize an understanding of the disease process, its effects, and treatment.

VIII. Cardiac arrest

A. **Description: sudden, unexpected cessation of the heart's pumping action and effective circulation**

B. **Etiology and incidence**

1. Ventricular fibrillation is the major cause of cardiac arrest; possible precipitating factors include:
   a. MI
   b. Congenital heart disease
   c. Heart failure
   d. Pulmonary embolus
   e. Anesthetics, antiarrhythmic drug overdose
   f. Electrical shock
   g. Electrolyte imbalances
   h. Near drowning
   i. Hypothermia
   j. Ventricular irritation due to cardiac pacing during cardiac catheterization or angiography
   k. Acute hemorrhage
   l. Hypoxia or acidosis
   m. Myocarditis

2. Asystole also may trigger cardiac arrest; precipitating factors include:
   a. Drug overdose
   b. Hemorrhage
   c. Anaphylaxis
   d. Respiratory acidosis or hypercapnia
   e. Left-ventricular heart failure

3. Cardiac arrest also can result from electromechanical dissociation stemming from:
   a. Severe MI
   b. Heart wall rupture
   c. Cardiac tamponade
   d. Hemorrhage

4. Other possible causes of cardiac arrest include:
   a. Cardiac standstill resulting from severe hypoxia
   b. Circulatory collapse with acute hypotension due to vasodilation or hypovolemia

C. **Pathophysiology and management**

1. Cardiac arrest typically follows premonitory signs (e.g., hypotension, ECG monitor changes, respiratory failure).

2. It represents a medical emergency requiring immediate cardiopulmonary resuscitation (CPR) to restore heart function and circulation.

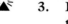

3. **Emergency treatment such as CPR must restore circulation within approximately 4 minutes after the onset of cardiac arrest to prevent irreversible brain damage.**

D. **Assessment findings**

1. Clinical manifestations of cardiac arrest include:

a. Immediate loss of consciousness

b. **Absence of palpable pulses and heart sounds; *absence of carotid pulse is the most reliable sign***

c. Apnea or gasping respirations

d. Ashen-gray skin

2. Because of the life-threatening nature of cardiac arrest, prompt identification of arrest and initiation of CPR is essential. The nurse should not waste valuable time assessing blood pressure or listening for a heartbeat.

E. **Nursing diagnoses**

1. Decreased Cardiac Output

2. Impaired Gas Exchange

F. **Planning and implementation**

1. Begin resuscitation measures immediately to prevent irreversible brain damage.

2. Summon assistance, and establish a patent airway.

3. Provide artificial ventilation by mouth-to-mouth resuscitation or with an Ambu bag; start oxygen as soon as possible.

4. Provide artificial circulation through external cardiac compression.

5. Defibrillate using direct-current countershock for ventricular fibrillation or tachycardia.

6. Establish a patent IV line if not already in place.

7. Administer emergency drugs as ordered.

8. Provide emotional support to family members or significant others and other clients as necessary.

9. Teach family members or significant others:

a. Steps of CPR

b. Basic pathophysiology of the underlying disease process

G. **Evaluation**

1. The client responds to resuscitation.

2. Family members or significant others verbalize an under-

standing of CPR and the pathophysiology of underlying disease.

3. The client and family members or significant others display decreased anxiety.

IX. Endocarditis

A. **Description: infection of endocardium or heart valves resulting from invasion of bacteria or other organisms; may be acute, subacute, or chronic**

B. **Etiology and incidence**

    1. Causative organisms include:
        a. Bacteria (e.g., *Streptococcus viridans, Staphylococcus aureus, Enterococci*)
        b. Fungi (e.g., *Candida albicans, Aspergillus*)
        c. Rickettsiae

    2. Predisposing factors include:
        a. History of valvular heart disease
        b. Prosthetic valve replacement surgery
        c. Debilitation
        d. Indwelling catheter placement
        e. Prolonged IV antibiotic therapy
        f. IV drug abuse
        g. Dental surgery

C. **Pathophysiology and management**

    1. Ineffective organisms travel through the bloodstream and are deposited on heart valves or other portions of the endocardium.

    2. This triggers fibrin and platelet aggregation, which engulfs the organisms, forming friable verrucous vegetations.

    3. The vegetations typically form on valves but also may extend to the endocardium.

    4. Vegetations covering the valve surface can lead to ulceration and necrosis, with subsequent deformity and dysfunction of the valve leaflets.

    5. Management options include antibiotic therapy.

D. **Assessment findings**

    1. Signs and symptoms of endocarditis include:
        a. Weakness, fatigue
        b. Weight loss, anorexia
        c. Fever, chills, diaphoresis
        d. Cough
        e. Arthralgia
        f. Splenomegaly
        g. Petechiae of the anterior trunk, conjunctivae, and mucosa
        h. Splinter hemorrhages in nail beds

           i.   Roth's spots, Osler's nodes, Janeway's lesions
           j.   New heart murmur or a change in an existing murmur, especially in the presence of fever

    2.   Laboratory and diagnostic studies may reveal:
       a.   Blood cultures positive for causative organisms
       b.   Elevated WBC count and erythrocyte sedimentation rate (ESR)
       c.   Anemia
       d.   Valvular damage identified on echocardiogram
       e.   ECG changes indicating arrhythmias, cardiomegaly

E. Nursing diagnoses
    1.   Activity Intolerance
    2.   Decreased Cardiac Output
    3.   Knowledge Deficit
    4.   Pain

F. Planning and implementation
    1.   Administer antibiotics as prescribed; observe for side effects or signs and symptoms of allergic reaction.
    2.   Monitor temperature at regular intervals.
    3.   Draw blood for serial cultures to evaluate the effectiveness of therapy.
    4.   Monitor ECG for arrhythmias.
    5.   Observe for signs and symptoms of congestive heart failure.
    6.   Prepare the client for possible valve replacement as ordered.
    7.   Provide psychosocial and emotional support.
    8.   Provide client and family teaching, covering:
       a.   The need for prophylactic antibiotics before dental work; childbirth; genitourinary, GI, or gynecologic procedures; or any procedure or event that can cause transient bacteremia
       b.   Signs and symptoms of complications to watch for and report
       c.   The need for regular temperature monitoring

G. Evaluation
    1.   The client demonstrates stabilization of the inflammatory process.
    2.   The client reports reduced pain.
    3.   The client exhibits increased tolerance with activity progression.
    4.   The client displays decreased anxiety.
    5.   The client and family members or significant others verbalize an understanding of the disease process, its effects, and treatment.

X. Pericarditis

   A. Description: inflammation of the pericardium, the fibroserous sac that surrounds the heart; may be acute or chronic

   B. Etiology and incidence

   1. Pericarditis—particularly the acute form—may be idiopathic.
   2. Identified causes include:
      a. Bacterial, fungal, or viral infection
      b. Neoplasms
      c. Connective tissue disorders
      d. Hypersensitivity reactions
      e. Injury to the pericardium (e.g., MI, trauma, cardiac surgery)
      f. Drugs such as hydralazine and procainamide
      g. High-dose radiation therapy to the chest
      h. Uremia
      i. Aortic aneurysm with pericardial leakage
      j. Myxedema with cholesterol deposits in the pericardium

   C. Pathophysiology and management

   1. Acute pericarditis may be fibrinous or effusive, producing serous or hemorrhage exudate.
   2. Chronic constrictive pericarditis is marked by progressive fibrous pericardial thickening.
   3. Prognosis varies depending on the underlying cause and is generally favorable, unless constriction occurs.

   D. Assessment findings

   1. Common clinical manifestations include:
      a. Sharp, sudden pain over the precordium, radiating to the neck and left scapular region; may be aggravated by breathing or movement and typically decreases when the client sits and leans forward
      b. Dyspnea due to decreased cardiac output, orthopnea
      c. Tachycardia
      d. Pericardial friction rub
      e. Distant heart sounds
      f. Increased cardiac dullness on percussion
      g. Absent apical impulse
      h. In the presence of cardiac tamponade: pallor, cool and clammy skin, hypotension, pulsus paradoxus, jugular venous distention
   2. Characteristic laboratory and diagnostic study findings include:
      a. Normal or elevated WBC count and erythrocyte sedimentation rate (ESR)
      b. Positive pericardial fluid culture

    c.   ECG changes: ST segment elevation, T-wave inversion, diminished QRS voltage with effusion

    d.   Echocardiography showing free space echo between the ventricular wall and pericardium

E.   **Nursing diagnoses**

   1.   Decreased cardiac output

   2.   Pain

F.   **Planning and implementation**

   1.   Maintain the client on bedrest.

   2.   Administer pain medication as prescribed. For example, meperidine or morphine may be prescribed for pain relief during the acute phase; salicylates relieve pain and hasten reabsorption of fluid; corticosteroids may be prescribed to control symptoms, and hasten resolution of the inflammatory process.

   3.   **Remember to taper corticosteroid dosage as the client completes therapy so that the adrenal gland will resume normal functioning.**

   4.   Place the client in an upright position, and administer oxygen as necessary to help relieve dyspnea.

   5.   Monitor for signs and symptoms of cardiac tamponade: hypotension, muffled heart sounds, pulsus paradoxus.

   6.   Prepare the client for possible pericardiocentesis as ordered.

   7.   Provide reassurance and emotional support.

   8.   Provide client and family teaching, covering:

       a.   Basic pathophysiology of pericarditis, its effects, and treatment

       b.   Progression of activity, with bedrest if pain, fever, or friction rub occur

       c.   Proper use of medications: purpose, action, dosage, side effects

G.   **Evaluation**

   1.   The client displays decreased anxiety, increased pain relief, and increased tolerance with activity.

   2.   The client and family members or significant others verbalize an understanding of the disease process, its effects, and treatment.

XI.   **Pacemaker implantation**

   A.   **Description**

      1.   A cardiac pacemaker is an electronic device that provides electrical stimuli to the heart muscle to initiate and maintain cardiac contractions when the heart's natural pacemakers are unable to do so; the device may be temporary or permanent.

      2.   Pulses are generated from a battery-operated pacer unit and transmitted to the heart through electrodes placed in direct contact with the heart muscle wall.

3. Universal pacemaker classification involves a three-letter identification code:
   a. The first letter identifies the chamber paced: A (atrium), V (ventricle), D (dual).
   b. The second letter identifies the chamber sensed: A (atrium), V (ventricle), D (dual).
   c. The third letter identifies the mode of response: T (triggered), I (inhibited), D (both).

B. **Pacing modes**
1. In the *asynchronous* (fixed) mode, the rate and rhythm of pacer beats is unaffected by spontaneous heart beats; the pacing electrode is in a ventricle.
2. In the *demand* (standby) mode, the pacer fires only when the rate of spontaneous beats drops below the preset minimum rate; the sensing and pacing electrodes usually are placed in a ventricle.
3. The *synchronous* mode uses a sensing circuit to detect atrial activity prior to ventricular activity; the sensing electrode is placed in an atrium, the pacing electrode in a ventricle.
4. In the *A–V sequential* mode, sensing and pacing electrodes are placed in both the atria and the ventricles.

C. **Indications**
1. Temporary pacemaker
   a. Diagnostic testing (hemodynamic assessment, antiarrhythmic drug evaluation)
   b. Acute MI
   c. Acute and chronic AV block
   d. Overdrive suppression of arrhythmia
   e. Symptomatic bradycardia or tachycardia
2. Permanent pacemaker
   a. Stokes-Adams syncope
   b. Sinus node dysfunction
   c. AV conduction abnormalities
   d. Chronic bundle branch block
   e. Recurrent tachyarrhythmias

D. **Insertion routes**
1. Temporary pacemaker
   a. Transvenous
   b. Transthoracic (usually emergency)
2. Permanent pacemaker
   a. Transvenous
   b. Epicardial
   c. Generator implantation usually under the skin in the pectoral region

E. Nursing diagnoses
1. Anxiety
2. Fear
3. Risk for Infection
4. Knowledge Deficit
5. Impaired Physical Mobility
6. Pain
7. Chronic Pain

F. Planning and implementation
1. For a client with a temporary pacemaker:
    a. **Place the client in an electrically safe environment. Make sure that all electrical equipment in the area is properly grounded.**
   b. Assess pacemaker function, heart rate, and rhythm frequently; note deviations from settings.
   c. Ensure that all connections are secure.
   d. Promote comfort.
   e. Provide reassurance and emotional support.
   f. Assess the insertion site daily, and provide site care according to protocol.
2. For a client with a permanent pacemaker:
   a. Assess pacemaker function, heart rate, and rhythm frequently; note deviations from settings.
   b. Assess the insertion site for bleeding, hematoma, or infection.
   c. Note data about model, date, and time of insertion; location of pulse generator; stimulus threshold; and pacer rate on the client's chart and at the head of the bed.
   d. Provide reassurance and emotional support.
   e. Teach the client to carry a card specifying important pacemaker information at all times; monitor pulse daily, and report any deviations to the physician; comply with prescribed physical activity limitations; watch for and promptly report signs and symptoms of complications; keep scheduled appointments for regular pacemaker check-up; avoid electromechanical devices that could interfere with pacing.
3. For all clients, monitor for problems and complications, including:
   a. Failure to pace
   b. Failure to sense
   c. Muscle stimulation due to cardiac perforation
   d. Infection
   e. Electromagnetic interference

G. **Evaluation**
1. The client demonstrates stabilization of cardiac rhythm with proper pacemaker pacing and sensing.
2. The client and family members or significant others verbalize understanding of pacemaker function and proper care and pulse monitoring techniques.
3. The client displays decreased anxiety.
4. The client reports reduced pain.
5. The client remains free from infection at the insertion site, as evidenced by normal body temperature and no local redness or drainage.

XII. Heart surgery
A. **Description: surgery performed on the heart either with (open-heart surgery) or without (closed-heart surgery) cardiopulmonary bypass or extracorporeal circulation**
B. **Types**
1. Coronary artery bypass grafting (CABG)
2. Aneurysm excision
3. Valvular repair or replacement
4. Septal closure
5. Heart transplantation
C. **Indications**
1. CAD
2. Acute MI
3. CHF
4. Rheumatic valvular dysfunction
5. Congenital abnormalities
6. Incompetent cardiac muscle
D. **Assessment**
1. Health history should focus on:
   a. Cardiac history, particularly arrhythmias
   b. Pulmonary history
   c. The client's emotional state and knowledge level
2. Physical assessment techniques depend on the underlying cardiac disorder but should always include:
   a. Vital signs
   b. ECG for cardiac rate and rhythm
   c. Monitoring of cardiovascular status, evidence of MI, effects of drugs
E. **Nursing diagnoses: postoperative**
1. Anxiety
2. Decreased Cardiac Output
3. Fear
4. Impaired Gas Exchange

     5. Risk for Infection

     6. Knowledge Deficit

     7. Pain

F. **Planning and implementation (*Note:* See Chapter 24, Perioperative Nursing, for more details on general nursing interventions.)**

    1. Preoperative

       a. Reinforce the surgeon's explanation of the procedure; go over expected events on the day of surgery.

       b. Provide reassurance and emotional support, and encourage the client and family members or significant others to express feelings and concerns.

       c. Obtain baseline laboratory data as requested.

       d. Orient the client and family members or significant others to the critical care unit.

       e. Administer sedatives as prescribed.

       f. Demonstrate and have the client practice postoperative activities: coughing, deep breathing, incision splinting, and turning in bed.

    2. Postoperative

       a. Secure the endotracheal tube, and maintain an adequate airway.

       b. Suction as necessary to ensure optimal ventilation.

       c. Ensure proper connection and functioning of all lines and tubes.

       d. Monitor physiologic parameters frequently.

       e. Administer pain medication as prescribed.

       f. Monitor for and take measures to prevent complications.

       g. Provide client and family teaching, covering guidelines for activity limitations and progression of activity; proper use of medications (purpose, action, dosage, side effects); dietary restrictions; wound hygiene; resumption of sexual activity; signs and symptoms of complications to watch for and report; referral to an outpatient rehabilitation program.

G. **Evaluation**

    1. The client demonstrates stabilization of cardiac rhythm, vital signs, and hemodynamic parameters.

    2. The client displays decreased anxiety, as evidenced by freedom in expressing feelings.

    3. The client and family members or significant others verbalize an understanding of the condition and postoperative care.

    4. The client displays increased tolerance to activity progression.

    5. The client remains free of infection at the incision site, as evi-

denced by normal body temperature and proper healing at
site with no unusual redness or drainage.

181

6. The client reports decreased pain.

Bibliography

AACN (American Association of Critical Care Nurses). (1991). *Core curriculum for critical care nursing* (4th ed.). Philadelphia: W. B. Saunders.

Bolander, V. R. (1994). *Luckmann & Sorensen's medical-surgical nursing: A psychophysiologic approach* (3rd ed.). Philadelphia: W. B. Saunders.

Clark, J., Queener, S. & Karb, V. (1990). *Pharmacological basis of nursing practice*. St. Louis: C. V. Mosby.

Darovic, G. O. (Ed.). (1995). *Hemodynamic monitoring* (2nd ed.). Philadelphia: W. B. Saunders.

Kinney, M. R., et al. (1995). *Comprehensive cardiac care.* (8th ed.). St. Louis: C. V. Mosby.

Nettina, S. (1996). *The Lippincott manual of nursing practice* (6th ed.). Philadelphia: Lippincott-Raven Publishers.

Smeltzer, S. C., & Bare, B. G. (1996). *Brunner and Suddarth's textbook of medical-surgical nursing* (8th ed). Philadelphia: Lippincott-Raven Publishers.

Springhouse Corporation. (1993). *Nursing student's guide to drugs.* Springhouse, PA: Springhouse Corp.

Woods, S. L., et al. (1995). *Cardiac nursing* (3rd ed.). Philadelphia: J. B. Lippincott.

STUDY QUESTIONS

1. In assessing a client with angina, which of the following would be considered a precipitating factor for pain?
   a. exposure to warmth
   b. smoking
   c. leaning forward
   d. eating a light meal

2. A female client diagnosed with an acute inferior myocardial infarction is stabilized and admitted to ICU. She denies pain and her vital signs and heart rhythm are stable but she appears agitated and uses her call light more often. Which of the following actions would be the best first step to address the client's needs?
   a. Assess her blood pressure more frequently.
   b. Explain that another episode is unlikely.
   c. Encourage her to discuss her feelings about the MI.
   d. Tell the client not to worry, she is in ICU.

3. Which of the following data would indicate that a client diagnosed with congestive heart failure is being compliant with the various aspects of discharge teaching?
   a. demonstrating better nutrition habits by gaining 10 lbs
   b. returning to the hospital as an inpatient less frequently
   c. significantly improving his or her activity level
   d. attending all the classes

4. A client is scheduled for transvenous temporary pacemaker implantation. To ensure an electrically safe environment for the client, the nurse should
   a. Remove all electrical equipment from the room.
   b. Remind staff not to touch the bed rail when adjusting pacemaker settings.
   c. Plug no more than one electrical cord into each two-plug outlet.
   d. Make sure that all electrical equipment is properly grounded.

5. The nursing assessment of a client diagnosed with congestive heart failure reveals moderate dyspnea; clammy, very pale skin; and cough producing frothy, blood-tinged sputum. Based on these findings, the nurse would suspect that the client is experiencing:
   a. angina
   b. early congestive heart failure
   c. pulmonary edema
   d. cardiac tamponade

6. The priority nursing intervention for the client experiencing severe pulmonary edema would be
   a. Call the physician.
   b. Assess airway patency, and administer oxygen via face mask.
   c. Prepare rotating tourniquets in case they are needed to decrease venous return.
   d. Administer an extra dose of digitalis

7. After coronary artery bypass graft surgery, a client becomes withdrawn and expresses anger and hostility toward his family, criticizing everything that they do. Which of the following diagnoses would be most appropriate for this client?
   a. Impaired Adjustment
   b. Ineffective Denial
   c. Risk for Violence
   d. Fear

8. While performing discharge teaching for a client with chronic congestive heart failure (CHF), the nurse should be sure to stress which of the following topics?
   a. the need for a structured exercise program
   b. the use of high sodium and low-potassium foods
   c. signs and symptoms of pulmonary edema
   d. possible surgical procedures

9. A 63-year-old, 4-day post-MI client progresses from a first-degree atrioventricular (AV) block to a second-degree AV block of the Mobitz II type over 6 hours. Although the client is asymptomatic, the nurse would anticipate which of the following interventions?
  a. assisting with pacemaker implantation
  b. administering digitalis
  c. administering lidocaine by IV bolus
  d. increasing IV fluid infusion to 175 mL/hr

10. After assisting with insertion of a temporary transvenous pacemaker, the nurse's priority in documentation would be which of the following?
  a. the client's cardiovascular response to the pacemaker
  b. the emotional state of the client
  c. the client's activity level
  d. the pacemaker information (e.g., type, settings) that has been given to the family

11. Transient bacteremia can cause endocarditis in clients with prosthetic heart valves. A client who has such a valve and whose nursing diagnoses include "Knowledge Deficit" would most need to know about which of the following?
  a. the need to report promptly any cold or flu-like symptoms
  b. antibiotic prophylaxis for invasive procedures such as dental work
  c. the need to assess the pulse rate daily
  d. staying on bedrest for any chest pain

12. A male client has end-stage congestive heart failure and exhibits signs of impending cardiac arrest. The client requests a full code even though he knows it probably won't save his life. The client's physician explains to the nurse that there is no reason to call a "code" because the client has no viable heart muscle left. What would be the nurse's most appropriate course of action in this situation?

  a. Do what the physician requests and not call a code.
  b. Follow through with a code if cardiac arrest occurs.
  c. Intervene on behalf of the client and persuade the physician to initiate a code.
  d. Ignore the situation.

13. In assessing a client's radial pulses, the nurse finds them to be irregular, with the apical pulse rate about 10 beats faster than the radial pulse rate. These findings point to which of the following cardiac arrhythmias?
  a. atrial fibrillation
  b. second-degree AV block
  c. ventricular tachycardia
  d. sinus bradycardia

14. Three days after CABG surgery a female client becomes disoriented and combative, and experiences hallucinations. Her pulse rate and blood pressure increase. The nursing assessment leads to a nursing diagnosis of Sensory/Perceptual Alterations. The nurse would therefore conclude the client is most likely experiencing:
  a. ICU psychosis
  b. repressed emotional problems
  c. acute CVA tenderness
  d. memory loss

15. The nursing assessment for a 46-year-old client with coronary artery disease reveals noncompliance with the medication regimen and three hospitalizations in the last 6 months for CHF. When planning discharge teaching, the nurse's best course of action for this client would be to
  a. Reteach the client about the medication schedule, and give pamphlets to read.
  b. Collect more data to help identify reasons for noncompliance.
  c. Teach the family about the medication schedule and the importance of compliance.
  d. Arrange for outpatient follow-up to ensure compliance.

16. Before discharge, the client who is recovering from an MI should be able to do which of the following activities?
   a. Remain on bedrest, except for sitting up in chair twice a day.
   b. Walk the hallway twice daily.
   c. Perform isometric exercises.
   d. Walk up and down two flights of stairs.

For additional questions, see
Lippincott's Self-Study Series Software
Available at your bookstore

ANSWER KEY

1. *Correct response: b*
   Any activity, such as smoking, that increases myocardial oxygen demands can lead to anginal pain. Smoking also causes vasoconstriction that can precipitate anginal attacks.
   a. Exposure to cold (constriction) may precipitate anginal pain, not exposure to warmth (dilation).
   c. Leaning forward usually relieves the pain of pericarditis.
   d. Light meals are recommended; heavy meals should be avoided because increased oxygen is needed to digest food.
   Knowledge/Physiologic/Assessment

2. *Correct response: c*
   Because her vital signs are stable, the client is most likely exhibiting anxiety related to the ventricular fibrillation episode. Encouraging the client to express her feelings is an appropriate first step in decreasing anxiety.
   a. Checking blood pressure more frequently will tend to increase anxiety rather than reassure the client.
   b and d. False or empty reassurances do not meet the client's needs.
   Comprehension/Psychosocial/ Implementation

3. *Correct response: b*
   Fewer hospitalizations indicate that the client is maintaining better heart function.
   a. Weight gain may indicate fluid gain and noncompliance with the regimen.
   c. A client with CHF usually cannot significantly increase activity level.
   d. Merely attending sessions does not necessarily signal compliance with the therapeutic regimen.
   Analysis/Health promotion/Evaluation

4. *Correct response: d*
   If electrical equipment is not grounded, the client could receive a shock directly to the heart.
   a, b, and c. These actions are not nec-
   essary to ensure electrical safety for the pacemaker client.
   Application/Safe care/Planning

5. *Correct response: c*
   Frothy, blood-tinged sputum is an indicator of pulmonary edema with interstitial fluid overload in the lungs due to left ventricular failure.
   a, b, and d. These conditions do not produce such sputum.
   Knowledge/Physiologic/Assessment

6. *Correct response: b*
   The first priority is to relieve respiratory difficulties. After ensuring a patent airway, the physician can be called.
   a. In most situations a nurse can do something before calling a physician.
   c and d. These interventions would be performed later, and only if prescribed by the physician.
   Application/Physiologic/Implementation

7. *Correct response: d*
   A client's psychoemotional status is typically fragile after surgery; anger often represents an attempt to mask fear.
   a, b, and c. These other diagnoses are not supported by this scenario.
   Analysis/Psychosocial/Analysis (Dx)

8. *Correct response: c*
   The client must be aware of signs and symptoms that would require immediate medical attention. Without medical treatment pulmonary edema will progress to death.
   a. A structured exercise program could be discussed within the limitations of the client's health but it is not most important.
   b. The diet should include salt-poor, potassium-rich foods, especially if the client is on diuretic therapy.
   d. Discussion of potential surgical procedures would not be appropriate in a teaching plan for a client with CHF.
   Comprehension/Health promotion/ Evaluation

9. Correct response: a
Progression of AV block in the presence of an anterior MI is indication for a pacemaker.
b. Digitalis possibly would potentiate the AV block.
c. Lidocaine is indicated for treatment of ventricular arrhythmias.
d. Increasing IV fluid infusion in the presence of an MI could precipitate heart failure.
Application/Physiologic/Planning

10. Correct response: a
The client's telemetry, pulse, and blood pressure should be closely monitored to make sure the pacemaker is capturing and beating at the specified rate.
b, c, and d. These should be assessed and documented but they are not priority. The client's activity level would most likely be restricted to bedrest.
Analysis/Health promotion/Evaluation

11. Correct response: b
The client should be instructed to notify all health care professionals who may perform invasive procedures that the client has a prosthetic heart valve and that prophylactic antibiotics should be given before the procedure to prevent transient bacteremia.
a. The client should report unexplained fever, not cold or flu-like symptoms.
c. There is no need to assess the pulse rate for valve replacement; this should be taught to clients with a pacemaker.
d. The need for bedrest usually is associated with MI.
Comprehension/Health promotion/ Implementation

12. Correct response: c
Every client has a right to receive his or her choice of care. As the client advocate in this situation, the nurse should work to ensure that the client's needs and wishes are met whenever possible.

a, b, and d. These actions would not be appropriate for this client.
Application/Safe care/Planning

13. Correct response: a
The rhythm of atrial fibrillation is irregular, with up to a 10-beat difference between apical and radial pulse.
b, c, and d. The findings do not point to any of these arrhythmias.
Comprehension/Physiologic/Assessment

14. Correct response: a
These signs and symptoms are indicative of ICU psychosis. The etiology is not known.
b, c, and d. These manifestations do not point to any of these disorders.
Analysis/Safe care/Analysis (Dx)

15. Correct response: b
The client may have a valid reason for noncompliance that can be identified and addressed.
a. Reteaching probably would not be effective for a client with a history of noncompliance.
c and d. Teaching his family and ensuring outpatient follow-up might work but may cause the client to lose a sense of control over his condition and its management.
Analysis/Health promotion/ Implementation

16. Correct response: b
This activity is a realistic cardiac rehabilitation goal for a post-MI client before being discharged.
a. The client should not be on bedrest except in the ICU. Cardiac rehabilitation starts upon admission.
c. Isotonic exercises are recommended, not isometric exercises which involve straining the heart, such as in Valsalva's maneuver.
d. A post-MI client would not be able to tolerate two flights of stairs.
Application/Safe care/Evaluation

Peripheral Vascular Disorders

I. Peripheral circulation

A. Structures

  1. Arteries

    a. The aorta, the first vessel carrying blood out of the heart, branches into arteries, then into arterioles, to distribute blood to the body.

    b. Arterioles end in microcirculation, or capillaries.

    c. Capillaries, thin-walled vessels through which nutrients and waste products pass, consist of a layer of endothelial cells and basement membrane surrounded by a pericapillary sheath of connective tissue.

    d. All other blood vessels (including veins) consist of an outer layer of connective tissue (tunica adventitia), a middle layer of muscle (tunica media), and an inner layer of endothelial cells (tunica intima).

    e. The thick arterial muscle layer can withstand higher pressures than can veins and can dilate or constrict depending on messages sent to it.

  2. Veins

    a. Blood travels from microcirculation into a system of collecting vessels known as veins.

    b. Small veins join to form progressively larger veins until they reach the right atrium of heart as the superior and inferior vena cavae.

    c. Valves in veins (except for the vena cavae and the portal, cerebral, intraabdominal, and pulmonary veins) break the hydrostatic column of blood into smaller units, facilitating movement of blood in one direction and with reduced pressures.

  3. Lymphatics

    a. Lymphatics are small, thin, veinlike vessels that conduct lymph through the body; they tend to lie near veins.

      b.   Valves and smooth muscle contractions act to direct lymph in one direction by way of the right lymphatic duct (draining the right side of the head, neck, thorax, and upper arms) and thoracic duct (draining most of the rest of the body) to the right and left brachio-cephalic veins.

      c.   Lymph nodes are small, oval bodies through which lymph flows on its way to veins.

      d.   Lymphoid tissue also is located in walls of the intestinal tract and in the spleen and thymus.

B.   **Functions**

    1.   Arteries

      a.   Arteries supply nutrients and oxygen to tissues.

      b.   An adequate supply of arterial blood to extremities produces normal-appearing skin and nails and good tissue healing.

      c.   Regulatory mechanisms from the nervous system and local tissues provide for vasodilation and vasoconstriction as needed.

    2.   Veins

      a.   Veins carry deoxygenated blood and waste products of cellular metabolism to the heart.

      b.   Normal venous pressure is much lower than arterial pressure and is lower in the right atrium than in the feet.

      c.   This pressure gradient enables veins to channel blood from capillaries to the heart's right side.

      d.   Venous volume and pressure are regulated actively by neurogenic venoconstriction caused by alpha-adrenergic nerves, and passively by elastic recoil of the vein wall after distending pressure falls below the level necessary to hold the vein in a rounded shape.

      e.   Inspiration creates an intrathoracic vacuum and facilitates blood flow to the right atrium.

    3.   Lymphatics

      a.   The lymphatics collect lymph from tissues and return it to the blood.

      b.   This system helps protect the body from infection by microorganisms.

II.   **Overview of peripheral vascular disorders**

    A.   **Assessment**

      1.   The nurse should explore the client's health history for risk factors for atherosclerosis, a primary cause of peripheral vascular disorders (see Chapter 7, Section II.A.1).

      2.   Physical assessment should focus on:

a. Skin color and temperature changes: coolness, possibly indicating deficient blood supply; pallor, also associated with diminished blood supply; blanching, which may indicate diminished arterial pressure in a body part; rubor, which may occur with chronic ischemia; cyanosis, resulting from insufficient blood oxygen and, if localized, indicating poor circulation in that area

b. Pain due to tissue ischemia

c. Necrosis and ulceration, which can occur in both arterial and venous disorders, with symptoms depending on cause

d. Muscle atrophy, loss of strength and joint mobility, which occurs in chronic ischemia

e. Exercise tolerance (especially important in arterial disorders)

f. Pulse volume; peripheral pulse grading: 0 = absent, 1+ = weak and thready, 2+ = normal, 3+ = full and bounding

g. Bruits: heard most easily during systole; pitch correlates with degree of stenosis

h. Capillary refill time, indicating peripheral perfusion and cardiac output; acceptable time, less than 3 seconds

i. Blood pressure, both standard arm pressure measurement and ankle arm index (ankle systolic pressure divided by arm systolic pressure): normal ankle arm index is greater than 1.0; 0.5 to 0.7 indices found in clients with claudication, 0.4 to 0 indices in clients with resting pain

B. **Laboratory studies and diagnostic tests**

1. Noninvasive procedures include:

a. Doppler ultrasound, a simple, inexpensive, highly reliable procedure used to obtain qualitative and quantitative information electronically about blood flow in arteries or veins

b. Plethysmography, involving measurable changes in calf volume which correspond to changes in blood volume; test procedure used to assess changes in venous volume and carotid artery blood flow

c. Treadmill test, an exercise test done to evaluate total extremity blood flow after exercise and to detect pain occurring with exercise or signs of activity intolerance, such as shortness of breath

d. Digital subtraction angiography (DSA) or digital intravenous angiography, a radiologic technique that uses an image-intensifier video system to display vessels on a television monitor

   2. Invasive procedures include:
- a. Phlebography (venography), involving radiologic visualization of veins after injection of contrast medium
- b. Angiography, involving radiologic visualization of arteries after injection of contrast medium
- c. ^{125}I-fibrinogen uptake test, a sensitive, though costly and time consuming, screening for acute calf vein thrombosis; involves injection of radioactive iodine

C. **Psychosocial implications**

   1. A client with a peripheral vascular disorder may experience problems in coping related to:
- a. The chronic and debilitating nature of the disorder
- b. Fear of loss of body part or function

   2. The client also may have self-concept concerns related to fear of:
- a. Role changes toward increasing dependence
- b. Rejection
- c. Body image changes with disease progression

   3. Concerns related to lifestyle changes may be associated with potential changes in:
- a. Physical ability and activity level
- b. Work performance and potential job loss
- c. Economic security

   4. The client also may be concerned about changes in social interaction leading to:
- a. Isolation
- b. Depression

D. **Medications used to treat peripheral vascular disorders (additional medications may be included with specific diseases)**

   1. *Vasodilators,* which dilate vessels and improve blood flow by relaxing vascular smooth muscle and decreasing peripheral vascular resistance
- a. Examples: hydralazine (Apresoline), minoxidil (Minodyl)
- b. Selected nursing considerations

   𝒏 ▸ Because medication lowers blood pressure, do not administer if client's blood pressure drops below 90/60.
   ▸ Instruct client to monitor blood pressure frequently.

   2. *Anticoagulants,* which disrupt the coagulation pathways, thereby preventing platelet aggregation in the compromised arteries
- a. Examples: heparin, typically used on an inpatient basis, and coumarin derivatives, such as warfarin sodium (Coumadin), for outpatient use

b. Selected nursing considerations

- ▶ During heparin therapy, monitor activated partial thromboplastin time (APTT), which should be 1.5 to 2 times the normal value of 30 to 40 sec.
- ▶ During coumarin therapy monitor prothrombin time (PT), which should be 1.5 to 2.5 times the normal value of 12 sec.
- ▶ Instruct client to report any prolonged or unexplained bleeding.

3. *Antilipemic* agents, which lower high serum cholesterol levels by binding bile salts in the bowel and forming an insoluble complex that is excreted in the stool
   a. Examples: cholestyramine (Colybar)
   b. Selected nursing considerations

- ▶ Mix medication with 60 mL water or fruit juice to mask the unpleasant flavor.
- ▶ Instruct client to increase fluid intake to prevent constipation.

4. *Thrombolytics,* which dissolve fibrin deposits (thrombi)
   a. Examples: alteplase (t-PA), streptokinase (Streptase), urokinase (Abbokinase)
   b. Selected nursing considerations

- ▶ Administer IV as prescribed.
- ▶ Monitor for internal bleeding every 15 to 30 minutes for the first 8 hours and then every 4 hours throughout therapy.

5. *Adrenergic blockers*, which control hypertension by blocking response to sympathetic nerve impulses or circulating catecholamines, by dilating peripheral vessels, and by depressing adrenergic activity
   a. Examples: atenolol (Tenormin), clonidine (Catapres), guanethidine (Ismelin), methyldopa (Aldomet), metoprolol (Lopressor), nadolol (Corgard), prazosin (Minipres), propranolol (Inderal)
   b. Selected nursing considerations

- ▶ Monitor blood pressure frequently.
- ▶ Monitor intake and output and daily weight gain, suggesting signs of congestive heart failure.

III. Peripheral arterial occlusive disease

A. Description: a form of arteriosclerosis involving occlusion of arteries, most commonly in the lower extremities; may be acute or chronic

B. Etiology and incidence

1. Acute occlusion may result from trauma, thrombosis, or embolism; about 90% occur in the lower extremities.
2. Possible causes of chronic occlusion include:
   a. Atherosclerosis
   b. Inflammation
   c. Thrombosis
   d. Embolism
   e. Trauma
   f. Autoimmune response

C. Pathophysiology and management

1. Narrowing of the arterial lumen or damage to the endothelial lining can result from such factors as:
   a. Atherosclerotic buildup of lipid deposits
   b. Arteriosclerosis obliterans, causing arterial occlusion
2. This leads to reduced or absent peripheral blood flow and, if unchecked, tissue ischemia and eventual necrosis.
3. Acute arterial occlusion results in immediate decrease in arterial flow distal to the occlusion with a resultant decrease in nutrient and oxygen supply to perfused tissue.
4. In chronic arterial occlusion, gradual onset allows for some development of collateral circulation around areas of occlusion; chronic nutrient and oxygen deficit causes more trophic changes than acute occlusion.
5. Effects of arterial occlusion in the lower extremities may include:
   a. Aortoiliac arterial stenosis and occlusion
   b. Femoropopliteal arterial stenosis and occlusion
   c. Arterial ulcers of distal toes, anterior tibia, and lateral malleolus
   d. Distal arterial embolization of large or small vessels of the feet
6. Effects in the upper extremities may include:
   a. Subclavian steal syndrome, resulting in arm ischemia from blockage of the subclavian artery with subsequent incomplete perfusion from the carotid artery
   b. Thoracic outlet syndrome, resulting from pinching of the subclavian artery by muscle, the first rib, or the clavicle
7. Among management options are medication administration and supportive care.

D. **Assessment findings**

1. Clinical manifestations of acute arterial occlusion are commonly termed the *"six Ps"*:
    a. *Pain* or loss of sensory nerves secondary to ischemia
    b. *Paresthesias* and loss of position sense
    c. *Poikilothermia* or coldness
    d. *Paralysis*
    e. *Pallor* due to empty superficial vessels (can progress to mottled, cyanotic, cadaverous cold leg)
    f. *Pulselessness*
2. The most important clinical manifestations of chronic arterial occlusion are:
    a. Intermittent claudication (calf muscle pain occurring when muscle is forced to contract without adequate blood supply, such as after walking a certain measurable distance; alleviated with rest)
    b. Resting pain (pain at rest when limited blood flow cannot meet even very low tissue requirements)
    c. Trophic changes in skin and nails: dryness, scaling, and thinning of skin; decreased or absent hair growth; and brittle and thickened nails
3. Additional assessment findings may also include:
    a. Decreased or absent peripheral pulses
    b. Coldness, pallor, rubor, or cyanosis
    c. Arterial ulcers and cellulitis
    d. Gangrenous changes marking death and decay of tissues

E. **Nursing diagnoses**

1. Activity Intolerance
2. Altered Nutrition: More than body requirements
3. Pain
4. Chronic Pain
5. Impaired Skin Integrity
6. Altered Tissue Perfusion: Peripheral

F. **Planning and implementation**

1. Provide proper positioning:
    a. Place the client's legs in a dependent position in relationship to the heart to improve peripheral blood flow.
    b. Avoid raising the client's feet above heart level unless specifically prescribed by the physician (e.g., as part of Burger-Allen exercises).
    c. Keep the client in a neutral, flat, supine position if in doubt about nature of peripheral vascular problems.
2. Promote vasodilation:

    a.   Provide insulating warmth with gloves, socks, and other outer wear as appropriate.

    b.   Keep room temperatures comfortably warm.

    c.   Instruct the client to warm himself or herself with warm drinks or warm baths.

    d.   Never apply a direct heat source to the extremities; limited blood flow combined with possible paresthesias can lead to tissue damage from heat earlier than would occur in a client with normal circulation.

    e.   Teach the client about the vasoconstrictive effects of nicotine and caffeine, emotional stress, and chilling; discuss ways to avoid or minimize these risk factors.

    f.   Teach the client to avoid constricting clothes such as garters, knee-high stockings, and belts.

3. Promote comfort:

    a.   Use measures to increase circulation to extremities to help alleviate pain.

    b.   Administer analgesics as ordered, preferably nonnarcotics to prevent dependency in chronic occlusive disorders.

4. Promote and teach skin and foot care:

    a.   Teach the client with chronic disease the need for scrupulous daily foot care.

    b.   Provide gentle daily washing and drying of feet with mild soap and warm water.

    c.   Inspect affected limbs (such as feet) daily for areas of injury, broken skin, trophic changes, pulselessness.

    d.   Apply lanolin to dry areas.

    e.   Use lamb's wool between overlapping toes.

    f.   Trim nails straight across with clippers, not scissors.

    g.   Use cotton or wool socks to absorb moisture.

    h.   Avoid injury to affected extremity from scratching, home treatment of corns and blisters and injury sites, improper nail cutting, and walking in shoes that do not fit.

    i.   Never use razor blades or harsh commercial products.

    j.   Warn against going barefoot or wearing high heels, tight shoes, shoes with pointed toes, and shoes that cause feet to sweat.

    k.   Do not use heating pads to warm cold feet.

    l.   Seek medical help for treatment of corns, calluses, and ingrown toenails.

    m.   Notify the physician of the first signs of injury.

5. Promote activity and mobility:

    a.   Prevent hazards of immobility with proper turning, positioning, deep breathing, and isometric and range-of-motion exercises.

b. Use an orthoframe, a trapeze, a foot cradle, or a padded foot board to promote healing and protect skin.

c. For a client with decreased arterial function but without activity-limiting tissue damage, encourage a program of balanced exercise and rest to promote development of collateral circulation.

d. Instruct the client to use pain or intermittent claudication as a guide to limiting activity during exercise (i.e., view onset of pain as a signal to stop and rest).

6. Provide client and family teaching, covering:
   a. The nature of the disorder and its treatment
   b. Proper foot care
   c. Risk factors and the importance of complying with the therapeutic regimen
   d. Prevention of circulatory complications by avoiding injury
   e. The need for ongoing follow-up care

7. As prescribed, administer medications, such as vasodilators, anticoagulants, antilipemic agents, or thrombolytics. Also as prescribed administer other medications, for example, aspirin and pentoxifylline, which prevent platelet aggregations leading to thrombosis or emboli (see Section II.D).

8. Provide care for a client undergoing angiography or percutaneous transluminal angioplasty (PTA):
   a. Preprocedure, provide information related to the procedure; validate that informed consent has been obtained; mark peripheral pulses; obtain diagnostic data as ordered; and withhold food and fluids as prescribed.
   b. Postprocedure, maintain bedrest as prescribed, keeping the involved extremity extended; monitor vital signs and assess peripheral pulses and circulation every 15 minutes for 2 hours then every hour for 4 hours; assess for bleeding, hematoma, or swelling at catheter insertion site; encourage oral fluids; and monitor urine output.

9. Provide care for a client receiving an autogenous saphenous vein or a synthetic (expanded polytetrafluoroethylene [PTFE] or Gore-Tex) bypass graft:
   a. **Prepare the client for surgery, and mark the site of the peripheral pulses.**
   b. Monitor client carefully after procedure (especially for the first 24 hours) for signs of graft occlusion as manifested by decreased arterial perfusion.

    c.   Position the involved extremity in the position prescribed by the physician to prevent constricted arterial flow and edema.

    d.   Monitor for development of compartment syndrome (swelling of calf muscles), which can impede circulation and necessitate fasciotomy (incision in fascia to relieve pressure on vessels).

    e.   Be alert for embolization with ischemia of foot and lower leg.

    f.   Anticipate and take steps to prevent complications of any surgical procedure involving general anesthesia, particularly respiratory problems and infection.

10.   Provide care for a client who has received axillofemoral or axillobifemoral bypass graft:

    a.   Avoid positioning the client on the side of the graft following the procedure.

    b.   Warn the client not to wear tight clothing, which can lead to graft occlusion.

11.   Provide care for a client undergoing endarterectomy, sympathectomy, or amputation.

G. **Evaluation**

   1.   The client demonstrates increased arterial blood supply to extremities, as evidenced by:

    a.   Warm skin

    b.   Improved skin color

    c.   Decreased muscle pain with exercise

    d.   Palpable peripheral pulses

   2.   The client maintains proper positioning.

   3.   The client exhibits decreased venous congestion, as evidenced by decreased edema in extremities.

   4.   The client complies with measures to promote vasodilation and prevent vasoconstriction, including:

    a.   Protecting extremities from cold

    b.   Avoiding smoking, constricting clothing and appliances, and crossing the legs

    c.   Participating in a stress management program

   5.   The client reports freedom from pain and increased activity tolerance.

   6.   The client exhibits good tissue integrity and adheres to the foot care regimen.

   7.   The client performs self-care activities.

IV. **Deep venous thrombosis (DVT)**

   A. Description: blood clot formation in the deep veins of the lower extremities or in the pelvic veins

   B. Etiology and incidence

   1. Thrombus formation occurs when two of three conditions of Virchow's triad are present:
      a. Venous stasis
      b. Hypercoagulability
      c. Injury to the venous wall
   2. Conditions contributing to venous stasis include surgery, obesity, pregnancy, and congestive heart failure.
   3. Conditions associated with hypercoagulability include malignant neoplasms, dehydration, blood dyscrasias, and oral contraceptive use.
   4. Vein wall trauma may result from:
      a. IV injection
      b. Thromboangiitis obliterans (Buerger's disease)
      c. Fractures and dislocations
      d. Chemical injury from sclerosing agents
      e. Injection of radiopaque media for imaging studies
      f. Use of certain antibiotics (e.g., chlortetracycline)

   C. Pathophysiology and management

   1. A clot forms when platelets adhere to the vein lining or endothelium, release adenosine diphosphate (ADP), and begin the process of platelet aggregation, platelet plug, and clot formation.
   2. As a clot enlarges, it may block blood flow through the vein and obstruct venous drainage from the area distal to the clot.
   3. Within 24 to 48 hours after formation, the clot may dislodge and travel to the pulmonary artery (pulmonary embolism), a life-threatening emergency.
   4. Chronic venous insufficiency, or postphlebotic syndrome (PPS), results from dysfunctional valves that reduce venous return, increase venous pressure, and cause venous stasis; it follows most severe cases of DVT and may take 5 to 10 years to develop.
   5. Management may rely on medications and/or surgery.

   D. Assessment findings

   1. DVT may be asymptomatic, or may produce some or all of the following clinical manifestations:
      a. Swelling (usually unilateral), erythema, and warmth of calf or thigh associated with inflammation of phlebitis
      b. Pain in calf muscle on dorsiflexion (Homans' sign) due to stretching of inflamed vein

      c.   Tenderness in calf or thigh

      d.   Low-grade fever

   2. **Hallmarks of postphlebotic syndrome PPS include:**

      a.   **Chronic swollen limbs**

      b.   **Thick, coarse, brownish skin around the ankles**

      c.   **Venous stasis ulcers**

E. **Nursing diagnoses**

    1.   Fear

    2.   Impaired Physical Mobility

    3.   Pain

    4.   Chronic Pain

    5.   Impaired Tissue Integrity

    6.   Altered Tissue Perfusion: Peripheral

F. **Planning and implementation**

    1.   Provide proper positioning:

      a.   Elevate the client's legs above the level of the heart and have the client avoid prolonged standing or sitting to promote venous return.

      b.   Instruct the client to avoid activities or positions that produce pressure on leg muscles.

      c.   Maintain the client in a flat, supine position (bedrest may be used to facilitate healing) if in doubt regarding positioning.

    2.   Promote venous return in the unaffected leg:

      a.   Instruct the client to maximize the effects of the calf muscle pump to augment venous return by walking with a heel-toe gait and doing similar exercises if confined to bed.

      b.   Postsurgery, encourage deep-breathing exercises and early ambulation to promote venous return and help prevent DVT.

      c.   Elevate the foot of the bed about 6 inches while the client is sleeping to promote venous return.

    3.   Maximize comfort:

      a.   Decrease discomfort through measures that promote venous return.

      b.   Apply warm packs to the legs to reduce pain.

      c.   Administer mild sedatives or analgesics as needed; avoid certain antiinflammatory agents, which increase bleeding (such as aspirin or ibuprofen) for a client receiving anticoagulant therapy.

    4.   Provide care associated with medical and surgical interventions as appropriate:

      a.   Assess postoperative clients and clients with decreased activity and a history of DVT for signs of thrombophlebitis.

b. Observe the lower extremities for skin changes.

c. Monitor APTT and APT in clients receiving anticoagulant therapy (see Section II.D).

d. Avoid performing IM injections, invasive procedures, and other minor types of trauma for a client receiving anticoagulant therapy.

 e. **Never give aspirin to a client receiving heparin or a coumarin derivative; doing so may induce bleeding.**

f. Instruct the client to report any unexplained bleeding to physician such as bleeding gums, nosebleeds, or blood in urine and to wear medical identification such as a bracelet or necklace.

g. Instruct the client not to go barefoot, to wear gloves when gardening, to use an electric razor, and to be careful when using sharp objects. If a cut should occur, tell the client to apply direct pressure for 5 minutes without interruption, and if bleeding does not stop to go to an emergency room.

h. Be aware that heparin acts almost immediately to interfere with blood clotting, whereas the effects of warfarin and other coumarin derivatives do not begin for 24 to 48 hours.

i. Keep antidotes for heparin (protamine sulfate) and for coumarin derivative (vitamin K) overdose on hand. Green leafy vegetables that are high in vitamin K should be used in moderation because it is the antidote for warfarin.

j. Monitor a client receiving thrombolytic therapy (e.g., streptokinase) for bleeding from body orifices or into any body organ or cavity.

k. Carefully monitor venous and arterial function in the affected extremity following an invasive vein procedure such as phlebography, thrombectomy, embolectomy, vein ligation or stripping, or interruption of the vena cava with a filter or other device to prevent emboli.

l. Assess for hemorrhage, infection, nerve damage, and DVT after surgical removal of varicose veins.

5. Provide client and family teaching, covering:

a. Avoiding sources of pressure above the knees (e.g., crossing the legs, sitting in chairs that are too high, wearing garters and knee-high stockings)

b. Initiating proper positioning and exercises to promote venous return

      c.   Using antiembolism stockings

      d.   Recognizing signs and symptoms of DVT and chronic venous insufficiency and reporting them promptly

      e.   Taking precautions during anticoagulant therapy

G. **Evaluation**

  1. The client demonstrates restored skin integrity.

  2. The client verbalizes understanding of measures to avoid trauma to legs.

  3. The client demonstrates knowledge of proper positioning to promote circulation.

  4. The client increases physical mobility, gradually progressing to an optimal activity level while controlling pain-inducing activity.

V. **Venous stasis ulcers**

A. **Description: excavation of the skin surface resulting from sloughing of inflamed necrotic tissue, usually in the lower extremities**

B. **Etiology and incidence**

  1. Causes of venous stasis ulcers include:

      a.   Postphlebotic syndrome and venous stasis (the most common cause)

      b.   Deep venous obstruction from abdominal tumor or pregnancy

      c.   Valvular incompetency in the ileofemoral vein

      d.   Major burns

      e.   Sickle cell disease

      f.   Neurogenic disorders

      g.   Hereditary factors

  2. Incidence is increasing, especially in the elderly population.

C. **Pathophysiology and management**

  1. Over time, incompetent valves in veins result in excessive venous pressure and subsequent rupture of small skin veins and venules.

  2. Chronic changes of subcutaneous fibrosis, cutaneous atrophy, and lymphatic obstruction associated with stasis contribute to tissue breakdown and infection in local tissues.

  3. Once the skin breaks down and venous ulcers develop, healing is prolonged and difficult. The problem may be lifelong.

  4. Management includes prevention, special interventions, and possibly surgical measures.

D. **Assessment findings**

  1. Common clinical manifestations include:

      a.   Visible skin ulcers

      b.   Dark pigmentation

      c.   Eczema or stasis dermatitis

      d.   Normal arterial pulses

    2. The client may report varying degrees of pain, ranging from mild discomfort to dull, aching pain, typically relieved by leg elevation.

E. Nursing diagnoses

    1. Risk for Infection

    2. Impaired Physical Mobility

    3. Pain

    4. Chronic Pain

    5. Impaired Skin Integrity

F. Planning and implementation

    1. Provide for ulcer debridement and healing:

        a. Remove dead or damaged material from the wound, using wet-to-dry dressings with saline solution and coarse-mesh gauze filled with cotton.

        b. Use whirlpool therapy to debride the ulcer bed.

        c. Consider using an enzymatic debrider, such as Debrisan or Elase, to aid removal of debris.

        d. Prepare for surgical debridement if necessary.

        e. Assist in application of Unna's boot (dressing of medicated gauze covered with elastic wrap) as ordered.

    2. See Section IV.F.1–3 for additional nursing interventions related to promoting venous return, maximizing comfort, promoting healing, and providing client education.

G. Evaluation (see Deep venous thrombosis, Section IV.G)

VI. Varicose veins

A. Description: abnormally dilated veins with incompetent valves occurring most commonly in the lower extremities and lower trunk, usually in the great and small saphenous veins

B. Etiology and incidence

    1. Common causative factors include:

        a. Congenital valve or vein wall defects

        b. Valve damage from trauma, obstruction, DVT, or inflammation

        c. Chronic venous distention associated with occupations requiring prolonged standing, obesity, or pregnancy

        d. Systemic conditions that interfere with venous return

        e. Loss of vein wall elasticity with aging

    2. Varicose veins are fairly common, affecting about 15% of the adult population; incidence is about three times greater in women than in men.

C. Pathophysiology and management

    1. Weakened vein walls cannot withstand normal pressure and dilate with pooling of blood.

    2. Vein dilation prevents the valve cusps from meeting, resulting in increased backup pressure in lower vein segments.

    3. Increased dilation increases valve stretching and worsens the condition.

    4. Problems associated with varicose veins include:

        a. Unsightly appearance

        b. Concomitant venous insufficiency of deep veins

        c. Rarely, hemorrhage with abrasion of a vein surface

    5. Treatment of mild cases may involve teaching the client to take measures to promote venous return.

    6. Severe cases may require surgical ligation and removal of varicose veins.

D. Assessment findings

    1. The most obvious manifestation is dilated, twisting, discolored veins, usually of the legs but possibly on the lower trunk.

    2. Many people experience few symptoms beyond dilated leg veins and mild leg aching after prolonged standing.

    3. Others experience more serious effects, such as:

        a. Easy leg fatigue

        b. Cramping (especially nocturnal) and a feeling of heaviness in the legs

        c. Ankle edema

        d. Signs and symptoms of deep venous insufficiency

        e. Rarely, bleeding with abrasion of a vein surface

E. Nursing diagnoses

    1. Activity Intolerance

    2. Chronic Pain

    3. Altered Tissue Perfusion: Peripheral

F. Planning and implementation

    1. Promote venous return in the unaffected leg:

        a. Instruct the client to maximize the action of the calf muscle pump in augmenting venous return by walking with a heel-toe gait or doing similar exercises if confined to bed.

        b. Encourage deep breathing exercises and early ambulation in postsurgical clients as a means of promoting venous return and preventing DVT.

        c. Elevate the foot of the bed 6 inches while the client is sleeping to promote venous return.

    2. Provide care associated with medical and surgical interventions as appropriate:

        a. Prepare the client for surgery, if scheduled.

        b. Postoperatively, observe for skin changes; monitor venous and arterial function carefully; and assess for hemorrhage, infection, nerve damage, and DVT.

3. Provide client and family teaching, covering:
   a. The need to avoid anything that can increase pressure above the knees (e.g., crossing the legs, sitting in chairs that are too high, wearing garters and knee-high stockings)
   b. Proper positioning and exercise to promote venous return
   c. The use of antiembolism stockings (TED hose), support hose, or elastic stockings. Instruct the client to put on stockings while lying down with legs in air to promote venous return. Apply the stockings to clean, dry legs. The stockings may be removed once or twice daily and should be washed and air-dried regularly.

G. Evaluation
1. The client demonstrates restoration of tissue perfusion.
2. The client verbalizes precautions to avoid trauma to legs.
3. The client practices proper positioning to promote circulation.
4. The client increases physical mobility, gradually progressing to an optimal activity level while controlling pain-inducing activity.

VII. Lymphedema
A. Description: tissue swelling caused by obstructed lymph flow in an extremity

B. Etiology and incidence
1. Primary lymphedema (also known as lymphedema of unknown origin or idiopathic lymphedema) may be congenital (present at birth), praecox (developing early in life), or tardia (developing late in life); it may be associated with:
   a. Aplasia (no lymph vessels)
   b. Hypoplasia (smaller or fewer lymph vessels than normal)
   c. Hyperplasia (larger or more numerous lymph vessels)
2. Lymphedema praecox is the most common type, with peak incidence occurring in the second decade of life and most commonly affecting females.
3. Secondary lymphedema results from damage or obstruction of the lymph system by disease or procedure, such as:
   a. Trauma
   b. Neoplasms
   c. Mosquito-transmitted filariasis, caused by the filarial nematode *Wuchereria bancrofti* and others
   d. Inflammation
   e. Surgical excision of axillary, inguinal, or iliac lymph nodes
   f. High-dose radiation therapy

C. **Pathophysiology and management**
1. Collection of lymph distal to a blocked lymphatic results in increased intralymphatic pressures, causing lymphatic wall dilation and valve incompetency.
2. Resultant backward lymph flow produces lymphatic dilation and valve incompetency in distal lymphatics and, if unchecked, eventually in even the smallest peripheral lymphatics.
3. Increased intralymphatic pressure leads to protein accumulation in the interstitial spaces.
4. Protein accumulation increases colloid osmotic pressures in the tissues, resulting in fluid retention and edema.
5. Chronic lymph congestion leads to fibrosis, formation of dense connective tissue in subcutaneous tissue.
6. Management involves measures to promote lymphatic drainage and prevent thrombi.

D. **Assessment findings**
1. Clinical manifestations of primary lymphedema commonly include:
   a. Nonpitting edema
   b. Dull, heavy sensation
   c. Absence of pain
   d. Roughened skin without ulceration of skin or cellulitis
   e. Marked limb enlargement
2. Secondary lymphedema related to filariasis may produce:
   a. Intermittent episodes of high fever with chills
   b. Malaise and fatigue
   c. Tender regional lymphadenopathy
   d. Severe muscle pain
   e. Areas of erythema with increased edema and elephantiasis (severe edema)
3. Secondary lymphedema related to neoplasms commonly causes nonpainful lymph node enlargement or edema.

E. **Nursing diagnoses**
1. Body Image Disturbance
2. Risk for Altered Body Temperature
3. Fatigue
4. Fluid Volume Excess
5. Anticipatory Grieving
6. Impaired Physical Mobility
7. Pain
8. Chronic Pain

F. **Planning and implementation**
1. Assess for lymphedema:
   a. Measure and compare extremities for enlargement in all clients at risk.

  b. Assess for coexisting symptoms of lymphedema (initially pitting then brawny and nonpitting edema, no pain, and absence of infection) to rule out venous disorder as cause of edema.

 2. Promote lymphatic drainage:

  a. Coordinate physical therapy for arm or leg lymphedema: mechanical or manual squeezing of tissue followed by specific active and passive exercises to press stagnant lymphatic fluid into the blood stream.

  b. Elevate the affected extremity (e.g., elevate the arm on a pillow with the elbow higher than the shoulder and the hand higher than the elbow).

  c. Apply an elastic sleeve or stocking if prescribed for chronic lymphedema.

  d. Administer diuretics. These agents increase urine output which leads to decreased blood volume, which in turn will decrease edema.

  e. **During diuretic therapy, monitor the client's intake and output and potassium level. Also measure the circumference of the affected extremity with a tape measure to assess the client's progress.**

  f. As prescribed, administer anticoagulants (see Section IV.F.4.c–i for nursing interventions).

  g. Prepare the client for excisional removal of edematous subcutaneous tissue, if planned.

 3. Instruct the client and family to observe for and report red streaks on the affected extremity, fever and chills, penetrating wounds, and enlarged and tender lymph nodes.

 4. Provide emotional support:

  a. Assist the client with a diagnosis of neoplastic disease in coping with associated problems.

  b. Encourage the client to express fears and concerns, for example of altered body image; listen actively.

  c. Assist a client experiencing altered body image to select concealing clothing and take other measures to emphasize positive aspects of body image.

G. **Evaluation**

 1. The client reports reduced pain and discomfort.

 2. The client exhibits reduced edema with proper positioning of extremity.

 3. The client demonstrates increased activity tolerance as edema subsides.

 4. The client demonstrates compliance with prescribed positioning and exercise program and relates the date and time of the next scheduled follow-up appointment.

5. The client projects an improved self-concept, as evidenced by:
   a. Acknowledgement of positive changes in body image
   b. Expressions of self as a whole person
   c. Participation in social interaction

VIII. Lymphadenitis

A. **Description: an inflammatory condition of the lymph nodes; can be acute or chronic**

B. **Etiology and incidence**

1. Acute lymphadenitis occurs most commonly in the cervical region in association with infections of the teeth or tonsils, or in the axillary or inguinal regions secondary to infection in an extremity.

2. Generalized lymphadenopathy (involving two or three regionally separated lymph node groups) may result from inflammation, neoplasm, or immunologic reactions.

3. Chronic lymphadenitis results from longstanding infection and scarring with fibrous tissue replacement.

C. **Pathophysiology and management**

1. Lymph nodes act as defensive barriers and are secondarily involved in almost all systemic infections and in many neoplastic disorders.

2. Acute lymphadenitis involves one of two pathologic processes:
   a. Suppuration in lymph nodes due to infection with pyogenic organism
   b. Hyperplasia, edema, and leukocytic infiltration of lymph nodes in nonpyogenic infection (e.g., spirochetes, rickettsiae, and viruses)

3. Management measures may include drug therapy and comfort interventions.

D. **Assessment findings**

1. Clinical manifestations include:
   a. Enlarged, tender, warm, and reddened lymph nodes
   b. Generalized symptoms of infection such as fever and malaise

2. The infectious process also may produce red streaks from wounds or areas of cellulitis toward regional lymph nodes.

E. **Nursing diagnoses**

1. Anticipatory Grieving
2. Risk for Infection
3. Pain

F. **Planning and implementation**

1. Promote resolution of infectious processes:
   a. Obtain cultures, and administer antibiotics as prescribed.
   b. Provide instruction in proper use of antibiotics for diag-

nosed infections. Emphasize the need to take the full amount prescribed.

    c.   Assess for signs of lymphangiitis (acute inflammation of lymphatic channels) in clients exhibiting signs and symptoms of infections or with penetrating injuries.

  2. See Lymphedema, Section VII.F, for additional interventions related to client teaching and emotional support.

G. Evaluation

  1. The client demonstrates resolution of infectious process with use of prescribed medications and absence of signs and symptoms of infection.

  2. The client reports reduction in or absence of pain.

  3. The client projects an improved self-concept, as evidenced by:

    a.   Acknowledgment of changes in body image

    b.   Expressions of self as a whole person

    c.   Participation in social interaction

IX. Extremity amputation

A. Description: surgical resection of a limb or a part of a limb

B. Indications

  1. Life-threatening situations; for example:

    a.   Severe toxicity due to gangrene, usually secondary to chronic arterial occlusion

    b.   Malignant tumors

    c.   Severe osteomyelitis

  2. Intractable limb pain from such conditions as:

    a.   Chronic infections

    b.   Trophic ulcers

  3. Chronic and severe functional impairment due to a damaged extremity, as in:

    a.   Injury, including crushing wounds

    b.   Congenital deformities

    c.   Chronic ischemia from extensive peripheral vascular disease

C. Types of amputation

  1. *Open* or *guillotine* amputation is usually performed on an infected limb since it allows the wound to drain freely; a second surgery for stump revision and closure is done once infection has been eradicated (see Fig. 8-1).

  2. *Closed* or *flap* amputation is performed when there is no evidence of infection and no need for draining (see Fig. 8-1).

D. Types of prostheses

  1. A total-contact rigid dressing sometimes is applied in the operating room (immediate prosthetic fitting) to protect the

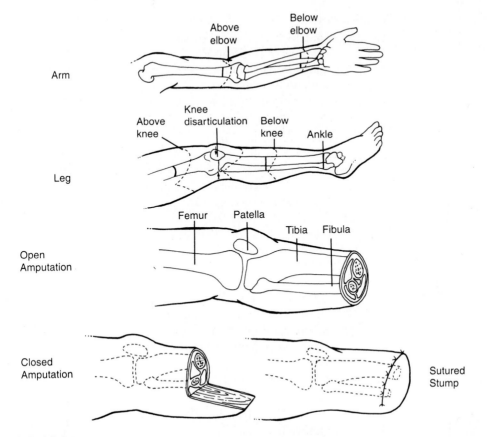

FIGURE 8-1.
Sites and types of amputations. The most common amputations of the extremities occur at landmarks and are known generally as below the elbow (BE), above the elbow (AE), at the ankle (also called Syme's operation), below the knee (BK), and above the knee (AK). The operations are usually called *open amputation*, indicating that the wound remains open for drainage until infection resolves and the wound can be closed, or *closed* or *flap amputation*, indicating no infection to contraindicate closing the wound immediately after the operation.

stump from injury and prevent stump swelling by gently compressing tissue.

2. A permanent leg prosthesis is a rigid dressing that connects to an adjustable pylon and foot-ankle assembly to permit walking. This prosthesis must be changed three to four times before application of a permanent prosthesis since the stump shrinks with healing.

3. In cases when immediate prosthetic fitting is not possible—as after open amputation—fitting may be delayed until stump healing is complete.

E. Complications

    1.   Infection, bleeding, skin breakdown, and pain are common complications of amputation.

    2.   Immediate prosthetic fitting is thought to reduce problems of infection and bleeding.

F. Psychosocial and rehabilitation considerations

    1.   Amputation affects self-image and may be difficult to accept, particularly by a young person.

    2.   On the other hand, a person suffering chronic pain—due to chronic ischemia, for example—may welcome amputation.

    3.   In most cases, a cooperative, committed person with good coordination and energy can attain independent function with the use of a prosthesis.

    4.   Conditions and factors that can preclude prosthesis fitting and ambulation include:

        a.   Severe neurologic disease

        b.   Severe renal failure

        c.   Altered mentation (e.g., disorientation, senility, psychosis, severe mental retardation)

        d.   Severe cardiopulmonary disease

        e.   High risk of gangrene in the opposite leg

        f.   Poor stump healing

        g.   Lack of motivation

G. Nursing diagnoses

    1.   Body Image Disturbance

    2.   Anticipatory Grieving

    3.   Risk for Infection

    4.   Knowledge Deficit

    5.   Impaired Physical Mobility

    6.   Pain

    7.   Chronic Pain

    8.   Altered Tissue Perfusion: Peripheral

H. Planning and implementation

    1.   Provide proper positioning, and take measures to prevent contractures; for example:

        a.   Avoid elevating the stump on a pillow for more than 48 hours following surgery.

        b.   Avoid positioning the stump in an externally rotated, abducted position to prevent contractures.

        c.   Prevent abduction contractures by adducting the stump on a regularly scheduled basis.

        d.   Perform range-of-motion (ROM) exercises (active or passive) at least three times a day.

        e.   Position the client prone for several hours each day.

        f.   If amputation involved a leg, place a footboard on the

        end of the bed to prevent footdrop in the remaining leg.

    g.   Initiate exercises to prevent contractures as soon as possible (ideally, on the first or second postoperative day), including active ROM for the remaining leg, strengthening exercises for the arms, and hyperextension of the stump.

    h.   Have the client who received a prosthesis immediately walk as early as the first postoperative day to help prevent contractures (using a rigid cast prevents hip and joint contractures).

2.   Promote skin integrity

    a.   Inspect the stump and all bony prominences daily for evidence of skin breakdown or infection.

    b.   Provide a high-protein diet with vitamin and mineral supplements.

    c.   Keep the client well hydrated with oral or IV fluids.

3.   Keep in mind that phantom limb sensation occurs in 1% to 10% of all clients with amputations, especially in above-knee amputations, for some time after amputation. Keep the client active to help decrease phantom limb pain.

4.   Administer analgesics as needed. Narcotics may be needed to control severe incisional and phantom pain; propoxyphene (Darvon) is usually sufficient to control pain in a client who received an immediate prosthesis fitting.

5.   **Believe the client who reports phantom pain. The pain phenomenon is real to the client.**

6.   Monitor for excessive bleeding. Outline blood stains on dressings with a pen and observe every 10 minutes for 24 hours for increase in size; report excessive bleeding at once.

7.   Keep a large tourniquet at the bedside in case of massive hemorrhage.

8.   Assess for hematoma formation, which will delay wound healing and provide a culture medium for bacterial growth. Assist the surgeon with hematoma aspiration as necessary.

9.   Take steps to prevent stump edema:

    a.   Elevate the stump on a pillow for 24 to 48 hours to improve venous return, prevent edema, and promote comfort. (*Note:* Do not elevate the stump for more than 48 hours, which could lead to hip contracture.)

    b.   Apply a plaster cast sock or elastic compression stocking to the stump immediately after surgery.

10.   Encourage self-care and independent mobility, and promote a positive self-concept; observe carefully for signs of depression or despondency.

11. Assess for and intervene as necessary to prevent or control general postoperative complications that prolong healing and delay a return to self-care.
12. Assess the client's and family's adaptation to the amputation.
13. Provide client and family teaching, covering:
    a. Stump care: Wash with mild soap, rinse carefully, and dry thoroughly, and perform careful daily inspection with a mirror for redness, blistering, or abrasions.
    b. Point out the need to avoid putting adhesive bandages or tape on the stump; they may irritate the skin and cause sores and infection when pulled off.
    c. Advise the client to avoid applying any creams or lotions (softens skin excessively) or alcohol (dries the skin, leading to cracking) to the stump.
    d. Discuss the importance of wearing a woolen stump sock without holes or darned areas and washed in cool water and mild soap to prevent shrinkage.
    e. Proper prosthesis use: Put prosthesis on immediately on arising and keep it on all day to prevent stump swelling.
    f. Prosthesis care: Clean the prosthesis socket daily with a damp cloth—being careful never to pour water into the socket, which may damage leather parts and cause metal parts to rust—and dry it thoroughly to prevent skin irritation.
    g. Stress the importance of never adjusting or mechanically altering the prosthesis without professional help.
    h. Urge the client to schedule a yearly appointment for follow-up evaluation of the prosthesis and necessary adjustments.

I. **Evaluation**
   1. The client demonstrates reduced pain.
   2. The client participates in self-care and rehabilitative activities.
   3. The client maintains skin integrity with no evidence of infection.
   4. The client projects good self-esteem and a positive self-concept.
   5. The client demonstrates resolution of the grieving process.
   6. The client achieves independence in self-care; for example:
      a. Balances during transfers and position changes
      b. Performs transfers safely
      c. Uses assistive devices properly
      d. Verbalizes satisfaction with ability to perform ADLs
   7. The client achieves the highest level of independent mobility possible.

X. Hypertensive vascular disease

A. Description: intermittent or sustained elevation in systolic or diastolic blood pressure; occurs as two major types: primary (essential) hypertension and secondary hypertension

B. Etiology and incidence

1. About 20% of the adult population develops hypertension; more than 90% of these cases have no identifiable medical cause (primary hypertension).
2. Identified risk factors for primary hypertension include:
   a. Family history
   b. Stress
   c. Obesity
   d. High dietary intake of sodium or saturated fats
   e. Excessive caffeine, alcohol, or tobacco use
   f. Oral contraceptive use
   g. Sedentary lifestyle
   h. Aging
3. Incidence of primary hypertension is higher in men than in women and is twice as high in blacks as in whites.
4. In about 10% of cases, hypertension is secondary to an identifiable medical diagnosis (secondary hypertension).
5. Conditions associated with secondary hypertension include:
   a. Renal vascular disease
   b. Renal parenchymal disease
   c. Primary hyperaldosteronism
   d. Cushing's syndrome
   e. Pheochromocytoma
   f. Coarctation of the aorta
   g. Thyroid, parathyroid, or pituitary dysfunction
   h. Pregnancy

C. Pathophysiology and management

1. Onset of primary hypertension typically begins as a labile (intermittent) process in clients who are in the late 30s to early 50s. The disease process gradually becomes permanent.
2. Occasionally, severe hypertension develops abruptly and takes an accelerated or "malignant" course with rapid deterioration; acute elevation (diastolic pressure usually over 130 mmHg), known as *hypertensive crisis,* can rapidly produce irreversible neurologic, cardiac, and renal damage.
3. In hypertension, sensitivity to norepinephrine released at postganglionic nerve fibers of the sympathetic nervous system results in vasoconstriction.
4. Cortisol and other steroids from the adrenal cortex contribute to this vasoconstrictive response.

5. Vasoconstriction results in reduced blood flow to the kidney, triggering release of renin and leading to formation of angiotensin, a potent vasoconstrictor; secretion of aldosterone by the adrenal cortex; and retention of sodium and water by the renal tubules.

6. The combination of vasoconstriction and sodium and water retention results in elevated blood pressure.

7. Uncontrolled hypertension increases the risk of various complications, including stroke, coronary artery disease, congestive heart failure, renal failure, and eye changes.

8. Management measures focus on medication therapy and lifestyle modifications.

D. Assessment findings

1. Hypertension usually produces no symptoms until vascular changes occur in the heart, brain, or kidneys.

2. Diagnosis of hypertension is confirmed by serial blood pressure readings above 140/90 mmHg in persons under age 50 or 160/90 mmHg in persons over age 50.

3. Because many people experience transient blood pressure elevations during examination (so-called white coat hypertension), remeasurement after about 10 minutes is recommended to obtain a more accurate reading.

4. Diagnostic studies associated with hypertension are those that evaluate cardiac, cerebral, and renal function; for example:
   a. Urinalysis
   b. Intravenous pyelography
   c. Serum potassium, BUN, and creatinine
   d. ECG
   e. Chest x-ray

E. Nursing diagnoses

1. Knowledge Deficit
2. Noncompliance

F. Planning and implementation

1. Not all persons with primary hypertension need medication to achieve and maintain blood pressure control. A nonpharmacologic approach is helpful for individuals with mild hypertension and is an effective adjunctive therapy for those receiving medications. A nonpharmacologic approach consists primarily of teaching, and its success depends on the client's compliance with necessary lifestyle modifications.

2. Teach the client and family the following:
   a. Reduce weight by restricting caloric intake (especially cholesterol and fats).
   b. Restrict sodium intake (refer to dietitian, if possible).

    c.   Reduce or avoid alcohol and caffeine intake (caffeine stimulates the sympathetic nervous system).

    d.   Conduct a regular physical activity and exercise program (exercise enhances sense of well-being, provides an outlet for emotional tension, raises serum levels of high-density lipoproteins (HDL), aids in weight control). Recommend a gradually progressive program of aerobic activity such as walking, jogging, or swimming; discourage isometric exercises such as weightlifting.

    e.   Urge the client to stop smoking if applicable. This is one lifestyle modification in which there can be no compromise.

    f.   Promote relaxation techniques (progressive relaxation, meditation, autogenic training, biofeedback, and yoga).

    g.   Monitor blood pressure regularly. Teach the client how to take blood pressure, keep a record of the readings, and take the record to future medical appointments.

    h.   Discuss the importance of lifelong medical follow-up. Remind the client that the disease is known as the "silent killer" because severe organ damage can occur even if the client is asymptomatic.

    i.   **Evaluate the client's compliance (after teaching about the disease process, factors contributing to symptoms and risks, and the importance of effective management).**

3.   Instruct the client in and supervise the use of prescribed anti-hypertensive medications. The "stepped-care" approach for primary hypertension progresses through the following medications: thiazide, loop, and potassium-sparing diuretics; calcium-channel blockers; adrenergic inhibitors; and vasodilators.

    a.   Thiazide diuretics (e.g., chlorthalidone and hydrochlorothiazide) slightly inhibit the mechanisms that affect water absorption and increase urine volume.

    b.   Loop diuretics (e.g., furosemide) inhibit sodium and chloride reabsorption in the ascending loop of Henle in the nephron.

    ▶ **Because therapy with thiazide and loop diuretics can lead to hypokalemia, instruct the client to notify the physician of muscle cramping (especially the calf muscles), dry mouth, and dizziness.**

    ▶ **Show the client how to get up slowly from a sitting or lying position to prevent orthostatic hypotension.**

    ▶ **Monitor the client's potassium level and offer instruction about taking a potassium supplement or eating potassium-rich foods.**

c. Potassium-sparing diuretics (e.g., spironolactone or triamterene) help minimize or prevent hypokalemia by decreasing renal potassium excretion, but their use can precipitate hyperkalemia.

n ▸ Monitor the client's potassium level.
▸ Instruct the client to *avoid* potassium-rich foods.

d. Calcium-channel blockers (diltiazem [Cardizem], nifedipine [Procardia]) inhibit calcium ions from crossing myocardial and vascular smooth muscle, thereby producing vasodilation and decreased myocardial contractility.

n ▸ Do not administer when blood pressure is less than 90/60 or apical pulse is less than 60.

e. Angiotensin-converting enzyme (ACE) inhibitors (captopril [Capoten]) prevent angiotensin I from converting to angiotensin II, a potent vasoconstrictor, thereby decreasing peripheral vascular resistance.

n ▸ Do not give if blood pressure is below 90/60.
▸ Teach about orthostatic hypotension.

f. For clients receiving an adrenergic blocker (see Section II.D):

n ▸ Monitor the client's blood pressure and condition regularly if blood pressure falls below 90/60.
▸ Inform the client that the medication may cause orthostatic hypotension, drowsiness, mental confusion, and impotence.
▸ Do not discontinue medication abruptly; doing so can lead to hypertensive crisis.

g. For clients receiving a vasodilator (see Section II.D):

n ▸ Monitor client's blood pressure, which may drop.
▸ Instruct client to rise slowly from sitting or lying position to prevent orthostatic hypotension.
▸ Advise client not to discontinue medication abruptly; doing so can lead to hypertensive crisis.

4. Advise the client always to take medications on time, not to skip doses, and never to take a larger dose of medication than prescribed without first consulting the physician. Instruct client to report any unusual effects.
5. Intervene in hypertensive crisis:
    a. Monitor IV drug administration, and assess blood pressure and heart rate often.
    b. Assess for target organ damage as manifested by restlessness, confusion, somnolence, coma, seizures, blurred vi-

sion, headache, nausea, vomiting (signs of hypertensive encephalopathy); signs of left ventricular failure and myocardial ischemia; and azotemia, oliguria, protein, sediment, and red blood cells in urine in renal damage.

G. **Evaluation**

1. The client exhibits no signs or symptoms of progressive vascular changes.
2. The client verbalizes understanding of the disease process, potential complications, and treatments.
3. The client demonstrates compliance with the prescribed therapeutic regimen, including scheduled follow-up evaluations.

Bibliography

Bates, B. (1995). *A guide to physical examination* (6th ed.). Philadelphia: J. B. Lippincott.

Bolander, V. R. (1994). *Luckmann and Sorensen's basic nursing: A physiologic approach* (3rd ed.). Philadelphia: W. B. Saunders.

Clark, J., Queener, S., & Karb, V. (1990). *Pharmacologic basis of nursing practice* (4th ed.). St. Louis: C. V. Mosby.

Hargrove-Huttel, R. A. (1991). Arterial hypertension. *Advancing Clinical Care, 6*(1), 4–9.

Nettina, S. (1996). *The Lippincott manual of nursing practice* (6th ed.). Philadelphia: Lippincott-Raven Publishers.

Smeltzer, S. C., & Bare, B. G. (1996). *Brunner & Suddarth's textbook of medical-surgical nursing* (8th ed.). Philadelphia: Lippincott-Raven Publishers.

Springhouse Corporation. (1992). *Nursing student's guide to drugs* Springhouse, PA: Springhouse Corp.

STUDY QUESTIONS

1. The nurse evaluates the client 4 hours after a right femoral angiogram. The nurse notes that the right leg and foot are cool and pale, and no pulses are palpable in the foot. Which of the following nursing actions would be appropriate?
   a. Reassure the client that this is a common complication after angiography and it will improve within 24 hours.
   b. Notify the client's physician immediately with the findings.
   c. Elevate the leg, and give the client an analgesic.
   d. Ambulate the client to restore circulation to the foot.

2. A client has been admitted for evaluation of severe right leg lymphedema of idiopathic origin. The nurse's plan of care will be addressing the client's reaction to the problem. Why is this important?
   a. Lymphedema signals cancer.
   b. The infection results from inadequate bathing.
   c. Leg swelling can cause severe limb disfigurement.
   d. Altered circulation may necessitate leg amputation.

3. Immediate postoperative nursing interventions for the client who has undergone a closed below-the-knee amputation of the right leg due to gangrene of the right foot include
   a. carefully monitoring for bleeding and wound healing
   b. explaining the need for a second surgery in several weeks to prepare the stump for prosthesis fitting
   c. placing the stump in a dependent position immediately after surgery to enhance blood flow and healing
   d. positioning the stump in an externally rotated, abducted position to prevent contractures

4. At a blood pressure screening clinic, an elderly client exhibits a reading of 169/94 mmHg. Which of the following statements by the clinic nurse would be most appropriate?
   a. "Your blood pressure is normal. Please have it checked again in 1 year."
   b. "Your blood pressure is elevated a little above normal. Please have it checked again within 6 months."
   c. "Your blood pressure is elevated a little above normal. Please make an appointment to see your doctor within the next 2 weeks."
   d. "Your blood pressure is dangerously elevated. Please have it evaluated by your doctor immediately, within 1 week or less."

5. On which of the following areas should the nurse focus during assessment of a client with calf leg pain associated with exercise?
   a. leg color, temperature, pulses, pain description
   b. smoking history, deep vein thrombosis history, presence of edema
   c. allergy and medication history, usual activity pattern
   d. menopausal state, occupation, and socioeconomic status

6. For a client with chronic arterial occlusive disease of the lower extremities, placing the legs lower than the heart is an intervention associated with which of the following nursing diagnoses?
   a. Activity Intolerance
   b. Altered Tissue Perfusion: Peripheral
   c. Pain
   d. Risk for Disuse Syndrome

7. A female client is admitted to the hospital for abdominal surgery. Which of the following assessment data indicate that this client is at increased risk for developing deep venous thrombosis following surgery?
   a. She is 5'7" tall and weighs 125 lb.
   b. She walks 2 miles daily for exercise.

c. She has had three pregnancies.

d. She will be immobile during and for a short time after the surgery.

8. Nursing interventions for the client diagnosed with peripheral vascular disease include
   a. providing and teaching about proper foot care
   b. warning against alcohol ingestion
   c. promoting a low-residue diet
   d. encouraging the use of heavy, snug, support stockings

9. Three days after femoral-popliteal bypass surgery a client has a positive Homans' sign, with no edema, redness, or excessive warmth of the skin of the calf, and vital signs within normal limits. Of the following statements evaluating these data, which is most appropriate?
   a. A positive Homans' sign indicates the presence of acute arterial insufficiency.
   b. Deep venous thrombosis is unlikely without calf swelling.
   c. Deep venous thrombosis is highly possible, and physician assessment is indicated.
   d. Calf muscle cramping associated with ambulation is probable, and bedrest is indicated.

10. The client is diagnosed with deep vein thrombosis of the right leg. About 12 hours after a heparin infusion has been started, the client reports that her gums bleed when she brushes her teeth. The nurse's most appropriate initial action would be to
    a. Discontinue the heparin infusion immediately.
    b. Notify the physician of the client's symptoms.
    c. Administer a coumarin derivative to reverse the effects of heparin.
    d. Reassure the client that this is a normal response to heparin.

11. A client complains of severe pain in the foot that was amputated 3 days ago. The client can't understand why the missing foot hurts so much. The nurse's most appropriate response would be to
    a. Assess the stump for bleeding, and administer anticoagulants.
    b. Reassure the client that phantom pain commonly occurs and eventually should subside. Then administer an analgesic.
    c. Reassure the client that phantom pain is common and will soon disappear, and administer a sedative medication.
    d. Monitor the client carefully for infection in the stump, and elevate the stump for 72 hours.

12. The client is being discharged to a rehabilitation unit after a below-the-knee amputation secondary to peripheral vascular disease. Which of the following data would best meet the expected outcome of absence of infection?
    a. The client demonstrates urinary output within normal limits.
    b. The client reports pain relief from pain medication.
    c. The client demonstrates respiratory rate within normal limits.
    d. The client maintains body temperature within normal range.

13. A woman diagnosed with essential hypertension reports that she never eats salt but doesn't like to take her pills because they "make me dizzy and I go to the bathroom all night." Based on this information, which of the following nursing diagnoses would be most appropriate for this client?
    a. Noncompliance with the self-care program related to negative effects of prescribed therapy
    b. Knowledge Deficit related to the relationship between the treatment regimen and control of the disease process
    c. Noncompliance with the self-care program related to recent short-term memory loss
    d. Knowledge Deficit related to rela-

tionship of medication side effect to therapeutic effects

14. The client diagnosed with essential hypertension has blood pressure of 224/118 mmHg, pulse rate of 74, and respiration rate of 22. Knowing that complications can result from high blood pressure, which additional assessment data should the nurse collect before notifying the physician of the findings?

   a. most recent blood glucose level
   b. most recent bowel movement
   c. presence of chest pain
   d. presence of leg cramps

15. Of the following, which would be the most important indicator that a female client with essential hypertension understands and can comply with the therapeutic regimen to achieve long-term control of hypertension?

   a. She states an understanding of the need to take antihypertensive medications for the rest of her life.
   b. She relates the importance of never discontinuing a prescribed medication without the physician's permission.
   c. She independently adjusts the dose of her antihypertensive medication.
   d. She states the need to continue taking her prescribed antihypertensive medication even if side effects develop.

16. Assessment data that support the diagnosis of varicose veins include

   a. dilated, twisting, discolored veins and nocturnal cramping
   b. intermittent claudication and nonpalpable pedal pulses
   c. positive Homans' sign and edematous, reddened calf
   d. marked limb enlargement and nonpitting edema

For additional questions, see
Lippincott's Self-Study Series Software
Available at your bookstore

ANSWER KEY

1. Correct response: b

The findings indicate an acute occlusion of the arterial circulation, possibly by an embolus or thrombus following angiography and necessitating immediate intervention to restore circulation to the leg.

a. This is not a usual or a normal response.

c. Although pain medication would be appropriate, elevating the leg would further impede arterial circulation to the foot.

d. Ambulation and calf muscle exercise would cause further tissue ischemia.

Analysis/Physiologic/Implementation

2. Correct response: c

Lymphedema praecox is the most common group of idiopathic lymphedema types and results in nonpitting edema with mild to severe enlargement of the limb.

a. Cancer is not a cause of idiopathic lymphedema; however, lymphedema can be associated with neoplasms.

b. Lymphedema is not an infection although it may result from one.

d. Extremity amputation would not be indicated in this case.

Knowledge/Psychosocial/Planning

3. Correct response: a

Bleeding and infection are common postoperative complications after amputation.

b. A second surgery is done for open or guillotine amputations, not for closed amputations.

c. The stump should be elevated for 24 to 48 hours postoperatively to control edema.

d. External rotation and abduction of the stump can cause contractures.

Comprehension/Safe care/Planning

4. Correct response: c

Although elevated, it is not a dangerous elevation, but follow-up evaluation by the client's physician should take place within 2 months.

a and b. These answers are incorrect; physician evaluation should occur earlier.

d. This is not an urgent problem necessitating physician evaluation.

Application/Health promotion/Implementation

5. Correct response: a

Calf leg pain associated with exercise or intermittent claudication is symptomatic of ischemia caused by arterial occlusive disorders of the legs. These parameters can be used to ascertain clinical symptoms of arterial problems.

b. Nicotine can cause vasoconstriction, but edema and deep venous thrombosis typically do not cause intermittent claudication.

c and d. These answers are incorrect because the listed parameters are not considered urgent in assessment of a client experiencing claudication.

Knowledge/Physiologic/Assessment

6. Correct response: b

Altered tissue perfusion is enhanced as blood flows to the extremities in a dependent position in relationship to the heart.

a, c, and d. These other diagnoses do not address the basic problem of chronic arterial occlusive disease.

Comprehension/Health promotion/Analysis (Dx)

7. Correct response: d

The immobility and resultant venous stasis associated with surgery and a general anesthetic represent one of the three conditions necessary for thrombus formation.

a and c. Although obesity and pregnancy are associated with hypercoagulability (another of the three conditions), the client is neither obese nor pregnant.

b. A history of regular exercise is not identified as either a preventive or risk factor for thrombus formation associated with surgery.

Analysis/Health promotion/Assessment

8. *Correct response: a*

The hallmark of peripheral vascular nursing, proper foot care, is necessary to prevent further tissue injury and possible amputation.

b. Alcohol is a vasodilator and not specifically prohibited in arterial occlusive disease.

c. A controlled-calorie, low-fat diet is appropriate, not a low-residue diet.

d. Tight garments can inhibit arterial circulation; support stockings are indicated for venous, not arterial, insufficiency.

Application/Safe care/Planning

9. *Correct response: c*

Because of the risk of pulmonary embolism, calf pain or tenderness in a postoperative client must be considered a sign of thrombophlebitis until ruled out by physician analysis.

a. A positive Homans' sign is not associated with assessment for acute arterial insufficiency.

b. Early thrombophlebitis may not have resulted in obvious tissue swelling.

d. Before assuming another cause for the pain, thrombophlebitis must be ruled out.

Analysis/Physiologic/Evaluation

10. *Correct response: b*

Bleeding from body orifices is a side effect of heparin that could indicate excessive anticoagulation, necessitating further physician evaluation, including activated partial thromboplastin time (APTT) monitoring.

a. The prescribed dose of heparin might be therapeutic and not excessive. A drug may be discontinued only following physician's order to do so.

c. Protamine sulfate, not coumarin derivative, is the reversal agent for heparin.

d. APTT evaluation and assessment of other potential sources of bleeding must be done before concluding that the symptom is not serious.

Application/Safe care/Implementation

11. *Correct response: b*

Phantom pain occurs in up to 10% of all clients who have undergone amputation; it may persist for 2 to 3 months. It is real pain, and analgesic medication is needed for pain control.

a. Bleeding is not considered the cause for the pain.

c. Sedation will not alleviate the pain and may interfere with mobility and rehabilitation.

d. Infection is not considered a cause for phantom pain, and elevation is contraindicated postoperatively because it can promote development of contractures.

Application/Physiologic/Implementation

12. *Correct response: d*

Body temperature combined with improving wound pain and absence of drainage or induration of the wound are data to support the expected outcome of absence of infection.

a and c. Good urinary output and normal respiratory rate are not specific indicators pointing to absence of wound infection.

b. Pain medication requirement is not the most specific listed indicator of wound infection.

Analysis/Physiologic/Evaluation

13. *Correct response: a*

Medication side effects are keeping the client from taking the pills, resulting in uncontrolled hypertension.

b and c. The data do not reflect lack of knowledge of the treatment regimen or a short-term memory loss problem.

d. This answer is incorrect because it implies the need to tolerate side effects to achieve therapeutic effects, which is not now considered necessary in most cases.

Analysis/Psychosocial/Analysis (Dx)

14. *Correct response: c*

   Cardiac changes, including angina, can result from hypertension.

   a, b, and d. These answers are incorrect; none are considered complications of hypertension although they may have an effect on the degree of blood pressure elevation.

Application/Physiologic/Assessment

15. *Correct response: b*

   Life-threatening hypertensive crisis can result from sudden withdrawal from medication in an unsupervised setting.

   a. Antihypertensive agents constitute a cornerstone of intervention, yet some clients achieve control with other means.

c. Independent adjustment of antihypertensive medications is not a recognized self-care principle.

d. The available antihypertensive agents and blood pressure management regimens are so varied that individualized treatment regimens can be devised to minimize or eliminate discomforting side effects.

Application/Health promotion/ Evaluation

16. *Correct response: a*

   The most obvious manifestations of varicose veins are dilated, twisting, discolored veins, usually of the legs but possibly on the lower trunk.

   b. These are signs and symptoms of arterial occlusive disease.

   c. These are signs and symptoms of deep venous thrombosis.

   d. These are signs and symptoms of lymphedema.

Knowledge/Physiologic/Assessment

Gastrointestinal Disorders

I. Gastrointestinal system

A. Structures

1. The GI system consists of the mouth, esophagus, stomach, small intestine, large intestine, and associated structures.

2. *Mouth* structures include lips, teeth, gingivae and oral mucosa, tongue, hard palate, soft palate, and pharynx.

3. A muscular tube extending from the pharynx to stomach, the *esophagus* consists of several layers:

    a. External layer: fibrous tissue

    b. Muscular layer: striated muscle in the upper esophagus, smooth muscle in the remainder

    c. Submucosal layer: loose connective tissue, blood and lymphatic vessels, and nerves

    d. Mucosal layer (innermost layer): mucus-secreting glands that lubricate the food bolus to facilitate passage

4. *Esophageal openings* include the upper esophageal sphincter (UES) at the cricopharyngeal muscle, and the lower esophageal sphincter (LES), or cardiac sphincter, which normally remains closed and opens only to pass food into the stomach.

5. A muscular pouch situated in the upper abdomen under the liver and diaphragm, the *stomach* consists of three anatomic areas: the fundus, body (or corpus), and antrum (or pylorus).

6. The stomach wall has four tissue layers:
   a. Fibroserous coat: outer layer
   b. Muscular coat: produces peristaltic activity
   c. Submucosal coat: contains blood and lymph vessels and nerves
   d. Mucosal lining: epithelial lining of stomach in longitudinal folds (rugae), which allow distention and increase surface area; contains many glands that secrete gastric juice

7. The LES or cardiac sphincter allows food to enter the stomach and prevents reflux into the esophagus. The pyloric sphincter regulates flow of stomach contents (chyme) into the duodenum.

8. The *small intestine*, a coiled tube approximately 22 ft long and 1 inch in diameter, extends from the pyloric sphincter to the ileocecal valve at the large intestine; sections include the duodenum, the jejunum, and the ileum.

9. Tissue layers are similar to those of the stomach. Numerous villi—tiny, finger-like projections in the mucosal layer—provide a vast surface area for secretion, digestion, and absorption.

10. A shorter, wider tube (5 to 6 ft long, 2 to $2\frac{1}{2}$ inches in diameter) beginning at the ileocecal valve and ending at the anus, the *large intestine* consists of three sections:
    a. Cecum: a 2- to 3-in blind pouch, extending from the ileocecal valve to the vermiform appendix
    b. Colon: the main portion of the large intestine, divided into four anatomic sections: ascending, transverse, descending, and sigmoid
    c. Rectum: 7 to 8 in long, extending from the sigmoid colon to the anus

B. Function

1. **The GI system performs two major body functions:**
   a. **Digestion of food and fluid, with absorption of nutrients into the blood stream**
   b. **Elimination of waste products through defecation**

2. Digestion begins in the mouth with chewing and the action of ptyalin, an enzyme contained in saliva that breaks down starch.

3. Swallowed food passes through the esophagus to the stomach where digestion continues through several processes:
   a. Secretion of gastric juice, containing hydrochloric acid

and the enzymes pepsin and lipase (and, in infants, renin)

    b.   Mixing and churning through peristaltic action

4.   From the pylorus, the mixed stomach contents (chyme) pass into the duodenum through the pyloric valve.

5.   In the small intestine, food digestion is completed and most nutrient absorption occurs. Digestion results from the action of numerous pancreatic and intestinal enzymes (e.g., trypsin, lipase, amylase, lactase, maltase, sucrase) and bile.

6.   In the large intestine, the cecum and ascending colon absorb water and electrolytes from the now completely digested material; the rectum stores feces for elimination.

II. Overview of gastrointestinal disorders

A. Assessment

1.   Health history should focus on:

    a.   History of the present illness and chief complaint, which can provide sufficient information for diagnosis in about 80% of clients

    b.   Appetite and food intolerance; usual food intake with 24-hour recall

    c.   Pain: character, location, timing (e.g., before meals or after meals), alleviating measures

    d.   Bowel elimination patterns: frequency, color, consistency, laxative use (Table 9-1)

    e.   Presence of any of following: dark urine, jaundice, weight loss, nausea and vomiting

    f.   Previous GI tract surgery

2.   Physical assessment should reveal the following normal findings:

    a.   Mouth: mucosa of mouth smooth, pink, moist; symmetric movement of all structures

    b.   Teeth and gingivae: natural teeth present with dental caries filled or well-fitting dentures; no gingival redness or swelling

    c.   Tongue: pink and velvety

    d.   Throat: no redness or swelling

    e.   Abdomen: see Chapter 1, Nursing Process and Health Assessment, Section IV.S.

B. Laboratory studies and diagnostic tests

1.   Blood and serum studies to evaluate GI function include:

    a.   Albumin-globulin ratio and total protein: responsible for oncotic pressure; decreased in malabsorption and malnutrition

    b.   Alkaline phosphatase: measures enzyme activity in bone, intestine, liver, biliary systems; elevated in liver disorders

TABLE 9-1.
Constipation and Diarrhea

DESCRIPTION	SIGNS AND SYMPTOMS	NURSING INTERVENTIONS
Constipation		
Elimination pattern characterized by hard, dry stools which result from delayed passage of food residue	▶ Decresed frequency of defecation ▶ Hard, formed stool ▶ Reported sensation of rectal fullness ▶ Straining at stool ▶ Painful defecation ▶ Abdominal distention	▶ Urge client to increase intake of dietary fiber. ▶ Encourage increase in water or other fluid intake. ▶ Recommend regular exercise. ▶ Advise establishing a regular time for bowel movement. ▶ Administer laxatives judiciously.
Diarrhea		
Frequent passage of loose, fluid, unformed stools	▶ Loose, fluid stools ▶ Increased frequency of defecation ▶ Additional bowel sounds ▶ Increased stool volume ▶ Reported abdominal discomfort and cramping	▶ Provide instruction on proper and safe preparation and storage of food products such as fruits, vegetables, dairy products, and meat. ▶ Teach client how to clean cooking utensils and food containers properly to prevent epidemic diarrhea. ▶ Assess client for dehydration. ▶ Encourage increased oral fluid intake. ▶ Administer antidiarrheal medications as prescribed.

    c.   Bilirubin: both unconjugated (direct) liberated from RBCs, and conjugated (indirect) not yet passed through the liver; elevated with impaired biliary excretion or increased RBC production

    d.   Cholesterol: measures circulating free cholesterol; provides information on liver metabolism and synthesis

    e.   Miscellaneous tests to evaluate absorptive activity of GI tract (e.g., iron, calcium, cholesterol, prothrombin time, carotenes, vitamin A)

2.   Urine and fecal studies include:

    a.   Urine urobilinogen: normally present in small amounts; increased when liver fails to reabsorb, decreased in malabsorption

    b.   Fecal urobilinogen: normally present in feces, providing normal color to feces; decreased in biliary obstruction

    c.   Fecal fat (two different evaluations): qualitative evaluation measures fat content as either neutral (such as ingested mineral oil) or fatty acid (such as lipids); in quantitative evaluation, the client eats a diet with a prescribed amount of fat, and stool is collected for 72 hours

    d.   Stool guaiac: detects occult blood in stool, indicating GI bleeding

3.   Important radiographic studies of the GI system include:

    a.   Upper GI or barium swallow: visualization via fluoroscopy of esophagus and stomach after client swallows barium; serial radiographs show outline of structures

    b.   Lower GI or barium enema: instillation of barium into the large intestine, with fluoroscopy and filming to visualize structures and determine the efficiency of emptying

    c.   Cholecystogram: radiopaque dye taken by mouth on the evening before radiographic examination; agent excreted in bile

4.   Motility studies use manometric catheters to measure intraluminal pressure in GI structures. Esophageal manometry evaluates peristaltic contractions and sphincter integrity; rectal manometry measures internal and external sphincter pressures.

5.   Endoscopic studies provide direct visualization of internal GI structures (and a means to obtain biopsy samples) using a long, flexible tube containing a fiberoptic light source; types include esophagoscopy, gastroscopy, colonoscopy, sigmoidoscopy, and esophagogastroduodenoscopy.

6.   Other useful studies include:

    a.   Ultrasonography

    b.   Computed tomography (CT) scanning

    c.   Magnetic resonance imaging (MRI)

    d.   Scintigraphy, to detect bleeding when endoscopy is not possible

    e.   Gastric analysis, to determine the nature of secretions

C.   **Psychosocial implications**

1.   Clients with GI disorders may experience coping difficulties related to:

    a.   Fear of rejection

    b.   Uncertainty about the disease process and prognosis

2.   Self-concept concerns commonly related to GI disorders include:

    a.   Rejection by others

    b.   Body image changes

3.   Changes in social interaction related to GI disorders can lead to such problems as:

    a.   Isolation

    b.   Depression

4. GI disorders also can entail lifestyle concerns related to potential changes in:
   a. Physical abilities
   b. Activity level
   c. Work performance and the potential loss of job

D. Medications used to treat GI problems (additional medications may be included with specific diseases)

1. *Antacids,* which neutralize gastric acidity
   a. Examples: aluminum hydroxide (Amphojel), calcium carbonate (Tums), dihydroxyaluminum sodium carbonate (Rolaids), magaldrate (Riopan), magnesium hydroxide (Milk of Magnesia)
   b. Selected nursing considerations

   ▶ **Instruct client taking suspension form of drug to shake medication well and take alone or with small amount of water.**
   ▶ **Advise client to take other medications 1 or 2 hours before or after taking antacid.**

2. *Antiemetics,* which relieve nausea and vomiting by inhibiting medullary chemoreceptor triggers; drug choice depends on the cause of vomiting
   a. Examples: scopolamine (Transderm-Scop), dimenhydrinate (Dramamine), diphenhydramine (Benadryl), promethazine (Phenergan), chlorpromazine (Thorazine), metoclopramide (Reglan), benzquinamide (Emete-Con)
   b. Selected nursing considerations

   ▶ **Advise the client that this medication may cause drowsiness.**
   ▶ **Because the medication may cause chemical irritation, administer by deep IM injection into a large muscle mass.**

3. *Emetics,* such as syrup of ipecac, which induces vomiting to treat some poisonings and drug overdoses
4. *Cytoprotective agents,* which produce an ulcer-adherent complex that hastens healing
   a. Examples: sucralfate (Carafate)
   b. Selected nursing considerations

   ▶ **Instruct client to take medication 1 hour before meals and at bedtime.**
   ▶ **Advise client to take medication 1 hour before or after taking an antacid.**

5. *Histamine (H$_2$) receptor antagonists,* which suppress the stimulus for gastric acid production
   a. Examples: cimetidine (Tagamet), famotidine (Pepcid), ranitidine (Zantac)
   b. Selected nursing considerations
   ► Instruct client to continue taking medication even after pain subsides.
   ► If appropriate, urge client to stop smoking (smoking increases gastric acid).

6. *Laxatives,* which induce defecation
   a. Examples

   ► Bulk laxatives, such as psyllium (Metamucil), which absorb water and increase fecal bulk
   ► Stimulant laxatives, such as bisacodyl (Dulcolax), cascara sagrada (Cas-Evac), and castor oil (Alphamul), which stimulate peristalsis through mucosal irritation
   ► Stool softeners, such as docusate sodium (Colace), which ease stool passage by facilitating the mixing of water with the fecal mass
   ► Saline, or osmotic, laxatives, such as magnesium hydroxide (Milk of Magnesia), which retain and increase water in the feces

   b. Selected nursing considerations
   ► Administer a bulk laxative with fluid and give immediately before it congeals.
   ► Avoid overuse which causes laxative dependence.
   ► Administer only as directed.

7. *Anticholinergics,* which inhibit the actions of acetylcholine at cholinergic receptor sites, thereby decreasing gastric secretions
   a. Examples: belladonna alkaloids, such as atropine; anisotropine (Valpin 50); scopolamine (Transderm-Scop), propantheline (Pro-Banthine)
   b. Selected nursing considerations
   ► Advise the client that side effects include drowsiness and dry mouth.
   ► Encourage increased fluid intake.
   ► For safety's sake, caution the client to avoid activities, such as driving, that require alertness and concentration until the effects of the drug are known.

8. *Antidiarrheals,* which absorb excess water from stool
   a. Examples: kaolin-pectin mixtures (Kaopectate), diphenoxylate-atropine (Lomotil), loperamide (Imodium), paregoric

b.   Selected nursing considerations

 ▸ To assess effectiveness of agent, record number and consistency of stools.

III.   Stomatitis

A.   Description: inflammation of the oral mucosa from various causes

B.   Etiology and incidence

1.   Stomatitis may be caused by infection, trauma, excessive dryness, chemical irritants and toxic agents, or hypersensitivity.

2.   Infectious agents that can produce stomatitis include:

a.   Viruses (e.g., the herpes simplex virus, which causes acute herpetic stomatitis)

b.   Fungi (e.g., *Candida albicans,* which causes candidiasis, or thrush)

3.   Damage from mechanical trauma (e.g., irritation from jagged teeth, cheek-biting, mouth-breathing, use of a too-stiff toothbrush) can cause characteristic lesions.

4.   Irritants that can produce stomatitis include strong mouthwashes or toothpastes, tobacco, and chemotherapeutic agents.

5.   Causes of aphthous ulcer ("canker sore") remain unclear; suspected predisposing factors include stress, allergy, vitamin deficiency, and viral infection.

C.   Assessment findings

1.   Clinical manifestations vary with the type of stomatitis.

2.   Acute herpetic stomatitis is marked by small, clear vesicles in single or multiple eruptions, commonly preceded by sore throat, headache, nausea and vomiting, and malaise; usually lasts about 1 week.

3.   Candidiasis produces characteristic raised white patches and ulcers; infection may spread to other areas of the GI tract, the skin, or the respiratory system.

4.   Manifestations of mechanical trauma vary with the cause; small lacerations or abrasions with bleeding or exudate are common.

5.   Chemical irritation typically produces generalized redness and swelling; chemotherapy may cause swollen, easily bruised mucosa and possibly ulcerations with exudate.

6.   Aphthous ulcer appears as a well-circumscribed lesion with a white center and a reddish ring around the periphery.

D.   Nursing diagnoses

1.   Risk for Fluid Volume Deficit

2.   Risk for Infection

3.   Altered Nutrition: Less than body requirements

      4. Altered Oral Mucous Membrane
      5. Pain

E. Planning and implementation
    1. Promote meticulous oral hygiene, instructing the client to:
       a. Brush and floss teeth and massage gums several times daily.
       b. When pain prevents use of a toothbrush, use gauze or a sponge toothette to cleanse the oral mucosa.
       c. Use water, saline, or a dilute solution of hydrogen peroxide instead of toothpaste or mouthwash.
    2. If the client has a fungal infection, administer an antifungal agent, such as nystatin (Mycostatin).
       a. Instruct the client to "swish and swallow" to coat the oral mucosa.
       b. **First make sure client's mouth is free of debris before giving drug; then have client hold suspension in mouth for at least 2 minutes.**
    3. Promote adequate food and fluid intake; suggest:
       a. A bland diet, avoiding spicy and acidic foods
       b. Use of topical or systemic analgesics
       c. Eating food and fluids served lukewarm or cold, which may minimize discomfort and result in increased intake

F. Evaluation
    1. The client displays intact oral mucosa with no evidence of inflammation.
    2. The client demonstrates appropriate oral hygiene.
    3. The client is free of pain and discomfort.
    4. The client maintains a nutritionally balanced diet.
    5. The client remains free of systemic infection.

IV. Esophagitis
  A. Description: inflammations of the esophageal mucosa; may be acute or chronic
  B. Etiology and incidence
    1. Esophagitis most commonly results from recurrent reflux of gastric contents into the distal esophagus.
    2. Reflux may result from:
       a. Incompetent LES
       b. Gastric or duodenal ulcers
       c. Prolonged nasogastric intubation
  C. Pathophysiology and management
    1. Normally, the LES blocks reflux of gastric juice into the esophagus. Defects in the LES mechanism (e.g., decreased resting LES pressure, LES relaxation, transient increase in intraabdominal pressure) can lead to reflux.

        2. Persistent reflux can lead to esophageal ulcer formation, bleeding, and scarring.

  D. **Assessment findings**

        1. Common clinical manifestations include:

            a. Heartburn, acid regurgitation, belching

            b. Dysphagia

            c. Esophageal pain possibly radiating to the arms, neck, back, jaw, and substernal area; may be precipitated by increased abdominal pressure as can occur from bending, straining, obesity, or pregnancy

        2. Diagnostic tests may include:

            a. Esophagoscopy, barium swallow

            b. Bernstein acid-perfusion test

            c. Acid-reflux test

            d. Esophageal manometry

  E. **Nursing diagnoses**

        1. Knowledge Deficit

        2. Altered Nutrition: Less than body requirements

        3. Pain

  F. **Planning and implementation**

        1. Promote adequate nutritional intake; instruct the client to:

            a. Eat small, frequent meals of mostly bland foods.

            b. Chew food thoroughly before swallowing.

            c. Drink fluids to aid swallowing and food passage down the esophagus.

            d. Avoid irritants such as spicy or acidic foods, alcohol, caffeine, and tobacco.

            e. Do not lie down after eating, and avoid eating within 3 hours of bedtime.

        2. Elevate the head of the client's bed with blocks to help minimize reflux.

  G. **Evaluation**

        1. The client verbalizes measures to promote good nutrition.

        2. The client verbalizes understanding of the causes and treatment of esophagitis.

        3. The client reports reduced regurgitation and pain.

V. **Hiatal hernia (diaphragmatic hernia)**

  A. **Description: protrusion of an upper portion of the stomach through an area of weakness in the diaphragm**

  B. **Etiology and incidence**

        1. Hiatal hernia usually results from diaphragmatic muscle weakening or diaphragm malformations; predisposing factors include aging, trauma, surgery, and disorders such as esophageal cancer and kyphoscoliosis.

    2. The disorder may occur in 10% to 20% of the population; approximately half of those affected experience no symptoms. Incidence is higher in women than in men and increases with age.

C. **Pathophysiology and management**

    1. Hiatal hernia develops when the muscular collar around the esophageal–diaphragmatic junction weakens and loosens.

    2. This loosening allows the upper portion of the stomach to protrude into the chest when intraabdominal pressure increases, as may result from obesity, ascites, pregnancy, bending, straining, coughing, constrictive clothing, or extreme physical exertion.

    3. Medical treatment is the preferred choice, but about 15% of clients with hiatal hernia require surgery.

D. **Assessment findings**

    1. Signs and symptoms of hiatal hernia may include:

        a. Heartburn occurring 30 to 60 minutes following a meal

        b. Substernal pain due to reflux; worsens when lying down

        c. Belching, regurgitation of sour-tasting secretions

        d. Feeling of abdominal fullness

    2. Diagnostic tests include:

        a. Esophagoscopy

        b. Barium swallow

E. **Nursing diagnoses**

    1. Knowledge Deficit

    2. Pain

F. **Planning and implementation**

    1. Teach the client measures to prevent hiatal hernia or minimize symptoms:

        a. Avoid bending, lifting heavy objects, straining (Valsalva's maneuver), reclining after meals, and tight clothing.

        b. Avoid spicy and acidic foods, alcohol, and tobacco.

        c. Eat small, frequent, bland meals.

        d. Eat a high-fiber diet to help prevent constipation and thus minimize straining on defecation.

        e. Administer antacid agent to neutralize gastric acid and decrease the direct acid irritation of the stomach mucosa (see Section II.D).

    2. If symptoms persist, prepare the client for surgical repair.

G. **Evaluation**

    1. The client verbalizes factors that precipitate symptoms and means of avoiding or minimizing these factors.

    2. The client reports decreased pain and other symptoms.

VI. **Peptic ulcer disease**
- **A.** Description: ulcers—circumscribed breaks in the mucosa—occurring in the stomach, the duodenum, and, less commonly, the distal esophagus and the jejunum
- **B.** Etiology and incidence
  1. Peptic ulcer disease is thought to be related to *H. pylori* infection; contributing factors are related to gastric acid secretion and include:
     a. Altered gastric acid and serum gastrin levels
     b. Tobacco smoking and alcohol use
     c. Use of aspirin, other nonsteroidal antiinflammatory drugs, and steroids
     d. Genetic predisposition
     e. Psychosomatic factors (e.g., chronic anxiety, type A personality)
  2. Peptic ulcer disease occurs in 5% to 10% of the population; only about one half of the cases are diagnosed. Duodenal ulcers are three times more common than gastric ulcers.
  3. Peak incidence for duodenal ulcers is between ages 25–50.
  4. Peak incidence for gastric ulcers is over age 50; incidence is about equal in men and women.
- **C.** Pathophysiology and management
  1. The basic problem in peptic ulcer disease is excessive secretion of hydrochloric acid in relation to the protective effects of mucus secretion and acid neutralization.
  2. Normally, tightly packed epithelial cells protect the gastric mucosa from irritation. Back-diffusion of acid through damaged mucosa may cause gastric ulcers.
  3. Hypersecretion of acid, possibly related to overactive vagal stimulation, contributes to duodenal ulcer formation.
  4. Possible complications of peptic ulcer disease include perforation, hemorrhage, and pyloric obstruction.
  5. Management involves medications and lifestyle modification.
- **D.** Assessment findings
  1. Peptic ulcer disease may be asymptomatic in up to 50% of persons affected.
  2. Gastric ulcers may produce:
     a. Pain, commonly described as burning, aching, or gnawing in the upper epigastrium; occurring 30 minutes to 1 hour following meals (rarely at night); and unrelieved by eating
     b. Epigastric tenderness
  3. Signs and symptoms of duodenal ulcers may include:
     a. Pain, described as burning, aching, or gnawing in the right epigastrium; occurring 2 to 3 hours after meals,

possibly causing the client to awaken at night; and relieved by eating
   b. Belching, nausea, and vomiting
   c. GI bleeding, either a slow oozing manifested by melena or a sudden, rapid loss of large amounts of blood through hematemesis
   d. Epigastric tenderness
4. Important diagnostic tests include:
   a. Barium swallow
   b. Gastroscopy

E. Nursing diagnoses
1. Knowledge Deficit
2. Altered Nutrition: Less than body requirements
3. Pain

F. Planning and implementation
1. Teach the client methods to minimize symptoms while still maintaining adequate nutrition, such as:
   a. Avoiding caffeine, alcohol, and spicy and acidic foods
   b. Avoiding other foods that previously have caused pain; specific dietary restrictions will vary from client to client
   c. Eating small, frequent, bland meals
2. As prescribed, administer medications which may include antacids; anticholinergics, such as atropine or anisotropine; histamine (H_2) receptor antagonists, such as cimetidine; and cytoprotective agents, such as sucralfate (see Section II.D).
3. Teach the client about necessary lifestyle modifications aimed at decreasing stress and maximizing effective coping.
4. Recent research reveals that antibiotic therapy to destroy *H. pylori* not only aids healing of initial ulcers but also prevents ulcer recurrence.
5. Prepare the client for surgery if indicated; possible procedures include:
   a. Vagotomy and pyloroplasty
   b. Distal subtotal gastrectomy

G. Evaluation
1. The client reports reduced pain.
2. The client verbalizes appropriate diet modifications.
3. The client demonstrates compliance with the prescribed medication regimen.

VII. Appendicitis
A. Description: inflammation of the vermiform appendix
B. Etiology and incidence
1. The precipitating event in appendicitis is obstruction of the

appendix lumen, which can result from fecalith, kinking of appendix, inflammation, or neoplasm.

    2. Appendicitis occurs in about 7% of the population and affects males more often than females; peak incidence is between ages 10 and 30.

C. **Pathophysiology and management**

    1. Obstruction of the appendix lumen causes increased intraluminal pressure and triggers an inflammatory process that can lead to infection, necrosis, and perforation.

    2. Perforation and rupture can cause peritonitis, a life-threatening complication.

D. **Assessment findings**

    1. Common clinical manifestations include:

        a.   Acute abdominal pain, usually in the right lower quadrant (McBurney's point); rebound tenderness

        b.   Nausea and vomiting

        c.   Low-grade fever

    2. Laboratory evaluation may reveal leukocytosis.

E. **Nursing diagnoses**

    1. Fluid Volume Deficit

    2. Risk for Infection

    3. Altered Nutrition: Less than body requirements

    4. Pain

F. **Planning and implementation: prompt surgery is indicated to prevent perforation; provide general preoperative and postoperative care (see Chapter 24, Perioperative Nursing, for details)**

G. **Evaluation**

    1. The client reports reduced pain.

    2. The client remains free of infection.

    3. The client exhibits adequate fluid status; drinks six to eight glasses of water daily.

    4. The client demonstrates appropriate choices in dietary intake.

VIII. **Diverticulitis**

A. **Description: a condition involving inflammation of diverticula, small saccular herniations in the colonic wall**

B. **Etiology and incidence**

    1. Formation of diverticula is associated with increased intraluminal pressure due to such factors as low-fiber diet, chronic constipation, and obesity.

    2. Diverticula develop in about 50% of persons over age 60 in the United States; incidence is greatest in men.

    3. Diverticulitis occurs in about 25% of persons with diverticula.

C. **Pathophysiology and management**

    1. Diverticula form as the colonic mucosa pushes through the muscular coat at weak points; increased intraluminal pressure is the apparent precipitating factor.

2. The diverticula gradually fill with undigested food matter and bacteria; as they enlarge, they become more susceptible to irritation and inflammation.

3. Management calls for rest, medication, and dietary modifications in hopes of avoiding complications.

4. Even a minute perforation of an inflamed diverticulum can lead to bacterial or fecal contamination of pericolic tissues.

5. Inflamed bowel tissue may adhere to the bladder or another pelvic organ; fistula formation may occur.

6. Repeated inflammation causes the colonic wall to thicken, narrowing the lumen and possibly causing acute obstruction.

7. Other dangerous complications include peritonitis and hemorrhage.

D. Assessment findings

1. Clinical manifestations may include:
   a. Change in bowel habits
   b. Dull, steady or episodic pain in the left lower abdominal quadrant or the epigastrium (depending on location of the diverticulitis)
   c. Rectal bleeding
   d. Anorexia
   e. Low-grade fever

2. Laboratory evaluation may reveal leukocytosis.

3. Studies performed to aid differential diagnosis may include:
   a. Colonoscopy
   b. Proctoscopy
   c. Barium enema

E. Nursing diagnoses

1. Constipation
2. Knowledge Deficit
3. Altered Nutrition: Less than body requirements
4. Pain
5. Chronic Pain

F. Planning and implementation

1. **Inform the client that all nursing interventions for diverticulitis are aimed at moving the stool through the colon as easily and with as little irritation as possible.**

2. During an acute exacerbation, which results when food or bacteria in the diverticula cause inflammation:
   a. Provide measures to rest the colon: keep client NPO, administer IV fluids, institute nasogastric suctioning, and keep client on bedrest.

IN b. Before administering prescribed broad-spectrum antibiotics, such as cephalexin (Keflex), to treat infection of the diverticulum, check client's drug allergy history.

IN c. As prescribed, administer agents, such as propantheline or oxyphencyclimine, which decrease gastric smooth muscle spasms before meals and at bedtime.

3. As symptoms subside:
    a. Slowly increase oral intake until the client is drinking between six and eight glasses of water daily.
    b. Offer a low-fiber diet until signs of infection decrease; then gradually increase fiber until the client is eating a high-fiber diet.
    c. Help restore the client's normal bowel elimination pattern by administering one or more of the following: bulk laxatives; stimulant laxatives; stool softeners, typically used for elderly clients because they are gentle and less likely to cause laxative dependence; saline laxatives; and at least 8 oz of water with any agent (see Section II.D).

4. Encourage daily exercise, such as walking, which will increase bowel peristalsis.

5. If surgical bowel resection is indicated, provide appropriate preoperative and postoperative care (see Chapter 24, Perioperative Nursing, for more information).

G. **Evaluation**
    1. The client reports absence of pain.
    2. The client exhibits return to normal elimination pattern, marked by:
        a. No abdominal cramping
        b. Passage of soft, formed stool
    3. The client demonstrates appropriate choices in dietary intake.

IX. Peritonitis

A. **Description: acute or chronic inflammation of the peritoneum, the membrane lining the abdominal cavity and covering the viscera**

B. **Etiology and incidence**
    1. Peritonitis usually results from bacterial (commonly, *Escherichia coli* or *Streptococcus faecalis*) invasion of the peritoneum due to such causes as:
        a. Ruptured appendix
        b. Diverticulitis
        c. Perforated gastric or duodenal ulcer
        d. Mesenteric thrombosis

          e.   Peptic ulcer disease
          f.   Neoplasm
          g.   Bowel strangulation
          h.   Ulcerative colitis
          i.   Penetrating abdominal wound

2. Other possible causes include:
    a.   Chemical irritation, as can result from ruptured bladder, ovary, or fallopian tube
    b.   Bile spillage into the peritoneal cavity, as can result from ruptured gallbladder or gangrenous cholecystitis
    c.   Contamination of the peritoneal cavity with surgical glove powder, talc, particles of suture material, or lint from surgical drapes

C. Pathophysiology and management

1. Peritoneal contamination may be localized in an abscess or diffused throughout the peritoneum, depending on its origin and on the effectiveness of the client's defenses.
2. The infectious process shunts blood to the inflamed area, leading to fluid shifts.
3. Paralytic ileus develops in early stages; as ileus and fluid shifting progress, dehydration and, possibly, acidosis occur.
4. Life-threatening complications of peritonitis include bowel obstruction, renal failure, respiratory insufficiency, shock, and, in some cases, liver failure. Management calls for treating the infection.

D. Assessment findings

1. Onset of peritonitis typically is marked by severe localized or diffuse abdominal pain, with or without guarding and rebound tenderness.
2. Paralytic ileus produces abdominal distention, usually with nausea and vomiting and possibly with diarrhea; bowel sounds are decreased or absent.
3. Fever, tachycardia, and chills point to sepsis.
4. Shallow, guarded respirations suggest diaphragmatic involvement.
5. Late manifestations include signs of dehydration and acidosis.
6. Laboratory analysis indicates leukocytosis, possibly leukopenia in severe cases.
7. Diagnostic tests include:
    a.   Paracentesis, to identify the causative organism
    b.   Abdominal radiograph, which may reveal the location of the perforation

E. Nursing diagnoses

1. Ineffective Breathing Pattern
2. Risk for Altered Body Temperature

      3. Risk for Fluid Volume Deficit
      4. Risk for Infection
      5. Pain

F. Planning and implementation

      1. Monitor respiratory status closely.

      2. Position the client to maximize comfort; assess pain frequently.

      3. Take steps to reduce and prevent the spread of infection.

      4. Monitor fluid and electrolyte balance.

      5. Administer analgesics and antibiotics as prescribed.

      6. If surgery is indicated, provide general preoperative and postoperative care (see Chapter 24, Perioperative Nursing, for more information).

G. Evaluation

      1. The client remains free of infection.

      2. The client reports absence of pain or control of pain with analgesics.

      3. The client exhibits normal breathing pattern.

      4. The client maintains adequate fluid status; drinks six to eight glasses of water daily.

      5. The client registers normal body temperature.

      6. The client exhibits normal bowel sounds.

X. Gastroenteritis

A. Description: inflammation of the stomach and small intestine

B. Etiology and incidence

      1. Gastroenteritis is a generic term for various common specific and nonspecific intestinal disorders.

      2. Among the many possible causes of gastroenteritis are:

         a. Bacterial food poisoning (e.g., *Staphylococcus aureus, Salmonella, Shigella*)

         b. Amoebae (e.g., *Entamoeba histolytica*)

         c. Adenoviruses, enteroviruses, and coxsackieviruses

         d. Parasites (e.g., *Ascaris, Enterobius*)

         e. Nonbacterial food poisoning from toxins in plants (e.g., mushrooms), seafood, or contaminated food

         f. Side effects of certain drugs (e.g., antibiotics)

C. Pathophysiology and management

      1. In healthy adults, gastroenteritis usually is a self-limiting problem producing minor GI symptoms that are more inconvenient than dangerous.

      2. In young children, elderly adults, and debilitated persons, however, these GI symptoms can produce serious—possibly even life-threatening—fluid and electrolyte losses.

D. **Assessment findings**
1. Clinical manifestations vary with the cause and the level of the GI tract involved; common signs and symptoms include:
   a. Abdominal cramping
   b. Nausea and vomiting
   c. Diarrhea
2. Other possible findings include fever, malaise, and borborygmi.

E. **Nursing diagnoses**
1. Fluid Volume Deficit
2. Pain
3. Risk for Impaired Skin Integrity

F. **Planning and implementation**
1. Provide measures designed to allow the GI tract to rest (e.g., keep the client NPO and maintain bedrest).
2. As symptoms subside, gradually provide clear liquids.
3. Closely monitor intake, output, and fluid and electrolyte status; increase fluid intake with IV infusion if necessary.
4. Provide additional perianal skin care for a client with severe diarrhea.
5. Administer antiemetics as prescribed (see Section II.D).

G. **Evaluation**
1. The client demonstrates return to normal elimination pattern, marked by:
   a. No abdominal cramping
   b. Passage of soft, formed stool
2. The client maintains skin integrity.
3. The client maintains adequate fluid status; drinks six to eight glasses of water daily.

XI. **Malabsorption syndromes**
A. **Description: various disorders resulting from impaired absorption of nutrients in the small intestine**
B. **Etiology and incidence**
1. The many possible causes of malabsorption can be divided into two categories: impaired digestion and impaired absorption.
2. Impaired digestion can result from:
   a. Postgastrectomy (especially with gastrojejunostomy), causing decreased pancreatic stimulation due to bypass of the duodenum, decreased mixing of food with digestive enzymes, and decreased intrinsic factor
   b. Impaired function of the liver and biliary tract or pancreas, resulting in lack of digestive enzymes

3. Impaired absorption can result from inadequate absorptive surface due to:
    a. Massive intestinal resection following vascular insult or inflammatory bowel disease (short bowel syndrome)
    b. Jejunal bypass for morbid obesity
    c. Inflammation of the bowel wall causing decreased surface for absorption
4. Postgastrectomy, stagnation of contents in the proximal small bowel can lead to bacterial overgrowth, which breaks down bile salts and impairs fat absorption
5. Impaired absorption also can result from excessively rapid transit time due to:
    a. Lactase deficiency
    b. Mucosal disruption
    c. Crohn's disease
    d. Infections that alter intestinal villi
    e. Gluten intolerance
6. Radiation exposure can affect rapidly proliferating cells in the GI mucosa, leading to inflammation, edema, and ischemic changes through the entire thickness of the bowel wall (radiation enteritis); may appear within days (acute) or months to years (chronic) following radiation treatment.

C. Pathophysiology and management: pathology varies depending on the cause (Table 9-2)

D. Assessment findings

1. Clinical manifestations vary widely depending on cause (see Table 9-2).
2. Common symptoms in many malabsorption syndromes include:
    a. Diarrhea
    b. Steatorrhea—pale, soft, bulky, malodorous stools
    c. Abdominal distention and cramping
    d. Weakness
    e. Dry skin and hair
    f. Weight loss
3. Laboratory studies and diagnostic test results also vary but may include:
    a. Decreased serum albumin and total protein
    b. Decreased hemoglobin and RBC count
    c. Altered electrolyte levels
    d. Decreased serum carotene level
    e. Thickened intestinal mucosa, demonstrated on barium swallow or barium enema

TABLE 9-2.
Comparison of Normal Absorption With Malabsorption States

| | NORMAL ABSORPTION | | MALABSORPTION | |
SMALL BOWEL	NUTRIENT	ALSO REQUIRES	CAUSE	CLINICAL S AND S
Duodenum	Iron	Gastric acid	Lack of gastric acid (gastrectomy)	Pallor, anemia
	Calcium	Vitamin D parathyroid	↓Vitamin D ↓fat digestion	Chvostek, Trousseau, tetany, bone pain, pathologic fracture
Jejunum	Protein	Pancreatic secretions	↓amt. panc. sec. or inadequate absorptive surface (SBS)	Weakness, fatigue, edema, cachexia
	Carbohydrate	Pancreatic secretions	↓amt. panc. sec (SBS)	Diarrhea, flatulence, abd. distention
	Fat	Pancreatic lipase bile	↓amt. panc. sec.	Steatorrhea, diarrhea, weight loss
			↓bile acid ↓synthesis-liver ↓amt. to duodenum ↓ileal absorption	Jaundice, pruritis
	Vitamin A	Bile salts	Lack of bile salts	Night blindness, dry skin and conjunctiva
	Vitamin D	Bile salts	Lack of bile salts	Osteomalacia, bone pain
	Vitamin E	Bile salts	Lack of bile salts	Rare to have S and S
	Vitamin K	Bile salts	Lack of bile salts	Easy bruisability, bleeding
	Folic acid		Impaired mucosal absorption	Diarrhea, weight loss, irritability, forgetfulness
Ileum	Vitamin B_{12}	Intrinsic factor	Gastric resection, ↓amt. panc. sec. ileal resection	Neuropathy, glossitis anorexia
Colon	Water		↓length of colon →↓absorption →↑excretion	Watery diarrhea

E. Nursing diagnoses
   1. Diarrhea
   2. Risk for Fluid Volume Deficit
   3. Altered Nutrition: Less than body requirements
   4. Risk for Impaired Skin Integrity

F. Planning and implementation
   1. Assist with initiation and maintenance of total parenteral nutrition, if indicated.
   2. Instruct the client in general nutritional concepts, including:
      a. Basic groups in the food pyramid

      b.   Foods to be avoided—depends on cause of malabsorption (e.g., grain products in gluten intolerance, lactose in lactase deficiency)

    3.   Encourage meticulous perianal skin care; clean and dry skin thoroughly after each episode of diarrhea.

G.   **Evaluation**

    1.   The client maintains adequate nutritional and hydration status.

    2.   The client maintains perianal skin integrity.

XII.   **Regional enteritis (Crohn's disease)**

    A.   **Description: a slowly progressive, persistent granulomatous disease anywhere in the GI tract (but most commonly in the terminal ileum) that extends through the entire thickness of the mucosal wall**

    B.   **Etiology and incidence**

        1.   The exact cause is unknown; contributing factors may include:

            a.   Allergies and other immune disorders

            b.   Lymphatic disorders

            c.   Infection

            d.   Genetic predisposition

        2.   Crohn's disease is most prevalent between ages 20 and 40, and occurs equally in both sexes. Incidence is highest in Jews and lowest in blacks.

    C.   **Pathophysiology and management**

        1.   Pathology typically includes:

            a.   Marked thickening and inflammation of the intestinal wall

            b.   Swollen mesenteric lymph nodes

            c.   Focal granulomas

            d.   Cobblestone patches of edematous, reddish-purple tissue interspersed with patches of normal tissue

            e.   Strictures secondary to scarring

        2.   Possible complications include intestinal obstruction, abscess and fistula formation, and perforation.

        3.   Treatment measures include dietary modifications, medications, and, possibly, surgery.

    D.   **Assessment findings**

        1.   Clinical effects vary; the most prominent manifestations commonly include:

            a.   Abdominal tenderness and pain; typically colicky and increasing after meals

            b.   Diarrhea, flatulence, steatorrhea

          c.   Signs of nutritional deficits (e.g., poor skin turgor, weight loss, anemia)

          d.   Perianal fistulas and abscesses

          e.   Systemic effects (e.g., fever, malaise, anorexia)

    2.   Other manifestations can affect the liver, kidneys, skin, joints, and eyes.

    3.   Important laboratory studies and diagnostic tests include:

          a.   Barium enema

          b.   Proctosigmoidoscopy

          c.   Colonoscopy

          d.   Stool analysis

          e.   Hemoglobin and hematocrit analysis

E.   **Nursing diagnoses**

    1.   Diarrhea

    2.   Fluid Volume Deficit

    3.   Knowledge Deficit

    4.   Altered Nutrition: Less than body requirements

    5.   Pain

    6.   Risk for Impaired Skin Integrity

    7.   Impaired Social Interaction

F.   **Planning and implementation**

    1.   For a client experiencing diarrhea, provide an easily accessible bedpan or commode.

    2.   Provide meticulous skin care to the perianal area.

    3.   Administer antidiarrheal drugs as prescribed (see Section II.D).

    4.   Monitor intake and output, and weigh the client daily.

    5.   Assess for fluid and electrolyte imbalance, particularly for dehydration; administer IV fluids and electrolytes as indicated.

    6.   Promote good nutrition by:

          a.   Offering bland, easily digested foods

          b.   Providing small, frequent meals

    7.   Assist the client with pain management; administer analgesics as needed.

    8.   Provide client teaching, covering:

          a.   The importance of good nutrition and adequate fluid intake

          b.   Stress-management techniques

          c.   Perianal skin care

          d.   The need for follow-up visits to the physician

    9.   If surgery is indicated, provide appropriate preoperative and postoperative care (see Chapter 24, Perioperative Nursing, for more information).

G.   **Evaluation**

    1.   The client maintains adequate nutrition and fluid status.

2. The client reports relief of pain.
3. The client exhibits manageable bowel elimination patterns.
4. The client verbalizes appropriate self-care practices (e.g., medications, diet).

XIII. Ulcerative colitis

A. **Description: an inflammatory disorder affecting the colonic mucosa and submucosa**

B. **Etiology and incidence**

1. Etiology is unclear; possible predisposing factors include:
   a. Family history
   b. Bacterial infection
   c. Allergic reaction
   d. Autoimmune disorder
   e. Emotional stress
2. Ulcerative colitis occurs primarily between ages 15 and 40, and affects both sexes about equally. A higher-than-average incidence has been reported in the Jewish population.

C. **Pathophysiology and management**

1. Ulcerative colitis is characterized by inflammation and ulceration involving the mucosal and submucosal layers only.
2. It typically begins in the rectum or sigmoid colon and spreads upward, possibly extending throughout the entire colon.
3. Inflammation produces congestion, edema, and ulcerations that develop into abscesses.
4. Mild ulcerative colitis may produce only localized symptoms; however, a severe, fulminant case can result in perforated colon, leading to life-threatening peritonitis.

D. **Assessment findings**

1. **The cardinal sign of ulcerative colitis is diarrhea containing pus, blood, and mucus; may or may not contain liquid feces.**
2. Other common symptoms include:
   a. Abdominal cramping and tenderness
   b. Anorexia and weight loss
   c. Fever
3. Laboratory studies and diagnostic tests are the same as for Crohn's disease (see Section XII.D).

E. **Nursing diagnoses: same as those for Crohn's disease (see Section XII.E)**

F. **Planning and implementation: nursing interventions similar to those for Crohn's disease (see Section XII.F)**

G. **Evaluation: refer to evaluation criteria for Crohn's disease (see Section XII.G)**

XIV. Irritable bowel syndrome (IBS)

A. Description: a common functional disorder of GI motility not associated with anatomic changes; also known as spastic colon or irritable colon

B. Etiology and incidence

    1. IBS is generally associated with such factors as:

        a. Psychologic stress

        b. Prediverticular disease with changes in the bowel wall

        c. Low-residue diet

    2. It accounts for approximately half of all cases of GI illness in the United States; incidence is greater in women than in men.

C. Pathophysiology and management

    1. IBS develops in the absence of organic disease or anatomic abnormality.

    2. Emotional stress may disturb autonomic nervous system function, leading to disrupted intestinal motility and transit time.

    3. Treatment measures include medications and dietary modifications.

D. Assessment findings

    1. The typical triad of findings in IBS includes:

        a. **Abdominal pain with tenderness on palpation**

        b. **Altered bowel habits: diarrhea or constipation**

        c. **Absence of detectable disease**

    2. Abdominal pain may be localized in the lower left quadrant, constant or intermittent, and relieved by passing gas or stool.

    3. Diarrhea often alternates with constipation; stools may contain increased mucus but seldom blood.

    4. Symptoms often mimic those of other conditions, hindering differential diagnosis. Diagnosis must first rule out any organic GI disease or abnormality.

    5. The client may report recent emotional disturbance.

    6. Dietary history may reveal a low-residue diet.

    7. Laboratory studies and diagnostic tests commonly reveal:

        a. Normal sigmoidoscopy findings

        b. Normal complete blood count

        c. Normal stool analysis

E. Nursing diagnoses

    1. Ineffective Individual Coping

    2. Diarrhea or Constipation

    3. Knowledge Deficit

    4. Pain

F. **Planning and implementation**

1. Teach the client measures to reduce symptoms, such as:
   a. Eating a high-fiber diet and avoiding gas-forming foods
   b. Adhering to a schedule of regular work and rest periods
   c. Avoiding or minimizing stress-producing situations
   d. Drinking six to eight glasses of water daily to prevent constipation
2. Encourage the client to comply with any prescribed medication regimen, which may include anticholinergics, such as atropine (Donnatal); antispasmodic medication, such as propantheline (Pro-Banthine), which inhibits gastric smooth muscle spasms; and/or bulk laxatives (see Section II.D).
3. Provide the client with reassurance and emotional support to help decrease anxiety and increase his or her sense of control over the situation and its management.

G. **Evaluation**

1. The client remains symptom-free.
2. The client complies with prescribed dietary and activity modifications.

Bibliography

Beam, E. (1995). *Helicobacter pylori* and peptic ulcer disease. *Clinical Reviews, 5*(6), 51–62.

Bolander, V. R. (1994). *Sorensen & Luckmann's basic nursing: a physiologic approach* (3rd ed.). Philadelphia: W. B. Saunders.

Carpenito, L. J. (1995). *Nursing diagnosis: Application to clinical practice* (6th ed.). Philadelphia: J. B. Lippincott.

Clark, J., Queener, S., & Karb, V. (1990). *Pharmacologic basis of nursing practice* (4th ed). St. Louis: C. V. Mosby.

Gordon, M. (1995). *Manual of nursing diagnosis 1995–1996*. St. Louis: C. V. Mosby.

Nettina, S. (1996). *The Lippincott manual of nursing practice* (6th ed.). Philadelphia: Lippincott-Raven Publishers.

Phipps, W. J., Long, B. C., & Woods, N. F. (1994). *Medical-surgical nursing: Concepts and practice* (5th ed). St. Louis: C. V. Mosby.

Smeltzer, S. C., & Bare, B. G. (1996). *Brunner & Suddarth's textbook of medical-surgical nursing* (8th ed). Philadelphia: Lippincott-Raven Publishers.

Society of Gastroenterology Nurses and Associates. (1993). *SGNA gastroenterology nursing: A core curriculum*. St. Louis: C. V. Mosby.

Springhouse Corporation. (1992). *Nursing student's guide to drugs*. Springhouse, PA: Springhouse Corp.

STUDY QUESTIONS

1. Steatorrhea may occur in which of the following conditions?
   a. malabsorption syndromes
   b. gastritis
   c. irritable bowel syndrome
   d. duodenal ulcer

2. Nursing interventions for the client admitted with acute diverticulitis include
   a. administering bulk laxatives and increasing fluid intake
   b. encouraging high-fiber diet and inserting rectal tube
   c. keeping the client NPO and initiating nasogastric suctioning
   d. administering antidiarrheal medications and encouraging low-fiber diet

3. Nursing assessments for the client with esophagitis include
   a. midepigastric pain and tenderness
   b. abdominal distention and fever
   c. abdominal cramping and nausea/vomiting
   d. heartburn and dysphagia

4. When assessing a client admitted with a bleeding gastric ulcer, the nurse would expect to find which of the following stool characteristics?
   a. coffee-ground color
   b. clay colored
   c. black, tarry
   d. bright red

5. When developing a client teaching plan for a client with a hiatal hernia, the nurse should be sure to include instructions to
   a. Eat three large meals per day with no restrictions.
   b. Lie down immediately following a meal.
   c. Gradually increase the amount of lifting done.
   d. Eat frequent, small, bland meals with high fiber content.

6. A 17-year-old client comes into the emergency room complaining of severe abdominal pain in the right lower quadrant and nausea and vomiting in the last 6 hours. The client has a temperature of 100.4°F. Based on these data, the nurse would suspect
   a. diverticulitis
   b. appendicitis
   c. regional enteritis
   d. ulcerative colitis

7. A client has developed a malabsorption problem after receiving radiation therapy to the head, neck, and abdomen 6 months ago. Discharge teaching about the cause and ways to decrease symptoms should focus on which of the following areas?
   a. teeth and tongue
   b. sigmoid and rectum
   c. small intestine
   d. large intestine

8. Which of the following would be appropriate outcomes for interventions aimed at preventing or minimizing constipation?
   a. The client eats a high-fiber diet.
   b. The client avoids physical exercise.
   c. The client drinks one to two glasses of water daily.
   d. The client maintains a sedentary lifestyle.

9. For planning at-home reporting criteria for a client with malabsorption syndrome, which of the following stool characteristics would be most valuable in identifying diarrhea?
   a. quantity
   b. constituents
   c. color
   d. consistency

10. Which of the following statements best describes regional enteritis (Crohn's disease)?
    a. It involves continuous lesions, ultimately spreading throughout the entire large intestine.
    b. It typically appears as patches of normal colon between areas of inflammation.

   c. It involves only the mucosa and submucosa of the bowel wall.

   d. Its cardinal sign is malabsorption.

11. Irritable bowel syndrome (IBS) can best be described as

   a. an inflammatory process

   b. the result of longstanding GI disease

   c. a functional disorder

   d. an inherited trait

12. Nursing care of a client with gastroenteritis should include which of the following interventions?

   a. Encourage optimal nutritional intake.

   b. Alleviate abdominal pain and cramping.

   c. Administer an oral antiemetic every 2 hours.

   d. Monitor intake and output and electrolyte levels.

13. A client with alopecia and stomatitis resulting from chemotherapy complains of an inability to eat because of "mouth sores." The client also reports feeling embarrassed by hair loss and abandoned by being excluded from certain activities. Based on these data, which of the following nursing diagnoses best reflects the nurse's identification of the problem most likely to impair the client's healthful progress.

   a. Impaired Tissue Integrity

   b. Social Isolation

   c. Grieving

   d. Altered Nutrition: Less than body requirements

14. Which of the following nursing actions demonstrates the nurse's understanding of one of the primary complications for peritonitis?

   a. Provide small, frequent meals.

   b. Frequently assess respiratory status.

   c. Assess skin integrity regularly.

   d. Evaluate stools for color and consistency.

ANSWER KEY

1. **Correct response: a**
   Steatorrhea—bulky, fatty stools—indicates decreased fat absorption.
   b, c, and d. Steatorrhea is not associated with any of these disorders.
   Comprehension/Physiologic/Assessment

2. **Correct response: c**
   During acute diverticulitis the bowel must be put totally at rest, so the client must be kept NPO; nasogastric suctioning will decompress the bowel.
   a. Bulk laxatives and increased fluid intake will help prevent an exacerbation of diverticulosis.
   b. A high-fiber diet would further irritate the bowel, and a rectal tube is not required for diverticulitis.
   d. Usually diarrhea does not accompany diverticulitis. The client should be NPO during acute exacerbation and should gradually resume eating a low-residue diet after pain subsides.
   Application/Physiologic/Implementation

3. **Correct response: d**
   Common clinical manifestations of esophagitis include heartburn, acid regurgitation, belching, dysphagia, and esophageal pain radiating to arms, neck, and jaw.
   a, b, and c. These are clinical manifestations of peptic ulcer disease (a), peritonitis (b), ar. ! gastroenteritis (c).
   Comprehension/Physiologic/Assessment

4. **Correct response: c**
   Melena, or black, tarry stools, is a sign of bleeding high in the GI tract. The action of the digestive enzymes turns the bright red blood black and tarry before defecation occurs.
   a, b, and d. Clay-colored stools would be expected with biliary obstruction; bright red blood would indicate bleeding from low in the GI tract.
   Comprehension/Physiologic/Evaluation

5. **Correct response: d**
   Eating small, bland meals with high fiber helps diminish reflux and decrease constipation (to prevent straining).
   a, b, and c. The client with hiatal hernia should avoid bending, lifting heavy objects, reclining after meals, eating spicy foods, and using alcohol and tobacco.
   *Comprehension/Health promotion/
   Implementation*

6. **Correct response: b**
   Severe right lower quadrant pain (McBurney's point), nausea/vomiting, and a low-grade fever are all common clinical manifestations of appendicitis.
   a, c, and d. These clinical manifestations do not support the diagnostic criteria for these disease processes.
   Comprehension/Physiologic/Assessment

7. **Correct response: c**
   The small bowel (duodenum, jejunum, and ileum) is responsible for the absorption of most of the major nutrients.
   a, b, and d. Although an abnormality of the large bowel could affect water reabsorption, and abnormalities of the teeth and tongue could alter the ability to ingest food, it is the small intestine that supports nutrient absorption.
   *Analysis/Health promotion/
   Implementation*

8. **Correct response: a**
   A high-fiber diet induces rapid movement through the colon and a large, soft stool.
   b, c, and d. Sedentary lifestyle is a predisposing factor in constipation. Regular physical exercise, a high-fiber diet, and plenty of water all contribute to regular elimination.
   *Application/Health promotion/
   Implementation*

9. *Correct response: d*
Increased fecal fluid content is most descriptive for diarrhea.
a, b, and c. It also is important to assess stool color and presence of mucus. The quantity becomes important only when it represents a change from the person's usual elimination pattern.
Application/Safe care/Planning

10. *Correct response: b*
Crohn's disease generally exhibits a characteristic "cobblestone" appearance involving the entire bowel wall, with patches of normal colon between areas of inflammation.
a, c, and d. None of these statements characterizes Crohn's disease.
Analysis/Physiologic/Planning

11. *Correct response: c*
Irritable bowel syndrome is a functional disorder of motility (i.e., no anatomic changes are present).
a, b, and d. None of these responses describes IBS.
Knowledge/Physiologic/Assessment

12. *Correct response: d*
Vomiting and diarrhea put the client at risk for fluid volume deficit and electrolyte imbalance.

a, b, and c. Usually, the GI tract is allowed to rest by omitting all oral intake. The cause of pain cannot be alleviated.
Application/Safe care/Implementation

13. *Correct response: c*
Grief is an important process in the progression toward healthy resolution.
a, b, and d. These diagnoses all would have an impact on the client's physical or emotional health but grieving will affect the progress toward healthful resolution.
Analysis/Health promotion/ Analysis (Dx)

14. *Correct response: b*
The infectious process can progress to respiratory complications.
a and d. Paralytic ileus commonly occurs, so feeding this client is inappropriate—as is assuming that diarrhea will occur.
c. Impaired skin integrity is not a primary potential complication specific to this disease; rather, it can occur in any client on bedrest.
Application/Safe care/Implementation

Endocrine and Metabolic Disorders

I. Endocrine and metabolic system

A. Hormones

1. Hormones are chemical substances secreted by endocrine glands directly into the blood stream to act on specific target cells; types include:

    a. Protein or peptide hormones (e.g., insulin, vasopressin, growth hormone [GH], adrenocorticotropic hormone [ACTH]): generally act on cell membranes by binding to receptors

    b. Amine and amino acid derivatives (e.g., epinephrine, norepinephrine): act on cell membranes

    c. Steroids (e.g., cortisol, estrogen, testosterone): act intracellularly to modify protein synthesis

2. Hormones regulate growth and development, fluid and electrolyte balance, reproduction, adaptation to stress, and metabolism.

3. Hormone secretion is regulated through feedback mechanisms (i.e., increased levels of a specific hormone or its cations or metabolites inhibit secretion, and decreased levels stimulate secretion).

B. Pituitary gland

1. Located at the inferior aspect of the brain within the sella turcica (a small recess in the sphenoid bone), the pituitary gland consists of anterior and posterior lobes.

2. The *anterior lobe* synthesizes and releases hormones, including:

   a. GH: affects growth of bones and muscles; influences protein, lipid, carbohydrate, and calcium metabolism

   b. Prolactin (PRL): affects mammary glands to stimulate milk production

   c. Thyroid-stimulating hormone (TSH): stimulates thyroid hormone production

   d. ACTH: stimulates the adrenal cortex to produce steroids (primarily cortisol)

   e. Follicle-stimulating hormone (FSH): stimulates ovaries to develop follicles and secrete estrogen; stimulates testes to develop seminiferous tubules and perform spermatogenesis

   f. Luteinizing (or interstitial cell-stimulating) hormone (LH): stimulates ovaries to form corpus luteum, initiate ovulation, and produce progesterone; stimulates testes to secrete testosterone

3. Anterior pituitary hormone release is regulated by the hypothalamus, which secretes releasing and inhibiting hormones.

4. The *posterior lobe* stores and releases hormones synthesized in the hypothalamus, including:

   a. Oxytocin: stimulates uterine and mammary gland contractions

   b. Antidiuretic hormone (ADH, vasopressin): acts on the distal renal tubule to increase water reabsorption; rate of release is regulated by plasma osmolality

C. **Thyroid gland**

1. A butterfly-shaped gland located in the neck behind the trachea, the thyroid produces three hormones:

   a. Thyroxine (T_4) and triiodothyronine (T_3)—produced predominantly from peripheral conversion of T_4 to T_3: regulate cellular metabolic activity; secretion is under the control of TSH

   b. Thyrocalcitonin: secreted in response to high blood calcium levels; lowers blood calcium levels by inhibiting bone resorption

D. **Parathyroid glands**

1. These small glands, usually four, surround the posterior thyroid tissue; they are often difficult to locate and may be removed accidentally during thyroid or other neck surgery.

2. In response to low blood calcium level, the parathyroids produce parathormone (PTH), which raises blood calcium levels by increasing calcium resorption from kidneys, intestines, and bones.

E. Adrenal glands

1. Located at the upper poles of both kidneys, the adrenals contain two distinct types of endocrine tissue.
2. The adrenal medulla, in the center of the gland, reacts to autonomic nervous system signals to release catecholamines:
   a. Epinephrine (80%): prepares the body for the fight-or-flight response by converting glycogen, stored in the liver, to glucose and increasing cardiac output
   b. Norepinephrine (20%): exerts effects similar to epinephrine and produces extensive vasoconstriction
3. The outer portion, the adrenal cortex, is stimulated by ACTH to produce corticosteroids:
   a. Mineralocorticoids (primarily aldosterone): released in response to angiotensin II and ACTH; increase sodium reabsorption and potassium loss primarily through the renal tubules
   b. Glucocorticoids (primarily cortisol): released in response to ACTH; increase blood glucose by stimulating gluconeogenesis and lipolysis and decrease protein synthesis; suppress the inflammatory response; promote sodium retention and potassium loss
   c. Adrenal sex hormones (androgens and estrogen): govern development of certain secondary sex characteristics

F. Pancreas

1. A slender, elongated organ lying horizontally in the posterior abdomen behind the stomach, the pancreas functions as both an endocrine and an exocrine gland.
2. Exocrine functions involve secretion of pancreatic digestive enzymes by specialized cells.
3. Endocrine functions are controlled by the alpha, beta, and delta cells of the islets of Langerhans:
   a. Alpha cells secrete glucagon, which increases blood glucose through gluconeogenesis.
   b. Beta cells secrete insulin, which regulates protein, carbohydrate, and fat metabolism by facilitating glucose, amino acid, and fatty acid transport; also promotes glycogen, protein, and triglyceride synthesis.
   c. Delta cells secrete somatostatin (inhibitory hormone) and gastrin.

G. Gonads

1. The gonads consist of the ovaries and testes.
2. Although the gonads exert some systemic metabolic effects, their primary function is in reproduction (see Chapter 11, Reproductive and Sexual Disorders).

II. Overview of endocrine and metabolic disorders

A. Assessment

1. Nursing health history should focus on:
   a. Changes in the client's usual health patterns and behavior (e.g., mental status, sensory function, nutrition, elimination, activity tolerance, and sleep patterns)
   b. Family history of endocrine disorders
   c. Any past or present health problems, procedures, or treatments that can put the client at risk for developing an endocrine disorder (e.g., radiation therapy to the head or neck)
2. Important physical assessment aspects include:
   a. Stature, fat distribution, shape of face
   b. Color, texture, and turgor of skin; surgical scars; unusual bruising
   c. Protruding or sunken eyes, lid lag or retraction
   d. Hair distribution
   e. Presence of goiter
   f. Vital signs
   g. Heart sounds
   h. Lung sounds
   i. Body weight
   j. Bowel sounds

B. Laboratory studies and diagnostic tests

1. Measurement of hormones in blood and urine reflects production and activity of hormones related to specific endocrine and metabolic disorders. Specific tests are discussed under the appropriate disorder in this chapter; types of testing include:
   a. Static (present time) measurement: detects elevated or depressed hormone levels; diagnostic for certain disorders
   b. Dynamic testing: involves administration of a stimulating or suppressing agent, followed by measurement of hormone response; requires close collaboration with laboratory personnel to ensure correct sequence of timed specimens
2. Imaging tests assist in identifying causative factors; studies include:
   a. Scans
   b. Computed tomography (CT) scan
   c. Magnetic resonance imaging (MRI)
   d. Bone mineral densitometry
3. Other important studies include:
   a. Visual field testing
   b. Selective venous sampling

C. Psychosocial implications

1. A person with an endocrine or metabolic disorder may experience difficulty coping with the disease process related to such factors as:
   a. Chronic nature of the disorder
   b. Sense of loss of control
   c. Fear of complications or death
2. Common self-concept concerns are related to fears of:
   a. Body image changes
   b. Rejection
   c. Sexual dysfunction
   d. Emotional instability
3. Endocrine and metabolic disorders commonly produce lifestyle concerns related to potential changes in:
   a. Physical and mental functioning (elderly persons at increased risk because declines in physical and mental functioning may be erroneously attributed to aging)
   b. Work performance, with potential for loss of job
4. A client with an endocrine or metabolic disorder also may experience changes in social interaction due to:
   a. Isolation
   b. Depression

D. Medications used to treat endocrine and metabolic problems (additional medications may be included with specific diseases)

1. Medications that suppress the release of growth hormone and prolactin
   a. Example: bromocriptine (Parlodel)
   b. Selected nursing considerations

    ▸ Administer with meals to minimize GI distress.
   ▸ Instruct client to report vision problems, severe nausea/vomiting, acute headaches.
   ▸ Advise client to limit use of alcohol.

2. Medications that suppress the release of growth hormone, insulin, and glucagon
   a. Example: octreotide (Sandostatin)
   b. Selected nursing considerations

    ▸ Monitor blood glucose levels.
   ▸ Administer subcutaneously; rotate injection sites.
   ▸ Explain that drug may cause dizziness, drowsiness. Use caution until response to medication is known.

3. *ADH replacement agents,* which conserve renal water by increasing urine osmolality and decreasing urine flow rate

a. Examples: desmopressin (DDAVP), vasopressin (Pitressin)

b. Selected nursing considerations

𝕟 ▸ **Administer intranasally or deep IM.**
▸ **Instruct client to report signs of water intoxication (drowsiness, lethargy, headache, sudden weight gain, severe nasal congestion); caution against adjusting dosage without consulting physician.**

4. *Antithyroid agents*, which interfere with conversion of iodine into thyroglobulin, thereby inhibiting thyroid hormone synthesis

a. Examples: propylthiouracil (PTU), methimazole (Tapazole)

b. Selected nursing considerations

𝕟 ▸ **Advise client to report flulike symptoms and fever immediately; they may be drug-induced.**
▸ **Report signs and symptoms of hyper/hypothyroidism.**
▸ **Caution client not to use products containing iodine, such as cough medicines, iodized salt, or shellfish.**

5. *Beta-adrenergic blockers*, which relieve sympathomimetic symptoms (e.g., tachycardia) of hyperthyroidism by regulating sympathetic nervous system activity

a. Examples: propranolol (Inderal), reserpine (Serpasil)

b. Selected nursing considerations

𝕟 ▸ **Explain safety precautions for dealing with orthostatic hypotension.**
▸ **Caution client to avoid discontinuing abruptly; doing so can exacerbate angina or MI.**

6. *Iodine-containing agents*, which inhibit release of stored thyroid hormone and retard hormone synthesis

a. Examples: potassium iodide (SSKI), Lugol's solution

b. Selected nursing considerations

𝕟 ▸ **Administer short term before thyroidectomy.**
▸ **Administer through straw with fluids.**

7. *Glucocorticoids*, which are used for replacement therapy and to block conversion of T_4 to T_3

a. Examples: hydrocortisone sodium succinate (Solu-Cortef), cortisone (Cortone), methylprednisolone (Medrol), dexamethasone (Decadron), prednisone (Deltasone)

b. Selected nursing considerations

𝕟 ▸ **Inform client that medication cannot be stopped abruptly but should be discontinued gradually to pre-**

vent withdrawal symptoms and, possibly, shock or death.
- ▶ Identify signs and symptoms of cushingoid effects to report including weight gain, moon face, buffalo hump, hirsutism.

8. *Thyroid hormone,* which raises metabolic rate, promotes gluconeogenesis, increases use of stored glycogen, stimulates protein synthesis, and affects protein and carbohydrate metabolism and cell growth
   a. Examples: levothyroxine (Synthroid)
   b. Selected nursing considerations

   m ▶ Administer in morning to avoid bedtime insomnia.
   - ▶ Instruct client to notify physician of signs and symptoms of hypo/hyperthyroidism.
   - ▶ Monitor cardiac response to increased metabolic rate and oxygen requirements.

9. *Adrenocortical steroid inhibitors,* which decrease cortisol production
   a. Examples: ketoconazole (Nizoral), aminoglutethimide (Cytadren), mitotane (Lysodren)
   b. Selected nursing considerations

   m ▶ Administer in divided doses to reduce nausea and vomiting, and instruct client to continue taking medication despite discomfort.
   - ▶ Inform client to take safety precautions because medication may cause drowsiness and orthostatic hypotension (dizziness and lightheadedness upon standing).

10. *Mineralocorticoids,* which are used for hormone replacement
    a. Examples: fludrocortisone (Florinef)
    b. Selected nursing considerations

    m ▶ Explain that additional doses may be needed in times of stress.
    - ▶ Instruct client to report weight gain and severe headache.

11. *Oral hypoglycemic agents,* which reduce blood glucose levels by stimulating pancreatic insulin production
    a. Examples: tolbutamide (Orinase), acetohexamide (Dymelor), chlorpropamide (Diabinese), glipizide (Glucotrol), Glyburide (Diabeta)
    b. Selected nursing considerations

    m ▶ Instruct client to take medication daily and to continue other measures (diet, exercise) to decrease blood glucose levels.

> ► Advise client that insulin may be needed during times of increased stress.
> ► Forewarn that possible side effects may include hypoglycemia and incompatibility with alcohol.

12. *Insulin*, which replaces endogenous insulin and maintains blood glucose levels by regulating protein, carbohydrate, and fat metabolism
   a. Examples: Ultralente/U, PZI, long-acting; NPH/N, Lente/L, intermediate-acting; Regular/R, Semilente/S, fast-acting; Humulin 70/30 (70% NPH and 30% R), combination agent
   b. Selected nursing considerations

> ► Discuss dosage schedule, explaining that fast-acting insulin has peak effect 2–4 hours after administration, intermediate-acting insulin has peak effect in 6–8 hours, long-acting insulin has peak effect in 14–16 hours, and combination insulins have peak effect depending on their components. For example, Humulin 70/30 contains 70% NPH and 30% regular insulin.
> ► Teach and demonstrate preparation; administration techniques; injection sites and rotation; insulin and equipment care, storage, and disposal.

III. Anterior pituitary dysfunction

A. Description: undersecretion or oversecretion of anterior pituitary hormones (ACTH, TSH, GH, LH, PRL)

B. Etiology and incidence
   1. Causes of undersecretion (hypopituitarism) include:
      a. Pituitary gland infarction
      b. Surgical removal of the pituitary
      c. Genetic disorders or replacement with tumor tissue
   2. Oversecretion (hyperpituitarism) commonly results from a secretory adenoma, which stimulates the target gland (adrenal, thyroid) or tissue.

C. Pathophysiology and management
   1. Hypopituitarism affects thyroid, adrenal, and gonadal function (see Section VI, Hypothyroidism, and Section XI, Adrenal hypofunction, for more information).
   2. Hyperpituitarism commonly results in altered ACTH or GH secretion, leading to Cushing's syndrome or acromegaly (see Section X, Cushing's syndrome, for more information).

D. Assessment findings
   1. Clinical manifestations of excessive GH secretion (acromegaly in adults) may include:
      a. Coarse features (e.g., broad skull, protruding jaw, prognathism, broadening of hands and feet)

        b.   Thickened heel pads

        c.   Thick tongue

        d.   Change in ring and shoe size

        e.   Dental changes

        f.   Hypertension

        g.   Diabetes mellitus

        h.   Headache, visual disturbances

        i.   Lethargy

        j.   Sinus congestion

        k.   Decreased libido

2. Diagnostic tests for excessive GH secretion may reveal:

        a.   Elevated GH and somatomedin-C levels

        b.   Diminished visual fields

        c.   Tumor visualized on radiologic examination, such as CT scans

3. Signs and symptoms of excessive PRL secretion include:

        a.   Breast discharge

        b.   Decreased libido

        c.   Amenorrhea

        d.   Impotence

        e.   Headache, visual disturbances

        f.   Lethargy

4. In excessive PRL secretion, diagnostic tests may reveal:

        a.   Elevated serum PRL level

        b.   Decreased visual fields

        c.   Tumor visualized on radiologic examination, including CT scans

E. Nursing diagnoses

1. Risk for Injury

2. Knowledge Deficit

3. Self Esteem Disturbance

4. Sexual Dysfunction

F. Planning and implementation

1. Encourage the client to verbalize feelings about the disorder and its effects on his or her body.

2. Discuss the disorder's effects on sexual functioning with the client and partner.

3. Administer prescribed medications, which may include bromocriptine to lower prolactin level (see Section II.D).

4. If pituitary irradiation is indicated, prepare the client for therapy.

5. If surgical removal of a pituitary tumor is indicated, reinforce the surgeon's explanation of the procedure.

6. Monitor a postsurgical client for signs of complications, such as:

  a. Hemorrhage

  b. Transient diabetes insipidus (DI)

  c. Rhinorrhea, which may indicate cerebrospinal leak

  d. Adrenal insufficiency (see Section XI) and thyroid insufficiency (see Section VI)

  e. Infection, particularly meningitis (marked by fever, nuchal rigidity, headache)

  f. Visual disturbances, particularly decreased visual fields

G. **Evaluation**

 1. The client verbalizes a sense of well-being.

 2. The client resumes usual sexual practices.

 3. The client verbalizes understanding of the treatment regimen.

 4. The client takes medications as prescribed.

 5. The client remains free of surgical complications.

 6. The client demonstrates restoration of normal endocrine function.

 7. The client exhibits no visual deficits.

IV. Posterior pituitary dysfunction

A. **Description**

 1. Dysfunction of the posterior pituitary involves either oversecretion or undersecretion of antidiuretic hormone (ADH).

 2. Specific disorders include:

  a. DI, caused by undersecretion of ADH, resulting in excessive dilute urine production

  b. Syndrome of inappropriate ADH (SIADH), involving oversecretion of ADH and resulting in excessive water conservation

B. **Etiology and incidence**

 1. Possible causes of DI include:

  a. Posterior pituitary destruction from tumors

  b. Vascular accidents

  c. Surgery or hypothalamic damage

  d. Certain drugs that can interfere with ADH secretion or action (e.g., phenytoin, alcohol, lithium carbonate)

 2. Nephrogenic DI, either familial or arising from various renal disorders, occurs when the distal renal tubules do not respond to ADH.

 3. SIADH can result from:

  a. Central nervous system disorders

  b. Stimulation due to hypoxia or decreased left atrial filling pressure

  c. Pharmacologic agents (e.g., chemotherapy, chlorpropamide)

  d. Overuse of vasopressin therapy

       e.   Ectopic ADH production associated with some cancers

       f.   Nausea or narcotic use, which can stimulate ADH secretion

C. **Assessment findings**

    1. Clinical manifestations of DI include:

       a.   Profoundly increased output (5 to 20 L/day) of dilute urine

       b.   Nocturia

       c.   Extreme thirst

       d.   Weight loss

       e.   Possible tachycardia, hypotension, and weakness

    2. Laboratory and diagnostic tests for DI may reveal:

       a.   Elevated plasma osmolality and serum sodium level

       b.   Water deprivation test demonstrating inability of the kidneys to concentrate urine despite increased plasma osmolality and low plasma vasopressin level

       c.   Vasopressin test demonstrating that the kidneys can concentrate urine after administration of ADH; differentiates central (pituitary or hypothalamic) DI from nephrogenic DI

    3. Signs and symptoms of SIADH include:

       a.   Decreased urine output

       b.   Weight gain

       c.   Altered mental status (e.g., headache, confusion, lethargy, seizures and coma in severe hyponatremia)

       d.   Delayed deep tendon reflexes

    4. In SIADH, laboratory study results may include:

       a.   Decreased serum sodium and osmolality

       b.   Elevated urine sodium and osmolality

       c.   Elevated ADH level

D. **Nursing diagnoses**

    1. Fluid Volume Deficit (in DI)

    2. Fluid Volume Excess (in SIADH)

    3. Risk for Injury

    4. Knowledge Deficit

    5. Sleep Pattern Disturbance

E. **Planning and implementation**

    1. For both DI and SIADH:

       a.   Monitor intake and output, and weigh the client daily.

       b.   Monitor vital signs.

       c.   Assess skin turgor and mucous membranes.

       d.   Provide meticulous skin and mouth care.

    2. For DI:

       a.   Replace fluids as indicated; assess for and report any illness, injury, or other problem that could prevent adequate fluid intake.

b. Encourage the client to drink fluids in response to thirst.

c. Administer prescribed ADH replacement agents such as vasopressin (see Section II.D).

   3. For SIADH:

a. Restrict fluid intake as indicated.

b. Regularly assess mental status.

c. Modify the client's environment as necessary to reduce the risk of injury.

m   d. **Administer lithium as prescribed. Lithium increases free water loss. It must be administered with plenty of water and food to minimize GI upset. Blood levels must also be monitored. Therapeutic level is 1.0 to 1.5 mEq/L.**

m   e. **Administer phenytoin (Dilantin) as prescribed. Phenytoin inhibits the release of ADH which, in turn, increases urine output. Give with food to minimize GI distress; promote good oral hygiene to reduce gingival sensitivity; monitor serum level of drug (normal level: 10–20 µg/mL).**

  F. Evaluation

    1. The client has fluid balanced restored.

    2. The client verbalizes understanding of the treatment regimen.

    3. The client demonstrates compliance with the prescribed medication regimen.

    4. The client reports absence of nocturia (in DI).

    5. The client demonstrates return to previous level of mental functioning (in SIADH).

    6. The client remains injury-free (in SIADH).

V. Hyperthyroidism

  A. Description: a metabolic imbalance resulting from excessive thyroid hormone production; Graves' disease the most common form

  B. Etiology and incidence

    1. Autoimmune dysfunction is the most common cause of Graves' disease; autoantibodies apparently mimic TSH, leading to hypersecretion of thyroid hormones.

    2. Genetic factors seem to play a role.

    3. Other possible causes include:

      a. Toxic nodular goiter

      b. Exposure to iodine

   c. TSH-secreting pituitary tumor (rare)

   d. Thyroiditis

  4. Incidence is greatest between ages 30 and 40 and is higher in women than in men.

C. **Pathophysiology and management**

  1. Excessive secretion of thyroid hormone leads to increased metabolic rate, excessive heat production, and increased responsiveness to catecholamines.

  2. These actions lead to profound changes in many organ systems.

  3. Effective treatment usually can control symptoms.

  4. However, severe, acute exacerbation—thyroid storm—may be a life-threatening emergency.

D. **Assessment findings**

  1. Clinical manifestations of hyperthyroidism may include:

   a. Nervousness, irritability, hyperactivity, emotional lability, and decreased attention span

   b. Weakness, easy fatigability, exercise intolerance

   c. Heat intolerance

   d. Weight change (loss or gain), increased appetite

   e. Insomnia, interrupted sleep

   f. Frequent stools, diarrhea

   g. Menstrual irregularities, decreased libido

   h. Warm, sweaty, flushed skin with a velvety-smooth texture, spider telangiectasias

   i. Tremor, hyperkinesia, hyperreflexia

   j. Exophthalmos, retracted eyelids, staring gaze

   k. Hair loss

   l. Goiter

   m. Bruits over the thyroid gland

   n. Elevated systolic blood pressure, widened pulse pressure, S3 heart sound

  2. Laboratory findings may include:

   a. Increased T_4 and T_3 levels

   b. Nondetectable TSH

   c. Presence of antithyroid antibodies and thyroid-stimulating immunoglobulins (TSI), increased radioactive iodine uptake

  3. Thyroid storm is marked by hyperthermia, hypertension, delirium, vomiting, abdominal pain, and tachyarrhythmias.

  4. Elderly persons with hyperthyroidism often present with heart failure, atrial fibrillation, and few, if any, of the classic symptoms listed above.

E. **Nursing diagnoses**

  1. Activity Intolerance

2. Decreased Cardiac Output

3. Hyperthermia (in thyroid storm)

4. Risk for Injury

5. Knowledge Deficit

6. Altered Nutrition: Less than body requirements

F. Planning and implementation

    1. Assist the client and family members or significant others in exploring treatment options. (Include family members or significant others because the client's attention span deficit may impair his or her retention of information.) Options include:

        a. Pharmacotherapy with drugs that interfere with thyroid hormone synthesis or release (see V.F.2, below, and Section II.D)

        b. Radioactive iodine therapy, which permanently limits thyroid hormone secretion by destroying thyroid tissue; hypothyroidism, requiring lifelong replacement therapy, usually develops at some point after this treatment

        c. Surgery (thyroidectomy), which is seldom done; thyroid levels must be lowered preoperatively to prevent thyroid storm

    2. Administer *antithyroid drugs* as ordered, which may include propylthiouracil (PTU) and methimazole (Tapazole); beta adrenergic blockers, such as propranolol; iodine-containing agents, such as potassium iodide solution; or glucocorticoids (see Section II.D).

    3. Promote a calm environment conducive to rest and relaxation.

    4. Minimize the client's energy expenditure by assisting with activities as necessary and encouraging the client to alternate periods of activity with rest.

    5. Monitor nutritional status; provide increased calories and other nutritional support as needed.

    6. Assess the client's mental status and decision-making ability; intervene as needed to ensure safety.

    7. Provide eye protection for a client with exophthalmos: patches, drops, artificial tears; instruct regarding use.

    8. Monitor vital signs and hemodynamic parameters (for an acutely ill client) for signs of heart failure.

    9. Reduce body temperature with a cooling mattress and acetaminophen; avoid aspirin, which may displace thyroid hormone from its carrier protein and increase hormone levels.

    10. Supply sufficient fluids to offset losses from diaphoresis.

    11. Provide appropriate comfort measures for the febrile client.

    12. Recognize that drug turnover rates may be greatly accelerated in hyperthyroid states.

      13. Emphasize the importance of complying with the medication regimen and long-term medical follow-up plans.

      14. Reassure the family that any abrupt changes in the client's behavior likely are disease related and should subside with antithyroid therapy.

G. **Evaluation**

      1. The client reports adequate energy to perform activities of daily living (ADLs).

      2. The client maintains adequate nutritional intake to meet metabolic demands.

      3. The client demonstrates stable vital signs, including body temperature.

      4. The client verbalizes understanding of the prescribed medication regimen and of long-term treatment options.

      5. The client verbalizes understanding of the importance of long-term health care follow-up.

VI. **Hypothyroidism**

    A. **Description: a state of insufficient serum thyroid hormone**

    B. **Etiology and incidence**

      1. Primary hypothyroidism results from pathologic changes in the thyroid gland due to:

        a. Autoimmune thyroiditis (Hashimoto's disease)

        b. Thyroidectomy

        c. Radioactive iodine therapy

        d. Antithyroid medication therapy

      2. Secondary hypothyroidism results from failure of the pituitary gland to secrete adequate TSH, possibly due to tumor, surgical removal, or irradiation.

      3. Hypothyroidism is most prevalent in persons between ages 40 and 50 and affects more women than men.

    C. **Pathophysiology and management**

      1. Inability of the thyroid gland to secrete sufficient amounts of thyroid hormone leads to decreased cellular metabolic activities, decreased oxygen consumption, and decreased heat production.

      2. These actions produce mild to marked effects in all organ systems.

      3. A person with hypothyroidism is at risk for life-threatening myxedema coma, which can develop gradually over the years or acutely in response to precipitating factors such as infection, cold exposure, or sedative use.

    D. **Assessment findings**

      1. Signs and symptoms of hypothyroidism include:

        a. Sluggishness, lethargy, depression, apathy, fatigue, exercise intolerance

      b.   Memory impairment
      c.   Muscle aches, numbness and tingling in hands
      d.   Cold intolerance
      e.   Constipation
      f.   Weight gain, decreased appetite
      g.   Menstrual irregularities, infertility, decreased libido
      h.   Dry skin, brittle nails, dry hair
      i.   Edema—nonpitting and periorbital
      j.   Husky voice, hoarseness
      k.   Possible goiter
      l.   Possible neck scar from previous thyroid surgery
      m. Delay in muscle contraction and relaxation of tendon reflexes
      n.   Diastolic hypertension
      o.   Bradycardia

  2. Laboratory studies may reveal:
      a.   Decreased T_4 and T_3 levels
      b.   Increased TSH (primary)
      c.   Presence of antithyroid antibodies (autoimmune)
      d.   Elevated cholesterol and CPK

  3. Affected elderly persons may display few, if any, symptoms of hypothyroidism.

  4. Myxedema coma is marked by:
      a.   Hypotension
      b.   Hypoventilation
      c.   Hypothermia
      d.   Stupor possibly progressing to coma

E. **Nursing diagnoses**
  1. Activity Intolerance
  2. Decreased Cardiac Output
  3. Constipation
  4. Hypothermia (in myxedema coma)
  5. Knowledge Deficit

F. **Planning and implementation**
  1. Administer thyroid hormone as prescribed (see Section II.D).
  2. Recognize that thyroid hormone administration may precipitate adrenal insufficiency in a previously undiagnosed client, possibly necessitating glucocorticoid administration.
  3. Keep in mind that a client with hypothyroidism is very sensitive to narcotics, anesthetics, and sedatives; drug degradation is delayed, and respiratory depression can develop.
  4. Encourage the client to alternate periods of activity with rest.
  5. Administer fluids cautiously—the client may not be able to excrete a heavy water load. If the client has hypoglycemia, infuse a concentrated source of glucose.

6. Provide relief of constipation as indicated.
7. **To prevent vascular collapse in a hypothermic client, refrain from aggressive rewarming.**
8. Institute respiratory assistance when necessary.
9. Implement infection-prevention measures.
10. Instruct the client (and family members or significant others, when applicable) in the prescribed medication regimen, including purpose, dosage schedule, and signs of over- and under-replacement.

G. **Evaluation**
1. The client reports adequate energy to perform ADLs.
2. The client exhibits stable vital signs, including body temperature.
3. The client reports restoration of normal bowel function.
4. The client and family members or significant others verbalize understanding of the prescribed medication regimen and of health care follow-up plans.

VII. **Other thyroid dysfunctions**
A. **Description**
1. Subacute thyroiditis: self-limiting thyroid inflammation
2. Autoimmune (Hashimoto's) thyroiditis: chronic inflammatory disorder
3. Simple goiter: thyroid enlargement not associated with inflammation or neoplasm
4. Thyroid cancer: papillary, follicular, medullary, and anaplastic carcinomas

B. **Etiology and incidence**
1. Associated with viral infection, subacute thyroiditis commonly follows mumps, influenza, or coxsackievirus or adenovirus infection.
2. The most common form of thyroiditis, autoimmune thyroiditis, results from antibodies to thyroid antigens in the blood.
3. Simple goiter may result from:
   a. Compensation for dietary iodine deficiency (rare in the United States)
   b. Use of certain drugs (e.g., iodine-containing agents, lithium) in susceptible clients
   c. Compensatory response to excessive TSH secretion, such as results from thyroid hormone hyposecretion
4. Thyroid cancer may be associated with history of exposure to external head and neck radiation.

C. **Pathophysiology and management**
1. Subacute thyroiditis may be accompanied by transient hyper-

thyroidism; inflammation and hyperthyroidism usually resolve spontaneously with no residual effects.

2. In autoimmune thyroiditis, chronic thyroid inflammation leads to lymphocytic infiltration with fibrosis and diminished hormone secretion. These changes produce thyroid enlargement and, in some cases, hypothyroidism.

3. Goiters may be diffuse and symmetric or nodular. Depending on the cause and degree of enlargement, treatment may not be necessary.

4. In thyroid cancer, prognosis depends on cell type. Papillary and follicular adenocarcinoma generally are associated with good prognoses and medullary carcinoma with a less favorable prognosis. Anaplastic carcinoma, most common in older adults, carries a very poor prognosis.

5. Management measures may include medications and/or surgery.

D. Assessment findings

1. Subacute thyroiditis may produce moderate thyroid enlargement, some pain, and mild dysphagia.

2. Autoimmune thyroiditis typically produces painless thyroid enlargement. Diagnosis is confirmed by needle biopsy demonstrating antithyroid antibodies.

3. In goiter, thyroid enlargement ranges from slight to gross. Massive goiter can produce respiratory difficulty and dysphagia due to compression of the trachea and esophagus.

4. Manifestations of thyroid cancer may include:
   a. Reports of respiratory distress, sensation of lump in throat, dysphagia
   b. Palpable, hard, painless nodule in the thyroid
   c. Needle biopsy positive for cancer
   d. Thyroid scan showing area of decreased uptake

E. Nursing diagnoses

1. Anxiety
2. Ineffective Breathing Pattern
3. Risk for Injury
4. Knowledge Deficit
5. Pain
6. Impaired Swallowing

F. Planning and implementation

1. For subacute thyroiditis, provide symptomatic treatment directed at reducing inflammation.

2. For autoimmune thyroiditis, administer thyroid hormone as prescribed (see Section II.D).

3. Treatment for goiter may not be indicated. If appropriate, as-

sist with thyroid suppression therapy or prepare the client for surgery.

    4. Support the client and family members or significant others as they explore the nature and prognosis of thyroid cancer. Reinforce the importance of long-term follow-up to ensure the most favorable prognosis possible.

    5. If surgery is indicated for thyroid cancer, plan interventions for subtotal or total thyroidectomy, including:

        a. Providing preoperative instruction and emotional support

        b. Providing postoperative comfort measures (e.g., analgesics, adequate head support, semi-Fowler's position, humidification)

        c. Monitoring for complications (e.g., respiratory obstruction, hemorrhage, tetany)

        d. Ensuring adequate fluid intake as tolerated

        e. Preparing the client for total body scan to detect any remaining thyroid tissue; radioactive iodine may be given to eradicate tissue after total thyroidectomy

        f. Reinforcing the importance of taking thyroid hormone replacement exactly as prescribed

  G. **Evaluation**

    1. The client and family members or significant others verbalize knowledge of diagnosis, prognosis, and treatment plan.

    2. The client exhibits stable vital signs, with absence of respiratory difficulty and dysphagia.

    3. The client reports absence of pain.

    4. The client verbalizes the importance of complying with the prescribed medication regimen and plans for long-term follow-up care.

VIII. **Hyperparathyroidism**

  A. **Description: overproduction of parathyroid hormone (PTH); results in high blood calcium levels and bone demineralization**

  B. **Etiology and incidence**

    1. Primary hyperparathyroidism is a common condition usually occurring after age 60 and affecting women more often than men. About 80% of cases are linked to a single adenoma of the parathyroid gland; remaining cases are due to parathyroid hyperplasia. (*Note:* The following sections apply to clients with primary hyperparathyroidism.)

    2. Secondary hyperparathyroidism results from an adaptive increase in PTH secretion associated with problems involving chronic hypocalcemia.

  C. **Pathophysiology and management**

    1. PTH is critical to normal calcium homeostasis. Insufficient circulating calcium level stimulates PTH production, which acts to raise calcium level; when calcium level rises to normal, PTH secretion is inhibited.

2. A parathyroid adenoma or other problem can produce excessive PTH despite normal serum calcium, causing the abnormalities of primary hyperparathyroidism.

3. Treatment is usually medical and surgical.

D. **Assessment findings**

1. Hyperparathyroidism may be asymptomatic or may produce such clinical manifestations as:

    a. Fatigue, muscular weakness, listlessness

    b. Height loss and frequent fractures

    c. Renal calculi

    d. Anorexia, nausea, abdominal discomfort, constipation

    e. Memory impairment

    f. Polyuria, polydipsia

    g. Back and joint pain

    h. Hypertension

2. Laboratory and diagnostic studies may reveal:

    a. Elevated total and ionized serum calcium levels

    b. Decreased serum phosphate level

    c. Hypercalciuria and hyperphosphaturia

    d. Bone demineralization on radiograph or bone mineral densitometry

    e. Elevated PTH level

    f. Possible abnormal parathyroid scan

    g. Possible uremia secondary to nephrocalcinosis

E. **Nursing diagnoses**

1. Activity Intolerance

2. Constipation

3. Risk for Injury

4. Altered Nutrition: Less than body requirements

5. Pain

6. Altered Urinary Elimination

F. **Planning and implementation**

1. Prepare the client for surgical treatment of primary hyperparathyroidism: adenoma removal, hyperplastic gland resection. Care is similar to that for thyroidectomy (see Section VII.F.5).

2. Provide preoperative care:

    a. Force fluids to prevent dehydration, constipation, and kidney stone formation.

    b. Reduce added calcium by eliminating over-the-counter antacids, which may contain calcium; thiazide diuretics, which interfere with renal calcium excretion; and excessive intake of dairy products.

𝕟 c. **As prescribed, administer a diuretic, such as furosemide (Lasix) if necessary, and monitor potassium level. Assess for signs and symptoms of hypokalemia (e.g., muscle cramping), and keep accurate intake and output records.**

𝕟 3. **As indicated, provide aggressive calcium supplementation after surgery to compensate for "hungry bone" syndrome. Observe the client for symptoms of hypercalcemia (e.g., nausea, vomiting, headache, mental confusion, anorexia).**

4. Assess for renal calculi; report hematuria or flank pain as necessary.

5. Take measures to protect the client from injury, including:
   a. Assisting with ADLs and ambulation as necessary
   b. Encouraging weight-bearing to reduce calcium loss from bones
   c. Instructing about strategies to minimize falls, which may lead to fractures

6. Provide relief of constipation as indicated.

7. Monitor nutritional status and intervene as necessary.

8. Provide comfort measures and analgesics as needed.

𝕟 9. **If prescribed, administer digitalis preparations with caution in hypercalcemic clients. Observe for toxicity (nausea, vomiting, yellow haze). Do not administer if apical pulse falls below 60; monitor digoxin level for possible toxicity (>2).**

10. Instruct nonsurgical candidates in phosphate or estrogen therapy as indicated.

11. Teach the client about postoperative calcium carbonate supplementation, if prescribed.

12. Reinforce the health care follow-up schedule.

G. Evaluation

1. The client reports adequate energy to perform ADLs.

2. The client maintains normal bowel function.

3. The client remains injury-free and displays normal surgical wound healing, if applicable.

4. The client reports absence of pain or adequate pain control with oral analgesics.

5. The client displays no evidence of tetany.

6. The client maintains adequate food and fluid intake.

7. The client verbalizes the importance of complying with the prescribed medication regimen and plans for follow-up care.

IX. Hypoparathyroidism

A. **Description: PTH deficiency characterized by hypocalcemia, hyperphosphatemia, and neuromuscular hyperexcitablity**

B. **Etiology and incidence**

    1. Hypoparathyroidism may be iatrogenic, caused by accidental removal of or trauma to parathyroid glands during thyroidectomy, parathyroidectomy, or radical head or neck surgery.

    2. It also can result from an autoimmune genetic dysfunction (affects women more often than men).

    3. A reversible form may be associated with hypomagnesemia, which interferes with PTH secretion.

C. **Pathophysiology and management**

    1. Reduced PTH production slows bone resorption, increases neuromuscular irritability, decreases serum calcium level, and increases serum phosphate level.

    2. In chronic hypoparathyroidism, calcification can occur in some organs (e.g., the eyes [cataracts] and basal ganglia [possibly causing permanent brain damage]).

    3. Supportive care, medication therapy, and regular follow-up care are significant management measures.

D. **Assessment findings**

    1. Clinical manifestations include:

        a. Anxiety, irritability

        b. Numbness, tingling, cramps in extremities

        c. Dysphagia

        d. Photophobia

        e. Evidence of neuromuscular hyperexcitability: positive Chvostek's and Trousseau's signs, carpopedal spasms, bronchospasms, laryngeal spasms, arrhythmias, convulsion

        f. Paradoxical calcification in eyes

    2. Laboratory studies may reveal:

        a. Low ionized and total calcium levels

        b. Elevated blood phosphate level

        c. Low PTH level

E. **Nursing diagnoses**

    1. Risk for Injury

    2. Knowledge Deficit

F. **Planning and implementation**

    1. Intervene for life-threatening tetany as indicated:

        a. **Administer IV calcium gluconate to prevent calcium depletion. Calcium is essential for capillary integrity and normal functioning of the nervous, muscular, and skeletal systems. Administer the amount pre-**

scribed slowly through a large vein to avoid infiltration (which may cause severe necrosis and sloughing of tissue). Keep client on bedrest at least 1 hour after drug administration to prevent orthostatic hypotension.

b. **Expect to administer oral calcium and vitamin D supplement after crisis resolves. Observe client for symptoms of hypercalcemia (e.g., nausea, vomiting, headache, mental confusion, anorexia).**

c. Be alert for possible laryngeal spasm and resulting respiratory obstruction; keep a tracheostomy set available.

d. Institute seizure precautions.

e. Minimize environmental stimuli.

f. After the crisis resolves, closely monitor calcium levels; keep IV calcium gluconate in the client's room.

2. For chronic hypoparathyroidism treatment may include:

a. Diet high in calcium and low in phosphorus

b. **Vitamin D and, typically, magnesium supplementation. *Note:* In clients receiving magnesium, observe for symptoms of hypermagnesemia (hypotension, respiratory depression, muscle weakness, confusion).**

c. Oral calcium preparations, such as calcium gluconate, to supplement the diet

3. Teach the client about the medication regimen, including purpose, dosage schedule, and signs and symptoms of hypocalcemia and hypercalcemia. Inform the client that dosage will be adjusted periodically based on laboratory findings.

4. Emphasize the importance of regular follow-up evaluation and care.

G. Evaluation

1. The client exhibits no signs of tetany.

2. Serum calcium level is within normal range.

3. The client verbalizes understanding of the medication schedule and follow-up plans.

4. The client verbalizes signs and symptoms of hypocalcemia and hypercalcemia to watch for and report.

X. Cushing's syndrome

A. Description: a syndrome involving excessive production of adrenocortical hormones, primarily cortisol but also androgens and mineralocorticoids

B. Etiology and incidence

1. The most common cause of Cushing's syndrome is bilateral adrenal hyperplasia (Cushing's disease).

2. Other causes include:
  a. Adrenal adenomas and carcinomas
  b. Ectopic ACTH production by tumors in other organs, such as the lungs and pancreas
  c. Glucocorticoid therapy
3. Incidence is higher in women than in men.

C. Pathophysiology and management
  1. Regardless of etiology, impaired regulation of adrenocortical hormones results in excessive hormone levels.
  2. Manifestations of Cushing's syndrome result from the effects of excessive adrenocortical hormone levels on various body systems and functions.
  3. Treatment may involve medical and surgical interventions.

D. Assessment findings
  1. Clinical manifestations depend on the adrenocortical hormones involved and may include:
    a. Weight gain and altered fat distribution (e.g., central obesity with round [moon] face and buffalo hump)
    b. Muscle weakness, proximal muscle wasting, fatigue
    c. Frequent infections and poor wound healing
    d. Symptoms of hyperglycemia
    e. Mental status changes, mood swings
    f. Menstrual disturbances (amenorrhea)
    g. Diminished libido
    h. Skin changes: striae, bruises, acne, thinning of scalp hair
    i. Hypertension
    j. Hirsutism
    k. Susceptibility to compression fractures
    l. Edema
  2. Laboratory studies may reveal:
    a. Hypokalemia or hyperglycemia
    b. Depressed eosinophil and lymphocyte counts
    c. Elevated plasma cortisol and 24-hour urine cortisol results
    d. Abnormal dexamethasone suppression test findings (morning cortisol level above 5 g/dL after administration of 1.0 mg of dexamethasone the night before)
    e. Elevated ACTH (indicative of ACTH-mediated Cushing's syndrome)
  3. Selective venous sampling can differentiate between pituitary and ectopic ACTH production. In this procedure, catheters are inserted into each petrosal sinus draining the pituitary gland and peripheral vein, then ACTH levels are measured after administration of corticotropin-releasing hormone (CRH).

4. Selected radiographic and computerized axial tomography (CAT) studies may be done to determine the site of ectopic ACTH production (e.g., bronchogenic oat cell carcinoma).

E. Nursing diagnoses

1. Activity Intolerance
2. Ineffective Individual Coping
3. Risk for Injury
4. Knowledge Deficit
5. Self Esteem Disturbance

F. Planning and implementation

1. Teach the client and family members or significant others about disease pathology and its influence on the client's body and mental status.
2. Encourage them to ask questions and verbalize any concerns.
3. Take measures to protect the client from injury and infection, including:
   a. Assessing skin integrity regularly
   b. Avoiding agents that can damage skin (e.g., tape, strong soaps)
   c. Promoting good hygiene
   d. Modifying the environment to remove or minimize hazards
4. Monitor vital signs, and weigh the client daily.
5. Schedule activities to allow adequate rest periods, helping prevent fatigue.
6. If surgery is indicated, prepare the client for the scheduled procedure, which may include:
   a. Adrenalectomy, if the cause is adrenal adenoma
   b. Transsphenoidal hypophysectomy, if the cause is pituitary adenoma
   c. Tumor resection
7. If surgery is not indicated, instruct the client and family members regarding prescribed adrenocortical steroid inhibitors which decrease cortisol production (see Section II.D).
8. Keep in mind that any treatment modality will cause temporary (permanent with bilateral adrenalectomy) adrenal insufficiency.

G. Evaluation

1. The client exhibits increased ability to carry out self-care activities.
2. The client and family members or significant others verbalize correct understanding of the treatment plan.
3. The client remains infection- and injury-free.

4. The client openly discusses feelings about the disorder's effects on his or her body image.
5. The client decreases or maintains body weight.
6. The client verbalizes increased self-esteem.
7. The client complies with the prescribed medication regimen.

XI. Adrenal hypofunction

A. **Description: deficiency of adrenocortical hormones; either primary (Addison's disease) or secondary to another problem**

B. **Etiology and incidence**

1. Addison's disease can result from:
   a. An autoimmune process
   b. Hemorrhage into the adrenal gland
   c. Adrenalectomy
   d. Neoplasm
   e. Fungal infection
   f. Tuberculosis
2. Secondary adrenal insufficiency is associated with:
   a. Suppression of the hypothalamic–pituitary axis secondary to exogenous steroid use
   b. Pituitary destruction or removal
   c. Inadequate cortisol replacement, especially during times of stress
3. Adrenal hypofunction occurs in all age groups and affects both sexes about equally.

C. **Pathophysiology and management**

1. Any problem causing adrenal cortex hypofunction results in deficiencies of adrenocortical hormones.
2. Hormone deficiency produces various fluid, electrolyte, and metabolic disturbances.
3. Hormone replacement therapy is the main treatment.

D. **Assessment findings**

1. Common clinical manifestations include:
   a. GI complaints (anorexia, nausea, vomiting, abdominal pain, diarrhea)
   b. Fatigue, muscle weakness, arthralgias
   c. Decreased alertness, confusion
   d. Weight loss
   e. Dry skin, decreased body hair, possible increased pigmentation in excessive ACTH stimulation
   f. Hypotension
   g. Hyperthermia
   h. Tachycardia
2. Suggestive laboratory findings include:
   a. Low blood glucose and serum sodium levels
   b. Increased serum potassium level

       c.   Low 24-hour urinary 17-ketosteroids

       d.   Increased eosinophils

  3.   Definitive laboratory findings include:

       a.   Low cortisol and high ACTH levels in primary adrenal failure; low to normal levels in secondary (pituitary) failure

       b.   On the ACTH stimulation test, low to normal cortisol response in secondary failure and flat or absent response in primary failure

       c.   Low plasma aldosterone in primary failure

E. **Nursing diagnoses**

  1.   Fluid Volume Deficit

  2.   Knowledge Deficit

F. **Planning and implementation**

  1.   Monitor vital signs, daily weight, and intake and output.

  2.   Assess skin turgor and mucous membrane hydration.

  3.   Administer IV fluids to correct fluid deficiency as indicated.

  4.   Administer replacement glucocorticoids; hydrocortisone is usually the drug of choice for adrenocortical replacement because it has both glucocorticoid and mineralocorticoid properties. The physician prescribes the lowest dosage that will correct adrenal hypofunction with minimal side effects.

       a.   **Instruct client to take the medication for life and not to discontinue abruptly because doing so may cause severe withdrawal symptoms leading to possible shock and death.**

       b.   **Explain that dosage may need to be increased during times of increased stress; instruct client to carry or wear medical identification.**

  5.   As prescribed, administer mineralocorticoids for partial replacement of steroid hormones (an exogenous glucocorticoid must be administered for adequate control; see Section II.D).

  6.   Discuss hormone therapy including its purpose, side effects, duration of therapy, symptoms of abnormalities to report to healthcare manager, and the need to inform all health care providers about the steroid replacement therapy.

  7.   If overreplacement of glucocorticoids is indicated, inform the client of the purpose of therapy and possible side effects—cushingoid appearance, weight gain, acne, hirsutism, peptic ulcer, diabetes mellitus, osteoporosis, infection, muscular weakness, mood swings, cataracts, hypertension.

  8.   Help prevent adrenal crisis by ensuring that hospitalized, acutely ill clients on long-term glucocorticoid therapy receive additional doses to compensate for stress.

G. Evaluation

1. The client exhibits restoration of fluid and electrolyte balance.
2. The client demonstrates absence of orthostasis.
3. The client and family members or significant others verbalize understanding of the treatment plan.
4. The client and family members or significant others verbalize appropriate actions to take during periods of increased stress.

XII. **Diabetes mellitus**

A. **Description**

1. Diabetes mellitus is a disorder of carbohydrate metabolism resulting from deficiency of or resistance to available insulin and characterized by hyperglycemia.
2. It is classified as:
   a. IDDM, or insulin-dependent diabetes mellitus Type I, accounting for 5% to 10% of cases and characterized by insulin deficiency and risk of ketosis
   b. NIDDM, or noninsulin-dependent diabetes mellitus Type II, accounting for 90% of cases and characterized by defects in insulin release and use, insulin resistance, and little risk of ketosis
   c. Impaired glucose tolerance: an asymptomatic, subclinical stage characterized by blood glucose level that is abnormal but does not meet the diagnostic criterion for diabetes
   d. Gestational diabetes: a transitory glucose intolerance during pregnancy that resolves after delivery; associated with increased risk of developing overt diabetes later in life
   e. Diabetes mellitus associated with other conditions: glucose intolerance caused by other diseases, drugs, or agents

B. **Etiology and incidence**

1. IDDM typically occurs in persons under age 25; its exact cause is unknown, but it may result from an autoimmune process possibly triggered by virus, with genetic factors playing a part.
2. NIDDM most commonly affects persons over age 40; causative factors include obesity and genetic susceptibility.
3. Diabetes mellitus affects approximately 6% of the U.S. population (about 11 million people) and is the third-leading cause of death from disease.

C. **Pathophysiology and management**

1. In diabetes mellitus, insulin secretion is disproportionate to blood glucose levels as a result of:

    a.   Deficient insulin production by beta cells

    b.   Lack of adequate insulin secretion in response to high blood glucose level

    c.   Inactivation of insulin in circulation

2. Defective regulation of alpha and beta cell hormone release causes gluconeogenesis, resulting in mobilization rather than storage of proteins and fats.

3. Lack of adequate number of insulin receptors on cell surfaces impairs glucose absorption by cells, resulting in excessive blood glucose level.

4. Acute complications of diabetes mellitus include:

    a.   Diabetic ketoacidosis (DKA): severe hyperglycemia and acidosis resulting from a combination of insulin deficiency (relative or absolute) and increased levels of insulin antagonistic hormones (glucagon, cortisol, GH, epinephrine), associated with failure to take insulin as prescribed, new diagnosis of IDDM diabetes, or increased physical stress (e.g., infection, surgery)

    b.   Hyperglycemic hyperosmolar nonketotic coma (HHNK): a combination of severe hyperglycemia and hyperosmolality with little or no acidosis, occurring most often in older adults with undiagnosed or NIDDM and associated with stress (e.g., infection, surgery, hyperalimentation) or ingestion of certain drugs (e.g., thiazide diuretics, glucocorticoids, phenytoin, sympathomimetics)

    c.   Hypoglycemia: excessive insulin to blood glucose ratio linked to excessive use of hypoglycemic agents (insulin, oral agents), decreased food intake, increased physical activity, excessive alcohol consumption, or renal failure (secondary to decreased insulin degradation)

5. **Diabetes mellitus also can produce chronic complications, including:**

    a.   **Microangiopathy: thickening of capillary basement membrane, most prominently in the retina and glomerulus**

    b.   **Macroangiopathy: atherosclerotic changes accelerated by lipid abnormalities exacerbated by elevated blood glucose level**

    c.   **Neuropathy: abnormal nerve function possibly caused by alteration in enzyme system affecting nerve sheaths or neural cell function**

    d.   **Increased susceptibility to infection resulting from impaired ability of granulocytes to respond to infectious agents**

D. **Assessment findings**
1. Common clinical manifestations of diabetes mellitus include:
   a. Polyuria, polydipsia, and polyphagia
   b. Weight loss
   c. Fatigue and weakness
   d. Visual disturbances
   e. Recurrent skin, vulva, and urinary tract infections
2. Diagnosis is based on fasting blood glucose level above 140 mg/dL or postprandial blood glucose level above 200 mg/dL measured on more than one occasion; oral glucose tolerance tests are rarely recommended for diagnosis.
3. Other useful laboratory tests include:
   a. Glycosylated hemoglobin (includes hemoglobin A1C), to assess average blood glucose level over the previous 2 to 4 months
   b. Other glycosylated proteins (glycated albumins and serum fructosamine), to assess blood glucose control over the previous 1 to 3 weeks
   c. Urine tests for sugar (random, 24-hour) and ketones
4. Clinical manifestations and laboratory findings in DKA include:
   a. Dehydration
   b. Tachycardia
   c. Kussmaul's respirations
   d. Acetone breath
   e. Decreased level of consciousness (LOC)
   f. GI disturbances (nausea, vomiting, abdominal pain)
   g. Elevated serum potassium level
   h. ABG values indicating acidosis
5. HHNK is marked by:
   a. Dehydration
   b. Decreased LOC
   c. Tachycardia
   d. Hypotension
   e. Blood glucose >700 mg/dL
   f. Blood osmolality >330 mOsm/kg
   g. Absence of ketosis, but possible mild lactic acidosis
   h. Azotemia
   i. Electrolyte disturbances (hypernatremia, hypokalemia)
6. Manifestations of hypoglycemia include:
   a. Blood glucose 70 mg/dL
   b. Cool, moist skin or pallor
   c. Tachycardia
   d. Tremor, paresthesias, confusion
   e. Headache progressing to loss of consciousness or seizures

E. Nursing diagnoses
1. Ineffective Individual Coping
2. Knowledge Deficit
3. Noncompliance

F. Planning and implementation
1. Assess the client's and family members' or significant others' knowledge of diabetes and its management, and develop an individualized teaching plan that covers (as appropriate):
   a. Possible causes and basic pathophysiologic concepts
   b. Use of oral hypoglycemics (such as tolbutamide or glipizide) in NIDDM to lower the blood glucose level by stimulating insulin release from functioning beta cells and by increasing cellular sensitivity to insulin (see Section II.D)
   c. Use of insulin in IDDM (or uncontrolled NIDDM with oral hypoglycemics), which is the replacement for endogenous insulin (see Section II.D)
   d. Techniques for prescribed monitoring methods: blood glucose, urine glucose, or ketones; including frequency, care and disposal of equipment, record keeping, and reporting of results
   e. Prescribed dietary modifications: typically low fat, low cholesterol, low sodium, and high fiber, based on the food exchange system developed by the American Diabetes Association or some other structured meal plan and with an emphasis on consistent meal schedules and food amounts
   f. Appropriate exercise program
   g. Hygiene and safety measures: foot care and protection, care of minor wounds, the importance of medical identification cards and jewelry, avoidance of noxious substances (e.g., alcohol, smoking), annual ophthalmologic follow-up
   h. Management of acute illness: continuing taking insulin or oral hypoglycemics as prescribed, increasing self-monitoring frequency, testing urine ketones, notifying the physician, maintaining adequate fluid and caloric intake
   i. Signs and symptoms of acute and chronic complications to watch for and report
2. Assess and promote the client's compliance with the prescribed therapeutic and monitoring regimens. Monitor indicators of glycemic control: glycosylated hemoglobin and other proteins, blood glucose level, and presence of complications.

3. Enhance the client's and family members' or significant others' coping skills by:
   a. Encouraging open discussion of feelings and concerns
   b. Encouraging questions and answering them honestly
   c. Involving family members or significant others in teaching and planning
   d. Making referrals to support persons or groups as appropriate
4. Intervene as indicated for a client exhibiting signs and symptoms of DKA:
   a. Restore fluid and electrolyte balance by administering IV fluids and electrolytes (Na, Cl, K, phosphorus).
   b. Reverse acidosis; administer sodium bicarbonate for severe acidosis (pH < 7.0).
   c. Monitor urine ketones.
   d. Restore carbohydrate, protein, and fat metabolism by administering regular insulin (usually continuous low-dose IV).
   e. Monitor vital signs.
   f. Monitor blood glucose levels.
   g. Maintain accurate intake and output records.
   h. Prevent complications (e.g., hypokalemia or hypoglycemia [add glucose when blood glucose 300 mg/dL], cerebral edema [monitor LOC]).
   i. Assess for precipitating factors.
5. Intervene as indicated to manage HHNK:
   a. Restore fluid volume, usually with isotonic IV solutions.
   b. Restore electrolyte balance; administer potassium replacement when urine output is adequate.
   c. Prevent complications (e.g., hypoglycemia [add glucose to IV solutions when blood glucose drops], hypokalemia, thrombus formation).
   d. Assess for precipitating factors.
6. For a client experiencing hypoglycemia:
   a. Monitor blood glucose level.
   b. Replace glucose through oral (15 g carbohydrate) or IV glucose (50% dextrose) or glucagon (IM or SQ); *do not force oral fluids in a client with impaired consciousness.*
   c. Protect the client from injury, and observe closely until he or she is fully recovered.
   d. Administer a source of long-acting carbohydrate to prevent subsequent episodes.
   e. Assess for precipitating factors.
   f. Keep in mind that a person with longstanding diabetes may develop a defect in counterregulatory hormones, which impairs awareness of hypoglycemic symptoms and

puts the person at increased risk for brain damage due to prolonged, untreated hypoglycemia.

    g.   Recognize that beta-blocker therapy also can blunt sympathetic symptoms of hypoglycemia, interfering with detection.

7.   Monitor for signs and symptoms of chronic complications, and intervene as indicated.

G.   **Evaluation**

1.   The client and family members or significant others verbalize understanding of the disorder and the therapeutic regimen.

2.   The client complies with the prescribed medication regimen.

3.   The client exhibits adequate glycemic control.

4.   The client achieves or maintains body weight goals.

5.   The client participates in a regular exercise program, as tolerated.

6.   The client and family members or significant others openly discuss their feelings and concerns regarding diabetes and its management.

7.   The client practices precautions aimed at preventing acute and chronic complications.

8.   The client exhibits no signs of acute or chronic complications.

Bibliography

American Diabetes Association. (1986). National standards and American Diabetes Association review criteria for diabetes patient education programs. *Diabetes Care, 9*(4), XXXVI–XLIII.

American Diabetes Association. (1989). Standards of medical care for patients with diabetes mellitus. *Diabetes Care, 12*(5), 365–368.

Bolander, V. R. (1994). *Sorensen & Luckmann's basic nursing: A physiologic approach* (3rd ed.). Philadelphia: W. B. Saunders.

Carpenito, L. J. (1995). *Nursing diagnosis: Application to clinical practice* (6th ed.). Philadelphia: J. B. Lippincott.

Clark, J., Queener, S., & Karb, V. (1990). *Pharmacologic basis of nursing practice* (4th ed). St. Louis: C. V. Mosby.

Galuk, D. (1991). Diabetes mellitus Types I and II. *Advancing Clinical Care 6*, 5.

Gordon, M. (1995). *Manual of nursing diagnosis 1995–1996*. St. Louis: C. V. Mosby.

Karch, A. (1995). *Lippincott's nursing drug guide*. Philadelphia: J. B. Lippincott.

Kurtz, S. S. (1990). Adherence to diabetes regimens: Empirical status and clinical applications. *Diabetes Educator, 16*(1), 50–56.

Smeltzer, S. C., & Bare, B. G. (1996). *Brunner & Suddarth's textbook of medical-surgical nursing* (8th ed.). Philadelphia: Lippincott-Raven Publishers.

Springhouse Corporation. (1992). *Nursing student's guide to drugs*. Springhouse, PA: Springhouse Corp.

Steil, C. F., & Deakins, D. A. (1992). Oral hypoglycemics . . . what you and your patient need to know. *Nursing 92, 22*, 34, 44.

STUDY QUESTIONS

1. Which of the following assessment findings would help identify transient diabetes insipidus (DI) in a client who underwent transsphenoidal surgery?
   a. polyuria, polydipsia, and polyphagia
   b. urine output, tented skin turgor, urine specific gravity
   c. nervousness; weakness; warm, sweaty, flushed skin
   d. constipation, cold intolerance, sluggishness

2. Fluid management in the client with syndrome of inappropriate antidiuretic hormone (SIADH) should include
   a. rapid IV fluid infusion
   b. fluid restriction
   c. increasing oral fluid intake
   d. administering glucose-containing IV fluids

3. The client receiving propylthiouracil (PTU) should be instructed to stop the medication immediately and call the physician if which of the following occurs?
   a. diarrhea
   b. palpitations
   c. fever
   d. weight gain

4. Which of the following statements about analgesic therapy for a client with hypothyroidism is correct?
   a. Increased dosages will be needed because the client is overweight.
   b. Analgesics are not needed because the client already is lethargic.
   c. Decreased dosages will be needed due to prolonged drug degradation rates.
   d. Increased dosages will be needed because of the hypermetabolic state.

5. In the postoperative parathyroidectomy client, "hungry bone" syndrome is manifested by
   a. carpopedal spasms
   b. weakness
   c. back pain
   d. polyuria

6. Discharge instructions for the hypoparathyroid client should include which of the following?
   a. Avoid diuretics in order to minimize calcium loss.
   b. Use any over-the-counter vitamin D preparation.
   c. Supplement calcium intake.
   d. Avoid strenuous exercise because of fracture risk.

7. The nursing diagnosis Body Image Disturbance would most likely be associated with which of the following medical conditions?
   a. Addison's disease
   b. thyroiditis
   c. diabetes insipidus
   d. Cushing's syndrome

8. Preoperative care for a client receiving long-term glucocorticoid therapy should include
   a. holding the glucocorticoid because the client is NPO
   b. administering an increased dose parenterally
   c. administering the usual dose intramuscularly
   d. administering the usual dose with a sip of water

9. Discharge instructions for the client receiving levothyroxine (Synthroid) would include
   a. Check serum glucose level twice daily.
   b. Take medication at night to avoid insomnia.
   c. Notify physician if diarrhea, nervousness, or increased heart rate occur.
   d. Have blood test to monitor glycosylated hemoglobin every 3 months.

10. Which of the following represents the best indication of good overall diabetes control?
    a. The client reports urine glucose levels indicating no glucosuria.
    b. The client displays glycosylated he-

moglobin level within control range.

c. The client reports urine ketone levels reflecting no ketonuria.

d. The client records home glucose test results daily.

11. Which of the following represents the best advice to give a diabetic client about eye examinations?

a. Examinations should be scheduled every year.

b. Examinations should be scheduled every 2 years.

c. Changes in vision do not necessitate immediate medical attention.

d. Examinations should be performed by an optometrist.

12. Knowledge deficit is a common nursing diagnosis for the client with insulin-dependent diabetes mellitus. Which of the following client behaviors would best support this diagnosis?

a. recent weight gain of 15 lb

b. failure to monitor blood glucose level

c. skipping insulin doses when feeling ill

d. crying whenever diabetes is mentioned

13. Blood glucose monitoring reveals that a client is hyperglycemic before breakfast. Which of the following insulin adjustments would indicate that the client has a good understanding of the effects of both NPH and regular insulin?

a. The client increases the morning dose of regular insulin.

b. The client increases the evening dose of NPH insulin.

c. The client increases the morning dose of NPH insulin.

d. The client increases the evening dose of regular insulin.

14. When planning care for a diabetic client with end-stage renal disease, the nurse should expect that the client's insulin requirements most likely would:

a. increase

b. remain the same

c. decrease

d. fluctuate greatly

15. The nursing assessment data reveal that the client has thickened heel pads, a thick tongue, and a change in ring and shoe size. Which of the following would the nurse expect to be probable explanations for the client's symptoms?

a. excessive growth hormone secretion

b. undersecretion of antidiuretic hormone

c. excessive adrenocorticosteroid production

d. undersecretion of beta cells

16. Altered LOC commonly accompanies hyperglycemic hyperosmolar nonketotic coma. Which of the following nursing diagnoses reflects the pathophysiologic process accounting for this complication?

a. Altered Nutrition: Less than body requirements

b. Impaired Gas Exchange

c. Fluid Volume Deficit

d. Fluid Volume Excess

ANSWER KEY

1. **Correct response: b**
   Urine output, signs of dehydration (tented skin turgor), and urine specific gravity all are indicators of antidiuretic deficiency.
   a, c, and d. Theses are signs and symptoms of diabetes mellitus, hyperthyroidism, and hypothyroidism.
   Knowledge/Physiologic/Assessment

2. **Correct response: b**
   Treatment is geared toward reducing water retention.
   a, c, and d. Administration of fluids only increases water intoxication.
   Application/Physiologic/Implementation

3. **Correct response: c**
   Fever may be indicative of infection, and infection may be caused by agranulocytosis.
   a and b. Diarrhea and palpitations are symptoms of hyperthyroidism.
   d. Weight gain is a common consequence of decreasing thyroid hormone levels.
   Application/Safe care/Planning

4. **Correct response: c**
   A client with hypothyroidism has increased sensitivity to all drugs because of altered metabolism and excretion, depressed metabolic rate and respiratory status.
   a. Weight is not a factor.
   b. Failure to administer analgesics when appropriate may cause unnecessary suffering.
   d. Increased dosages may lead to overdose.
   Analysis/Safe care/Planning

5. **Correct response: a**
   In "hungry bone" syndrome, the bones take up calcium at an accelerated rate, leading to hypocalcemia. Carpopedal spasm, caused by neuromuscular irritability, is a symptom of hypocalcemia.
   b and c. Weakness and back pain are unrelated to calcium balance.

   d. Polyuria is a symptom of hypercalcemia.
   Application/Safe care/Assessment

6. **Correct response: c**
   Chronic hypoparathyroidism requires calcium supplementation.
   a. Diuretic use is not necessarily discouraged—in fact, thiazide diuretics promote calcium resorption.
   b. Vitamin D is necessary for calcium absorption, but special prescription preparations may be needed.
   d. There is no contraindication to exercise since osteoporosis is rare in this group.
   Application/Safe care/Implementation

7. **Correct response: d**
   In Cushing's syndrome, excessive cortisol level causes fat redistribution with truncal obesity, moon face, and buffalo hump; excessive androgen levels cause hirsutism.
   a. In Addison's disease, the only body appearance alteration is excessive skin pigmentation.
   b and c. Thyroiditis and diabetes insipidus do not affect body habitus.
   Comprehension/Psychosocial/ Analysis (Dx)

8. **Correct response: b**
   During periods of stress, such as surgery, glucocorticoid dosages must be increased.
   a, c, and d. Decreased or usual doses may cause adrenal insufficiency.
   Application/Physiologic/Implementation

9. **Correct response: c**
   Diarrhea, nervousness, and increased heart rate (signs of hyperthyroidism) would indicate an overdose of medication.
   a and d. These would be appropriate for a client with diabetes mellitus.
   b. Levothyroxine (Synthroid) should be taken in the morning to prevent insomnia.

Knowledge/Physiologic/Assessment

10. *Correct response: b*
Glycosylated hemoglobin values reflect the average blood glucose level over a 2-month period.
a and c. Urine tests (glucose and ketones) reflect blood glucose control over only the past few hours.
d. Reports of home blood glucose tests may be helpful but studies have shown that they often are fabricated.

11. *Correct response: a*
Current standards of care published by the American Diabetes Association recommend annual eye examinations by an ophthalmologist. The standards also recommend immediate evaluation of any vision changes.
b. Annual examinations are recommended.
c. Any vision change merits immediate evaluation.
d. An ophthalmologist, not an optometrist, is the appropriate health care professional for this eye examination.

Knowledge/Health promotion/ Implementation

12. *Correct response: c*
During periods of illness, insulin injections should be continued even if food intake is decreased since physical stress increases blood glucose levels.
a and b. Weight gain and failure to monitor blood glucose level represent noncompliant behavior.
d. Crying demonstrates ineffective coping.

Comprehension/Health promotion/ Analysis (Dx)

13. *Correct response: b*
The NPH insulin taken at supper exerts its greatest effect during the night and at breakfast. The peak action of regular insulin occurs at 3 to 4 hours, so it could not affect breakfast-time blood glucose level. The morning dose of NPH will have dissipated long before breakfast.
a, c, and d. These dosage adjustments would be inappropriate.

Analysis/Health promotion/Evaluation

14. *Correct response: c*
Renal failure prevents the kidneys from degrading insulin normally; as a result, insulin is available longer.
a and b. This increased availability means that an increased or same dose of insulin may cause hypoglycemia.
d. Renal failure, by itself, does not cause increased fluctuation of insulin doses.

Analysis/Physiologic/Planning

15. *Correct response: a*
Thickened heel pads, thick tongue, and a change in ring and shoe size are all signs of excessive growth hormone secretion.
b, c, and d. These are not correct. These are SIADH, Cushing's disease, and diabetes mellitus, respectively.

Knowledge/Physiologic/Assessment

16. *Correct response: c*
Plasma hyperosmolality resulting from Fluid Volume Deficit causes decreased LOC.
a and b. Neither Impaired Gas Exchange nor Altered Nutrition is linked directly to altered LOC, although they both may be involved in the progression of this syndrome.
d. Fluid volume excess is not implicated in this complication.

Analysis/Physiologic/Analysis (Dx)

Reproductive and Sexual Disorders

11

I. **Reproductive system**
A. Sexual development
1. Development begins at conception.
 2. Sex is determined by the male XY chromosome and female XX chromosome; XX chromosome in combination with XY chromosome can equal either X from each parent (girl) or X from mother and Y from father (boy).
3. Gender development also involves psychosocial and behavioral factors.
B. Structures
1. Female
a. The external genitalia include the mons pubis, clitoris, labia majora, labia minora, Bartholin's glands, Skene's glands, and urethral meatus.

b.   The internal genitalia include the vagina, uterus, ovaries, and fallopian tubes.

c.   The perineum is an area of muscle, fascia, and ligaments between the vulva and rectum.

d.   The vagina is a muscular tube about $2\frac{1}{2}$ in (6 cm) long anteriorly and $3\frac{1}{2}$ in (9 cm) long posteriorly.

e.   The uterus is a pear-shaped organ separated from the vagina by the cervix and usually lying at a 90-degree angle to the vagina. The endometrium lines the uterus; the myometrium is the muscular uterine layer.

f.   The fallopian tubes terminate in fimbriae that surround the ovaries.

g.   Each almond-shaped ovary normally measures about $1\frac{1}{2}$ in (3.5 cm) by $\frac{3}{4}$ in (2 cm).

h.   The breasts contain mammary glands organized into lobules with collecting ducts that terminate in the nipples.

2.   Male

a.   The penis contains three columns of erectile tissue and the urethra, which terminates at the glans.

b.   The scrotum is divided by a septum; each scrotal sac contains a testis, epididymis, and vas deferens.

c.   Each testis measures about 2 in (5 cm) by 1 in (2.5 cm); it contains seminiferous tubules, in which spermatogenesis occurs, and interstitial cells, which produce testosterone.

d.   The vas deferens enters the ejaculatory duct in the prostate gland, which lies under the bladder and surrounds the urethra.

e.   A bundle of blood vessels, nerves, muscle fibers, and the vas deferens and muscle fibers, the spermatic cord extends from the testis through the inguinal canal to the abdominal cavity.

C.   Function

1.   Female

a.   Hormonally controlled, the menstrual cycle normally ranges from 22 to 34 days (average, 28 days).

b.   During the menstrual phase, comprising the first 5 days of the cycle, low estrogen and progesterone levels stimulate hypothalamic gonadotropin releasing hormone (GnRH) and pituitary follicle-stimulating hormone (FSH) and luteinizing hormone (LH) secretion.

c.   Estrogen secretion causes endometrial buildup during the proliferative phase. Ovulation occurs at midcycle due to a surge of LH.

d. During the luteal phase, the corpus luteum secretes estrogen and progesterone to maintain the endometrium. When conception does not occur, the corpus luteum degenerates, hormone levels decrease, and the cycle begins again.

e. Fertilization of the ovum by a sperm usually occurs in the distal third of the fallopian tube. About 5 days later, the zygote implants into the uterine endometrium.

f. Menopause occurs when menses cease (for at least 1 year), in most women between ages 40 and 55.

g. After menopause, the ovaries atrophy, estrogen levels fall, and changes occur in the vagina, cardiovascular system, skeletal system, and integumentary system.

h. Important female reproductive hormones include:

  ▸ Gonadotropin releasing hormone (GnRH), secreted by the hypothalamus: stimulates anterior pituitary secretion of FSH and LH
  ▸ Follicle stimulating hormone (FSH), secreted by the anterior pituitary: acts on an ovarian follicle to cause it to mature
  ▸ Luteinizing hormone (LH), secreted by the anterior pituitary: acts on ovarian follicle to secrete estrogen; surges at midcycle to produce ovulation; controls secretion of estrogen and progesterone by the corpus luteum
  ▸ Estrogen, secreted by the ovary (follicle, then corpus luteum): causes proliferation of the endometrium
  ▸ Progesterone, secreted by the corpus luteum: maintains the endometrium and causes it to become thick and secretory
  ▸ Human chorionic gonadotropin (HCG), secreted by chorionic villi in the endometrium of a pregnant female: stimulates the corpus luteum to secrete estrogen and progesterone until the placenta takes over

2. Male

a. Spermatogenesis begins at puberty and continues throughout life. It occurs in several stages:

  ▸ Spermatogonia grow and develop into primary spermatocytes, each containing 44 autosomes and 2 sex chromosomes, X and Y.
  ▸ Primary spermatocytes divide to become secondary spermatocytes, each containing 22 autosomes and 1 sex chromosome, either X or Y.
  ▸ Secondary spermatocytes divide to form spermatids, each retaining 23 chromosomes.
  ▸ Spermatids mature into spermatozoa.

b. Testosterone, secreted by testicular interstitial (Leydig) cells, is essential for the development and maintenance of male sex organs and secondary sex characteristics.

    c.   Testosterone secretion begins in utero and increases at puberty, controlled by LH and FSH secreted by the anterior pituitary.

    d.   The prostrate gland secretes fluid during sexual activity to add volume to semen, enhance sperm motility, and neutralize male urethral and vaginal acidity to enhance fertility.

  3. Sexual response patterns

    a.   According to sex researchers Masters and Johnson, both male and female sexual response is characterized by vasocongestion and myotonia.

    b.   Sexual desire is controlled by the limbic system of the brain and is mediated by the ratio of testosterone to estrogen.

    c.   The four phases of sexual response are excitement, plateau, orgasm, and resolution.

II. Overview of reproductive and sexual disorders

  A. **Assessment**

    1. Female

      a.   The nursing health history should focus on obtaining information about:

- Any pain, unusual discharge, irregular bleeding, fever, or urinary symptoms
- Menstrual history
- First day of last menstrual period (LMP)
- Pregnancy and delivery history
- Contraceptive use
- Fertility problems
- Sexual activity and use of safe sex practices
- History of sexually transmitted disease (STD)
- Past gynecologic surgery, disorders, or trauma
- Medication use
- Family history of gynecologic problems
- Breast self-exam (knowledge of, frequency of)
- Pap smear history
- Any other pertinent data from the physical examination

      b.   Physical examination is conducted with the client draped and in the supine position for breast and abdominal exam and in the lithotomy position for a pelvic exam.

      c.   Inspection and palpation of the breasts is done to note any asymmetry, skin dimpling, nipple discharge, tenderness, or masses. Client teaching for self-examination should be done during assessment.

      d.   The external genitalia are inspected before the internal gynecologic exam is performed. Discharge and lesions should be noted on both external and internal exam.

   e. The vagina should appear pink with plentiful rugae in the premenopausal woman.

   f. The cervix is pink to red, firm, nontender, with a round or slitlike orifice, and possibly with watery or mucoid discharge.

   g. Bimanual palpation of the uterus and adnexa should reveal no masses, enlargement, or tenderness.

2. Male

   a. The health history should include information about:

- Pain, discharge, lesions of the genitalia
- Any difficulty with erection or ejaculation
- Urinary function
- Fertility
- Medication use
- Family history
- Previous illnesses, surgery, or trauma of the genitourinary system
- History of STDs
- Chronic illnesses that may affect sexual functioning (e.g., diabetes mellitus, cardiovascular or neurologic disease)
- Past and current patterns of sexual activity; safe or unsafe sex practices; contraceptive use
- Testicular self-exam (knowledge of, frequency of)
- Any other pertinent data from the physical examination

   b. Preparation for physical exam involves urination (unless urine sample or urethral discharge specimen will be needed); disrobing from the waist down and draping; and explanation and reassurance and glove donning by the nurse.

   c. Inspection of the male genitalia involves the penis, scrotum, and inguinal area. The examiner notes skin color and integrity, presence of lesions, discharge from the urethral meatus, retractability of the foreskin in an uncircumcised male, pubic hair distribution, swollen lymph nodes, and bulges that may indicate hernias.

   d. Palpation of the testes should reveal two nontender, smooth, freely movable oval masses.

   e. Palpation of the inguinal area is done superficially to detect enlarged or tender lymph nodes, as well as by invaginating the finger through the scrotum into the external inguinal ring to check for hernia while the client bears down.

   f. The prostate is palpated during a rectal exam; it should be firm and nontender and not protrude into the rectum.

B. **Laboratory studies and diagnostic tests**
  1. The Papanicolaou (Pap) test involves cytologic analysis of a sample scraped from the cervix and other tissues to detect infections and malignant changes.
  2. Noninvasive tests to evaluate female internal reproductive organs include hysterosalpingography, computed tomography (CT) scan, and pelvic ultrasonography.
  3. Invasive female reproductive tract tests include colposcopy and laparoscopy.
  4. Diagnostic tests used to detect breast tumors include mammography, thermography, ultrasonography, and tissue biopsy.
  5. Tests to detect STDs include:
      a. Culture and sensitivity
      b. Gram stain
      c. Rapid plasma reagin (RPR)
      d. Serologic testing for syphilis
      e. Special enzyme or antibody tests
  6. Semen analysis evaluates male fertility by checking sperm motility and quantity.

C. **Psychosocial implications**
  1. The client with a reproductive system or sexual disorder may experience self-concept changes related to:
      a. Concern about the ability to perform sexually
      b. Body image changes
      c. Change in role perception as a sexual or reproductive partner
  2. Changes in social and interpersonal interaction may include:
      a. Isolation from sexual partner
      b. Depression over loss of or change in function
      c. Inability to alter perception of self as a viable sexual and procreative being
      d. Inability to find alternative and satisfying means of sexual expression
  3. The client may experience difficulty coping with the disease or condition, possibly manifested by:
      a. Fear of rejection
      b. Fear of death
      c. Anxiety about potential dysfunction
      d. Inability to live comfortably with uncertainty of future with altered sexual or reproductive function

  4. **When caring for a client with a reproductive or sexual disorder, the nurse should:**
      a. **Provide a therapeutic environment.**
      b. **Maintain confidentiality and privacy.**

    c.   Consider the client's sensitivity to sexual matters.

    d.   Maintain a nonjudgmental attitude to encourage more complete disclosure.

D.   **Medications used to treat reproductive disorders (additional medications may be included with specific diseases)**

    1.   *Antibiotics,* which kill infection-causing bacteria

        a.   Examples: penicillin G (Bicillin), for *Treponema pallidum;* ampicillin (Unasyn), for *Neisseria gonorrhoeae;* erythromycin (E-Mycin), azithromycin (Zithromax), for *Chlamydia trachomatis*

        b.   Selected nursing considerations

        ▶ Before administration, check client for history of antibiotic allergies. After initial administration, monitor client for at least 30 minutes in case of anaphylaxis.

        ▶ When administering by injection, give deep IM.

    2.   *Antivirals,* which inhibit viral replication

        a.   Example: acyclovir (Zovirax), for use against herpes simplex virus types 1 and 2 and other viral infections

        b.   Selected nursing considerations

        ▶ Inform client that medication will decrease severity and duration of disorder but will not cure and may exacerbate it.

    3.   Antiinfectives and antiprotozoals

        a.   Examples: metronidazole (Flagyl), for trichomoniasis; atovaquone (Mepron), for *Pneumocystis carinii* infection

        b.   Selected nursing considerations

        ▶ Advise client that sexual partner must be treated also.

        ▶ Caution client that alcohol and metronidazole do not mix. Side effects, such as nausea, vomiting, headache, may result.

    4.   *Oral contraceptive and other hormonal agents,* which prevent conception by inhibiting FSH secretion and thereby preventing ovulation and/or managing menstrual irregularities

        a.   Examples: *progestins* to treat abnormal uterine bleeding and amenorrhea include such agents as hydroxyprogesterone (Duralutin), medroxyprogesterone (Provera), ethinyl estradiol/norethindrone (Ortho-Novum), progesterone (Gestrol); and *estrogens* to treat abnormal uterine bleeding and menopausal symptoms include such agents as dienestrol (DV), diethylstilbestrol (DES), estrone (Estronol), and quinestrol (Estrovis)

        b.   Selected nursing considerations

🎵 ► Urge client to stop smoking to prevent precipitating possible thromboemboli.
  ► Advise client to take oral medications with food to minimize GI distress.
  ► Administer injectable preparations deep IM and rotate injection sites.

5. *Androgenic steroid,* which inhibits gonadotropin release and depresses FSH and LH; used to treat endometriosis.
   a. Example: danazol (Cyclomen)
   b. Selected nursing considerations

   🎵 ► Instruct client to keep an accurate record of the menstrual cycle and to report possible pregnancy immediately.

6. *Fertility agents* which induce ovulation
   a. Example: clomiphene (Anafranil)
   b. Selected nursing considerations

   🎵 ► Inform the client that medication increases likelihood of multiple pregnancy.

III. Sexually transmitted diseases (STDs)
A. Description
1. STDs are infections of the genitalia and reproductive organs (and other body tissues). They are transmitted by sexual activity. (Acquired immunodeficiency syndrome [AIDS], caused by the human immunodeficiency virus [HIV], also can be transmitted sexually, but this disorder of the immune system is discussed in Chapter 12, Section XI.)
2. Types include:
   a. Vulvovaginitis
   b. Cervicitis
   c. Urethritis
   d. Pelvic inflammatory disease (PID)
   e. Epididymitis
   f. Genital lesions
   g. Systemic infections

B. Etiology and incidence
1. Causative organisms include:
   a. For vulvovaginitis: *Trichomonas vaginalis* (trichomoniasis), a protozoan; *Sarcoptes scabiei* (scabies) and *Phthirus pubis* (pubic lice), two ectoparasites
   b. For cervicitis and urethritis (may ascend to cause PID and epididymitis): *Neisseria gonorrhoeae* (gonorrhea), *Chlamydia trachomatis* (chlamydial infections)

      c.   For genital lesions: herpes simplex virus (genital herpes); human papilloma virus (genital warts, condyloma acuminatum) *Molluscum contagiosum; Hemophilus ducreyi* (chancroid); *Chlamydia trachomatis* (lymphogranuloma venereum, or LGV)

      d.   For systemic infection: *Treponema pallidum* (syphilis); human T-lymphotropic viruses

 2.   STDs are the most prevalent form of infection in the United States; chlamydia is the most common STD. Incidence of all STDs is rising because of increased sexual activity, greater use of nonbarrier contraceptives, and the increasingly high cost of finding and treating partners.

C.   Pathophysiology and management

    1.   Infectious organisms enter through the skin and mucous membrane of the genital, oral, or anal regions.

    2.   They produce inflammation in surrounding tissue and in some cases ascend the reproductive tract, causing scarring and infertility (gonorrhea and chlamydial infection).

    3.   In syphilis, the organism travels via the bloodstream, and over many years, damages tissues such as the heart and nervous system.

    4.   In genital herpes, the virus ascends the peripheral nerve to the dorsal root ganglia, where it remains latent until factors such as fever, menses, stress, or pregnancy precipitate recurrent outbreaks.

    5.   Some STDs can be transmitted to the fetus through the placenta or the birth canal, causing spontaneous abortion or congenital infection of the newborn.

    6.   Management measures are mostly pharmacologic and hygienic.

D.   Assessment findings

    1.   History may reveal unprotected sexual activity with a new partner or one who has not been monogamous.

    2.   Vaginitis, cervicitis, and urethritis typically produce complaints of discharge and possibly irritation, itching, or dysuria. On physical exam, the discharge may vary:

      a.   Trichomoniasis: yellow and frothy, with a red, excoriated vulva and vagina (males are usually asymptomatic)

      b.   Gonorrhea: purulent, yellow

      c.   Chlamydia: watery to mucoid to purulent

    3.   Scabies and pubic lice may produce itching, excoriation, burrows, papules, or visible nits or lice.

    4.   Ascending infections are marked by fever as well as pelvic pain in women and testicular pain and swelling in men.

    5.   Genital lesions may be apparent on inspection of the skin and

mucous membranes of the genital, oral, and anal regions; other symptoms may or may not be present. Examples include:

    a.   Syphilis: nonpainful chancre with mild inguinal lymphadenopathy in primary syphilis; generalized rash, fever, and lymphadenopathy in secondary syphilis

    b.   Genital herpes: painful vesicles that erode to form ulcers with inguinal lymphadenopathy, possibly headache, milder recurrent outbreaks

    c.   Genital warts: nonpainful, soft, fleshy papillary or sessile masses

  6.   Laboratory findings may include:

    a.   Positive RPR or other serologic tests in syphilis

    b.   Positive Gram stain and culture and sensitivity for *N. gonorrhoeae*

    c.   Positive herpes simplex virus tissue culture or antibody test

    d.   Positive tissue culture or antibody test for *C. trachomatis*

    e.   Positive antibody test for HIV

E. Nursing diagnoses

  1.   Anxiety

  2.   Knowledge Deficit

  3.   Risk for Infection

  4.   Noncompliance

F. Planning and implementation

  1.   Reduce anxiety caused by embarrassment and fear by conveying a caring, nonjudgmental attitude; offering reassurance and support; and ensuring confidentiality.

  2.   Teach the client about the disorder and its treatment, principles of transmission, possible complications, and safer sex practices.

  3.   Administer medications as prescribed which may include antibiotic, antiprotozoal, antiinfective, or antiviral medications (see Section II.D).

  4.   Give pain medications as needed. They are prescribed for the individual client and the specific cause of pain.

  5.   Explain medication action, side effects, dosage schedule.

  6.   Teach comfort and hygiene measures, such as sitz baths and saline soaks.

  7.   Advise sexual abstinence until follow-up testing indicates cure or control.

  8.   Encourage treatment of sexual partners.

G. Evaluation

  1.   The client reports decreased pain and discharge.

2. The client demonstrates reduced lymphadenopathy and healing of genital lesions.
3. Laboratory cultures reveal no infection.
4. The client demonstrates appropriate self-medication techniques.
5. The client states the intention to abstain from sex for the prescribed period and to use safer sex practices in the future.
6. The client's sex partner(s) seek(s) treatment.

IV. Menstrual disorders

A. Description

1. Menstrual conditions include premenstrual syndrome (PMS), dysmenorrhea, amenorrhea, and abnormal uterine bleeding.
2. PMS is a cluster of symptoms occurring before onset of menstruation in the menstrual cycle.
3. Dysmenorrhea is painful menstruation. In primary dysmenorrhea, no pelvic pathology has been identified. In secondary dysmenorrhea, a pelvic condition causes pain.
4. Amenorrhea is absence of menstruation; it is either primary (delayed menarche) or secondary (occurring after menarche).
5. Abnormal uterine bleeding involves:
   a. Menorrhagia (excessive bleeding at the usual time of menstrual flow)
   b. Metrorrhagia (bleeding between periods or after menopause)

B. Etiology and incidence

1. Menstrual conditions may be caused by hormonal imbalance or pelvic pathology such as tumors or endometriosis.
2. Inadequate nutrition or excessive weight loss may cause amenorrhea.

C. Pathophysiology and management

1. A disruption in the feedback system between the ovarian, adrenal, thyroid, and pituitary hormonal secretions often occurs.
2. Pelvis pathology such as a uterine tumor or endometriosis may cause abnormal menstruation.
3. In PMS, the estrogen–progesterone ratio is increased during the luteal phase, causing characteristic estrogen-dependent symptoms.
4. In dysmenorrhea, excessive prostaglandin secretion causes uterine hypercontractility and arteriolar spasm.
5. Treatment measures are pharmacologic and supportive.

D. Assessment findings

1. In PMS, the client relates a history of headache, fatigue, mood swings, irritability, and full, tender breasts approximately 10 days before menses each cycle.

      2. In other menstrual conditions, history reveals abnormal menstruation in terms of how often, how long, how heavy, or how painful the menstruation is.

      3. Associated history findings may include weight loss, inadequate nutrition, or anorexia or bulimia.

      4. Physical exam may reveal a tender abdomen and possibly abdominal masses if underlying pelvic pathology is present.

      5. Diagnostic tests such as pelvic ultrasonography, hysterosalpingography, and laparoscopy may reveal pelvic pathology contributing to the menstrual problem.

      6. Complete blood count commonly reveals decreased hemoglobin and hematocrit with menorrhagia.

E. **Nursing diagnoses**

      1. Anxiety

      2. Ineffective Individual Coping

      3. Knowledge Deficit

      4. Pain

      5. Risk for Violence

F. **Planning and implementation**

      1. Offer reassurance and support.

      2. Teach self-administration of pain medication.

      3. Teach self-administration of oral contraceptives and similar agents (see Section II.D).

      4. Advise the client to keep a diary of the menstrual cycle, including occurrence and heaviness of flow and occurrence of pain and other symptoms.

      5. Encourage a well-balanced diet with adequate fluid and vitamin intake.

      6. Teach relaxation techniques to promote comfort and relieve tension.

G. **Evaluation**

      1. The client reports decreased emotional stress and improved pain relief.

      2. The client demonstrates appropriate use of medication.

      3. The client keeps a diary of the menstrual cycle.

      4. Hematocrit and hemoglobin values remain stable.

      5. The client eats a balanced diet and takes vitamin supplements.

V. **Gynecologic infections**

A. **Description**

      1. Gynecologic infections include:

         a. Vulvovaginitis

         b. Cervicitis

         c. Bartholinitis and Bartholin abscess

         d. Toxic shock syndrome (TSS)

         e. Pelvic inflammatory disease (PID)

   2. They may or may not be sexually transmitted (see Section III).

B. Etiology and incidence

   1. Gynecologic infections are caused by microorganisms such as bacteria and fungi. Vulvovaginitis is extremely common in women of all ages.

      a. Vulvovaginitis: *Candida albicans* (fungus) causes candidiasis or yeast vaginitis. *Gardnerella vaginalis* (bacteria) causes gardnerella vaginitis or nonspecific vaginitis; may be sexually transmitted

      b. Cervicitis and PID: *Chlamydia trachomatis* and *Neisseria gonorrhoeae* (sexually transmitted); *Escherichia coli,* streptococci, and staphylococci (not sexually transmitted)

   2. Atrophic vaginitis, an inflammatory condition caused by low estrogen levels in a postmenopausal woman, makes the vagina prone to infection by any organism.

   3. Bartholinitis and Bartholin abscess formation are caused by *N. gonorrhea* (sexually transmitted) as well as nonsexually transmitted bacteria surrounding the vulva (e.g., *E. coli,* streptococci, and staphylococci).

   4. Toxic shock syndrome (TSS) is caused by the toxins released by *Staphylococcus aureus.*

C. Pathophysiology and management

   1. Microorganisms invade the vulva and vaginal mucosa and may colonize and ascend the reproductive tract.

   2. Altered vaginal mucosal conditions (e.g., altered pH, disrupted normal vaginal flora, and low estrogen levels) alter resistance to infection.

   3. Childbirth, abortion, and some intrauterine procedures allow bacteria to gain intrauterine access by direct invasion and possibly by spreading through the blood and lymphatics.

   4. Menstruation provides a growth media for bacteria that may ascend upward to cause salpingitis and parametritis.

   5. In TSS, magnesium-absorbing fibers of tampons cause decreased magnesium levels, contributing to toxin production by bacteria in the lower reproductive tract.

   6. Management calls for pharmacologic measures.

D. Assessment findings

   1. Signs and symptoms of vulvovaginitis include:

      a. History of recent antibiotic use (may include risk factors for infection such as oral contraceptive use, diabetes mellitus, menopause, pregnancy, poor hygiene, synthetic or tight-fitting undergarments and clothing, frequent douching, or use of vulvovaginal products)

        b.   Complaint of vulvovaginal itching, irritation, fishy odor, and thick white to creamy grayish discharge

        c.   Reddened, swollen vulva and vagina

  2. Assessment findings for bartholinitis and abscess formation include:

        a.   Possible history of sexual activity with an infected partner

        b.   Acute pain between the labia, unilaterally

        c.   Possible fever

        d.   Red, swollen vulva unilaterally, possibly with drainage or visible abscess

  3. Assessment findings for PID include:

        a.   History of sexual activity with an infected partner; past episodes of infection; or recent childbirth, abortion, or intrauterine procedure

        b.   Complaints of lower abdominal pain, fever, nausea, and vaginal discharge

        c.   Unilateral or bilateral lower abdominal tenderness, cervical discharge, cervical motion tenderness, and adnexal tenderness on examination

        d.   Elevated white blood cell (WBC) count and positive culture results

  4. Assessment findings in TSS may include:

        a.   History of recent menses and tampon use

        b.   Complaints of sudden high fever, headache, vomiting, diarrhea, myalgias

        c.   Hypotension, possibly shock

        d.   A red, macular rash that desquamates in 7 to 10 days

        e.   Possibly decreased urine output and respiratory distress

        f.   Elevated WBC, blood, urea, nitrogen (BUN), bilirubin, and CPR levels

E. **Nursing diagnoses**

  1. Anxiety

  2. Hyperthermia

  3. Knowledge Deficit

  4. Pain

  5. Altered Tissue Perfusion

F. **Planning and implementation**

  1. Provide reassurance, confidentiality, and support to allay anxiety.

  2. Administer prescribed medications such as antibiotics and other antiinfective agents as indicated.

  3. **Teach self-administration of vaginal creams and/or irrigants as appropriate. When administering vaginal creams or suppositories advise client to lie down for 30 minutes**

after insertion and to wear a perineal pad to prevent soiling clothes. Instruct the client to wash hands before and after administration.

4. Explain the action, side effects, and interactions of all prescribed medications.
5. Maintain hydration with IV fluids for clients with nausea and vomiting, fever, and shock.
6. Promote comfort measures such as sitz baths and warm soaks as needed.
7. Teach the client to avoid risk factors for infection, if possible.
8. Promote safer sex practices and treatment of sex partner(s) as indicated.
9. Prepare the client with Bartholin's abscess for surgical drainage as indicated.
10. Ensure proper follow-up evaluation and care.

G. Evaluation

1. The client demonstrates decreased temperature, discharge, and tenderness and exhibits normal blood pressure.
2. The client reports adequate pain relief.
3. The client verbalizes understanding of the medication dosage schedule, method of administration, and side effects that warrant reporting.
4. The client states risk factors and sexual practices that can be altered to help prevent reinfection.
5. WBC count and other laboratory studies return to normal.

VI. Gynecologic tumors

A. Description

1. Gynecologic tumors include:
   a. Benign conditions such as ovarian cysts, uterine leiomyomas, and endometriosis
   b. Malignant conditions or cancer of the vulva, cervix, uterus, and ovary
2. Benign conditions usually do not predispose to malignancy.

B. Etiology and incidence

1. The exact cause of most gynecologic tumors is unknown.
2. The following factors have been associated with increased incidence of gynecologic tumors:
   a. Multiple sex partners and early sexual activity (cervical cancer)
   b. Estrogen therapy (uterine cancer)
   c. Diethylstilbestrol (DES) therapy by pregnant women (uterine cancer in their female offspring)
   d. Family history of ovarian cancer
3. Leiomyomas (also called fibroid tumors) occur in 20% of white women and 40% to 50% of black women.

    4. The incidence of endometriosis is increasing, possibly due to delayed childbearing. It is common in nulliparous 25- to 35-year-old women.

    5. The incidence of uterine cancer has been decreasing due to widespread annual Pap testing; however it remains a leading cancer in women.

C. **Pathophysiology and management**

    1. Ovarian cysts arise as normal ovarian constituents enlarge during the menstrual cycle (corpus luteal and follicular cysts) or as an ovum abnormally matures (dermoid cysts).

    2. In endometriosis, retrograde menstruation (transplantation theory) or retained remnants of embryonic epithelial tissue (metaplasia theory) cause aberrant proliferation of the endometrium, which bleeds and causes adhesions during menstruation.

    3. Many gynecologic tumors disrupt the normal menstrual cycle as they grow; some also may exert pressure on adjacent abdominal and pelvic structures.

    4. Management may include hormonal therapy, radiation, and surgery.

D. **Assessment findings**

    1. The client with an ovarian cyst may be asymptomatic or may experience such signs and symptoms as:

        a. Lower abdominal and back pain

        b. Dyspareunia (difficult or painful intercourse)

        c. Abnormal uterine bleeding

        d. Palpable ovarian mass

        e. Acute abdominal pain and guarding with rupture

        f. Rebound tenderness with rupture

        g. Ascites

    2. The client with leiomyomas may be asymptomatic or may exhibit the following findings:

        a. Pelvic pain, backache

        b. Constipation

        c. Urinary retention or urgency

        d. Dysmenorrhea, menorrhagia

        e. Palpable enlarged or irregular uterus

    3. Common assessment findings in endometriosis include:

        a. Dysmenorrhea starting 1 or 2 days before menstruation and persisting for 2 to 3 days

        b. Abnormal uterine bleeding

        c. Dyspareunia

        d. Infertility

        e. Tender palpable masses

4. Manifestations of cervical cancer may include:
   a. Vaginal discharge (early)
   b. Spotting (early)
   c. Chronic erosions of the cervix (early)
   d. Pain in the back and legs (late)
   e. Abnormal Pap smear findings
5. Assessment findings for endometrial cancer may include:
   a. Irregular vaginal bleeding and postmenopausal bleeding
   b. Abnormal Pap smear findings (in only 25% of clients)
6. Cancer of the vulva may be marked by:
   a. Pruritus (early)
   b. Vulvar bleeding, foul-smelling discharge, and pain
   c. Vulvar mass or ulceration
7. Assessment findings for ovarian cancer may include:
   a. Pelvic pain or backache (early)
   b. Irregular menses
   c. Premenstrual tension
   d. Postmenstrual bleeding
   e. Dyspepsia
   f. Acne
   g. Breast tenderness

E. Nursing diagnoses
   1. Anxiety
   2. Anticipatory Grieving
   3. Knowledge Deficit
   4. Pain
   5. Self Care Deficit
   6. Body Image Disturbance
   7. Sexual Dysfunction
   8. Altered Tissue Perfusion

F. Planning and implementation
   1. Relieve pain by administering prescribed pain medications.
   2. **Monitor respirations and blood pressure if narcotics are given.**
   3. Teach the client about side effects of hormonal therapy, and warn her to notify the physician if signs of thromboembolism occur (see Section II.D).
   4. For endometriosis, danazol may be prescribed.
   5. Prepare the client for surgery by offering information and reassurance and performing routine preoperative care (see Chapter 24).
   6. Provide appropriate postoperative care, monitoring for complications such as infection, urinary retention, paralytic ileus, fluid and electrolyte imbalance, and thromboembolism (see Chapter 24).

7. Monitor hemoglobin and hematocrit levels and transfuse blood products, as ordered, for a client with menorrhagia.
8. After a vulvectomy, perform vulvar irrigations to promote hygiene, comfort, and healing.
9. Educate the client about side effects of radiation therapy, if indicated for treatment of ovarian and some other cancers.
10. When caring for a client with a radiation implant, follow safety precautions for appropriate time and distance restrictions, discarding of linens, etc.
11. Provide emotional support, and encourage the client to express any concerns about sexual function, body image, fertility, and fear of death. Clear up any misconceptions the client may have.

G. Evaluation
1. The client reports adequate pain control.
2. The client displays reduced signs of anxiety (e.g., tachycardia, poor concentration, irritability, sweating, hyperventilation).
3. The client exhibits no fever, purulent wound drainage, wound swelling, or tenderness.
4. Hemoglobin and hematocrit remain stable.
5. The client verbalizes understanding of the effects of the disease process and treatment options.
6. Postoperatively, the client voids; bowel sounds resume; vital signs stabilize; and ambulation is attained.

VII. Structural disorders of the uterus and vagina

A. Description
1. Structural disorders of the vagina include:
    a. Vesicovaginal fistula
    b. Rectovaginal fistula
    c. Cystocele
    d. Rectocele
2. Structural disorders of the uterus include:
    a. Uterine displacement (retroversion and retroflexion)
    b. Uterine prolapse

B. Etiology and incidence
1. Structural disorders occur congenitally or as a result of pregnancy, delivery, surgery, or radiation therapy.
2. They become more common as aging weakens supporting tissues of the uterus and vagina.

C. Pathophysiology and management
1. With vaginal fistulas, an abnormal opening is formed through impaired tissue between the bladder or rectum and the vagina, allowing a trickle of urine or feces to flow through the vagina, causing irritation and infection.

2. Cystocele and rectocele develop as the pelvic floor muscles atrophy or weaken, allowing the bladder or rectum to bulge onto the anterior or posterior vaginal walls, interfering with urination and bowel elimination.

3. Normally, the uterus lies at a right angle to the vagina, inclined forward; however, in backward displacement of the uterus, the uterus has weakened supporting structures and thus tilts or is flexed backward.

4. Weakened supporting ligaments allow the uterus to work its way down the vaginal canal (prolapse) or outside the vaginal orifice (procidentia).

5. Surgery and hygienic measures may be helpful.

D. Assessment findings

1. The client commonly has a history of childbirth, pelvic surgery, or perineal or pelvic trauma.

2. Clinical manifestations may include:
   a. Pelvic pressure or pain, backache
   b. Urinary frequency, retention, or incontinence
   c. Fecal incontinence, constipation, flatus
   d. Leukorrhea (with fistulas)
   e. Visible uterine prolapse

3. Pelvic examination may reveal the structural disorder.

E. Nursing diagnoses

1. Bowel Incontinence
2. Risk for Infection
3. Knowledge Deficit
4. Pain
5. Impaired Tissue Integrity

F. Planning and implementation

1. Provide reassurance that structural disorders are not "normal" changes due to aging and that treatment will alleviate symptoms.

2. Provide and teach good perineal hygiene preoperatively and postoperatively to prevent infection, with perineal irrigations, douches, and sitz baths.

3. Explain surgical options, including possible postoperative complications (e.g., incisional infection and urinary retention; see Chapter 24).

4. Monitor urine output; insert a bladder catheter, if necessary.

5. Provide prescribed pain medications and ice packs postoperatively.

6. Teach the client how to apply and care for a pessary, if indicated.

7. Teach perineal muscle strengthening exercises to enhance support of pelvic structures and improve urinary continence.

8. Encourage good nutrition, heat application, and adequate rest to enhance fistula healing.

   G. **Evaluation**
1. The client reports relief of discomfort, urinary incontinence, and bowel incontinence.
2. The client remains free of urinary tract infection and incisional infection.
3. The client demonstrates proper hygiene.
4. The client demonstrates proper technique for perineal muscle strengthening exercises.

VIII. Breast tumors
   A. **Description**
1. Tumors of the breast are:
   a. Benign (e.g., fibrocystic disease, fibroadenoma, and intraductal papilloma)
   b. Malignant, including breast cancer and Paget's disease
2. Intraductal papilloma and Paget's disease affect the nipple.

   B. **Etiology and incidence**
1. Although the cause of breast cancer has not been elucidated, the effects of estrogen may play a role.
2. Risk factors include:
   a. Over age 40
   b. Familial history of breast cancer
   c. Early menarche
   d. Late menopause
   e. Nulliparous or birth of first child after age 34
   f. High-fat diet
   g. Oral contraceptive use
   h. Radiation exposure
   i. Presence of other cancer
3. Worldwide, breast cancer incidence is estimated at 1 million annually.

   C. **Pathophysiology and management**
1. In fibrocystic disease of the breast, small cysts are produced by overgrowth of fibrous tissue around the ducts.
2. In intraductal papilloma, a wartlike epithelial mass grows in a large collecting duct. It bleeds on trauma, and blood collects in the duct until areolar pressure expresses it out.
3. Paget's disease starts with an eczematoid condition of the nipple that spreads, erodes and ulcerates, and becomes cancerous.
4. Breast cancer, a primary carcinoma of breast tissue, attaches to the chest wall, invades surrounding tissue, and metastasizes by way of lymph channels.

5. Management includes regular checkups, comfort measures, surgery, radiation, and/or chemotherapy.

D. Assessment findings

1. Clinical manifestations of benign breast tumors may include:
   a. Breast pain and tenderness
   b. Change in mass size (larger and smaller) with menstrual cycle
   c. Palpable masses—firm, round, and freely movable
2. Assessment findings for conditions affecting the nipple include:
   a. Bloody nipple discharge (intraductal papilloma)
   b. Eczematous or ulcerated nipple (Paget's disease)
   c. Usually minimal pain
3. Signs and symptoms of breast cancer may include:
   a. A nontender lump, usually in an upper outer quadrant
   b. Pain (late)
   c. Axillary lymphadenopathy (late)
   d. Fixed, nodular breast mass (late)

E. Nursing diagnoses

1. Ineffective Coping
2. Fear
3. Anticipatory Grieving
4. Risk for Infection
5. Knowledge Deficit
6. Impaired Physical Mobility
7. Pain
8. Self Care Deficit
9. Body Image Disturbance
10. Sexual Dysfunction

F. Planning and implementation

1. Help allay the client's fears by offering information and support during the diagnostic process.
2. To minimize discomfort, teach a client with fibrocystic disease to wear a supportive bra, use analgesics, reduce methylxanthine intake, adhere to a low-salt diet, and apply warm or cool compresses.
3. Reinforce information the surgeon has told the client about treatment options, including breast reconstruction and prosthesis use.
4. After surgery for breast cancer, provide meticulous wound care to prevent infection and promote healing of grafts.
5. Postsurgery, elevate the arm on the affected side to promote drainage and enhance comfort.
6. Administer prescribed pain medications to reduce pain; monitor respirations and blood pressure with narcotic use.

7. Teach the client to avoid irritation or injury to the incision site or arm of the affected side, to help prevent infection stemming from reduced lymphatic circulation.
8. As indicated, provide referrals to self-help groups such as "Reach for Recovery," and for prosthesis or special garments.
9. Teach all women proper breast self-examination (BSE) technique.

G. **Evaluation**
1. The client expresses concerns about possible cancer, surgery, and effects on body image and sexuality.
2. The client reports pain relief.
3. The client participates in self-care activities.
4. The client demonstrates good recovery from surgery; ambulates and has improved ROM of affected arm.
5. The client displays good wound healing with no signs of incisional infection.
6. The client exhibits minimal arm edema.
7. The client demonstrates proper BSE technique.
8. The client states an intention to seek help from support groups.

IX. Infertility (male and female)

A. **Description**
1. Infertility refers to a couple's failure to achieve pregnancy within 1 to 2 years of unprotected intercourse.
2. It may be classified as primary or secondary.

B. **Etiology and incidence**
1. The cause of infertility may lie with the female, the male, or both.
2. Causes include uterine displacement, tumors, congenital abnormalities, and inflammation.
3. Causative factors and their approximate incidence include ovarian, 20%; tubal, 30%; cervical, 18%; and seminal, 30%.

C. **Pathophysiology and management**
1. Inflammation or structural abnormalities of the fallopian tubes or uterus can prevent the transportation of ovum and sperm or implantation of a fertilized ovum.
2. The ovaries may not produce and release ova regularly or secrete sufficient progesterone to produce an endometrium sufficient for implantation.
3. The pH of semen or vaginal secretions or conditions of cervical mucus may alter reception to sperm and prevent fertilization.
4. Sperm quantity, motility, or morphology may be inadequate for fertilization.

D. **Assessment findings**

1. The health history of an infertile woman may include STDs, reproductive tract surgery, abortions, PID, endometriosis, adhesions, displaced uterus, or an endocrine disorder.
2. History findings in an infertile man may include STDs, genital trauma, tuberculosis, mumps, orchitis, or cryptorchidism.
3. Pelvic examination may reveal structural disorders (uterine displacement) or inflammation (such as salpingitis).
4. Examination of the male genitalia may reveal structural disorders (cryptorchidism) or inflammation (epididymitis or orchitis).
5. Tubal insufflation may reveal poor tubal patency.
6. Postcoital cervical mucus test may be abnormal.
7. Sperm count or motility may be abnormal (fewer than 20 million).

E. **Nursing diagnoses**

1. Anxiety
2. Altered Role Performance
3. Sexual Dysfunction

F. **Planning and implementation**

1. Allay anxiety by providing information about the cause of infertility, diagnostic tests, and possible treatments.
2. Encourage both partners to express feelings related to loss and disappointment, altered roles, and sexual identity.
3. If indicated, assist with artificial insemination, instructing the client to lie flat for 30 minutes afterward.
4. Provide ongoing reassurance; most clients require repeated procedures, and success rate for infertility is only 25% to 50%.
5. Encourage the couple to explore other options, such as adoption.
6. Answer questions clients may have about clomiphene, a fertility agent used to induce ovulation. It may increase the likelihood of multiple pregnancy.

G. **Evaluation**

1. The client and partner verbalize feelings, understand treatment options, and cope with the outcome.
2. Pregnancy or a satisfactory alternative is achieved.

X. **Penile disorders**

A. **Description**

1. Conditions of the penis include phimosis and paraphimosis, priapism, and penile cancer.
2. In phimosis, the foreskin is constricted and cannot be retracted; in paraphimosis, the foreskin is retracted behind the glans and cannot be replaced.

   3. Priapism—uncontrolled, persistent erection—is a urologic emergency.

B. **Etiology and incidence**

   1. Poor hygiene of the uncircumcised penis plays a role in the development of phimosis and penile cancer.
   2. Priapism results from neural or vascular pathophysiology, such as sickle cell thrombosis, spinal cord tumors, or tumor invasion of the penis and its blood vessels.
   3. Cancer of the penis represents about 0.5% of malignancies in the United States and is more common in countries where circumcision is uncommon.

C. **Pathophysiology and management**

   1. In phimosis, normal secretions of the prepuce accumulate and cause balanitis, with subsequent scarring and calcification preventing foreskin retraction.
   2. In paraphimosis, once the foreskin is retracted, edema prevents reduction.
   3. In priapism, the corpora cavernosa become engorged with blood, and venous drainage is impaired; ischemia, fibrosis, gangrene, and impotence may result.

D. **Assessment findings**

   1. Phimosis is marked by a constricted, fixed foreskin over the glans.
   2. Paraphimosis typically involves sudden restriction of the foreskin behind the glans with edema of the penis distally.
   3. Common assessment findings in penile cancer include a painless, wartlike growth or ulcer on the glans or coronal sulcus.
   4. Priapism is characterized by persistent, painful erection in the absence of sexual desire.

E. **Nursing diagnoses**

   1. Fear
   2. Knowledge Deficit
   3. Pain
   4. Sexual Dysfunction

F. **Planning and implementation**

   1. Encourage bedrest, elevation of the penis, and ice application to reduce pain and swelling.
   2. Administer narcotics for pain relief, monitoring respirations and blood pressure.
   3. Prepare the client for circumcision, penectomy, or a blood shunting procedure as indicated.
   4. Postoperatively, monitor bleeding, administer analgesics, and change the petroleum gauze or pressure dressing as indicated.
   5. Offer reassurance to the client with penile cancer. Tell him

that he may still be able to participate in sexual intercourse after partial penectomy. Offer referral for counseling.

6. Teach uncircumcised clients proper cleansing of the glans and prepuce.

G. Evaluation

1. The client reports decreased pain.
2. Swelling is relieved, the foreskin is reducible, or erection subsides.
3. The client demonstrates proper cleansing of the penis.
4. The client remains free of bleeding or infection postoperatively.
5. The client expresses concerns about sexual activity and sexuality and seeks counseling as necessary.

XI. Impotence

A. Description

1. Impotence refers to the inability to achieve or maintain an erection sufficient to accomplish intercourse.
2. It may be classified as erectile or ejaculatory, and primary or secondary.

B. Etiology and incidence

1. Psychogenic causes include anxiety, fatigue, depression, and undue pressure to perform sexually.
2. Possible organic causes include:
   a. Occlusive vascular disease
   b. Endocrine conditions (e.g., diabetes, pituitary tumors, hypogonadism)
   c. Genitourinary conditions (e.g., prostatectomy)
   d. Hematologic disorders (e.g., Hodgkin's disease, leukemia)
   e. Neurologic disorders (e.g., neuropathy, parkinsonism)
   f. Genital trauma
   g. Alcohol and drug abuse
   h. Medication use (e.g., antipsychotics, anticholinergics, antihypertensives)
3. Incidence increases with age.

C. Pathophysiology and management

1. Pathologic processes are diverse but commonly involve decreased blood flow to the penis, altered nerve conduction, or decreased hormonal secretion.
2. Impotence may be partial or full, intermittent or constant, transient, selective for partners, and of sudden or gradual onset.

D. Assessment findings

1. The client history may reveal a chronic disease or condition, emotional or psychological problem, or use of an implicated medication.

    2. Nocturnal penile tumescence monitoring, Doppler studies of penile blood flow, and nerve conduction studies may be abnormal or normal.

E. Nursing diagnoses
    1. Anxiety
    2. Altered Role Performance
    3. Sexual Dysfunction

F. Planning and implementation
    1. Help reduce anxiety by maintaining privacy and confidentiality and encouraging the client to talk about sex- and role-related concerns.
    2. Encourage professional sex counseling if impotence is of apparent psychogenic origin.
    3. Encourage clients with chronic disease or who are on medications to follow up regularly and follow physician's orders, to prevent impotence as a complication. Encourage them to discuss any erectile dysfunction with their physicians; medications may be changed or treatment adjusted to promote sexual function.
    4. If a penile prosthesis is indicated, instruct the client on its use, and monitor for bleeding, infection, pain, or displacement after surgery.

G. Evaluation
    1. The client demonstrates and reports reduced anxiety.
    2. The client reports satisfaction in sexual relationships.

XII. Male reproductive infections

A. Description
    1. Male reproductive infections include prostatitis, orchitis, and epididymitis.
    2. Prostatitis may be acute or chronic.

B. Etiology and incidence
    1. Microorganisms such as bacteria, viruses, fungi, or parasites cause genitourinary infections.
    2. The most common bacterial offenders are gram-negative organisms.
    3. Sexually transmitted organisms also can cause these infections (see Section III).
    4. Noninfective inflammation of the prostate, epididymis, and testes may also result from trauma or chemical irritation.
    5. An estimated 35% of men older than age 50 suffer from chronic prostatitis.
    6. The cause of epididymitis in men younger than age 35 is usually *Chlamydia trachomatis*.

C. Pathophysiology and management

1. Microorganisms may be carried up the urethra to infect the prostate, epididymis, and testis, or they may be spread through the bloodstream.
2. Chemical irritation and inflammation of these organs results from extravasation of urine, possibly secondary to urethral stricture or prostatic hyperplasia.
3. Poor diffusion of antimicrobial medications into the prostate gland may cause relapsing infection in chronic prostatitis.
4. Treatment may rely on pharmacologic therapy and supportive measures.

D. Assessment findings

1. Signs and symptoms of prostatitis include:
    a. Sudden onset of fever and chills (acute prostatitis)
    b. Dysuria, urgency, frequency
    c. Perineal pain or low back pain
    d. Tender, swollen, warm indurated prostate on palpation
    e. Divided urine sample positive for bacteria and WBCs
2. Assessment findings in epididymitis include:
    a. Inguinal and scrotal pain
    b. Fever
    c. Tender, swollen epididymis
    d. Swollen, warm scrotum
    e. Possibly urine containing bacteria and WBCs
3. Common assessment findings in orchitis include pain and swelling of the testes.

E. Nursing diagnosis: Hyperthermia

F. Planning and implementation

1. Promote comfort by administering pain and antiinflammatory medications, baths, ice, bedrest, or scrotal elevation.
2. Administer antimicrobial medications as ordered; encourage the client to comply with lengthy therapy and follow-up to prevent relapse (see Section II.D). Administer pain medications as prescribed.
3. Discourage sexual activity until infection resolves. (However, sex may be beneficial with chronic prostatitis.) Encourage treatment for the client's sexual partner(s), if indicated.
4. Encourage adequate hydration to ensure adequate diffusion of antimicrobials.

G. Evaluation

1. Pain, fever, and swelling are resolved.
2. Urine cultures are negative.
3. Urine output is adequate.

4. The client complies with the treatment regimen and scheduled follow-up.

XIII. Prostate disorders

A. Description

1. Benign prostatic hyperplasia (BPH) is a benign enlargement of the prostate gland.
2. Prostate cancer is a malignant adenocarcinoma.

B. Etiology and incidence

1. Although their etiology is unknown, both conditions are hormone dependent.
2. Prostate cancer is the second most common cancer in men; incidence is greatest after age 50.

C. Pathophysiology and management

1. In both conditions, prostatic gland enlargement or the enlarging tumor obstruct urine outflow, leading to urinary retention, stasis, and infection.
2. Male sex hormones stimulate growth and enlargement.
3. Treatment measures may involve surgery, radiation, or hormonal therapy.

D. Assessment findings

1. Clinical manifestations may include:
   a. Symptoms of urinary obstruction (urgency, frequency, hesitancy, decreased urine stream, dribbling)
   b. Hematuria (cancer)
   c. On palpation, an enlarged, firm prostate (BPH) or a hard, fixed nodule (cancer)
2. Laboratory studies may reveal elevated acid phosphatase level (cancer) or abnormal renal function tests (advanced BPH).

E. Nursing diagnoses

1. Anxiety
2. Risk for Fluid Volume Deficit
3. Risk for Infection
4. Knowledge Deficit
5. Pain
6. Urinary Retention

F. Planning and implementation

1. Reduce anxiety by maintaining privacy, explaining all procedures and treatments, answering questions, and assuring the client.
2. Explain treatment options, which may include:
   a. Transurethral resection: suprapubic, perineal, or retropubic prostatectomy
   b. Radical prostatectomy and orchiectomy (for cancer only)

        c.   Radiation therapy

        d.   Hormonal therapy

3.   Provide preoperative and postoperative teaching, including complications such as bleeding, infection, and thrombosis.

4.   Maintain urinary catheter drainage to prevent urinary retention and infection. Postoperatively, maintain bladder irrigation to prevent hemorrhage. Monitor intake and output, bleeding, and vital signs.

5.   Administer pain medications as prescribed.

6.   Teach the client perineal muscle exercises to help regain urinary control; warn him to avoid the Valsalva maneuver until healing is complete.

7.   Provide information about sexual function.

G.   Evaluation

1.   The client verbalizes understanding of treatment, complications, and nursing care he will receive.

2.   The client exhibits no urinary retention, fever, or hemorrhage.

3.   The client reports adequate pain control.

4.   The client maintains urinary control and sexual function.

XIV.   Testicular tumors

   A.   Description

1.   Testicular cancers are classified as:

        a.   Germinal (seminomas, teratocarcinomas, embryonal carcinomas)

        b.   Nongerminal (epitheliomas)

2.   Hydrocele (collection of fluid in the tunica vaginalis of the testis) and varicocele (dilation of veins in the spermatic cord) are noncancerous masses.

   B.   Etiology and incidence

1.   Cryptorchidism, systemic infections, epididymitis, endocrine factors, and local trauma may play a role in the development of testicular tumors.

2.   Varicocele is a congenital condition.

3.   Although relatively rare, testicular cancer is the leading cause of cancer deaths in males aged 20 to 35.

   C.   Pathophysiology and management

1.   Testicular cancers arise from germinal or nongerminal cells of the testes as malignant tumors spread to regional lymph nodes and metastasize early.

2.   In hydrocele, fluid accumulates in the tunica vaginitis, possibly compromising testicular circulation, or it may become chronic.

3. In varicocele, enlargement or the spermatic vein may lead to infertility.
4. Management usually requires surgery.

D. Assessment findings

1. Signs and symptoms of testicular cancer may include:
   a. Painless enlargement of the scrotum
   b. Feeling of heaviness in the scrotum
   c. Backache, abdominal pain
   d. Weight loss, weakness
   e. Palpable firm, smooth testicular mass
   f. Elevated alpha-fetoprotein and HCG levels
2. Assessment findings in hydrocele and varicocele are minor but may include an enlarged scrotum and, in hydrocele, a testicular mass that transilluminates.

E. Nursing diagnoses

1. Anxiety
2. Body Image Disturbance
3. Knowledge Deficit
4. Sexual Dysfunction

F. Planning and implementation

1. Provide emotional support during the diagnostic process.
2. Explain treatment options, including:
   a. Orchiectomy, retroperitoneal lymph node dissection (RPLND), radiation therapy, or chemotherapy for testicular cancer
   b. Simple resection for symptomatic hydrocele or varicocele
3. Discuss client concerns about body image, sexual function, and fertility. Offer information about testicular prosthesis and sperm banking.
4. Administer prescribed pain medications postoperatively.
5. Provide ice and scrotal support postoperatively to reduce pain and swelling.
6. Teach the client to perform monthly testicular self-examination to aid early detection of testicular masses.

G. Evaluation

1. The client verbalizes understanding of the diagnosis, treatment, and prognosis.
2. The client reports adequate pain relief postoperatively.
3. The client verbalizes any concerns about sexuality.
4. The client demonstrates correct testicular self-examination technique.

Bibliography

Bolander, V. R. (1994). *Sorensen & Luckmann's basic nursing: A physiologic approach* (3rd ed.). Philadelphia: W. B. Saunders.

Clark, J., Queener, S., & Karb, V. (1990). *Pharmacologic basis of nursing practice* (4th ed.). St. Louis: C. V. Mosby.

Karch, A. (1995). *Lippincott's nursing drug guide*. Philadelphia: J. B. Lippincott.

Masters, W., and Johnson, V. (1966). *Human sexual response*. Boston: Little, Brown, & Co.

Nettina, S. (1996). *The Lippincott manual of nursing practice* (6th ed.). Philadelphia: Lippincott-Raven Publishers.

Smeltzer, S. C., & Bare, B. G. (1996). *Brunner & Suddarth's textbook of medical-surgical nursing* (8th ed.). Philadelphia: Lippincott-Raven Publishers.

Springhouse Corporation. (1992). *Nursing student's guide to drugs*. Springhouse, PA: Springhouse Corp.

STUDY QUESTIONS

1. Sexual development begins at conception when the male zygote unites with the female zygote. Which of the following will result in a female fetus?
   a. XX
   b. XY
   c. XXY
   d. YYX

2. Which uterine layer responds to hormonal stimulation, thickens during the proliferative phase of the menstrual cycle, and sheds during the menstrual phase?
   a. myometrium
   b. endometrium
   c. leiomyoma
   d. mucous membrane

3. The scrotum is divided by a septum into two sacs, each containing
   a. a testis, ejaculatory duct, and vas deferens
   b. a testis, epididymis, and vas deferens
   c. a testis, vas deferens, and prostate gland
   d. a testis, vas deferens, and inguinal gland

4. Ovulation occurs at the midpoint of the menstrual cycle as a direct result of secretion of which hormone?
   a. estrogen
   b. progesterone
   c. GnRH
   d. LH

5. For which of the following functions is testosterone *not* responsible?
   a. spermatogenesis
   b. development of male sex organs
   c. neutralization of urethral and vaginal acidity during intercourse
   d. maintenance of secondary sex characteristics

6. The human sexual response pattern, as described by Masters and Johnson, involves
   a. orgasmic, plateau, resting, and resolution phases
   b. excitement, plateau, orgasmic, and resolution phases
   c. excitement, resting, resolution, and resting phases
   d. excitement, orgasmic, resolution, and resting phases

7. Breast examination through inspection and palpation should reveal any abnormalities. Which of the following findings would most strongly indicate breast cancer?
   a. slight asymmetry of breasts
   b. fixed, nodular breast mass with dimpling of overlying skin
   c. bloody discharge from nipple
   d. multiple firm, round, freely movable masses that change with the menstrual cycle

8. Estrogens are used as oral contraceptives, as postmenopausal replacement therapy, and to treat inoperable prostatic cancer. Which of the following is a possible serious adverse reaction of estrogen therapy?
   a. thromboembolism
   b. weight gain
   c. diarrhea
   d. peptic ulcer disease

9. Which of the following STDs are caused by viruses and therefore will not respond to antibiotics?
   a. trichomoniasis and gonorrhea
   b. LGV and chlamydial cervicitis
   c. condyloma acuminatum (genital warts) and molluscum contagiosum
   d. syphilis and chancroid

10. Clinical manifestations of endometriosis include
    a. dysmenorrhea 1 to 2 days before and 2 to 3 days after menstruation and abnormal uterine bleeding
    b. foul-smelling vaginal discharge and vulvar mass or ulceration
    c. yellow and frothy discharge with a red excoriated vulva and vagina
    d. abnormal Pap smear findings and chronic erosions of the cervix

11. Teaching for the female client diagnosed with trichomoniasis and treated with metronidazole (Flagyl) includes
    a. drinking at least 8 oz of water with each dose and taking on an empty stomach
    b. not drinking any alcohol while taking medication and making sure sexual partner(s) is being treated
    c. stopping medication as soon as pain or itching subsides; storing medication in refrigerator
    d. encouraging client to lie down 30 minutes after taking medication and elevate lower extremities

12. Structural disorders of the uterus and vagina include displacement and prolapsed uterus and cystocele and rectocele. What medical treatment would be appropriate for such a disorder if surgery is contraindicated or refused?
    a. radiation therapy
    b. insertion of an intrauterine device (IUD)
    c. bedrest
    d. insertion of a pessary

13. One nursing intervention that can help decrease morbidity from gynecologic cancer is
    a. teaching women the importance of yearly Pap smears
    b. encouraging women to stop smoking
    c. encouraging women to breast-feed
    d. teaching women about contraception

14. Clinical manifestations of acute prostatitis include
    a. testicular pain and swelling
    b. inguinal and scrotal pain and edematous, warm scrotum
    c. hematuria and firm, enlarged prostate
    d. sudden onset of fever and chills and dysuria, urgency, and frequency

15. Although cancer of the penis is rare in the United States, a major etiologic factor in the cases that do occur is
    a. frequent urinary tract infections
    b. poor hygiene of the uncircumcised penis
    c. circumcision
    d. lack of sexual intercourse

16. Which of the following nursing interventions would be appropriate for a client with epididymitis?
    a. Apply ice and elevate the scrotum to relieve pain.
    b. Administer antiviral medications to fight the infection.
    c. Encourage sexual activity to relieve pressure.
    d. Discourage testing of sexual partners for STDs.

For additional questions, see
Lippincott's Self-Study Series Software
Available at your bookstore

ANSWER KEY

1. **Correct response: a**
   An X chromosome from each parent results in a female fetus (XX).
   b. An XY chromosome combination produces a male fetus.
   c and d. XXY results in a genetic defect, as does YYX.
   Knowledge/Physiologic/Not applicable

2. **Correct response: b**
   The endometrium responds to hormonal stimulation, thickens during the proliferative phase, and sheds during the menstrual phase.
   a. The myometrium is the muscular uterine layer.
   c. A leiomyoma is a benign tumor of the myometrium.
   d. There is no mucous membrane in the uterus.
   *Comprehension/Physiologic/
   Not applicable*

3. **Correct response: b**
   Each scrotal sac contains a testis, an epididymis, and a vas deferens.
   a, c, and d. The ejaculatory duct lies internally within the prostate gland, which lies below the bladder and surrounds the urethra. The inguinal canal separates the male pelvis from the abdominal cavity.
   Knowledge/Physiologic/Not applicable

4. **Correct response: d**
   LH surges at midcycle, after estrogen levels have peaked and stimulated a buildup of the endometrium.
   a. Estrogen levels peak early in the cycle.
   b. Progesterone is secreted in large amounts from the corpus luteum (after ovulation) during the secretory phase.
   c. GnRH secretion increases early in the menstrual cycle as a result of low estrogen and progesterone levels.
   Knowledge/Physiologic/Not applicable

5. **Correct response: c**
   Neutralization of urethral and vaginal acidity is accomplished through prostatic fluid secretion to enhance sperm performance during intercourse.
   a, b, and d. Testosterone is the primary male sex hormone that is responsible for spermatogenesis, development and maintenance of male sex organs, and secondary sex characteristics.
   *Comprehension/Physiologic/
   Not applicable*

6. **Correct response: b**
   According to Masters and Johnson, the human sexual response pattern consists of the excitement, plateau, orgasmic, and resolution phases.
   a, c, and d. These answers are rearrangements of the phases; "resting" is a coined term.
   *Comprehension/Physiologic/
   Not applicable*

7. **Correct response: b**
   A fixed nodular breast mass with dimpling of the overlying skin is a common late sign of breast cancer.
   a. Slight asymmetry of the breasts is often normal.
   c. Bloody discharge from the nipple occurs in intraductal papilloma, a benign condition.
   d. Multiple firm, round, freely movable masses that change in size with the menstrual cycle typically represent benign fibrocystic disease.
   Application/Physiologic/Assessment

8. **Correct response: a**
   Thromboembolism may result from prolonged estrogen therapy.
   b. Weight gain is an adverse reaction of estrogen but is not considered serious.
   c and d. Diarrhea and peptic ulcer diseases are not caused by estrogen.
   Application/Physiologic/Evaluation

9. *Correct response: c*
   Genital herpes is also caused by a virus.
   a. Trichomoniasis is caused by a protozoa.
   b and d. Gonorrhea, LGV, chlamydial cervicitis, syphilis, and chancroid are caused by bacteria.
   Comprehension/Physiologic/NA

10. *Correct response: a*
    Common assessment findings in endometriosis include dysmenorrhea starting 1 to 2 days before menstruation and persisting for 2 to 3 days; abnormal uterine bleeding; dyspareunia; infertility; and tender palpable masses.
    b, c, and d. These are signs and symptoms of cancer of the vulva, trichomoniasis, and cervical cancer, respectively.
    Application/Physiologic/Assessment

11. *Correct response: b*
    Metronidazole (Flagyl) should not be taken with alcohol and can cause a mild to severe reaction leading to unconsciousness, convulsions, and death. The sexual partner must be treated even if the partner has no symptoms. Abstinence should be observed until trichomoniasis is resolved.
    a, c, and d. All of these interventions are not applicable when taking metronidazole. Medication should be taken with food, and all medication should be taken even if symptoms subside. Lying down after administering vaginal creams or suppositories is encouraged.
    Application/Health promotion/Implementation

12. *Correct response: d*
    Insertion of a pessary can provide support to the uterus and vagina.
    a, b, and c. Radiation, insertion of an IUD, and bedrest are not appropriate therapies for structural disorders.
    Comprehension/Physiologic/NA

13. *Correct response: a*
    Annual Pap smears aid early detection of gynecologic cancer, enabling prompt treatment.
    b, c, and d. Although these responses are good nursing interventions, they will not result in decreased gynecologic cancer deaths.
    Application/Health promotion/Implementation

14. *Correct response: d*
    Signs and symptoms of acute prostatitis include sudden onset of fever and chills; dysuria, urgency, frequency; perineal pain or low back pain; and tender, swollen, warm indurated prostate on palpation.
    a, b, and c. These are clinical manifestations of orchitis, epididymitis, and benign prostatic hypertrophy, respectively.
    Application/Physiologic/Assessment

15. *Correct response: b*
    Poor hygiene of the uncircumcised penis is a major contributing factor to penile cancer.
    a, c, and d. Frequent urinary tract infections, circumcision, and lack of sexual intercourse do not lead to penile cancer.
    Comprehension/Health promotion/NA

16. *Correct response: a*
    Application of ice and elevation of the scrotum will help decrease pain and edema in the scrotal area.
    b, c, and d. Antibiotics will be administered; not antivirals. Encouraging sexual activity will not relieve pressure and is not appropriate for epididymitis (although it may be helpful with chronic prostatitis). Sexual partners should be tested for STDs since such an infection may have contributed to epididymitis.

Immunologic Disorders

I. **Immune system**
   A. Immune system components
   B. Immune mechanisms
   C. Nonspecific immunologic defense
   D. Specific immunologic defense
   E. Humoral immunity
   F. Cellular immunity
   G. Stages of cellular and humoral immunity
   H. Complement
   I. Hypersensitivity reactions
   J. Allergic disorders
   K. Autoimmune disorders
   L. Immune deficiency

II. **Overview of disorders**
   A. Significant assessment findings
   B. Important laboratory studies and diagnostic tests
   C. Psychosocial implications
   D. Medications used to treat immune problems

III. **Allergic rhinitis (hay fever)**
   A. Description
   B. Etiology and incidence
   C. Pathophysiology and management
   D. Assessment findings
   E. Nursing diagnoses
   F. Planning and implementation
   G. Evaluation

IV. **Allergic dermatoses**
   A. Description
   B. Etiology and incidence
   C. Pathophysiology and management
   D. Assessment findings
   E. Nursing diagnoses
   F. Planning and implementation
   G. Evaluation

V. **Asthma**
   A. Description
   B. Etiology and incidence
   C. Pathophysiology and management
   D. Assessment findings
   E. Nursing diagnoses
   F. Planning and implementation
   G. Evaluation

VI. **Anaphylaxis**
   A. Description
   B. Etiology and incidence
   C. Pathophysiology and management
   D. Assessment findings
   E. Nursing diagnoses
   F. Planning and implementation
   G. Evaluation

VII. **Rheumatoid arthritis**
   A. Description
   B. Etiology and incidence
   C. Pathophysiology and management
   D. Assessment findings
   E. Nursing diagnoses
   F. Planning and implementation
   G. Evaluation

VIII. **Lupus erythematosus (LE)**
   A. Description
   B. Etiology and incidence
   C. Pathophysiology and management
   D. Assessment findings
   E. Nursing diagnoses
   F. Planning and implementation
   G. Evaluation

IX. **Hypogammaglobulinemia**
   A. Description
   B. Etiology and incidence
   C. Pathophysiology and management

I. Immune system

A. Immune system components

1. The *lymphatic system*—lymph nodes and vessels—performs several important functions, including:
   a. Transporting lymph
   b. Filtering and phagocytizing (processing and killing) antigens
   c. Generating lymphocytes and monocytes
2. Major functions of the *spleen* include:
   a. Removing worn out erythrocytes from blood
   b. Storing blood and platelets
   c. Filtering and purifying blood
3. The *liver* is involved in:
   a. Phagocytosis by Kupffer cells (macrophages)
   b. Filtering and purifying blood
4. The *hematopoietic system*—bone marrow and lymphatic tissue—produces blood cells, including those involved in immunologic defense (leukocytes). Table 12-1 gives more information on types of leukocytes.

B. Immune mechanisms

1. Defense: resisting infection
2. Homeostasis: state of equilibrium of internal environment
3. Surveillance: recognition of self versus nonself
4. General immune responses include:
   a. Phagocytic: ingestion of foreign particles by white blood cells (WBCs)

TABLE 12-1.
Types of Leukocytes

CELL TYPE	NORMAL LEVEL	CHARACTERISTICS	FUNCTION
Granulocytes (polymorphonuclear leukocytes)	5000–10,000/mm^3	Formed in bone marrow Granular (under microscope)	Immediate response to cellular injury
Neutrophils	50%–70% of all leukocytes	12 hr life span; 2–4 hr life span with infection	Phagocytic First cell to site of cellular injury Contain lysosomes
Eosinophils	2%–4% of all leukocytes	Contain heparin histamine	Play role in hypersensitivity reaction
Basophils	<1% of all leukocytes	Granules filled with heparin; histamine	Play role in inflammatory response
Agranulocytes		Produced in lymphatic system Nongranular (under microscope)	Fight infection
Lymphocytes	25%–33% of all leukocytes	Classified as B cells or T cells	Phagocytosis Release of lymphokines Production of gamma globulins Cell-mediated reactions
Monocytes	4%–6% of all leukocytes	Circulate in blood but also settle in tissue where they are transformed into macrophages	Phagocytosis (can ingest larger particles than neutrophils; 5 times as many in 1 ingestion)

      b.   Humoral: formation of antibodies by plasma cells in response to foreign proteins

      c.   Cellular: attack of microbes by special killer T cells formed from lymphocytes

C. Nonspecific immunologic defense

    1.   This defense system provides the body's natural immunity.

    2.   External defenses consist of physical and chemical barriers (e.g., intact skin and mucous membranes, enzymes in tears and saliva, acidic gastric juices) that prevent entrance of foreign substances (antigens) or immunogens.

    3.   Internal defense systems, activated when antigens gain access to the internal environment, include phagocytosis by WBCs, inflammatory responses, and internal secretions (e.g., interferon).

D. **Specific immunologic defense**

1. *Active acquired immunity* involves production of antibodies and sensitized lymphocytes in response to an antigen or immunization.
2. Memory cells generated result in rapid immune response (defense) on reexposure to the antigen.
3. Adults require tetanus and diphtheria booster injection IM at least every 10 years; all health care workers should receive the hepatitis B vaccine.
4. *Passive acquired immunity* is a temporary immunity acquired by introduction of antibodies or sensitized lymphocytes from another source (e.g., antibodies through placental circulation to a fetus, gamma globulin, and antiserum from blood plasma of a person with acquired immunity); the body does not generate memory cells.
5. Both active and passive acquired immunity involve humoral (B-lymphocyte) and cellular (T-lymphocyte) immunity.

E. **Humoral immunity**

1. B lymphocytes (bursa derived) are involved in antibody (i.e., immunoglobulin) production.
2. Unsensitized B cells proliferate and mature into plasma cells after exposure to antigen.
3. Plasma cells differentiate into memory cells (which trigger B-cell response on subsequent exposure to same antigen) and antibodies.
4. Five types of antibodies are produced by the body:
    a. IgG (75% of total): activates complement, enhances phagocytosis, crosses placenta (passive immunity), active in second response (reinfection)
    b. IgA (15% of total): present in body fluids (blood, saliva, and tears; pulmonary, GI, prostatic, and vaginal secretions; and breast milk)
    c. IgM (10% of total): first antibody produced in the immune response; activates the complement system
    d. IgD (0.2% of total): role unclear; may be required on B-cell surface for transformation into plasma cells
    e. IgE (0.004% of total): associated with allergic and hypersensitivity reactions

F. **Cellular immunity**

1. T lymphocytes (thymus derived), on exposure to antigen, proliferate and differentiate into one of several types of T cells:
    a. Helper T cells (T4): assist B cells in humoral response to form antibodies

        b.   Suppressor T cells (T8): suppress B-cell synthesis of antibody production via feedback mechanism

        c.   Memory T cells: store future immune response to some antigen

        d.   Cytotoxic T cells: directly attack antigen, thus altering cell membrane with resultant cell lysis; also release chemical mediators known as lymphokines (i.e., interferon, migration inhibitory factor), which can attract and hold macrophages and lymphocytes to the site of injury

   2.   Cellular immunity functions primarily in:

        a.   Delayed hypersensitivity reactions

        b.   Rejection of transplants

        c.   Viral, fungal, and chronic infections

G. **Stages of cellular and humoral immunity**

   1.   Recognition: Circulating lymphocytes and macrophages recognize foreign material or antigens as "nonself."

   2.   Proliferation: Sensitized lymphocytes proliferate, differentiate, and mature into respective T and B cells.

   3.   Response: Antibody is produced with specific T-cell action.

   4.   Effector: Antigen is destroyed by antibody produced by B-cell or cytotoxic T-cell action.

H. **Complement**

   1.   Complement is a group of at least 20 circulating plasma proteins, made in the liver, that are sequentially activated in the presence of an antigen.

   2.   Functions include:

        a.   Cell lysis

        b.   Opsonization: making antigen more susceptible to phagocytosis

        c.   Chemotaxis: inducing phagocytes to antigen

        d.   Agglutination: clumping of antigens

        e.   Neutralization of viruses

        f.   Anaphylatoxin: stimulation of inflammatory response

   3.   Activation of complement can occur in one of two basic ways:

        a.   Classical: antigen–antibody complex activates C1 (first of circulating complement proteins)

        b.   Alternate: no antigen–antibody complex required; can be initiated by release of endotoxins; begins with C3

I. **Hypersensitivity reactions**

   1.   These reactions represent immune response to allergens that results in tissue destruction.

   2.   In Type I (anaphylactic) reactions, mediated by IgE antibody, most cell degranulation occurs, resulting in release of histamine.

3. Commonly involved organs in Type I reactions include GI tract, skin, and lungs. Common causative agents include drugs (penicillin and cephalosporins), insect venoms, blood products, and iodinated contrast mediums.

4. Type II (cytotoxic) reactions (e.g., hemolytic anemia) are mediated by IgG and IgM antibodies, which attach to self (usually circulating blood elements) and cause cell lysis.

5. Type III (immune complex) reactions (e.g., rheumatoid arthritis, Goodpasture's disease, serum sickness) are mediated by antigen–antibody complexes that deposit in the lining of blood vessels or on tissue surfaces.

6. Type IV (delayed hypersensitivity) reactions (e.g., contact dermatitis, transplant rejection) are mediated by lymphokines released from sensitized T-cell lymphocytes.

J. Allergic disorders

1. Interaction between antigen and antibody typically results in one or more manifestations of tissue injury.

2. Persons experiencing allergies are genetically predisposed to forming IgE antibodies.

3. Histamine and other mediators are released on reexposure to the allergen to which the person is sensitized.

K. Autoimmune disorders

1. In autoimmune disorders, the body no longer differentiates self from nonself.

2. Alterations in T cells or B cells produce autoantibodies and autosensitized T cells that cause tissue injury; these changes may involve one organ or many organ systems.

3. The cause remains unknown; many theories exist.

L. Immune deficiency

1. Immune deficiency is defined as a deficit in the immune system, either congenital or acquired, that makes the person susceptible to life-threatening opportunistic infection.

2. In congenital, or primary immunodeficiency, the body produces inadequate amounts of one or more immune cells. Deficits can be humoral (B cell), cell-mediated (T cell), or combined.

3. Acquired, or secondary, immunodeficiency is attributed to various etiologies, including:

   a. Immunosuppressive therapy: chemotherapeutic agents, corticosteroids, nonsteroidal antiinflammatory agents, irradiation

   b. Age: deterioration in thymus gland and T-cell functioning; decreased number of suppressor T cells and helper T cells

       c.   Disruption of skin integrity as occurs with burns and trauma

       d.   Nutritional deficits

       e.   Malignant processes such as leukemia, lymphoma

       f.   Infectious processes such as sepsis and AIDS

    4.   Manifestations vary according to the part(s) of the immune system affected. Humoral deficit predisposes to bacterial infections; cell-mediated deficit, to viral, fungal, and protozoan infections.

II. Overview of disorders

    A.   **Significant assessment findings**

        1.   General

            a.   Overall health status

            b.   Recurrent infections

            c.   Seasonal symptoms

            d.   Weight loss

            e.   Fever

        2.   Integumentary system: rashes and lesions

        3.   Head

            a.   Eyes: itching, burning, watering, vision problems, infections

            b.   Ears: recurrent infections, drainage

            c.   Nose: rhinitis, sneezing

            d.   Mouth: oral lesions, infections, sore throat

        4.   Neck: adenopathy

        5.   Respiratory

            a.   Cough

            b.   Wheeze

            c.   Dyspnea

            d.   Recurrent infection

        6.   Cardiovascular: palpitations, pain, Raynaud's phenomenon

        7.   Gastrointestinal: nausea, vomiting, diarrhea

        8.   Genitourinary: recurrent infections, dysuria, hematuria

        9.   Musculoskeletal

            a.   Weakness and fatigue

            b.   Joint pain and altered range of motion (ROM)

            c.   Ability to perform activities of daily living (ADLs)

      10.   Neurologic

            a.   Orientation

            b.   Level of consciousness

            c.   Sensorium

            d.   Paresthesias

      11.   Lymphatic and hematologic: adenopathy, abnormal bleeding

    B.   **Important laboratory studies and diagnostic tests**

        1.   T- and B-lymphocyte assays

    2. Immunoglobulin assays

    3. Radioallergosorbent test of IgE (RAST)

    4. Serum complement assays

    5. Autoantibody tests

        a. Antinuclear antibodies (ANA)

        b. Rheumatoid factor (RF)

    6. HIV (human immunodeficiency virus) test

C. Psychosocial implications

    1. A client with an immunologic problem may experience coping difficulties related to:

        a. The chronic, progressive nature of the disorder

        b. Debilitating disease effects

        c. Loss of friends and loved ones from the disease (e.g., from AIDS)

        d. Fear of dying

    2. The client may express self-concept concerns related to:

        a. Body image changes with disease progression

        b. Rejection

        c. Loss of outlets for sexual expression

        d. Role changes toward increased dependence

    3. The client may need to adjust to lifestyle changes made necessary by altered:

        a. Physical capacity

        b. Self-care ability

        c. Work performance, with potential for job loss and economic insecurity

    4. Disease-related changes in social interaction can lead to isolation, depression, and hopelessness.

D. Medications used to treat immune problems (additional medications may be included with specific diseases)

    1. *Antihistamines,* which inhibit histamine release

        a. Examples: chlorpheniramine maleate (Chlor-Trimeton), diphenhydramine (Benadryl), terfenadine (Seldane)

        b. Selected nursing considerations

            ▸ **Caution client that antihistamines (but not terfenadine) initially cause drowsiness, which usually subsides with continued use.**

            ▸ **Caution client that alcohol and antihistamines do not mix.**

    2. *Adrenergics* (also called sympathomimetics), which relax smooth bronchial muscle and dilate airways

        a. Examples: isoetharine (Bronkosol), metaproterenol (Alupent), albuterol (Ventolin), terbutaline (Brethine), epinephrine (Bronkaid), isoproterenol (Isuprel)

        b. Selected nursing considerations

    ▸ Instruct client to inhale twice as follows: inhale once, wait 1 minute, and inhale once more.

3. *Xanthine derivatives,* which relax bronchial smooth muscle, in asthma

    a.   Examples: aminophylline (Phyllocontin), theophylline (Theo-Dur), ephedrine (Adrenalin, Primatene)

    b.   Selected nursing considerations

𝕟 ▸ **Monitor serum level of theophylline (normal level, 10–20 mcg/mL).**

    ▸ **Provide medication at regular intervals.**

    ▸ **Instruct client to notify physician of irritability, restlessness, headache, insomnia, dizziness.**

4. *Corticosteroids* (oral or inhalable), which are used in severe immune or inflammatory responses

    a.   Examples: oral—hydrocortisone (Cortef), methylprednisolone (Medrol), dexamethasone (Decadron), prednisone (Deltasone); inhalable—beclomethasone (Vanceril)

    b.   Selected nursing considerations

𝕟 ▸ **Instruct client to take medication exactly as directed and to taper discontinuation of drug rather than stop abruptly, which could cause serious withdrawal symptoms leading to adrenal insufficiency, shock, and death.**

    ▸ **Forewarn client that drug may cause reportable cushingoid effects (weight gain, moon face, buffalo hump, and hirsutism) and may mask signs and symptoms of infection.**

5. *Cromolyn sodium,* which has bronchodilating effect

    a.   Example: Intal

    b.   Selected nursing considerations

𝕟 ▸ **Teach client to insert capsule in nebulizer device, exhale completely, place mouthpiece between lips, inhale deeply and hold breath for 10 seconds, and then exhale.**

6. *Vasopressors,* which rapidly restore blood pressure in anaphylaxis by producing vasoconstriction and stimulating the heart

    a.   Examples: norepinephrine (Levophed), metaraminol (Aramine)

    b.   Selected nursing considerations

𝕟 ▸ **Monitor client's vital signs, intake and output, mental status, peripheral pulses, and skin color.**

7. *Salicylates,* which reduce fever, inflammation, and pain

    a.   Example: aspirin

    b.   Selected nursing considerations

m ► Explain that prolonged use can have an anticoagulant effect.
- ► Instruct client to report bleeding gums or signs of GI bleeding.
- ► Recommend aspirin with enteric coating, which resists breakdown by stomach acid.

8. *Nonsteroidal antiinflammatory drugs* (NSAIDs), which reduce inflammation and pain
   a. Examples: acetaminophen (Tylenol), ibuprofen (Motrin), indomethacin (Indocin), meclofenamate (Meclofen), naproxen (Naprosyn, Aleve)
   b. Selected nursing considerations

   m ► Advise client to take NSAID with food to minimize GI upset.

9. *Immunoglobulin,* which provides passive immunity via IgG antibodies to protect against infection
   a. Example: gamma globulin (Gamimune N)
   b. Selected nursing considerations

   m ► Before administering, obtain allergy and immunization response history.
   - ► After administering, monitor client closely for signs and symptoms of allergic reaction.

10. *Antimicrobial agents,* for example, antibiotics, as prescribed for specific disorder or problem; obtain allergy history before administration and monitor client closely after administration.

11. *Antipruritic agents,* which may be topical steroids or anesthetics used to relieve or prevent itching
    a. Examples: topical steroids—desoximetasone (Topicort), hydrocortisone (Dermacort), triamcinolone (Kenalog); topical anesthetics—benzocaine (Americaine), dibucaine (Nupercainal)
    b. Selected nursing considerations

    m ► Advise client to wash hands before and after application.
    - ► Instruct client to clean affected area with warm water before application.

III. Allergic rhinitis (hay fever)

A. Description: an allergic reaction to inhaled airborne allergens, characterized by seasonal occurrences

B. Etiology and incidence

1. The most common form of respiratory allergy, hay fever is generally induced by airborne pollens.

    2. Common seasonal pollens include:
       a. Spring: tree pollens (e.g., oak, maple, birch)
       b. Summer: grass pollens (e.g., sheep sorrel, plantain)
       c. Fall: weed pollens (e.g., ragweed)
    3. Incidence occurs in all age groups but is especially high in children and adolescents.

C. Pathophysiology and management
    1. Allergic rhinitis occurs when IgE antibodies in the nasal mucosa combine with inhaled allergens on the mucosal surface.
    2. The resultant cell injury causes typical symptoms—sneezing, itching, and runny nose.
    3. Management measures are mostly pharmacologic.

D. Assessment findings
    1. Common clinical manifestations include:
       a. Itching, burning nasal mucosa
       b. Copious mucous secretions causing runny nose
       c. Red, burning, tearing eyes
       d. Sneezing
       e. Pale, boggy nasal mucosa
    2. The client may have a family history of allergies.
    3. Laboratory studies may reveal:
       a. Eosinophils in nasal secretions
       b. Lymphocyte count above $1200/\mu L$
       c. Elevated serum IgE
       d. Offending allergens identified by skin testing

E. Nursing diagnoses
    1. Ineffective Airway Clearance
    2. Knowledge Deficit
    3. Sleep Pattern Disturbance

F. Planning and implementation
    1. Obtain a comprehensive client history to try to determine the causative agent.
    2. Administer immunotherapy (usually by injection) as prescribed. If appropriate, advise client to avoid crowds and persons with known infections (see Section II.D).

G. Evaluation
    1. The client reports relief of symptoms.
    2. The client verbalizes understanding of the allergic reaction, its prevention, and treatment.
    3. The client complies with the prescribed medication regimen.

IV. Allergic dermatoses

    A. **Description:** a group of inflammatory conditions caused by skin reaction to irritating or allergenic materials; includes allergic contact dermatitis and atopic dermatitis

    B. **Etiology and incidence**

        1. Many substances can produce allergic contact dermatitis; common causes include exposure to poison ivy, topical medications, cosmetics, soaps, and industrial chemicals.

        2. The cause of atopic dermatitis is unknown, but it appears to be associated with a family history of allergic respiratory disorders (e.g., allergic rhinitis, asthma). Exacerbating factors appear to include irritants, infection, and certain allergens.

    C. **Pathophysiology and management**

        1. Allergic contact dermatitis involves delayed hypersensitivity and requires a latent period ranging from several days (for strong sensitizers such as poison ivy) to years.

        2. Although atopic dermatitis may appear at any age, it most commonly begins in infancy or early childhood. It may subside spontaneously, to be followed by unpredictable exacerbations throughout life.

        3. Management involves client education and medications.

    D. **Assessment findings**

        1. Common clinical manifestations include:

            a. Burning, itching, swelling, and erythema of skin

            b. Crusting, weeping lesions

        2. History may reveal known or suspected exposure to an allergen.

        3. The extent of rash depends on the allergen and exposure; rash may be local or generalized.

        4. Diagnosis may be made on the basis of skin eruptions and history of allergen exposure.

    E. **Nursing diagnoses**

        1. Risk for Infection

        2. Knowledge Deficit

        3. Pain

        4. Self Esteem Disturbance

        5. Impaired Skin Integrity

    F. **Planning and implementation**

        1. Provide symptomatic relief with antihistamines, antipruritics, or steroidal creams as prescribed (see Section II.D).

        2. Provide client and family teaching, covering:

            a. Basic pathophysiology of allergic reactions

            b. Methods to minimize exposure to offending allergens

            c. Comfort measures for symptomatic relief

        d.   Stress-reduction measures

        e.   Prescribed medications, including purpose, effects, dosage, administration, and possible side effects

G. **Evaluation**

    1.   The client displays clear skin free of rash, itching, burning, infection.

    2.   The client verbalizes understanding of the allergic reaction, its prevention, and treatment.

    3.   The client complies with the prescribed therapeutic regimen.

V. Asthma

A. **Description: a chronic reactive respiratory disorder producing episodic, reversible airway obstruction**

B. **Etiology and incidence**

    1.   Allergic asthma results from an immunologically mediated hypersensitivity to inhaled allergens such as airborne pollens and molds, dust, and animal danders.

    2.   Incidence is estimated at 3% to 8% of the population, with more than half the cases occurring in children under age 10.

C. **Pathophysiology and management**

    1.   Although the pathologic mechanisms of allergic asthma remain somewhat unclear, the fundamental process presumably involves a reaction of sensitized IgE antibodies to an inhaled allergen, with subsequent release of chemical mediators such as histamine, slow-reacting substance of anaphylaxis (SRS-A), and eosinophil chemotactic factor of anaphylaxis (ECF-A).

    2.   Obstruction results from constriction of bronchial smooth muscle, swelling of bronchial membranes, and hypersecretion of mucus.

    3.   Management focuses on prevention, relief of symptoms with medication, and client education.

D. **Assessment findings**

    1.   Clinical manifestations of asthma include:

        a.   Chest tightness

        b.   Prolonged, strenuous expirations

        c.   Wheezing on expiration

        d.   Cyanosis

        e.   Cough, nonproductive at first, followed by violent coughing that produces thin, gelatinous mucus and is relieved by a bronchodilator

        f.   Nausea and vomiting

        g.   Anxiety

    2.   Health history may reveal exposure to a known or suspected precipitating substance.

    3.   Pulmonary function studies reveal airway obstruction and decreased peak expiratory flow rate.

    4. Radiologic or bronchoscopic examination may be needed to rule out other causes of bronchial obstruction.

    5. Arterial blood gas (ABG) analysis typically reveals:

        a. Decreased PaO_2

        b. Initially, decreased $PaCO_2$ and increased pH

        c. Later, increased $PaCO_2$ and decreased pH

E. Nursing diagnoses

    1. Ineffective Airway Clearance

    2. Fear

    3. Knowledge Deficit

F. Planning and implementation

    1. Provide symptomatic relief by administering prescribed medications, particularly bronchodilators, such as a xanthine derivative (theophylline), isoetharine (Bronkosol), or cromolyn sodium (see Section II.D).

    2. As prescribed, administer corticosteroidal agents (see Section II.D) for asthma that fails to respond to other treatments.

    3. Administer oxygen as prescribed.

    4. Elevate the head of the bed, and lean the client forward to provide maximum lung expansion and ease respiratory effort.

    5. Monitor respiratory rate and depth, and auscultate lung sounds.

    6. Monitor ABGs to detect any changes from baseline.

    7. Provide reassurance to help relieve anxiety.

    8. Monitor for and take precautions to prevent complications, such as:

        a. Pneumothorax

        b. Pulmonary hypertension

        c. Right heart failure

        d. Respiratory failure

    9. Provide adequate hydration to liquefy secretions.

    10. Promote adequate rest to increase respiratory efficiency.

    11. Provide client and family teaching, covering:

        a. Basic pathophysiology of disease process, treatment, and prevention of further exacerbations

        b. Importance of strict compliance with the therapeutic regimen

        c. Purpose, effects, dosage, administration, side effects, and interactions of all prescribed medications

        d. Signs and symptoms of complications to watch for and report

        e. The need for increased fluid intake to thin bronchial secretions

        f. Activities allowed and discouraged

        g. Stress reduction methods

        h. The importance of follow-up care to monitor progress

G. Evaluation

1. The client displays relief of respiratory distress: absence of chest tightness, wheezing, cyanosis, cough, exaggerated expiratory effort.
2. The client uses appropriate coping mechanisms to control anxiety.
3. The client and family verbalize understanding of the disease process, prevention of acute asthma attacks, and treatment.
4. The client complies with the prescribed therapeutic regimen.

VI. Anaphylaxis

A. Description: an acute, life-threatening allergic reaction marked by rapidly progressive urticaria and respiratory distress

B. Etiology and incidence

1. Anaphylaxis results from ingesting or other systemic exposure to allergenic substances.
2. Possible causative substances include:
   a. Drugs, such as penicillin and other antibiotics, vaccines, hormones, salicylates, and local anesthetics
   b. Foods (e.g., legumes, nuts, berries, seafood, and egg albumin)
   c. Sulfite-containing food additives
   d. Insect venom (e.g., wasp, hornet, honeybee, certain spiders)

C. Pathophysiology and management

1. Anaphylactic reaction requires previous sensitization to the triggering allergen, with production of specific IgE antibodies that bind to mast cells and basophils.
2. On reexposure, IgE reacts immediately with the allergen and triggers release of potent chemical mediators (histamine, ECF-A) from basophils and mast cells.
3. Concurrently, IgG or IgM activates release of complement fractions, and two other chemical mediators—bradykinin and leukotrienes—trigger profound vascular changes that can lead to vascular collapse.

 4. **Anaphylaxis is considered a medical emergency because of the possibility of respiratory obstruction and vascular collapse. In severe cases, death may occur within 5 to 10 minutes of onset. Treatment includes establishing a patent airway, administering prescribed medications, and, later, teaching preventive measures.**

D. Assessment findings

1. Clinical manifestations depend on whether mediators remain local or are systemic.

2. Local effects include wheals with surrounding red flares and urticaria; usually not dangerous.
3. Systemic manifestations involve:
    a. Intense urticaria and edema at the site of injection or injury, rapidly spreading to the face, hands, and other body areas
    b. Respiratory distress from bronchospasm, coughing, sneezing, wheezing
    c. Arrhythmias, tachycardia or bradycardia, hypotension, and signs of circulatory collapse
    d. Nausea and vomiting, abdominal pain, diarrhea

E. Nursing diagnoses
  1. Decreased Cardiac Output
  2. Fear
  3. Impaired Gas Exchange

F. Planning and implementation
  1. Treat an anaphylactic attack as a medical emergency.
  2. Maintain an open airway.
  3. As prescribed, administer the following or combinations of the following:
      a. Antihistamines to suppress histamine release (see Section II.D)
      b. **Epinephrine, IM or subcutaneously, to constrict dilated blood vessels, raise the heart rate, improve myocardial contractility, and dilate the bronchioles. Use a tuberculin syringe to ensure exact dosage and monitor client closely after administration.**
      c. Vasopressors to increase blood pressure (see Section II.D)
      d. Corticosteroids to decrease inflammation (see Section II.D)
  4. Administer oxygen as indicated.
  5. Prepare to assist with emergency tracheotomy if necessary.
  6. Monitor vital functions, evaluating:
      a. Blood pressure, pulse, respirations
      b. ABG values
      c. ECG
      d. Urine output
  7. Establish a patent IV line for drug and fluid administration.
  8. Administer fluid replacement and volume expanders as prescribed.
  9. After an acute episode, promote rest and continue monitoring vital signs.
  10. Provide client and family teaching, covering:
      a. Basic pathophysiology of reaction and preventive measures

    b.   Identification and elimination of offending allergens
    c.   Importance of informing others of allergies, for example by wearing medical identification
    d.   The use of commercial "anti-sting" kits, if applicable

G. Evaluation

    1.   The client demonstrates relief of respiratory distress: absence of bronchospasm, wheezing, dyspnea.

    2.   The client maintains a regular pulse rate between 60 and 100 beats per minute.

    3.   The client exhibits no edema.

    4.   The client verbalizes understanding of anaphylactic reaction, prevention of recurrence, treatment of early signs and symptoms, and when to seek help.

VII. Rheumatoid arthritis

A. Description: a chronic, progressive disease involving inflammation of synovial joints

B. Etiology and incidence

    1.   Etiology is unknown although it apparently is an autoimmune disorder; exacerbations may be associated with increased physical or emotional stress.

    2.   Incidence is three times greater in women than in men. Peak age of onset is between age 30 and 60 although the disease can develop at any age.

C. Pathophysiology and management

    1.   Pathologic changes begin as inflammation and progress to destruction of joints, producing deformity and loss of motion.

    2.   The disease may affect only joints or may extend to body organs and blood vessels.

    3.   Therapy is supportive and pharmacologic.

D. Assessment findings

    1.   Common clinical manifestations include:
        a.   Swollen, warm, tender joints
        b.   Limited ROM in affected joints
        c.   Generalized edema or nodules around affected joints
        d.   Impaired mobility and ability to perform ADLs
        e.   Fatigue, weakness, anorexia
        f.   In later stages, weight loss, fever, anemia, muscle atrophy, Sjögren's syndrome

    2.   Laboratory and diagnostic findings may include:
        a.   Radiographic abnormalities: progressive joint damage
        b.   Increased immunoglobulin levels, increased complement levels
        c.   Increased RF titer
        d.   Increased erythrocyte sedimentation rate (ESR)

E. **Nursing diagnoses**
1. Knowledge Deficit
2. Impaired Physical Mobility
3. Altered Nutrition: Less than body requirements
4. Self Esteem Disturbance

F. **Planning and implementation**
1. Direct care at relieving pain, maintaining function, and preventing deformities.
2. Promote adequate rest; pay attention to maintaining proper body alignment and preventing contractures.
3. As appropriate, administer NSAIDs, aspirin, and/or corticosteroids (see Section II.D).
4. Apply hot or cold to affected joints according to the client's needs.
5. After the acute phase resolves, begin physical therapy.
6. Provide client teaching, covering:
   a. Basic pathophysiology of disease process and causes of exacerbation
   b. Importance of an activity program for self-care
   c. Principles of joint conservation and energy conservation
   d. Importance of maintaining optimum nutritional status
   e. Purpose, effects, dosage, administration, side effects, and interactions of all prescribed medications
   f. The need for follow-up care to monitor progress

G. **Evaluation**
1. The client maintains independence in activities of daily living (ADLs).
2. The client verbalizes relief of joint pain and discomfort.
3. The client maintains adequate nutrition.
4. The client maintains adequate muscle strength and ROM.
5. The client verbalizes understanding of the disease process, measures to prevent further decrease in function and movement, and prescribed medical treatments.
6. The client complies with the prescribed medical regimen.

VIII. **Lupus erythematosus (LE)**
A. **Description**
1. Systemic lupus erythematosus (SLE): a chronic systemic inflammatory disease affecting multiple body systems
2. Discoid lupus erythematosus (DLE): a form of lupus affecting the skin only

B. **Etiology and incidence**
1. SLE and DLE are thought to be autoimmune disorders.
2. SLE is the more common of the two; incidence is approximately 75 in 1 million people, with women affected at least 8

times more often than men and women of childbearing age particularly susceptible.

C. Pathophysiology and management

1. SLE involves markedly increased B-cell activity, hypergamma-globulinemia, autoantibody production, and decreased T-cell functions.
2. Symptoms result from immune complex invasion of body systems.
3. Disease progression is widely variable, characterized by recurring remissions and exacerbations.
4. Approximately 5% of clients with DLE develop SLE.
5. Prognosis is good with early detection and treatment; however, SLE can lead to potentially serious complications, including cardiovascular, renal, and neurologic problems and severe bacterial infections.
6. Treatment focuses on preventing complications and relieving inflammation.

D. Assessment findings

1. Clinical manifestations of SLE vary depending on the organs affected.
2. Early signs and symptoms may include:
   a. Fatigue, weakness
   b. Anorexia
   c. Occasional fever
   d. Joint stiffness
   e. Skin rash
3. Disease progression typically produces:
   a. Characteristic "butterfly" rash on face
   b. Skin eruptions on trunk or extremities
   c. Alopecia
   d. Photosensitivity
4. Associated manifestations may include:
   a. Raynaud's phenomenon
   b. Arthritis and deformity
   c. Polymyositis, peripheral vasculitis with hypertension
   d. Pericarditis, pericardial effusion
   e. Renal failure
   f. Nausea, vomiting, abdominal pain
   g. Signs and symptoms of pneumonitis, pleuritis, chronic obstructive pulmonary disease, interstitial fibrosis
   h. Psychosis, convulsions
5. DLE is marked by characteristic raised, red, scaling plaques, most commonly on the face, scalp, ears, neck, and other parts of the body exposed to sunlight.

      6. Laboratory studies may reveal:
         a. Anemia, thrombocytopenia, leukocytosis, or leukopenia
         b. LE cells in blood
         c. Positive anti-Sm and anti-DNA cell tests
         d. Proteinuria, cellular casts in urine
         e. False-positive rapid plasma reagin (RPR) test
         f. Increased ANA

E. **Nursing diagnoses**
    1. Body Image Disturbance
    2. Altered Tissue Perfusion: Renal
    3. Ineffective Breathing Pattern
    4. Decreased Cardiac Output
    5. Ineffective Individual Coping
    6. Risk for Fluid Volume Deficit
    7. Altered Nutrition: Less than body requirements
    8. Pain
    9. Altered Role Performance
    10. Self Esteem Disturbance
    11. Sensory and Perceptual Alterations
    12. Impaired Skin Integrity

F. **Planning and implementation**
    1. Aim interventions at retarding the inflammatory process.
    2. Administer nonsteroidal antiinflammatory drugs, salicylates, and corticosteroids as prescribed (see Section II.D).
    3. Keep skin clean and dry; apply topical ointments as prescribed.
    4. Inspect the skin for vasculitic lesions.
    5. Provide meticulous mouth care.
    6. Promote frequent rest periods to decrease fatigue.
    7. Convey empathy and reassurance to the client.
    8. Arrange for a dietary consult to ensure optimal nutrition while meeting the client's need for soft, easily tolerated foods.
    9. Relieve joint pain and stiffness by applying warm packs as needed.
    10. Maintain mobility and strength by instituting an appropriate exercise program.
    11. Provide client teaching, covering:
         a. Basic pathophysiology of the disease and its progression
         b. Purpose, effects, dosage, administration, side effects, and interactions of all prescribed medications
         c. Importance of follow-up care and of monitoring for and reporting new symptoms
         d. The need to consult a physician before receiving immunizations or taking birth control pills or over-the-counter drugs

    e.   Recommended and prohibited activities

    f.   Necessary lifestyle changes, such as avoiding sun and ultraviolet light exposure

    g.   Available community support groups

G. Evaluation

1. The client reports relief from joint pain and discomfort.
2. The client displays clean, dry skin with little or no itching, scaling, infections, or ulcerations.
3. The client reports acceptable energy level with minimal weakness and fatigue.
4. The client demonstrates adequate nutritional status.
5. The client verbalizes understanding of the disease process, prevention of infection, and treatment of exacerbations.

IX. Hypogammaglobulinemia

A. Description: primary humoral immunodeficiency marked by inadequate gamma globulin in the blood and associated with decreased resistance to infection

B. Etiology and incidence

1. X-linked hypogammaglobulinemia is a congenital disorder inherited via a gene located on the X chromosome.
2. The disorder affects male infants almost exclusively; incidence is about 1 in 50,000 to 100,000 births.
3. Unlike the X-linked form, acquired hypogammaglobulinemia is of unknown etiology, typically appears between ages 15 and 35, and affects males and females about equally.

C. Pathophysiology and management

1. In X-linked infantile hypogammaglobulinemia, B cells and B-cell precursors in the bone marrow and blood fail, for some unknown reason, to mature and secrete immunoglobulin.
2. In acquired hypogammaglobulinemia, most clients have a normal circulating B-cell count but deficient immunoglobulin synthesis or release.
3. Treatment involves infection prevention and medication therapy.

D. Assessment findings

1. Manifestations of hypogammaglobulinemia include:

    a.   Severe, recurrent bacterial infections; acute in X linked, chronic in acquired

    b.   Possibly signs and symptoms of associated SLE, rheumatoid arthritis, or vasculitis

2. Laboratory and diagnostic tests may reveal:

    a.   Low or absent IgG, IgA, IgM, IgE, IgD

    b.   Deficiency of B lymphocytes in congenital disease, no plasma cells in acquired disease

> c. Depleted B-cell germinal centers seen on lymph node biopsy

E. Nursing diagnosis: Risk for Infection

F. Planning and implementation

1. Prevent and treat bacterial infection as indicated.
2. Administer gamma globulin as prescribed (see Section II.D).
3. Administer antibiotics as prescribed (see Section II.D).
4. While the client is hospitalized, provide protective isolation to guard against nosocomial infections.
5. Provide client teaching, covering:
   a. Basic pathophysiology of immune deficiency
   b. Recognition and prevention of bacterial infections
   c. Signs and symptoms for which to seek medical assistance
   d. Purpose, effect, dosage, administration, side effects, and interactions of all prescribed medications
   e. The need for continued medical follow-up

G. Evaluation

1. The client demonstrates decreased incidence of recurrent bacterial infections.
2. The client verbalizes understanding of the disorder, infection prevention, and treatment.
3. The client complies with the therapeutic regimen.

X. Primary IgA deficiency

A. Description: a primary humoral immunodeficiency of IgA

B. Etiology and incidence

1. IgA deficiency seems to involve autosomal dominant or recessive inheritance.
2. It is the most common immunoglobulin deficiency, with incidence as high as 1 in 800 persons.

C. Pathophysiology and management

1. The primary mechanism in IgA deficiency appears to be abnormal terminal differentiation of IgA-bearing B cells.
2. Usually a benign disorder, IgA deficiency has been associated with increased incidence of:
   a. Bacterial infections
   b. Coexisting autoimmune disorders (e.g., SLE, rheumatoid arthritis)
   c. Allergic disorders (e.g., asthma, allergic rhinitis)
   d. Increased susceptibility to cancer
3. Treatment includes infection prevention, education, and medications.

D. Assessment findings

1. Many clients remain asymptomatic throughout a normal life-span.

       2. Possible manifestations include:
          a.   Chronic respiratory infection
          b.   Respiratory allergy
          c.   GI disorders (e.g., celiac disease, ulcerative colitis)
          d.   Signs and symptoms of autoimmune disorders
          e.   Signs and symptoms of malignant tumors (e.g., squamous cell carcinoma of the lungs, thymoma)
       3. Laboratory tests typically reveal:
          a.   Low IgA level (<5 mg/dL)
          b.   Normal IgG level
          c.   Normal or elevated IgM level

E. **Nursing diagnosis: Risk for Infection**
F. **Planning and implementation**
       1. See the sections of this text covering specific allergic disorders or autoimmune disorders as applicable.
       2. **Administer antibiotics as prescribed. Check for allergies.**
       3. Determine any known allergies before administering any medication or applying lotions, soaps, or creams.
       4. Provide client teaching, covering:
          a.   Basic pathophysiology of immune deficiency and associated autoimmune disorders
          b.   Ways to avoid exposure to allergens
          c.   How to recognize and prevent bacterial infections
          d.   Signs and symptoms to watch for and report
          e.   Purpose, effects, dosage, method of administration, side effects, and interactions of all prescribed medications
          f.   The importance of follow-up care
          g.   The increased susceptibility to anaphylaxis associated with blood transfusions
          h.   Early cancer detection measures

G. **Evaluation**
       1. The client remains free of bacterial infection.
       2. The client verbalizes understanding of the disorder, infection prevention, and treatment.
       3. The client complies with the therapeutic regimen.

XI. **Acquired immunodeficiency syndrome (AIDS)**
    A. **Description: severe immunodeficiency caused by the human immunodeficiency virus (HIV), which allows normally benign organisms to flourish and cause disease**
    B. **Etiology and incidence**
       1. **HIV is transmitted sexually and through direct contact with blood or blood products.**

2. Persons at risk for contracting HIV include:
    a. Anyone who engages in unprotected sexual activity with an infected partner
    b. Hemophiliacs and other recipients of transfused blood or blood components
    c. Intravenous drug abusers
    d. Children (perinatally) of mothers with HIV

C. Pathophysiology and management
1. HIV can be isolated from blood, semen, saliva, tears, breast milk, and cerebrospinal fluid.
2. After infection, the incubation period of HIV ranges from 6 months to 5 years, with an average of 2 years.
3. The clinical spectrum of AIDs encompasses:
    a. Persons who are HIV-seropositive and asymptomatic
    b. Persons with AIDS-related complex (ARC)
    c. Persons with AIDS who suffer from opportunistic diseases
4. To date, no cure or vaccine has been found. Treatment focuses on maintaining health and improving survival time.

D. Assessment findings
1. Health history findings may include recurring viral and bacterial infections.
2. Clinical manifestations may include:
    a. Fatigue
    b. Fever, night sweats
    c. Weight loss
    d. Generalized lymphadenopathy
    e. Nonproductive cough, shortness of breath
    f. Skin lesions, dry skin, pallor
    g. GI upset, chronic diarrhea
    h. Edema
    i. Visual impairment
    j. Painful oral lesions
    k. Bruising and bleeding tendencies
    l. Joint pain
3. Laboratory studies may reveal presence of HIV in serum.
4. Associated conditions may include:
    a. Opportunistic infections, such as *Pneumocystis carinii* pneumonia, mycobacterial infections, cryptococcus, toxoplasmosis, histoplasmosis, and cytomegalovirus
    b. Kaposi's sarcoma, AIDS-related lymphoma
    c. Neurologic deficits, AIDS dementia
    d. HIV wasting syndrome

E. **Nursing diagnoses**
1. Activity Intolerance
2. Ineffective Airway Clearance
3. Ineffective Individual Coping
4. Ineffective Family Coping
5. Diarrhea
6. Fear
7. Risk for Fluid Volume Deficit
8. Impaired Gas Exchange
9. Anticipatory Grieving
10. Altered Nutrition: Less than body requirements
11. Pain
12. Self Care Deficit
13. Self Esteem Disturbance
14. Impaired Skin Integrity
15. Social Isolation

F. **Planning and implementation**
1. Direct care toward maintaining optimal health and preventing complications.

 2. **Follow universal precautions to protect yourself from exposure to the client's blood or body fluids and to protect the client from cross-contamination.**
3. Monitor vital signs, ECG tracings, other vital functions as necessary.
4. Monitor respiratory functions: lung sounds, skin color, respiratory effort, sputum production.
5. Administer oxygen as prescribed.
6. Position the client to maximize lung expansion and ease breathing.
7. Administer prescribed medications as appropriate.
   a. Provide antimicrobial agents such as azidothymidine (AZT), an antiviral agent that inhibits HIV reproduction in cells, or trimethoprim-sulfamethoxazole (TMP/SMZ) (Bactrim) an antiinfective agent used to treat AIDS-related infections.
   b. **Give narcotic analgesics as prescribed to help decrease pain. Remember to monitor vital signs.**
   c. **Administer antianxiety agents such as alprazolam (Xanax), which depresses the central nervous system and decreases anxiety. Teach the client how to prevent or deal with orthostatic hypotension.**
   d. Deliver antipyretics (such as acetaminophen), which act on the hypothalamic heat-regulating center to decrease body temperature.

8. Monitor and record daily weight and intake and output.
9. Promote increased fluid intake; maintain IV fluid infusion if necessary.
10. Promote good nutrition; provide preferred foods, maintain tube feeding if necessary.
11. Administer antiemetics and antidiarrheals as requested.
12. Keep the client's skin clean and dry.
13. Turn or reposition the client every 2 hours; provide an antipressure mattress as necessary.
14. Apply protective barriers to the skin as necessary.
15. Help the client maintain as normal an environment as possible while hospitalized (e.g., pictures and items from home).
16. Allow the client adequate time to visit with family, friends, and other support persons; encourage open communication of feelings and fears.
17. Promote a balanced schedule of sleep, rest, and activity.
18. Provide for psychological and spiritual counseling as requested.
19. Support the client and others throughout the grieving process.
20. Teach the client and others about:
    a. Basic pathophysiology and progression of disease
    b. Purpose, effects, dosage, administration method, and side effects of all prescribed medications
    c. Principles of nutrition and the importance of maintaining optimal nutrition high in protein and calories
    d. Good hygiene practices and their importance
    e. Prevention and early detection of opportunistic infection
    f. Methods to prevent spread of HIV to others
    g. Signs and symptoms to report to the physician
    h. The importance of follow-up care
    i. Names and locations of local AIDS support groups

G. Evaluation
    1. The client remains free of opportunistic infection and respiratory problems.
    2. The client exhibits relief of symptoms such as fatigue, fever, night sweats, weight loss, diarrhea.
    3. The client maintains skin and oral mucosa integrity.
    4. The client maintains adequate nutritional status and fluid and electrolyte balance.
    5. The client reports relief of pain and discomfort, joint pain, nausea, abdominal pain.
    6. The client maintains an acceptable activity level without undue fatigue.
    7. The client exhibits decreased anxiety.

8. The client and family members or significant others verbalize understanding of the disease process, infection prevention measures, and treatments.
9. The client and family members or significant others progress through the grieving process.
10. The client and family members or significant others demonstrate appropriate coping mechanisms and use of support systems.
11. The client and family members or significant others verbalize acceptance of imminent death.
12. The client complies with the therapeutic regimen, including precautions to prevent disease transmission.

Bibliography

Bolander, V. R. (1994). *Sorensen & Luckmann's basic nursing: A physiologic approach* (3rd ed.). Philadelphia: W. B. Saunders.

Clark, J., Queener, S., & Karb, V. (1990). *Pharmacologic basis of nursing practice* (4th ed.). St. Louis: C. V. Mosby.

Cotran, R. S., Kumar, V., & Robbins, S. L. (1994). *Robbins pathologic basis of disease* (5th ed.). Philadelphia: W. B. Saunders.

Flaskerud, J. H., and Ungvarski, P. J. (1995). *HIV/AIDS: A guide to nursing care* (3rd ed.). Philadelphia: W. B. Saunders.

Guyton, A. C. (1992). *Human physiology and mechanisms of disease* (5th ed.). Philadelphia: W. B. Saunders.

Hood, G. H., & Dincher, J. R. (1992). *Total patient care: Foundations and practice* (8th ed.). St. Louis: C. V. Mosby.

Nettina, S. (1996). *The Lippincott manual of nursing practice* (6th ed.). Philadelphia: Lippincott-Raven Publishers.

Smeltzer, S. C., & Bare, B. G. (1996). *Brunner & Suddarth's textbook of medical-surgical nursing* (8th ed.). Philadelphia: Lippincott-Raven Publishers.

Sodeman, W. A., & Sodeman, T. M. (1985). *Pathologic physiology: Mechanisms of disease* (7th ed.). Philadelphia: W. B. Saunders.

Springhouse Corporation. (1992). *Nursing student's guide to drugs*. Springhouse, PA: Springhouse Corp.

STUDY QUESTIONS

1. Anaphylaxis is mediated by
   a. IgG
   b. IgM
   c. IgA
   d. IgE

2. A client diagnosed with *Pneumocystis carinii* pneumonia secondary to AIDS is crying over the loss of friends and family members who won't talk to the client anymore. Which of the following would be the nurse's best action?
   a. Advise the client not to worry and tell him everything will be all right.
   b. Ask the physician for a psychiatric consult to assess the client's mental functioning.
   c. Sit down and listen to the client's concerns and frustrations.
   d. Tell the client that the friends probably weren't true friends anyway if they would abandon the client like this.

3. Which of the following behaviors best demonstrates that a client diagnosed with primary IgA deficiency understands the instruction provided by the nurse?
   a. The client has no questions about home care.
   b. The client returns to the clinic the next time that signs and symptoms of a bacterial infection occur.
   c. The client calls at least twice weekly to report progress and ask questions.
   d. The client returns to the clinic regularly for follow-up and, although infections continue to occur, they are detected early and no hospitalization is required.

4. A client diagnosed with rheumatoid arthritis complains about joints that always hurt and says, "I just feel like staying in bed all day." Nursing interventions aimed toward maintaining as much function as possible would include

   a. refraining from exercise because it only aggravates the disease process
   b. applying elastic bandage wraps to all joints to increase the client's pain threshold
   c. maintaining a supine position most of the day so that the joints will not be stressed by weight bearing
   d. promoting aquatic (water) exercises to enhance joint mobility

5. When caring for a client with hypogammaglobulinemia, the nurse should anticipate preparing the client for which of the following diagnostic tests?
   a. erythrocyte sedimentation rate (ESR)
   b. antinuclear antibodies (ANA)
   c. lymph node biopsy
   d. skin biopsy for Kaposi's sarcoma

6. A client is started on immunotherapy for allergies. After the first injection the nurse notes a large red wheal on the client's arm, coughing, and expiratory wheezing. What should the nurse do first?
   a. Notify the physician of what is happening.
   b. Administer IM epinephrine per protocol for anaphylaxis.
   c. Begin oxygen by way of nasal cannula.
   d. Start an IV for medication administration.

7. Medication discharge teaching for the client who is using a steroidal cream for allergic dermatoses includes instructing the client to
   a. apply an occlusive dressing over the inflamed area after applying the cream
   b. wash hands before and after applying the cream
   c. not wash the inflamed area before applying the cream
   d. clean the inflamed area with alcohol before applying the steroidal cream

8. Which of the following nursing diagnoses would be most appropriate for a

client hospitalized with complications of SLE, such as vasculitis?
   a. Functional Incontinence
   b. Impaired Swallowing
   c. Urinary Retention
   d. Altered Tissue Perfusion: Renal

9. Protective clothing for a nurse assisting a physician with the insertion of a central line in a client with AIDS would include:
   a. gloves, mask, goggles (or face shield), and a gown or apron
   b. gown and gloves
   c. mask, gloves, and a gown or apron
   d. mask and gloves

10. A client diagnosed with hypogammaglobulinemia is scheduled for elective surgery to repair a ventral hernia. A priority nursing diagnosis during this client's hospitalization would be
   a. Fatigue
   b. Risk for Fluid Volume Deficit
   c. Risk for Infection
   d. Decreased Cardiac Output

11. A client who was stung by a bee now exhibits redness and swelling in the hand and forearm. The nurse should be sure to explain that
   a. Baking soda is the best treatment for a bee sting.
   b. The client may be hypersensitive to bee stings and might consider purchasing an anti-sting kit.
   c. The client shouldn't worry; people can't develop an allergy to bee stings.
   d. The client should have regular check-ups to determine the status of allergy to bee stings.

12. The nurse is about to administer an antiinfective agent, cefaclor (Ceclor), to a client who has primary IgA deficiency and otitis media. Before administration, the nurse should check

   a. the chest radiograph
   b. the client's history of previous illness
   c. the client's history for any known allergies
   d. the medical record for any other current infections

13. A client is complaining of a runny nose, itching, and burning eyes and sneezing since visiting a friend who had a cat in the home. These findings and symptoms are consistent with
   a. allergic rhinitis
   b. anaphylaxis
   c. bronchitis
   d. asthma

14. A client diagnosed with AIDS has had chronic diarrhea for the last 6 months and has lost 18 pounds in that time. Besides weight loss, assessment findings disclose tented skin turgor, dry mucous membranes, and listlessness. Which of the following nursing diagnoses focuses attention on the client's most immediate problem?
   a. Fluid Volume Deficit related to diarrhea and abnormal fluid loss
   b. Altered Nutrition: Less than body requirements
   c. Altered Thought Processes related to CNS effects of disease
   d. Diarrhea related to the disease process and acute infection

15. An AIDS client who has had chronic diarrhea, anorexia, a history of oral candidiasis, and weight loss needs dietary teaching. The teaching should focus on
   a. eating a low-protein, high-carbohydrate diet
   b. eating three large meals per day
   c. eating only unpasteurized diary products
   d. eating a high-protein, high-calorie diet

ANSWER KEY

1. **Correct response: d**
   IgE is associated with allergic and hypersensitivity reactions.
   a and b. IgG and IgM in Type II are associated with cytotoxic reactions.
   c. IgA is present in body fluids such as blood, saliva, and tears.
   Knowledge/Physiologic/Assessment

2. **Correct response: c**
   The client is beginning to express concerns to the nurse; active, nonjudgmental listening can help build a relationship of trust. The other choices are inappropriate.
   a. Providing false reassurance will not help the client cope.
   b. Further assessment is needed to determine whether a psychiatric consult should be considered.
   d. Discounting the client's feelings and giving advice would hinder development of a therapeutic relationship.
   Comprehension/Psychosocial/
   Implementation

3. **Correct response: d**
   The client is receiving follow-up care, and infections are detected early, indicating that the client understands the disease process.
   a. Not asking questions does not necessarily indicate understanding.
   b. Going in only after developing another bout of pneumonia may indicate that the client still does not understand the importance of early detection and prevention of infection.
   c. Constant questions could indicate the need for further explanation.
   Analysis/Health promotion/Evaluation

4. **Correct response: d**
   Water exercises are excellent because the water promotes buoyancy which eases joint movement.
   a and c. Persons with rheumatoid arthritis should maintain an active exercise program to strengthen and preserve muscle movement.
   b. Heat or cold applications, which promote circulation and reduce swelling, may help relieve pain, but elastic bandage wraps may not.
   Application/Safe care/Planning

5. **Correct response: c**
   A lymph node biopsy will show depleted B-cell germinal centers in hypogammaglobulinemia.
   a. ESR is used to detect inflammatory processes.
   b. ANA are measured to detect autoimmune disease.
   d. Kaposi's sarcoma is usually associated with AIDS.
   Knowledge/Physiologic/Assessment

6. **Correct response: b**
   Immediately give 0.2 to 0.5 mL of 1:1000 epinephrine IM.
   a, c, and d. These other interventions will follow.
   Comprehension/Physiologic/
   Implementation

7. **Correct response: b**
   The inflamed area is prone to infection. Before applying medication to it, the inflamed area and the hands should be washed. After application, the medication should be washed off the hands so that it will not be transferred to the eyes, skin, or other areas.
   a. The inflamed area is usually left open to air or a light gauze dressing is used (not occlusive).
   c and d. The inflamed area should be cleaned with water, not alcohol.
   Knowledge/Safe care/Planning

8. **Correct response: d**
   Decreased renal perfusion (as well as GI and peripheral perfusion) is typically present from vasculitis.
   a and b. Although problems associated with SLE commonly affect renal function, neither urinary reten-

tion nor incontinence typically occurs.

  c. Impaired swallowing is associated
with other diseases (e.g., myasthenia
gravis), not with SLE.

Comprehension/Physiologic/
Analysis (Dx)

9. **Correct response: c**
Although this is an invasive procedure,
it is not likely to generate droplets or
blood splashes; thus, protective goggles
may be advisable but not necessary.

  a. Goggles may be advisable but not
necessary.

  b and d. Do not include all the necessary protection.

Application/Safe care/Implementation

10. **Correct response: c**
A client with hypogammaglobulinemia
is at increased risk for nosocomial infections while hospitalized and therefore
should be in protective isolation.

  a, b, and d. These other diagnoses
would not be expected for this
surgery nor specifically for this
client.

Application/Health promotion/
Analysis (Dx)

11. **Correct response: b**
This client has experienced a moderate
reaction to the bee sting and may be
hypersensitive and should have access
to an anti-sting kit in the event she
should be stung again.

  a, c, and d. These interventions are all
inappropriate.

Application/Health promotion/Planning

12. **Correct response: c**
For a client with primary IgA deficiency, it is important to identify any allergies before administering medications.

  a, b, and d. Chest radiograph and history of illness or infection are irrele-
vant to medication administration.

Application/Safe care/Implementation

13. **Correct response: a**
This client most likely is suffering from
allergic rhinitis triggered by the friend's
cat.

  b. Anaphylaxis is an acute, life-threatening allergic reaction.

  c and d. Bronchitis and asthma produce symptoms in the lower respiratory tract.

Application/Physiologic/Assessment

14. **Correct response: a**
This client's most pressing problem is
dehydration due to the diarrhea.

  b, c, and d. These other problems, although they may occur, are of lower
priority than dehydration.

Analysis/Health promotion/
Analysis (Dx)

15. **Correct response: d**
Teaching should include this in addition to small, frequent meals and low-
microbial foods (e.g., pasteurized dairy
products, washed and peeled fruits and
vegetables, and well-cooked meats).

  a, b, and c. These instructions are all
inappropriate for this client.

Analysis/Physiologic/Planning

Integumentary Disorders

Note: This chapter does not discuss all disorders with significant skin involvement. Refer to the appropriate chapters in this text for information on the following skin disorders:

▶ Candidiasis: Chapter 20, Infectious Disorders
▶ Pressure sores: Chapter 22, Gerontologic Nursing

I. Integumentary system

A. Structures

1. **The body's largest organ, the skin has three layers:**
   a. **Subcutaneous layer, or hypodermis**
   b. **Dermis**
   c. **Epidermis**
2. Subcutaneous layer
   a. Consisting of loose connective tissue and fat cells, the hypodermis anchors the skin to bone and muscle.
   b. It also provides shock absorbing and insulating actions.
   c. Anatomic distribution of this layer is a secondary sex characteristic, different in women and men.
3. Dermis
   a. The layer beneath the epidermis, the dermis primarily comprises collagen fibrils, which provide mechanical strength to the skin.
   b. The dermis also contains blood vessels, nerves, lymphatics, hair follicles, and sebaceous and sweat glands.
4. Epidermis
   a. This thin, avascular, outermost layer of skin is nourished by diffusion from blood vessels in the dermis.
   b. The epidermis contains two main types of cells: *melanocytes* and keratinocytes.
   c. Scattered throughout the basal layer of the epidermis, melanocytes produce melanin, a pigment that shields deeper skin structures from sunlight. People of all races have basically the same number of melanocytes; differences in skin color are due to differences in the size and distribution of melanosomes produced by melanocytes.
   d. *Keratinocytes* develop from cells in the basal layer, then mature and move to the skin surface (stratum corneum), where they flatten, dehydrate, and become keratinized. Alterations in this process account for many dermatologic problems.
5. Epidermal appendages, formed from epidermal cells anatomically located in both the epidermis and dermis, include:
   a. Hair
   b. Nails
   c. Glands (apocrine, eccrine, sebaceous)

6. Hair
   a. Hair growth occurs in phases: resting (telogen), growth (anagen), and atrophy (catagen).
   b. Scattered patterns of these phases keep the total number of hairs relatively constant.
   c. Chemical, mechanical, or physiologic factors can convert all hair to the atrophic phase, resulting in baldness.
   d. Hair follicles are distributed on all skin surfaces except the palms and soles.
   e. No new hair-producing structures are produced after birth.
   f. Scalp hair grows about 1 cm per month.
7. Nails grow from nail matrix; they are made of a specialized keratin that becomes dry and firm.
8. Apocrine glands
   a. Located in the axillae, areolae, groin, perineum, and circumanal and periumbilical regions, these large sweat glands are rudimentary structures with no known useful purpose.
   b. They respond to autonomic, rather than thermal, stimulation to produce odorless, viscous, milklike droplets that cause a distinctive body odor when acted on by the bacteria normally present on the skin surface.
9. Eccrine glands
   a. These small sweat glands, distributed in the skin all over the body, are true secretory glands that produce sweat, which functions in thermoregulation and other processes.
   b. Sweat is a clear, aqueous solution containing 99% water and 1% solids. Hypotonic under normal conditions, a high rate of sweating may produce isotonic concentrations.
   c. Sweat moves to the skin surface by way of sweat ducts.
   d. Nerve fibers to sweat glands liberate acetylcholine. Atropine and other anticholinergics block receptor sites from responding, interfering with secretion.
   e. At environmental temperatures above 32°C, sweating occurs over the entire body; at lower environmental temperatures, sweat glands periodically secrete microscopic droplets as part of the body's total insensible water loss.
   f. Sweat provides the skin with an "acid mantle" (average pH 5.7 to 6.4); acidity retards growth of many bacteria that reside in the epidermal layer, glands, and hair follicles.

10. Sebaceous glands

    a.   Most prevalent and largest on the face, scalp, upper chest, and back (and absent from the palms and soles), sebaceous glands secrete sebum, a complex lipid mixture that empties into hair shafts.

    b.   The male hormone androgen initiates and sustains sebum production.

B. **Function**

    1. Protective functions

        a.   The skin forms a barrier between the internal organs and the external environment.

        b.   It is continuous with mucous membranes at external openings of the digestive, respiratory, and genitourinary systems.

        c.   The normally acidic skin and perspiration protect against invasion by bacteria and foreign matter.

        d.   The thickened skin of the palms and soles provides a tough covering to protect from the constant trauma to these areas.

    2. Percutaneous absorption

        a.   The epidermis is relatively impermeable to most chemical substances although various lipids (fatty substances) may be absorbed through the skin (e.g., vitamins A and D and steroid hormones).

        b.   Substances enter through the epidermis (transepidermal route) or through orifices of hair follicles (follicular holes).

        c.   Lipid-soluble substances absorb through the skin fairly rapidly and completely; absorption appears to be faster for substances that also are water soluble.

        d.   The rate of absorption is comparable to that for substances in the GI tract or injected subcutaneously.

        e.   Pharmacologic application of this absorption is currently the subject of intense research and development since certain drugs (e.g., dimethyl sulfoxide) are chemically linked with substances known to penetrate the skin.

    3. Sensory functions

        a.   Receptor endings of nerves in the skin provide constant monitoring of the immediate environment.

        b.   The primary functions of these receptors include sensing coldness, warmth, pain, and touch pressure.

        c.   Each type of receptor nerve ending responds to only one kind of cutaneous sensation.

        d.   The density of receptors varies in different body areas (e.g., the fingertips and lips are high-density areas compared to the back).

e. The skin contains various types of sensory endings:

- ▶ Naked nerve endings, which mediate all four sensory modalities
- ▶ Free nonmyelinated nerve endings, which mediate pain sensation
- ▶ Expanded tips on sensory nerve terminals, which mediate touch (Merkel's disks) and warmth (Tuffini endings)
- ▶ Encapsulated nerve endings, which mediate pressure (Pacinian corpuscles), touch (Meissner's corpuscles), and cold (Krause's end-bulbs)

4. Vitamin D production
   a. Endogenous production of vitamin D, necessary for the synthesis of vitamin D critical to bone metabolism, occurs in the epidermis.
   b. Only a few minutes of sun exposure on a small body area are needed for this production to occur.

5. Barrier function
   a. The skin prevents water and electrolyte loss and moistens subcutaneous tissues.
   b. Small amounts of water—approximately 500 mL/day in adults, varying with body and environmental temperatures—continuously evaporate from the skin surface as insensible perspiration.
   c. During immersion in water, the skin can accumulate up to three to four times its weight in water.
   d. The skin surface normally is covered with microorganisms, especially bacteria such as *Staphylococcus epidermis* and diphtheroids; infection occurs when the balance between host and microorganisms is upset.
   e. Healthy persons can develop bacterial skin infections, but predisposing factors such as moisture, obesity, skin disease, systemic steroids and antibiotics, chronic disease, and diabetes mellitus increase risk.

6. Thermoregulatory functions
   a. **The body continuously produces heat as a by-product of cellular metabolism; this heat is dissipated locally, primarily through the skin.**
   b. **The body's internal core temperature normally is maintained at a constant 37.6°C through a balance between heat production and heat loss.**
   c. Three primary processes are involved in heat loss from the body to the external environment:

- ▶ *Radiation:* the body's ability to give off its heat to another object of lower temperature situated at a distance

> ▸ *Conduction:* transfer of heat from the body to a cooler object in direct contact
> ▸ *Convection:* heat transferred by conduction to the air surrounding the body removed by bulk movement of warm air molecules away from the body

    d.   The rate of heat loss depends primarily on the skin's surface temperature, which in turn depends on skin blood flow, regulated by neural mechanisms. Increased blood flow results in delivery of more heat to the skin and a greater rate of heat loss from the body; when body temperature falls, the skin's blood vessels constrict to reduce heat loss from the body.

    e.   Perspiration facilitates heat loss from the body; it is regulated by body temperature, environmental temperature and humidity, and neurologic factors such as response to emotional stress.

7.   Immunologic functions

    a.   Wheal and flare reaction

> ▸ Involves swelling (wheal) and diffuse redness due to increased temperature in area from stimulus; dependent on local neurologic mechanisms; dilation of arterioles and venules (flare) constitutes normal reaction to injury
> ▸ Wheal caused by increased capillary permeability induced by trauma as protein-containing fluid leaks out of capillaries locally to produce edema
> ▸ Reaction associated with release of histamine, bradykinin

    b.   Immune complexes

> ▸ Major deposition sites of immune complexes include the dermal–epidermal junction and dermal vessels of the skin.
> ▸ Deposition of immune complexes leads to fixation and activation of complement at tissue sites.
> ▸ Vasodilation and increased permeability result from anaphylatoxin components of C3 and C5; neutrophils and monocytes attracted by complement-generated chemotactic factors result in acute and perhaps chronic inflammation.

8.   Circulatory function

    a.   Changes in the cutaneous vascular system contribute significantly to systemic circulatory status.

    b.   Skin color depends in part on the quantity of blood in the small vessels; skin temperature depends chiefly on the rate of blood flow through the skin.

    c.   Stimulation of sympathetic fibers supplying the skin causes vasoconstriction of cutaneous vessels; interruption of these fibers results in vasodilation of small arteries and arterioles.

        d.   The cutaneous circulatory system also responds to chemical agents, such as:

            ► Acetylcholine, which causes vasodilation
            ► Norepinephrine, epinephrine, and vasopressin, which cause vasoconstriction

    9. Esthetic function
        a.   The skin also contributes to each person's unique appearance and identity.
        b.   Skin defects or problems can have negative effects on a person's body image and self-esteem.

II. Overview of integumentary system disorders

A. Assessment

    1. Nursing health history should focus on obtaining information about:
        a.   Normal hygienic practices
        b.   Usual patterns of sun exposure
        c.   Exposure to irritants
        d.   Radiation exposure
        e.   Allergies
        f.   Nutritional status, especially intake of protein and vitamins A, B complex, C, and K
    2. Important aspects of physical examination include:
        a.   Assessing skin color, texture, and turgor
        b.   Inspecting the skin for abnormal growths, lesions, rashes, scars, or discoloration
        c.   Noting any areas of scaliness or dryness
        d.   Inspecting for signs of skin infection

B. Diagnostic procedures

    1. Skin cultures and microscopic examination can identify infectious organisms.
    2. Skin biopsy and histologic examination is done for cancer diagnosis.

C. Psychosocial implications

    1. A person with a serious skin disorder may have coping difficulties related to:
        a.   Short- and long-term skin disruptions
        b.   Chronicity of the disorder (e.g., burns)
        c.   Uncertain prognosis (e.g., cancer)
    2. The client may have self-concept concerns related to fear of:
        a.   Body image changes
        b.   Rejection by others
        c.   Loss of a body part
        d.   Role changes toward increased dependence

3. The client also may have lifestyle concerns related to potential changes in physical ability; independence; work performance, with possibility of job loss; and self-care ability.
4. Disease-related changes in social interaction patterns can lead to such problems as isolation, depression, and hopelessness.

D. Medications used to treat skin problems (Additional medications may be included with specific disease)

1. *Topical corticosteroids,* which relieve or prevent inflammation and itching
   a. Examples: desoximetasone (Topicort), hydrocortisone (Dermacort), triamcinolone (Kenalog)
   b. Selected nursing considerations

   ► **Advise client to wash hands before and after application.**
   ► **Instruct client to clean affected area with warm water before application.**

2. *Systemic corticosteroids,* which relieve inflammation
   a. Examples: hydrocortisone (Hydrocortone), methylprednisolone (Medrol), methylprednisolone acetate (M-Prednisol), prednisone (Prednicen-M), dexamethasone (Decadron)
   b. Selected nursing considerations

   ► **Instruct client to take medication exactly as directed and to taper discontinuation of drug rather than stop abruptly, which could cause serious withdrawal symptoms leading to adrenal insufficiency, shock, and death.**

3. *Topical antibiotics,* which suppress the growth of *Propionibacterium acnes* and reduce surface free-fatty-acid levels
   a. Examples: tetracycline (Topicycline), erythromycin (Akne-Mycin)
   b. Selected nursing considerations

   ► **Advise client to wash hands before and after application.**
   ► **Instruct client to clean affected area with water before application.**

4. *Systemic antibiotics,* which kill bacteria to treat or prevent infection
   a. Examples: the penicillins, cloxacillin (Tegopen), tetracycline (Achromycin)
   b. Selected nursing considerations

   ► **Check client history for drug allergies before administering.**
   ► **For tetracycline: Take medication 1 hour before or 2 hours after consuming food or dairy products.**

5. *Topical vitamin A,* which speeds cellular turnover thereby clearing keratin plugs from the pilosebaceous ducts
   a.   Examples: tretinoin (Retin-A)
   b.   Selected nursing considerations

   ► Caution client to avoid sun exposure (cover up, and wear a hat or sunscreen).
   ► Explain that noticeable improvement may take from 8 to 12 weeks during which skin redness and peeling are common.

6. *Other topical agents (e.g., coal tar products),* which may slow pathologic processes
   a.   Examples: *anthralin* preparations (Anthra-Derm, Dritho-Creme) which retard overactive epidermis without affecting other tissues
   b.   Selected nursing considerations

   ► Apply with tongue blade or gloved hand; do not apply to normal skin.
   ► Caution the client that anthralin, a coal tar derivative, will temporarily stain the skin and clothing.

III.   Seborrheic dermatitis

A.   Description: a chronic, inflammatory, scaling eruption characterized by periodic remissions and exacerbations

B.   Etiology and incidence

   1.   Seborrheic dermatitis is associated with genetic predisposition and aggravated by physical or emotional stress.
   2.   It most commonly develops in middle-aged or older people as multiple lesions occurring chiefly on the scalp, face, or trunk.

C.   Pathophysiology and management

   1.   Seborrhea refers to excessive production of sebum by sebaceous glands.
   2.   The typical clinical picture involves lifelong recurrences persisting for weeks, months, or even years.
   3.   Typical management measures involve prevention and supportive care.

D.   Assessment findings

   1.   Common clinical manifestations include:
      a.   Scaling (dry, moist, or greasy), predominantly in areas where glands are normally found in large numbers (e.g., trunk, face, scalp) and in skin folds
      b.   Patches of sallow, greasy-appearing skin with or without scaling and slight erythema
      c.   Pruritus and pain
   2.   Diagnosis must rule out psoriasis.

E.   Nursing diagnoses

   1.   Body Image Disturbance
   2.   Pain
   3.   Impaired Skin Integrity

F.   Planning and implementation

   1.   Remove any external irritants.
   2.   Instruct the client to avoid excessive heat and perspiration.
   3.   Tell the client to avoid scratching and rubbing affected areas.

G.   Evaluation: Client demonstrates absence of symptoms.

IV.   Noninfectious inflammatory dermatoses

A.   Description

   1.   *Psoriasis:* a chronic inflammatory disease marked by epidermal proliferation
   2.   *Exfoliative dermatitis:* a serious skin disorder characterized by progressive inflammation
   3.   *Pemphigus vulgaris:* a serous autoimmune skin disease marked by blisters on the skin and mucous membranes
   4.   *Toxic epidermal necrolysis (TEN):* a rare, potentially fatal skin disorder marked by epidermal erythema, necrosis, and skin erosions

B.   Etiology and incidence

   1.   Psoriasis appears to be a hereditary defect. It affects about 2% of the population in the United States; incidence is highest in whites.
   2.   The many possible causes of exfoliative dermatitis include:
      a.   A secondary or reactive response to an underlying skin disease
      b.   Lymphoma disease (may accompany or precede lymphoma)
      c.   Severe reaction to various drugs (e.g., sulfonamides, penicillins, anticonvulsants, analgesics)
   3.   Pemphigus vulgaris is an autoimmune disorder of unknown etiology.
   4.   The etiology of TEN is unknown but is probably related to immune function, as a reaction to drug ingestion or possibly secondary to viral infection.

C.   Assessment findings

   1.   Psoriasis is marked by:
      a.   Profuse, erythematous scales or plaques, often covering large areas of the body
      b.   Pruritus and sometimes pain
      c.   Possibly arthritic symptoms (e.g., joint stiffness)
   2.   Manifestations of exfoliative dermatitis include:
      a.   Skin effects: patchy or generalized erythematous erup-

tion (initially), followed by characteristic scaling, possibly with hair loss and nail shedding

    b.   Systemic effects: possible severe fluid and electrolyte imbalance, anemia, systemic infections

    3.   Pemphigus vulgaris produces:

        a.   Widespread bullae on the skin and mucous membranes that enlarge and rupture, leaving denuded areas that eventually form crusts

        b.   Possible fluid and electrolyte imbalance, systemic infection, or impaired nutrition, which may lead to critical illness requiring frequent hospitalization

    4.   Manifestations of TEN include:

        a.   Formation of large, flaccid bullae in some areas with shedding of large sheets of epidermis (along with toenails, fingernails, eyebrows, and eyelashes) in others

        b.   Possibly serious fluid and electrolyte imbalance and systemic infection that may lead to sepsis

D. **Nursing diagnoses**

    1.   Body Image Disturbance

    2.   Risk for Fluid Volume Deficit

    3.   Risk for Infection

    4.   Knowledge Deficit

    5.   Impaired Skin Integrity

E. **Planning and implementation**

    1.   Take steps to promote healing and prevent infection.

    2.   Relieve pain as indicated.

    3.   Maintain or restore fluid and electrolyte imbalance.

    4.   Teach the client about:

        a.   The nature of the disorder, its treatment, and prognosis

        b.   Prescribed medications

    5.   For the client with *psoriasis:*

        a.   Advise the client receiving systemic cytotoxic (e.g., methotrexate) therapy (inhibiting DNA synthesis in epidermal cells so as to speed the replacement of psoriatic cells) to continue taking the medication even if nausea and vomiting occur, to increase fluid intake to prevent nephrotoxicity, and to avoid alcoholic beverages.

        b.   Inform the client taking oral retinoids (such as vitamin A) that these agents modulate the growth and differentiation of epithelial tissue and show promise in treating psoriasis.

        c.   **Instruct the client to avoid sun exposure during photochemotherapy. This regimen of oral psoralens and phototherapy with ultraviolet A light (known as PUVA therapy) decreases cellular proliferation.**

PUVA therapy results in photosensitivity so the client should avoid exposure to sunlight during this time.

d. Show the client how to apply topical agents such as anthralin (see Section II.D).

6. For the client with *exfoliative dermatitis:*
   a. Explain how to take prescribed corticosteroids (see Section II.D).
   b. Provide instruction about prescribed antibiotics based on culture and sensitivity findings (see Section II.D).

7. For the client with *pemphigus vulgaris:*
   a. Discuss how to take prescribed high-dose corticosteroids to control the disease and keep the skin free of blisters (see Section II.D).
   b. Caution the client taking immunosuppressive agents, such as azathioprine (Imuran) or cyclophosphamide (Cytoxan) to report signs of serious organ dysfunction, such as flulike symptoms, clay-colored stools, or dark urine, to the physician. These medications are used to control disease and reduce the amount of corticosteroid therapy.
   c. If plasmapheresis is recommended, explain that this treatment is a reinfusion of specially treated plasma cells which temporarily decreases serum antibody concentration. The success rate of the process varies.

8. For the client with *TEN:*
   a. Administer systemic antibiotics to treat or prevent infection, which is the major cause of death in TEN.
   b. Also administer topical bacteriostatic agents, such as silver nitrate solution or nitrofurazone (Furacin) to prevent wound sepsis.

F. Evaluation
1. The client remains free of acute infection.
2. The client exhibits intact or only minimally disrupted skin integrity.
3. The client experiences fewer episodes of exacerbation.
4. The client demonstrates adequate fluid balance.
5. The client exhibits healthy adaptation to body image changes.

V. **Acne vulgaris**
   A. **Description: an inflammatory disease of the sebaceous follicles**
   B. **Etiology and incidence**
   1. Etiology appears to involve multiple factors, including genetics, hormonal factors, and bacterial infection.
   2. Diet does not affect incidence or severity.

   3. Incidence is highest at puberty although it may occur as early as age 8 and persist into adulthood in some people.
   C. **Pathophysiology and management**
   1. Acne eruptions are initiated by increased sebum production activated by androgenic hormones.
   2. Sebum is secreted into dilated hair follicles containing normal skin bacteria, such as *Propionibacterium acnes.*
   3. The bacteria secrete the enzyme lipase, which reacts with sebum to produce free fatty acids, which in turn trigger inflammation.
   4. At the same time, keratin produced by the hair follicles combines with sebum to form plugs in dilated follicles.
   D. **Assessment findings**
   1. Acne lesions may include closed comedones (whiteheads), open comedones (blackheads), papules, pustules, nodules, and cysts.
   2. Primary sites include the face, chest, shoulders, and upper back.
   E. **Nursing diagnoses**
   1. Body Image Disturbance
   2. Risk for Infection
   3. Impaired Skin Integrity
   F. **Planning and implementation**
   1. Encourage compliance with the prescribed topical therapy.
      a. **Point out that acne products containing benzoyl peroxide produce rapid and sustained reduction of inflamed lesions by depressing sebum production. Explain that these products initially cause skin redness and scaling but that the skin adjusts quickly.**
      b. Instruct the client about correctly using topical agents, such as vitamin A acid (Retin A) and antibiotics such as tetracycline (Akne-Mycin) (see Section II.D).
      c. Discuss use of any prescribed systemic antibiotics (see Section II.D).
   2. Advise the client that heat, humidity, and perspiration exacerbate acne.
   G. **Evaluation**
   1. The client exhibits resolution of acne lesions.
   2. The client remains free of infection.
VI. **Bacterial infections (pyodermas)**
   A. **Description and etiology**
   1. *Impetigo:* superficial skin infection caused by streptococci, staphylococci, or multiple bacteria; especially common in children living in poor hygienic conditions

2. *Folliculitis:* staphylococcal infection arising in hair follicles
3. *Furuncle (boil):* acute inflammation arising deep in one or more hair follicles and spreading into surrounding dermis
4. *Carbuncle:* abscess of skin and subcutaneous tissue representing extension of a large, deep-seated furuncle that has invaded several follicles

B. **Assessment findings**
1. *Impetigo* begins as small, red maculas and rapidly progresses to discrete, thin-walled vesicles; these vesicles rupture and become covered with a loosely adherent, honey-yellow crust.
2. *Folliculitis* produces single or multiple, superficial or deep papules or pustules close to hair follicles.
3. A *furuncle* is marked by tenderness, pain, surrounding cellulitis, and, after the furuncle localizes, a boggy center with a yellow or white head on the skin surface.
4. A *carbuncle* is marked by skin abscess along with such systemic symptoms as fever, pain, prostration, and leukocytosis.

C. **Nursing diagnoses**
1. Risk for Infection
2. Impaired Skin Integrity
3. Pain

D. **Planning and implementation**
1. Administer and teach about prescribed systemic antibiotics which treat or prevent infection after the first line of defense has been disrupted (see Section II.D).
2. Isolate drainage in severe cases of folliculitis, furuncles, or carbuncles.

E. **Evaluation**
1. The client reports reduction of pain.
2. The client remains free of infection.
3. The client's skin heals without inflammation.

VII. Herpes zoster (shingles)

A. **Description: an acute viral infection marked by painful vesicular skin eruptions**

B. **Etiology and incidence**
1. Herpes zoster is caused by the varicella-zoster virus (V-Z), which also causes varicella (chicken pox).
2. Incidence is greatest in adults older than age 50.

C. **Pathophysiology and management**
1. Herpes zoster results from reactivation of latent V-Z virus that has lain dormant since a previous episode of varicella. The cause of reactivation is unknown.
2. Treatment is medical and palliative.

D. **Assessment findings**
1. Herpes zoster is marked by painful vesicular eruptions along the route of inflamed nerves from one or more posterior ganglia.
2. Eruption is preceded and accompanied by itching and pain, which may radiate over entire region supplied by involved nerves.

E. **Nursing diagnoses**
1. Pain
2. Impaired Skin Integrity

F. **Planning and implementation**
1. Control pain with appropriate medications, and reduce itching with medications and topical lotions.

$\boldsymbol{m}$ **2. Administer acyclovir (Zovirax) systemically. This antiviral medication inhibits viral multiplication by affecting the DNA. Forewarn the client that the drug helps manage disease but does not cure it or prevent it from spreading.**

G. **Evaluation**
1. The client reports absence of pain.
2. The client displays intact skin without vesicular eruption.

VIII. **Parasitic skin diseases**

A. **Description and etiology**
1. Pediculosis—infestation by lice—involves three different parasites:
   a. *Pediculus humanus capitis* (head louse)
   b. *Pediculus humanus corporis* (body louse)
   c. *Phthirus pubis* (pubic or crab louse)
2. Scabies involves infestation by the itch mite, *Sarcoptes scabiei.*

B. **Pathophysiology and management**
1. Lice live on the host's skin surface and depend on the host for nourishment, feeding on human blood approximately five times daily.
2. They inject their digestive juices and excrement into the host's skin, and lay their eggs (nits) on hair shafts.
3. Adult itch mites burrow into the superficial layer of skin and lay two to three eggs daily for up to 2 months.
4. Eggs hatch in 3 to 4 days; clinical symptoms are related to a sensitivity reaction as larvae emerge to the skin surface.
5. Treatment involves killing the parasites and preventing their return.

C. **Assessment findings**
1. Manifestations of pediculosis include:
   a. Itching

      b.   Excoriation from scratching
      c.   Possibly small, red papules in infested areas
      d.   Tiny, gray-white nits on hair shafts

  2. Scabies is marked by:
      a.   Severe itching
      b.   Excoriated lesions possibly appearing as erythematous nodules
      c.   Possibly secondary bacterial infection

D. **Nursing diagnoses**
  1. Knowledge Deficit
  2. Pain
  3. Impaired Skin Integrity
  4. Social Isolation

E. **Planning and implementation**
  1. Teach the client with lice (or a parent if the client is a child) to shampoo with Kwell soap and remove nits with a fine-tooth comb.
  2. **Teach the client how to use a scabicide such as lindane (Kwell) or crotamiton (Eurax). Explain that the scabicide is directly absorbed by the parasites. Instruct client to wash scaling debris or crusts with warm, soapy water and dry area thoroughly before applying medication. Leave medication on for 12 to 24 hours then wash thoroughly.**
  3. Teach precautions to prevent future infestations.
      a.   Wash all bedding and clothing in hot water and dry on hot cycle of clothes dryer.
      b.   Never share hair brushes, combs, or hats.

F. **Evaluation**
  1. The client exhibits no sign of infestation.
  2. The client reports no discomfort.
  3. The client verbalizes important preventive measures to avoid reinfestation.

IX. **Skin cancer**

A. **Description and etiology**
  1. Basal cell carcinoma: localized, slow-growing cancer accounting for at least 75% of all skin cancers
  2. Squamous cell carcinoma: a primary lesion commonly surrounded by satellite nodules; more malignant and more clearly defined than basal cell carcinoma; grows rapidly in weeks or months and metastasizes readily
  3. Sweat gland carcinoma: a rare tumor usually occurring in the sixth and seventh decades of life but also reported in adolescents
  4. Kaposi's sarcoma: commonly associated with human immun-

odeficiency virus although etiology and pathogenesis have not been resolved

5. Melanoma: a rare malignant lesion originating in melanoblasts of skin

B. Assessment findings

1. Features of basal cell carcinoma include:
   a. Waxy, grayish-yellow, darkly pigmented or pink lesions; firm, but not indurated
   b. Lesions occurring in almost any body area, with the head and neck the most common sites
   c. Few signs of inflammation
2. Squamous cell carcinoma, commonly occurring on the lip, in paranasal folds, or in the axilla, typically appears as an ulcerated nodule with an indurated base.
3. A sweat gland carcinoma appears as a soft tissue mass present for many years.
4. Kaposi's sarcoma usually starts on the hands or feet as multiple plaques; reddish to purple in color; and flat, ulcerated, or polypoid in shape. Lymph nodes also may be involved. In terminal stages, tumors extend to the mucous membranes and portions of the GI tract.
5. Melanoma may develop in any area of the skin or pigmented region of the eye and occurs in three types:
   a. Superficial spreading melanoma: small, elevated, multicolored nodules with irregular margins
   b. Nodular melanoma: typically a polypoidal, darkly pigmented nodule somewhat resembling a blackberry
   c. Lentigo meligna melanoma: large, flat, darkly pigmented area with irregular margins and scattered black nodules

C. Nursing diagnoses

1. Body Image Disturbance
2. Ineffective Individual Coping
3. Ineffective Family Coping: Compromised
4. Fear
5. Knowledge Deficit
6. Pain
7. Impaired Skin Integrity

D. Planning and implementation

1. Review the treatment plan with the client and family or significant others; as indicated, discuss:
   a. Surgical excision with possible skin grafting
   b. Cryotherapy
   c. Curettage and electrodesiccation

         d.   Radiation therapy

         e.   Chemotherapy

  2. Prepare the client for scheduled treatments as indicated.

  3. Treat pain with analgesics as prescribed.

  4. Help reduce anxiety and facilitate coping by providing emotional support and reassurance and encouraging open expression of feelings and concerns.

  5. Teach the client and family or significant others about:

      a.   Postoperative wound care as appropriate

      b.   The need to limit sun exposure

      c.   Photoprotection methods

      d.   The importance of regular follow-up assessment to ensure early detection of any recurrence

      e.   Early signs of skin cancer to watch for and report

E. **Evaluation**

  1. The client and family demonstrate positive coping skills.

  2. The client demonstrates acceptance of altered body image and disease prognosis.

  3. The client states appropriate self-care measures.

  4. The client exhibits intact skin with no signs of infection.

  5. The client reports adequate pain control.

X. **Burns**

  A. **Description: skin injury resulting from heat, electric current, chemicals, friction, or excessive sunlight exposure**

  B. **Classification: depth of burn**

    1. Based on the standard depth of injury classification, burns are either first-, second-, or third-degree.

    2. Characteristics of *first-degree* burns (e.g., sunburn) include:

      a.   Superficial tissue destruction involving the epidermis only

      b.   Local pain and erythema; blisters absent for about 24 hours

      c.   Mild to absent systemic response

      d.   Requiring no treatment except in large burns of infants or elderly persons

      e.   Rapid healing (normally 3 to 5 days) without scarring

    3. Characteristics of *second-degree superficial partial-thickness* burns include:

      a.   Tissue destruction involving the epidermis and dermis

      b.   Skin appearing red to pale ivory and moist

      c.   Formation of wet, thin-walled blisters immediately after injury

      d.   Intact tactile and pain sensors

      e.   Healing in 21 to 28 days with variable amount of scarring

4. Characteristics of *second-degree deep partial-thickness* burns include:
   a. Tissue destruction involving possibly the entire dermis, leaving only skin appendages
   b. Mottled appearance with large areas of waxy white injury
   c. Dry surface
   d. Clinically indistinguishable from full-thickness burns at time of admission
   e. Healing spontaneously in about 30 days (However, current therapy indicates excision and skin grafting to diminish scarring and achieve early wound closure.)

5. Characteristics of *third-degree full-thickness* burns include:
   a. Involving the epidermis, dermis, and underlying subcutaneous tissue
   b. Injury appearing white, cherry red, or black; may or may not contain deep blisters or visible thrombosed veins
   c. Dry, hard, leathery appearance due to loss of epidermal elasticity
   d. Marked edema and decreased elasticity, which may necessitate escharotomies of circumferential burns within first few hours postinjury
   e. Painless to touch because of destruction of all superficial nerve endings in skin
   f. Requiring skin grafting with client's own skin (autograft) because all dermal elements have been destroyed and cannot regenerate

C. **Classification: extent of burn**
   1. The severity of burn injury can be classified according to American Burn Association criteria for minor, moderate uncomplicated, or major burn injuries.
   2. *Minor* burn injuries involve:
      a. Second-degree burn of <15% total body surface area (TBSA) in adults or <10% TBSA in children
      b. Third-degree burn of <2% TBSA not involving special care areas (eyes, ears, face, hands, feet, and perineum)
   3. *Moderate uncomplicated* burn injuries include:
      a. Second-degree burns of 15% to 25% TBSA in adults or 10% to 20% TBSA in children
      b. Third-degree burns of <10% TBSA not involving special care areas
   4. *Major* burn injuries involve:
      a. Second-degree burns of >25% TBSA in adults or >20% TBSA in children
      b. All third-degree burns of 10% TBSA or greater

       c.   All burns involving the hands, face, eyes, ears, feet, or perineum

       d.   All inhalation injury, electrical injury, and complicated burn injuries involving fractures or other trauma

       e.   All poor-risk clients with burn injury of any size

D. Nursing diagnoses

1. Ineffective Airway Clearance
2. Body Image Disturbance
3. Ineffective Breathing Pattern
4. Decreased Cardiac Output
5. Constipation
6. Ineffective Individual Coping
7. Diarrhea
8. Fluid Volume Deficit
9. Impaired Gas Exchange
10. Impaired Physical Mobility
11. Altered Nutrition: Less than body requirements
12. Pain
13. Sensory/Perceptual Alterations
14. Sexual Dysfunction
15. Impaired Skin Integrity
16. Sleep Pattern Disturbance
17. Impaired Tissue Integrity
18. Altered Tissue Perfusion: Peripheral
19. Altered Urinary Elimination

E. Planning and implementation

1. Eliminate the source of the burn, depending on cause:
   a. Flame: If clothes are smoldering, wet them using any available water; or smother flames using a blanket, rug, coat, etc.
   b. Scald: Pour cool liquid over area, and remove clothing.
   c. Chemicals: Remove clothing from involved areas and dilute chemical by flushing area with copious amounts of water; if eyes are involved, flush each eye with at least 1 L of lactated Ringer's other solution.
   d. Tar, asphalt, or melted plastic: Cool area by flushing with water; do not attempt to remove material unless the airway is compromised. (Solvents may be used after initial assessment to soften product and facilitate removal.)
   e. Electric current: Do not touch a person still in contact with an electrical source; if safe, move the person away from the electrical source without touching the source.
2. Ensure a patent airway; administer oxygen, if indicated.
3. Assess for and treat associated injuries.

4. Assess for and treat smoke inhalation injury; support pulmonary function through early intubation and volume ventilator-assisted respiration with optimal positive end expiratory pressure, large tidal volume, and lowest possible inspired oxygen concentration.

5. Assess for and treat carbon monoxide inhalation; administer 100% oxygen as prescribed until arterial blood gas results demonstrate adequate oxygenation, and perform frequent neurologic assessment until hypoxia resolves.

6. Monitor acid–base balance and electrolyte levels; intervene as necessary to correct imbalances.

7. Take special actions for electrical burns, including:

   a. Applying a cervical collar and placing the client on a spinal board as soon as possible (Severe contractions produced by electrical current passing through body may injure the spinal cord.)

   b. Monitoring for cardiac arrest or arrhythmias for at least 24 hours postinjury

   c. Assessing for and treating myoglobinuria resulting from massive soft tissue destruction accompanying major electrical injury; administering IV infusion of lactated Ringer's solution at a rate to maintain urine output at 100 mL/hour in adults or 2 mL/kg/hour in children until urine clears

   d. Preparing the client for early surgical exploration and wound debridement following cardiovascular stabilization, with debridement every 48 to 72 hours until wound closure is complete

   e. Preparing the client for amputation if indicated (Because of extensive deep damage caused by electrical current, amputation is necessary in more than 90% of electrical injuries.)

   f. Discussing potential late complications of electrical injury (e.g., corneal cataracts, ataxic gait abnormalities, and other associated neurologic problems)

8. Monitor for and treat burn shock, which occurs in all clients with major burn injury; sequence begins within minutes of injury and leads to death from hypovolemic shock unless treated appropriately.

9. Estimate burn size using either the Rule of Nines or the Lund and Browder chart (Fig. 13-1).

10. Provide appropriate fluid resuscitation, based on the Parkland formula (4 mL of lactated Ringer's solution × % TBSA burn × kg body weight = total fluid requirement for 24 hours postburn), with one half of total given in the first 8 hours post-

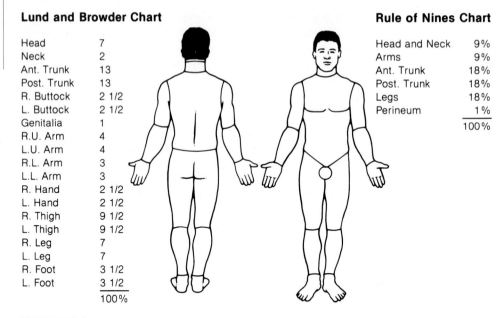

Lund and Browder Chart

Head	7
Neck	2
Ant. Trunk	13
Post. Trunk	13
R. Buttock	2 1/2
L. Buttock	2 1/2
Genitalia	1
R.U. Arm	4
L.U. Arm	4
R.L. Arm	3
L.L. Arm	3
R. Hand	2 1/2
L. Hand	2 1/2
R. Thigh	9 1/2
L. Thigh	9 1/2
R. Leg	7
L. Leg	7
R. Foot	3 1/2
L. Foot	3 1/2
	100%

Rule of Nines Chart

Head and Neck	9%
Arms	9%
Ant. Trunk	18%
Post. Trunk	18%
Legs	18%
Perineum	1%
	100%

FIGURE 13-1.
Two methods of charting burn injuries are known as the Lund and Browder chart and the Rule of Nines. These methods assign numerical values to body surface areas. The Rule of Nines chart assigns values in the amount of nine and multiples of nine. By both methods, the full body surface area totals 100%.

burn, one fourth of total given in second 8 hours postburn, and the last one fourth given in the third 8 hours postburn.

11. Estimate adequacy of fluid resuscitation based on urine output of 30 mL/hour; increase or decrease fluid to maintain hourly urine output.

12. Teach the client about planned skin grafting procedures as indicated.

13. Promote optimum recovery through such measures as:
   a. Ensuring optimum nutrition
   b. Providing meticulous wound management to prevent infection and achieve early wound coverage
   c. Initiating physical therapy to regain and maintain optimal range of motion and prevent contractures
   d. Providing psychosocial support to promote mental health
   e. Monitoring carefully to detect problems early and provide appropriate interventions to minimize complications
   f. Providing family-centered care to promote integrity of the family unit as it meets the demands of the rehabilitating burn client over several years

      g.   Encouraging postdischarge follow-up for several years of reconstructive therapy as needed

F. **Evaluation**

1. The client remains free of respiratory complications.
2. The client maintains or regains intact skin integrity.
3. The client remains free of infection at burn and harvest sites.
4. The client maintains optimal nutritional balance to promote healing.
5. The client participates in physical therapy to maintain optimal range of motion and function and prevent contractures.
6. The client remains free of late complications related to burns.
7. The client and family maintain an intact family unit.
8. The client and family make use of support services as needed.

Bibliography

Bolander, V. R. (1994). *Sorensen & Luckmann's basic nursing: A physiologic approach* (3rd ed.). Philadelphia: W. B. Saunders.

Carpenito, L. J. (1995). *Nursing diagnosis: Application to clinical practice* (6th ed.). Philadelphia: J. B. Lippincott.

Clark, J., Queener, S., & Karb, V. (1990). *Pharmacologic basis of nursing practice* (4th ed.). St. Louis: C. V. Mosby.

Lewis, S. M., & Collier, I. C. (eds.). (1992). *Medical-surgical nursing: Assessment and management of clinical problems* (2nd ed.). New York: McGraw-Hill.

Phipps, W. J., Long, B. C., & Woods, N. F. (1994). *Medical-surgical nursing: Concepts and practice* (5th ed.). St. Louis: C. V. Mosby.

Scherer, J. C., & Timby, B. K. (1995). *Introductory medical-surgical nursing* (6th ed.). Philadelphia: J. B. Lippincott.

Springhouse Corporation. (1992). *Nursing student's guide to drugs.* Spring House, PA: Springhouse Corp.

STUDY QUESTIONS

1. A relationship exists between the wide range of skin colors and the size and distribution of
   a. keratinocytes
   b. melanosomes
   c. stratum corneum
   d. melanin

2. A client is diagnosed with exfoliative dermatitis, and prednisone is prescribed. Client teaching for this medication includes
   a. taking the medication at night to prevent nocturia
   b. instructing the client not to discontinue the medication abruptly, but rather decrease the dosage gradually
   c. notifying the physician if the client loses weight or complains of muscle cramping
   d. instructing the client to stop taking the prednisone when the inflammation is gone

3. Evaluation of adequate fluid replacement in a burn client is based on the Parkland formula for fluid resuscitation. Which of the following outcome criteria is expected?
   a. The client received 2 mL/kg body weight × TBSA burned over the first 24 hours postburn.
   b. The client received 4 mL RL × % TBSA burn × kg body weight over the first 24 hours postburn.
   c. The client received 4 mL/kg body weight × % TBSA burned over the first 36 hours postburn.
   d. The client received 1 mL/kg body weight × % TBSA burned over the first 24 hours postburn.

4. Which skin layer primarily comprises collagen fibrils to provide the mechanical strength of skin?
   a. dermis
   b. epidermis
   c. hypodermis
   d. stratum corneum

5. Secretion of the apocrine glands would most likely occur in a client with which of the following nursing diagnoses?
   a. Altered Body Temperature
   b. Fear
   c. Impaired Tissue Integrity
   d. Impaired Physical Mobility

6. A client is diagnosed with acne vulgaris for which benzoyl peroxide is prescribed. Medication teaching would include
   a. taking the medication 1 hour before meals
   b. taking the medication with food to minimize gastric distress
   c. instructing client not to wash face with water before application
   d. explaining that initially the medication causes redness and scaling but that the skin will adjust quickly

7. The sensation of pain is elicited from
   a. free nonmyelinated nerve endings
   b. Merkel's disks
   c. Ruffini's endings
   d. Pacini's corpuscles

8. A client asks the nurse, "What is toxic epidermal necrolysis?" The nurse's best response is: "TEN is
   a. a rare, potentially fatal skin disorder that causes reddened, necrotic, eroded skin."
   b. an autoimmune disease that causes blisters on the skin and mucous membranes."
   c. an inflammatory disease of the sebaceous follicles."
   d. an acute viral infection marked by painful skin eruptions."

9. Using tepid sponge bathing to lower elevated core body temperature assists the skin in its thermoregulation function by way of which one of the following principles?
   a. radiation
   b. conduction
   c. convection
   d. dissipation

10. One of the immunologic functions of

the skin is the wheal and flare reaction. When evaluating a client's response to treatment, which of the following responses would indicate an immunologic rather than an infectious process?

a. reduced swelling (wheal) and diffuse redness
b. reduced dilation of arterioles and venules (flare)
c. resolution of the reaction associated with release of histamine
d. intact neurologic function

11. When evaluating the effectiveness of client teaching about health promotion and maintenance behaviors regarding skin care, the nurse would look for which of the following?

a. The client stays unprotected in the sun between noon and 4 p.m.
b. The client avoids repeated exposure to irritants and allergens.
c. The client has repeated low-dose radiation exposure.
d. The client avoids excessive sun exposure, if he or she is middle-aged.

12. For a previously healthy client presenting with erythema, bullae, and seborrhealike lesions, the nurse would obtain a nutritional history to determine whether symptoms may be associated with a dietary deficiency of the niacin and pyridoxine found in

a. vitamin B
b. vitamin C
c. vitamin K
d. vitamin A

13. At the scene of a burn injury, the first priority in treating a client who has sustained a partial thickness burn to the left hand would be

a. Apply ice packs to the burned area.
b. Apply Vaseline to the burned area.
c. Immerse the client's left hand in cool water.
d. Leave the burn alone and take the client to the emergency department immediately.

14. A furuncle has spread and now is being treated as a carbuncle. The client's treatment would be based on which of the following nursing diagnoses?

a. Risk for Infection
b. Altered Oral Mucous Membrane
c. Risk for Disuse Syndrome
d. Altered Tissue Perfusion: Peripheral

ANSWER KEY

1. **Correct response: b**
   Melanosomes are produced by melano-cytes.
   a. Keratinocytes are epidermal cells that produce keratin.
   c. The stratum corneum is the outer-most skin layer.
   d. Melanin is a pigment produced by melanocytes.
   Analysis/Physiologic/Assessment

2. **Correct response: b**
   Prednisone is a systemic corticosteroid. If stopped abruptly, adrenal insuffi-ciency may result and lead to shock and death. Dosage must be tapered off gradually.
   a and c. Prednisone will not cause in-creased urination, weight loss, or muscle cramping. Side effects of prednisone include moon face, weight gain, and other Cushingoid effects.
   d. This is contraindicated; the dosage must be decreased gradually.
   Application/Health promotion/
   Implementation

3. **Correct response: b**
   a, c, and d. These are incorrect for-mulas for fluid replacement.
   Application/Safe care/Evaluation

4. **Correct response: a**
   The dermis lies under the epidermis.
   b. The epidermis is the superficial vas-cular layer of skin.
   c. Hypodermis refers to below the skin.
   d. The stratum corneum is the horny, outermost layer of the epidermis.
   Knowledge/Physiologic/Assessment

5. **Correct response: b**
   The apocrine glands respond to auto-nomic nervous stimulation.
   a. The apocrine glands do not respond to thermal stimulation.
   c and d. Neither impairment of tissue

integrity nor mobility stimulates se-cretions from these glands.
Analysis/Physiologic/Analysis (Dx)

6. **Correct response: d**
   Benzoyl peroxide is a gel preparation that is administered once daily and ini-tially causes redness and/or scaling, but the skin adjusts quickly.
   a and b. The medication is a gel and has no effect on food intake.
   c. The client should wash and dry face thoroughly before application.
   Application/Health promotion/
   Implementation

7. **Correct response: a**
   Free nonmyelinated nerve endings me-diate pain sensation.
   b. Merkel's disks mediate touch.
   c. Ruffini's endings mediate warmth.
   d. Pacini's corpuscles are encapsulated nerve endings that mediate pressure.
   Knowledge/Physiologic/Assessment

8. **Correct response: a**
   Toxic epidermal necrolysis (TEN) is a rare, potentially fatal skin disorder marked by epidermal erythema, necro-sis, and skin erosions.
   b, c, and d. These are definitions of pemphigus vulgaris, acne vulgaris, and herpes zoster, respectively.
   Knowledge/NA/Evaluation

9. **Correct response: b**
   Conduction transfers heat from the body to a cooler object in contact, such as tepid water.
   a. Radiation involves the giving off of heat to cooler objects at a distance.
   c. Convection involves bulk removal of warm air away from body to air sur-rounding body.
   d. Dissipation is not a thermoregula-tory function.
   Comprehension/Physiologic/
   Implementation

10. **Correct response: d**
    An intact nervous system is required for an immunologic response.
    a, b, and c. All these responses can occur with either an immunologic or infectious process.
Analysis/Physiologic/Evaluation

11. **Correct response: b**
    Avoidance of exposure to irritants and allergens is recommended to prevent skin cancer and other skin disorders.
    a, c, and d. It is recommended that individuals of all ages have protection against the sun (sun block with a sun protection factor [SPF] of 15 or above) and that they avoid exposure to the sun during the time when the sun is strong, if possible. Any radiation (high or low) should be avoided or the person should use a protective lead shield.
Application/Health promotion/ Evaluation

12. **Correct response: a**
    Vitamin B is essential to complex metabolic functions.
    b and c. Vitamins C and K are essential for connective tissue formation and normal prothrombin synthesis, respectively.

    d. Vitamin A is essential for normal cell structure in the epithelium.
Comprehension/Health promotion/ Implementation

13. **Correct response: c**
    Immersing the left hand in cool water will give immediate and striking relief from pain, retard the burning process, and restrict local tissue edema and damage.
    a. Ice may worsen the tissue damage and lead to hypothermia in clients with large burns.
    b. Vaseline, ointments, and salves should not be used; they may cause further damage.
    d. The burn must be treated immediately to stop the burning process; then the client may be taken to the emergency department.
Application/Safe care/Implementation

14. **Correct response: a**
    Infection is very common, often resulting in abscess.
    b, c, and d. These other diagnoses would not be expected with this bacterial infection.
Analysis/Health promotion/ Analysis (Dx)

Neurologic Disorders

I. Nervous systems

A. Central nervous system: cranial

1. Structures
    a. The brain is enclosed within the bones of the cranium and covered by three meningeal layers: dura mater (outer), arachnoid mater, and pia mater (inner).
    b. Manufactured in the choroid plexus of the ventricular system, cerebrospinal fluid (CSF) circulates in the subarachnoid space.

c.   Ventricular structures include the lateral, third, and fourth ventricles; the aqueduct of Sylvius; and the foramina of Luschka and Magendie.

d.   The cerebrum is divided into left and right hemispheres by the falx, an indentation of the dura. Each cerebral hemisphere contains frontal, temporal, parietal, occipital, and limbic lobes.

e.   The cerebellum also is divided into left and right hemispheres, which are connected by the vermis.

f.   Brain stem structures include the medulla, pons, and midbrain.

g.   The basal ganglia encompass the caudate nucleus, putamen, globus pallidus, and substantia nigra.

h.   Other structures in the brain include the thalamus, hypothalamus, and pituitary gland.

i.   Supratentorial structures (above the dura fold) are known as the tentorium; infratentorial structures lie below the tentorium.

j.   Vascular supply to the brain is provided from the basilar artery, formed from the union of two vertebral arteries, and the internal carotids; these two systems join to form the circle of Willis.

2.   Function

a.   **According to the Monro Kellie principle, an increase in any one of three components (brain tissue, normally 88%; CSF, 9% to 10%; intravascular blood, 2% to 3%) results in increased intracranial pressure (ICP) because the skull bones do not allow for expansion from pressure buildup.**

b.   The meninges protect the brain from injury and infection.

c.   Between 500 and 700 mL of CSF is manufactured daily, but only 150 mL is circulating at any one time; excess CSF is absorbed through the arachnoid villi into the venous system.

d.   **Interference with CSF flow results in increased ICP.**

e.   The tentorium helps stabilize cranial structures within the skull.

f.   The frontal lobe, prerolandic, is the brain's center of foresight, abstract thinking, and judgment.

g.   The frontal lobe, postrolandic, controls voluntary motor movements.

h.   The temporal lobe is the center of memory and contains visual and auditory association areas.

i.   The parietal lobe controls sensory functions such as

recognition of pain, temperature, and pressure and sense of position of the body and limbs.

    j.   The occipital lobe is the center of visual function.

    k.   The limbic lobe is the center of emotions, drives, and basic survival functions.

    l.   The cerebellum is involved in coordination of muscle movements and maintenance of equilibrium and muscle tone.

    m.   The medulla oblongata contains several vital centers, including those for respiration, heart rate, vomiting, and hiccoughing.

    n.   In the pons, the pneumotaxic system controls respiratory patterns.

    o.   In the brain stem, the reticular activating system (RAS) maintains alertness.

    p.   The basal ganglia are involved in smooth muscle movement and processing of proprioceptive input.

    q.   The thalamus serves as the chief relay station for sensory fibers.

    r.   The hypothalamus helps regulate body temperature, fluid balance, and some endocrine functions.

    s.   The pituitary gland is the chief regulator of endocrine functions.

    t.   The brain uses about 20% of total cardiac output. An autoregulation mechanism maintains blood flow to the brain despite changes in systemic pressure; trauma can disrupt this mechanism.

    u.   The blood–brain barrier prevents many toxic substances in the blood stream from entering the brain.

B.   **Central nervous system: spinal cord**

    1.   Structure

        a.   The spinal cord is encased within the vertebral column, which consists of 31 vertebrae in cervical (C), thoracic (T), lumbar (L), sacral (S), and coccygeal segments.

        b.   The cervical, thoracic, and lumbar vertebrae are separated by disks. The disk's outer covering is termed the annulus; the inner part, the nucleus pulposus.

        c.   Like the brain, the spinal cord is covered by meninges (see Section I.A.1.a).

        d.   Vascular supply is provided from the radicular arteries and posterior and anterior spinal arteries.

        e.   Major descending tracts in the spinal cord include the lateral corticospinal (pyramidal), ventral corticospinal, reticulospinal, and vestibulospinal tracts.

        f.   Major ascending tracts include the lateral spinothalamic and ventral spinothalamic tracts and the posterior columns. Fibers of the lateral spinothalamic tract cross in the brain stem.

2. Function
   a. The vertebral column protects the cord and helps maintain an upright body position.
   b. The lateral corticospinal tract transmits impulses controlling voluntary motor movement.
   c. The lateral spinothalamic tract transmits pain and temperature impulses.
   d. The posterior columns carry tactile and kinesthetic impulses.

3. Neurologic dysfunction associated with cord damage depends on the level of injury:
   a. Below C4: loss of motor and sensory function from the neck down, including independent respiratory function and bowel and bladder control
   b. Below C6: loss of motor and sensory function below the shoulders; loss of bowel and bladder control; impaired intercostal muscle function
   c. Below C8: loss of motor control and sensation to parts of the arms and hands; loss of bowel and bladder control
   d. Below T6: loss of motor control and sensation below the midchest but with motor control and sensation preserved in the arms and hands; loss of bowel and bladder control
   e. Below T12: loss of motor control and sensation below the waist; loss of bowel and bladder control
   f. Below L2: loss of motor control and sensation in the legs and pelvis; loss of bowel and bladder control
   g. Below L4: loss of motor control and sensation in parts of the thighs and legs; loss of bowel and bladder control

C. **Peripheral nervous system**
   1. Structure
      a. The peripheral nervous system contains 12 pairs of cranial nerves and 31 pairs of spinal nerves.
      b. Cranial nerves, which are numbered, include the olfactory (CN I), optic (II), oculomotor (III), trochlear (IV), trigeminal (V), abducens (VI), facial (VII), acoustic (VIII), glossopharyngeal (IX), vagus (X), spinal accessory (XI), and hypoglossal (XII) nerves.
      c. The nuclei of many cranial nerves are located in the brain stem.
      d. Spinal nerves exit through vertebral foramina.

2. Function
   a. Spinal nerves contain both sensory and motor fibers.
   b. Motor fibers are of two types: *somatic,* which terminate in skeletal muscle, and *autonomic,* which innervate cardiac smooth muscle and glands.
   c. CNs III, IV, and VI control eye movement and pupil size.
   d. CN VII controls facial movements.
   e. CN IX controls the gag reflex.
   f. CN X controls many autonomic nervous system functions.

II. Overview of neurologic disorders

A. Assessment

 1. **Neurologic assessment involves assessing neurologic system intactness, with particular emphasis on sensation, motor ability (including coordination), alertness, and cognition (see Chapter 1, Section X, for details of a complete neurologic assessment).**

2. In the presence of specific disorders or nursing diagnoses, additional assessments or more in-depth assessment of specific areas may be done. The acuity of the client's condition determines the necessary frequency of "neuro" checks.

3. Various assessment tools (e.g., the Glasgow Coma Scale) may be used to assess the client's level of consciousness (LOC) (see Fig. 14-1).

4. The nurse assesses sensory function as follows:
   a. With the client blindfolded, touch all levels of each extremity, and ask him or her to identify the different pressure points.
   b. Ask if the client feels numbness, tingling, or other abnormal sensations.
   c. Assess whether the client with decreased arousal moves the extremities in response to pressure or more intense stimuli.
   d. Evaluate each extremity, and note any deficits.

5. Motor function assessment involves the following:
   a. Ask the client to grasp the examiner's hands with his or hers and to push against the examiner's palms with his or her feet; evaluate muscle strength.
   b. Have the client lift each arm and foot.
   c. Evaluate the client's ability to walk; assess posture, gait, and coordination.
   d. To assess fine motor coordination, have the client touch the examiner's fingertip, then his or her own nose.

ACTION	RESPONSE	SCORE
EYES OPEN	Spontaneously	4
	To speech	3
	To pain	2
	No response	1
BEST VERBAL RESPONSE	Oriented	5
	Confused	4
	Inappropriate words	3
	Incomprehensible sounds	2
	No response	1
BEST MOTOR RESPONSE	Obeys commands	6
	Localized pain	5
	Flexion withdrawal	4
	Abnormal flexion	3
	Abnormal extension	2
	Flaccid	1
	Total	

FIGURE 14-1.
The Glasgow Coma Scale is the standard scorecard for evaluating level of consciousness (LOC). In clients unable to respond verbally because of tracheal intubation, the score would contain a T rather than a numeral. In clients with eyes closed by swelling, the score would be noted by a C.

    e.   In a client with decreased arousal, assess movement in response to pressure or more intense stimuli.

6.   Assessing alertness (level of arousal and orientation) involves these steps:

    a.   Speak the client's name. If the client doesn't respond, speak louder, shake him or her, and finally apply a slightly painful stimulus; note whether the client opens his or her eyes or responds verbally.

    b.   Ask a responsive client to state his or her name, where he or she is, and the date, along with other questions that will provide data on level of orientation.

7. The nurse assesses a client's level of cognition (including judgment) by:
   a. Determining whether the client can follow commands
   b. Asking questions to evaluate memory (both recent and past)
   c. Determining the client's ability to calculate numerical problems
8. Pupil examination evaluates pupil size and response to light, along with equality of response.
9. Reflex assessment includes determining the presence or absence of the corneal and gag reflexes.
10. Neurologic assessment also should include assessment of vital signs and respiratory pattern.

B. **Laboratory studies and diagnostic tests**
   1. Magnetic resonance imaging (MRI) and computed tomography (CT) identify pathologies such as tumors, hematomas, and edema.
   2. Angiography, a radiologic test, allows the health care team to visualize vascular problems, tumors, and hematomas.
   3. Electroencephalography (EEG) evaluates the brain's electrical activity (alpha, beta, theta, and delta waves); used primarily in diagnosis of epilepsy and brain death.
   4. Ventriculography demonstrates the ventricular system by injection of contrast media (usually air) directly into a ventricle; used when infratentorial lesions are suspected.
   5. Lumbar puncture involves inserting a needle into the subarachnoid space to obtain data on CSF, CSF pressure, and possible infection. (Normal CSF is clear; contains 15 to 45 mg of protein per 100 mL, 50 to 80 mg glucose per 100 mL, and no red blood cells; and has a specific gravity of 1.007.)
   6. In myelography, radiographs taken after injection of a possibly irritating contrast medium into the spinal column detect tumors, disk abnormalities, or other spinal cord problems.

C. **Psychosocial implications**
   1. A client with a serious neurologic problem may experience coping difficulties due to such factors as:
      a. Chronic nature of the disorder
      b. Uncertain prognosis
      c. All-encompassing nature of limitations
   2. The client also may have self-concept concerns related to:
      a. Increased dependency, loss of independence
      b. Body image changes related to neurologic deficits
      c. Diminished outlets for sexual expression

3.   Lifestyle concerns may be related to potential changes in:
    a.   Physical ability
    b.   Work performance, with possibility of job loss
    c.   Self-care ability
    d.   Mental capacity
    e.   Economic stability
4.   The client also may be prone to changes in social interaction related to depression, isolation, and hopelessness.

D.   Medications used to treat neurologic problems (Additional medications may be included with specific disease)

1.   *Osmotic diuretics,* which decrease cerebral edema in head trauma by drawing water across intact membranes, thereby reducing the volume of brain and extracellular fluid
    a.   Example: mannitol (Osmitrol)
    b.   Selected nursing considerations

    ► **Monitor fluid and electrolyte balance.**
    ► **Maintain accurate intake and output records.**
    ► **Teach client how to prevent orthostatic hypotension.**

2.   *Corticosteroids,* which reduce inflammation and thereby increased ICP
    a.   Example: dexamethasone (Dexasone)
    b.   Selected nursing considerations

    ► **Administer IV during acutely increased ICP.**
    ► **Reduce dose gradually in long-term use to avoid abrupt withdrawal leading to adrenal insufficiency, shock, and death.**

3.   *Sedatives,* which depress CNS activity, thereby reducing restlessness and agitation, for example, in clients with cerebral aneurysm
    a.   Example: phenobarbital (Donnatal, Luminal)
    b.   Selected nursing considerations

    ► **Administer IV medication by large vein to avoid extravasation.**
    ► **Monitor vital signs closely because sedative drugs depress CNS and respiratory activity and may mask decreasing LOC.**
    ► **Institute safety precautions.**

4.   *Anticoagulants,* which prevent further clot extension in CVA by inhibiting coagulation
    a.   Example: warfarin (Coumadin)
    b.   Selected nursing considerations

    ► **Instruct the client to report any abnormal bleeding and bruising.**

> ▶ Advise the client to avoid or use caution handling sharp objects.

5. *Anticonvulsants,* which control seizure activity by an unknown mechanism
   a. Examples: carbamazepine (Tegretol), phenytoin (Dilantin), phenobarbital
   b. Selected nursing considerations

   n ▶ Inform client that medication may cause drowsiness, and advise avoiding activities that require mental alertness and coordination.
   ▶ Caution client not to stop medication abruptly as doing so may trigger seizure activity.
   ▶ Teach client to perform regular oral hygiene and seek regular dental care to control gingival problems and other oral side effects.
   ▶ Urge client to carry medical identification.
   ▶ Instruct client to report signs of serious side effects, such as rash or flulike symptoms.

6. *Antiparkinson agents,* which stimulate dopamine receptors to improve transmission of voluntary nerve impulses to the motor cortex
   a. Example: levodopa (L-dopa)
   b. Selected nursing considerations

   n ▶ Instruct client to report overdose signs, such as muscle or eye twitching, at once.
   ▶ Tell client not to take medication with food but to eat food 30 minutes after dose to minimize GI distress.
   ▶ Discuss precautions to take to prevent or minimize orthostatic hypotension.

7. *Anticholinergic agents,* which block cholinergic receptor sites to inhibit the action of acetylcholine
   a. Examples: trihexyphenidyl (Artane), procyclidine (Kemadrin), benztropine mesylate (Cogentin)
   b. Selected nursing considerations

   n ▶ Instruct client to take medication after meals to minimize GI upset.
   ▶ Advise client to increase fluid intake to prevent constipation (a side effect).
   ▶ Explain that this medication may cause drowsiness.

8. *Antihistamines,* which inhibit acetylcholine and have a mild sedative effect, thereby allaying tremors
   a. Example: diphenhydramine (Benadryl)
   b. Selected nursing considerations

► Direct client to take medications with food to minimize GI distress.
- ► Suggest client drink plenty of water, chew sugarless gum, or suck sour hard candy to relieve dry mouth.

9. *Cholinergic (anticholinesterase) agents,* which inhibit the breakdown of acetylcholine (a substance associated with muscle tone)
   a. Examples: pyridostigmine (Mestinon), neostigmine (Prostigmine)
   b. Selected nursing considerations

    ► Administer medication at same time daily to ensure maximum strength available for activity.
   - ► Administer medication with food to minimize GI distress.
   - ► In case of overdosage, have the antidote atropine on hand.

III. Head trauma
A. Description
1. Head trauma refers to direct or indirect impact to the head that produces some degree of brain injury.
2. Common types of head trauma include:
   a. Closed head injuries (concussion, contusion, laceration)
   b. Intracranial hemorrhage (epidural, subdural, or intracerebral hematoma)
   c. Skull fractures (open or closed)

B. Etiology and incidence
1. Common causes of head trauma include falls, automobile accidents, and beatings with blunt objects; intracerebral hematoma commonly results from missile injury (e.g., gunshot or stab wound).
2. Head trauma causes between 80,000 and 100,000 deaths each year in the United States; another 700,000 cases require hospitalization.

C. Pathophysiology and management

1. **Whatever the cause of head trauma, the most serious complication is increased ICP.**
2. Compensatory mechanisms for maintaining ICP within normal limits include:
   a. Increased CSF absorption
   b. Shunting of blood to the spinal subarachnoid space
   c. Decreased CSF production
3. Failure of these compensatory mechanisms results in the following sequence of events:

       a. Decreased cerebral blood flow with inadequate perfusion

       b. Increased PCO_2 and decreased PO_2, leading to hypoxia

       c. Vasodilation and cerebral edema

       d. Further increases in ICP

    4. Management of head trauma involves identifying and correcting the underlying cause of increased ICP and cerebral edema.

D. Assessment findings

    1. Clinical manifestations of head trauma depend on the type, site, and extent of injury.

    2. A common manifestation is loss of consciousness, ranging from a few minutes to an hour or longer.

    3. Signs and symptoms of increasing ICP include:

       a. Altered level of consciousness—particularly restlessness, a common early sign

       b. Pupil changes: fixed, dilated, slowed response, inequality

       c. Increasing systolic blood pressure with stable or falling diastolic pressure

       d. Bradycardia, widening pulse pressure

       e. Bradypnea, irregular breathing pattern

       f. Hyperthermia (late sign)

       g. Focal neurologic signs: visual changes (blurred or double vision, photophobia), muscle weakness or paralysis, decreased response to pain stimulus, positive Babinski's sign, decerebrate or decorticate posturing

       h. Headache

       i. Vomiting

    4. ICP monitoring detects increased ICP (generally >15 mmHg); the catheter can be placed in the ventricles, subdural space, or epidural space.

E. Nursing diagnoses

    1. Ineffective Airway Clearance

    2. Hyperthermia

    3. Risk for Infection

    4. Risk for Impaired Skin Integrity

    5. Altered Thought Processes

    6. Altered Tissue Perfusion: Cerebral

F. Planning and implementation

    1. Monitor neurologic status, including vital signs, level of consciousness, oculomotor nerve function, and motor and sensory status.

    2. Help maintain cerebral perfusion by:

       a. Administering prescribed osmotic diuretics to decrease

cerebral edema, corticosteroids to reduce inflammation, and sedatives to reduce restlessness (see Section II.D).

b. **Providing safety measures when administering sedatives and analgesics that may depress respirations and decrease LOC**
    c. Reducing or eliminating noxious stimuli
    d. Elevating the head of the bed 30 degrees
    e. Hyperventilating the client before suctioning
3. Maintain a patent airway; suction as needed, and position client to prevent airway obstruction.
4. Manage hyperthermia by:
    a. Providing only minimal bedcoverings and clothing
    b. Using a hypothermia blanket; avoid rapid cooling
    c. Administering antipyretics as prescribed
    d. Forcing fluids unless contraindicated
5. Prevent infection by using sterile technique for wound care and insertion of the ICP monitoring device and by keeping the monitoring system intact.
6. Maintain skin integrity by:
    a. Turning the client on regular schedule and protecting pressure points as needed
    b. Changing moist or wet linens immediately
    c. Lifting—not pulling—the client when changing position in bed
7. Provide passive range-of-motion (ROM) exercises to prevent contractures from prolonged immobility.
8. Help orient the client and reduce confusion by:
    a. Reducing external stimuli
    b. Providing for adequate rest
    c. Giving simple directions
    d. Providing familiar objects in the client's environment

G. Evaluation
    1. The client exhibits ICP within normal limits.
    2. The client demonstrates absence of lung infections or infiltrates.
    3. The client's body temperature is within normal range.
    4. The client's skin remains intact.

IV. Brain tumors
  A. Description
    1. Brain tumors are localized, space-occupying, intracranial neoplasms.
    2. Primary tumors (originating from brain tissue) include:
        a. Gliomas (astrocytomas, glioblastomas, ependymomas, medulloblastomas, oligodendrogliomas), accounting for 50% of primary brain tumors

    b.   Meningiomas, accounting for 13% to 18% of primary brain tumors

    c.   Pituitary adenomas

    d.   Neurinomas, accounting for about 8% of primary brain tumors

B. Etiology and incidence

    1.   The etiology of brain tumors remains unclear.

    2.   Incidence is approximately 4.5 per 100,000 persons in the United States; periods of peak incidence are before age 1 year, between ages 2 and 12 years, and between ages 40 and 60 years.

C. Pathophysiology and management

    1.   Arising from glial cells in the brain's connective tissue, gliomas tend to be fast-growing, infiltrative, and difficult to excise completely.

    2.   Meningiomas arise from the brain's dural covering; they are relatively slow growing and usually benign.

    3.   Pituitary adenomas may arise from various pituitary tissues and commonly affect endocrine function and vision.

    4.   Neurinomas arise from the coverings of any of the cranial nerves, most commonly from the acoustic nerve (CN VIII).

    5.   Metastatic tumors can migrate to the brain from other sites; common primary sites include the lung, breast, and colon.

    6.   Management includes surgery and other therapies.

D. Assessment findings

    1.   Signs and symptoms depend on tumor type, location, and rate of growth.

    2.   General manifestations include those related to increased ICP, such as headache, vomiting, papilledema, and altered sensorium.

    3.   Brain tumors also may produce focal neurologic effects, including motor abnormalities (e.g., weakness, paralysis, seizures) and sensory abnormalities (e.g., distorted vision, smell, hearing, touch).

    4.   CT scan or MRI can locate the tumor; other useful diagnostic studies may include angiography, ventriculography, and radionuclide scanning.

E. Nursing diagnoses

    1.   Anxiety

    2.   Body Image Disturbance

    3.   Hopelessness

    4.   Risk for Injury

    5.   Sensory/Perceptual Alterations: Visual, Auditory, Tactile

    6.   Risk for Impaired Skin Integrity

       7.   Altered Thought Processes

       8.   Altered Tissue Perfusion: Cerebral

F.   **Planning and implementation**

       1.   See Chapter 21, Cancer Nursing, for general nursing interventions appropriate to all cancer clients.

       2.   As applicable, prepare the client for craniotomy to remove the tumor or a portion of the tumor (see Chapter 24, Perioperative Nursing).

       3.   **Carefully monitor for signs of increased ICP and neurologic deficits.**

       4.   Provide information on tests, treatments, and other procedures to the client and family.

       5.   Provide eye care if the client experiences decreased corneal reflex.

       6.   If the client is confused, determine whether family members can stay with him or her; use restraints judiciously.

       7.   If the client experiences paresis or paralysis, provide needed assistance with mobility.

       8.   Assist with adaptation to sensory and perceptual changes (e.g., teach the client to turn or move his or her head to view the entire environment, to place needed items within his or her visual field, to face persons when talking, and to turn his or her head or position self so that he or she can hear well).

       9.   Assist the client with grooming and other self-care measures as needed.

   10.   Provide information on wigs and other items that can improve appearance as appropriate.

   11.   Teach the client and family stress management techniques such as progressive muscle relaxation, breathing techniques, guided imagery, and meditation.

   12.   Allow time for expression of feelings and concerns; if appropriate, encourage the client to keep a journal.

   13.   Refer the client and family to the chaplain or social services as appropriate.

   14.   Instruct the client and family in necessary home care measures.

   15.   Provide information on appropriate community resources and support groups.

G.   **Evaluation**

       1.   The client's ICP remains within normal range.

       2.   The client remains alert and well oriented.

       3.   The client remains injury-free.

       4.   The client maintains skin integrity.

       5.   The client and family members demonstrate low levels of anxiety.

      6.   The client interacts with others and participates in self-care.

      7.   The client and family acknowledge the client's condition; the client expresses positive statements of self-worth.

V. Cerebrovascular disorders

A. Description

1. This group of disorders involves disruption of blood supply to the brain.
2. Types include:
   a. Cerebrovascular accident (CVA, stroke)
   b. Transient ischemic attack (TIA)
   c. Cerebral aneurysm

B. Etiology and incidence

1. Causes of CVA include thrombosis (most common), embolism, and vessel rupture or spasm; the most common site is the middle cerebral artery.
2. CVA strikes more than 500,000 persons each year and is a leading cause of death in the United States. About half of the survivors sustain permanent neurologic deficits.
3. Considered a warning sign of CVA, TIA results from occlusion of an intracranial or extracranial artery, commonly associated with atherosclerosis. The most common site of TIA is at the bifurcation of the common carotid artery.
4. Cerebral aneurysm results from a weakness in a vessel wall due to a congenital defect or a degenerative process, such as hypertension or atherosclerosis. The most common type is berry aneurysm, and the most common site is in the anterior portion of the circle of Willis, usually at a vessel junction.

C. Pathophysiology and management

1. In CVA, sudden interruption of blood supply to areas of the brain results in cerebral anoxia and impaired cerebral metabolism, which damages brain tissue and produces focal neurologic deficits of varying severity.
2. In a TIA, temporary interruption of blood flow (lasting from seconds to hours) produces transient neurologic deficits that clear completely within 12 to 24 hours.
3. A cerebral aneurysm is prone to rupture, which causes blood to leak into the subarachnoid space (and sometimes into brain tissue, where it forms a clot), resulting in increased ICP and brain tissue damage.

D. Assessment findings

1. Clinical manifestations of CVA depend on the artery affected, the severity of damage, and the extent of collateral circulation that develops. Common signs and symptoms include:
   a. Hemiplegia and sensory deficits

      b.   Aphasia (Impairment may be in speaking, listening, writing, comprehending; most are mixed expressive and receptive.)

      c.   Homonymous hemianopia

      d.   Unilateral neglect of paralyzed side

      e.   Bladder impairment

      f.   Possible respiratory impairment

      g.   Impaired mental activity and psychologic effects

  2. Manifestations of TIA may include:

      a.   Temporary loss of consciousness or dizziness

      b.   Paresthesias

      c.   Garbled speech

  3. A client with a nonruptured cerebral aneurysm often is asymptomatic or reports nonspecific symptoms such as headache or blurred vision. Aneurysm rupture produces varying manifestations, which may include:

      a.   Signs and symptoms of increased ICP (see Section III.C)

      b.   Severe headache

      c.   Nuchal rigidity and pain on neck movement

      d.   Photophobia and possible blurred vision

      e.   Irritability and restlessness

      f.   Slight temperature elevation

E. Nursing diagnoses

  1. Impaired Verbal Communication

  2. Fatigue

  3. Impaired Physical Mobility

  4. Pain

  5. Altered Role Performance

  6. Self-Care Deficit: Feeding, Dressing and Grooming, Bathing and Hygiene

  7. Risk for Impaired Skin Integrity

  8. Social Isolation

  9. Unilateral Neglect

F. Planning and implementation

  1. Enhance communication by:

      a.   Using alternative means of communication as appropriate (e.g., gestures, pictures, alphabet board)

      b.   Giving simple commands with gestures; pointing to objects as you name them

      c.   Eliminating extraneous stimuli when communicating (e.g., turn off the television)

  2. Plan the client's care to allow for adequate periods of uninterrupted rest. Schedule therapy sessions after rest periods.

  3. Provide a balanced diet, and assist the client with eating if

necessary. Allow sufficient time for meals, place food so that the client can see it, and provide foods that are easy to handle.

4. Maximize the client's opportunities for social interaction.

5. Consider the client's interests when planning daily activities.

6. Teach the client how to use a walker, cane, or wheelchair as appropriate.

7. Instruct the client in the use of assistive devices, such as for putting on stockings.

8. Encourage the client to wear simplified clothing, such as with front opening snaps, secured.

9. Discuss necessary home adaptations (e.g., wheelchair ramps, shower seat, other bathroom modifications).

10. Assist the client with personal hygiene as necessary (e.g., hair washing and brushing, makeup application, shaving).

11. Teach and assist with or perform ROM exercises to help maintain muscle tone and prevent contractures.

12. Encourage the client to touch the paralyzed side and to participate in passive ROM exercises as appropriate.

13. When the client is in bed, position him or her on side with the hips slightly flexed in as natural a position as possible.

14. Reduce pain by:
   a. Administering analgesics as prescribed
   b. Positioning to decrease discomfort
   c. For a client with subarachnoid hemorrhage, reducing external stimuli, moving the client slowly, turning the neck gently

15. **Monitor the client after administering certain analgesics (e.g., narcotic analgesics), because these agents may depress respiration and mask decreasing LOC.**

16. Administer medications as prescribed, including osmotic diuretics to decrease cerebral edema, corticosteroids to reduce inflammation, sedatives to reduce restlessness, and anticoagulants to prevent cerebral blood clots (see Section II.D).

17. Prepare the client for surgical intervention as appropriate, which may include:
   a. Carotid enterectomy for a client experiencing TIA
   b. Craniotomy for surgical clipping of aneurysm

18. Teach the client's family:
   a. Effective communication techniques
   b. New ways of interacting with the client after discharge
   c. Ways to encourage the client in self-feeding
   d. Safety precautions (e.g., keeping the client's environment clear of obstacles)

G. Evaluation

1. The client demonstrates decreased frustration and increased ability to make his or her needs known.
2. The client exhibits the ability and sufficient energy to carry out necessary activities.
3. The client displays skin free of redness and breaks in integrity.
4. The client maintains interactions with others and seeks out social situations.
5. The client demonstrates the ability to use assistive devices or transfer himself or herself safely.
6. The client maintains weight within normal range with no undue weight loss.
7. The client exhibits appropriate personal hygiene and grooming and dresses appropriately.
8. The client does not have accidents and remains injury-free.
9. The client acknowledges his or her entire body and shows no evidence of unilateral neglect.
10. The client reflects absence of discomfort by facial expressions, body movements, and vital signs.

VI. Epilepsy

A. Description

1. Epilepsy refers to paroxysmal, uncontrolled, excessive firing of hyperexcitable neurons in the brain; not a disease entity in itself but rather an indicator of underlying pathology.
2. Types of seizures include:
   a. Tonic–clonic (grand mal)
   b. Absence (petit mal)
   c. Complex (temporal lobe; psychomotor)
   d. Jacksonian

B. Etiology and incidence

1. About 50% of cases of epilepsy are idiopathic, for which no underlying pathology can be identified.
2. Possible causes include:
   a. Birth trauma
   b. Head trauma
   c. Brain tumor
   d. Meningitis, encephalitis, or brain abscess
   e. Metabolic disorders (e.g., hypoglycemia, phenylketonuria)
   f. Cerebrovascular disorders
3. Approximately 2 million Americans have some form of epilepsy.

C. Pathophysiology and management

1. Seizure activity represents excessive, disordered firing of brain neurons.

    2. Seizures are classified as partial (complex, Jacksonian), arising from a localized area of the brain, or generalized (tonic–clonic, absence), marked by widespread electrical abnormality in the brain.

    3. Status epilepticus refers to continued seizure activity, a medical emergency treated with medications.

D. Assessment findings

    1. Tonic–clonic seizures are marked by:

        a. Generalized seizure activity with no focal onset, lasting about 2 minutes

        b. Possible prodrome of a vaguely uneasy feeling

        c. Loss of consciousness, with falling if upright at onset

        d. In the tonic phase, muscle contraction (including jaw clenching), possibly periods of apnea

        e. In the clonic phase, rhythmic, forceful movement of extremities; excessive salivation; rapid pulse

        f. Possible incontinence

        g. Stupor for 5 to 10 minutes after the clonic phase

    2. Features of absence seizures include:

        a. Generalized seizure activity with no focal onset, occurring primarily in children

        b. Momentary (10- to 30-second) loss of consciousness, marked by a glassy stare; usually no falling

        c. Possibly occurring repeatedly over the course of a day

    3. In a complex seizure, the client exhibits altered behavior (e.g., automatisms, unusual sensations, delusions) but is not aware of what is happening.

    4. A Jacksonian seizure begins in one part of the body (e.g., twitching of one side of the face or abnormal movements of one hand) and may progress to a generalized tonic–clonic seizure.

E. Nursing diagnoses

    1. Anxiety

    2. Risk for Injury

    3. Knowledge Deficit

    4. Impaired Social Interaction

F. Planning and implementation

    1. Observe and record the client's movements and behavior before, during, and after the seizure.

    2. Note the part(s) of the body affected by seizure activity.

    3. Note the duration of seizure activity.

    4. Administer anticonvulsants as prescribed and provide related instruction (see Section II.D).

    5. Provide client and family teaching, covering:

        a. Aura or indications of seizure

m   b.   **Care needed during seizure activity: protecting the head and extremities so that they do not hit objects during seizure; avoid restraining the client**

       c.   The need to provide for adequate rest after the seizure

       d.   Medication regimen, including side effects and signs of toxicity

       e.   Necessary lifestyle modifications such as getting adequate sleep, abstaining from alcohol, using relaxation techniques

       f.   The need for social interaction opportunities

   6.   Encourage family and friends not to be overprotective of the client.

   7.   Provide information on available community resources, including support groups.

G.   **Evaluation**

   1.   The client maintains blood level of medications within the therapeutic range.

   2.   The client exhibits no medication side effects, or if side effects do occur, they are detected early.

   3.   The client displays no bruises, fractures, or lacerations.

   4.   The client reports feeling rested and relaxed.

   5.   The client reports feeling good about social interactions and increased interactions.

VII.   **Spinal cord injuries**

A.   **Description: fractures, contusions, or compression of the vertebral column with damage to the spinal cord**

B.   **Etiology and incidence**

   1.   Causes of spinal cord injury include motor vehicle accidents, diving accidents, falls, sports injuries, and gunshot wounds.

   2.   Common sites of injury include the cervical spine and the junction of the thoracic and lumbar areas (T-12 and L-1).

C.   **Pathophysiology and management**

   1.   Spinal cord injuries can result from flexion, extension, rotation, compression, or a combination of these mechanisms.

   2.   Injury may directly damage the cord, or vertebral fracture or dislocation can be a potential source of cord injury, in which inappropriate movement can cause permanent damage.

   3.   Cord injury may be complete, involving total cord transection, or incomplete, with partial transection or other damage.

   4.   Damage ranges from mild transient cord concussion to immediate and permanent quadriplegia.

   5.   With cord damage, spinal shock may occur, with loss of motor, sensory, and autonomic activity below the level of injury. This condition may persist for several days to months after injury.

      6.   Management varies; usually rehabilitation is required.

D. **Assessment findings**

      1.   Common immediate symptoms of spinal cord injury include pain and paresthesias or, conversely, loss of sensation; altered motor function, ranging from paresis to paralysis; and possibly loss of consciousness.

      2.   Neurologic damage depends on the level of cord injury (see Section I.B.3); edema may temporarily increase deficits.

      3.   Spinal radiography can locate the area of cord damage.

E. **Nursing diagnoses**

      1.   Body Image Disturbance
      2.   Bowel Incontinence
      3.   Ineffective Individual Coping
      4.   Dysreflexia
      5.   Impaired Home Maintenance Management
      6.   Risk for Infection
      7.   Risk for Injury
      8.   Impaired Physical Mobility
      9.   Altered Sexuality Patterns
    10.   Risk for Impaired Skin Integrity
    11.   Altered Role Performance
    12.   Reflex Incontinence

F. **Planning and implementation**

      1.   Provide emergency treatment:

         a.   **Do not move the client until adequate personnel and equipment are available.**
         b.   Keep the neck aligned.
         c.   Immobilize the head and neck.

      2.   Using the Glasgow Coma Scale, perform frequent neuro checks to evaluate muscle strength, degree and type of movement, sensation, and warmth of all four extremities (see Figure 14-1).

      3.   Apply skeletal traction as prescribed; may use a Stryker or Circ-O-Lectric bed.

      4.   Explain aspects of care and positioning to the client and family.

      5.   Prepare the client for surgery, if appropriate—usually in fractures or dislocations to stabilize the spinal column (see Chapter 24, Perioperative Nursing, for more information).

      6.   Perform passive ROM exercises on paralyzed limbs to maintain joint mobility.

      7.   Teach the client active ROM exercises to maintain or increase strength and mobility in the upper extremities.

      8.   Work with other disciplines in securing needed assistive devices for ambulation and home maintenance management.

9. Teach the client transfer skills, if appropriate.
10. Provide for adequate rest periods.
11. Teach the client and family signs and symptoms of impending dysreflexic episodes.
12. Establish a regular bowel routine, and institute other measures to prevent constipation, such as:
    a. Setting a schedule for defecation, preferably 15 to 20 minutes after a meal
    b. Providing a warm liquid before defecation time
    c. Encouraging the client to ingest sufficient dietary roughage and adequate fluids, and to avoid foods that can cause constipation
    d. Encouraging the client to attempt defecation in the sitting position, if possible
13. Provide bladder care to prevent urine stasis, including:
    a. Scheduling frequent times for voiding
    b. Maintaining an adequate fluid intake but avoiding fluids before bedtime
    c. Identifying and using triggering mechanisms that can stimulate voiding
    d. Administering anticholinergic medications as prescribed
    e. Performing intermittent bladder catheterization as appropriate
14. Administer antihypertensive medications as prescribed to decrease blood pressure (see Chapter 8, Section X.F).
15. Collaborate with the client's family to identify ways to adapt the home environment to the client's needs.
16. Evaluate the client's and family members' coping strategies, and teach new strategies if needed.
17. As appropriate, provide information on alternative means for achieving sexual satisfaction.
18. Encourage the client and family members to verbalize concerns.

G. Evaluation
1. If neurologic deficit has resulted from injury, the client exhibits no increase in deficit.
2. If no deficit has occurred, the client develops no deficit.
3. The client demonstrates maximum use of remaining abilities in self-care and mobility.
4. The client maintains skin integrity.
5. The client expresses positive adaptation to deficits in psychologic and social realms.
6. The client verbalizes realistic expectations about the future and expresses feelings about his or her condition and its impact on his or her life.
7. Family members verbalize understanding of the client's con-

dition and demonstrate the willingness and ability to assist the client in functioning at his or her optimum level.

8. The client demonstrates adequate bowel and bladder control, with no constipation or urinary tract infections.
9. The client reports satisfaction with sexual expression.

VIII. Spinal cord tumors

A. Description: neoplasms of the spinal cord or its nerve roots; tumor types are the same as for intracranial tumors (see Section IV.A)

B. Etiology and incidence

1. The etiology of spinal cord tumors is unclear.
2. Incidence is rare compared to intracranial tumors (a ratio of about 1:4).

C. Pathophysiology and management

1. Tumors can develop anywhere along the spinal cord or its roots; the most common site is the thoracic area.
2. Primary cord tumors may be intramedullary (within the cord), extramedullary–intradural (within the subarachnoid space), or extradural (outside the dural membrane).
3. Effects depend on tumor type, site, and growth.
4. Tumors may invade the vertebral column; erosion of bone may cause collapse of vertebrae with resulting pressure on the spinal nerves and spinal cord.
5. Management may involve surgery and other treatments.

D. Assessment findings

1. Common clinical manifestations of spinal cord tumors include:
   a. Pain
   b. Motor dysfunction (e.g., muscle weakness and spasticity, decreased muscle tone, hyperreflexia, positive Babinski's sign)
   c. Sensory deficits (e.g., loss of pain, temperature, and touch sensation; paresthesias)
   d. Urinary retention and constipation
2. Neurologic deficits resulting from cord tumors often are similar to those associated with cord injury (see Section VII.D).
3. CT scan, MRI, myelography, and spinal radiography can determine tumor location and the extent of involvement.

E. Nursing diagnoses

1. Anxiety
2. Bowel Incontinence
3. Constipation
4. Impaired Physical Mobility
5. Pain

      6. Sexual Dysfunction
      7. Risk for Impaired Skin Integrity
      8. Urinary Elimination, Altered
      9. Urinary Retention

F. Planning and implementation

      1. Prepare the client for surgery, if appropriate (see Chapter 24, Perioperative Nursing).

      2. Prepare the client for radiation therapy, if prescribed (see Chapter 21, Cancer Nursing).

      3. Control pain with analgesics, proper body positioning, relaxation techniques, or transcutaneous electrical nerve stimulation (TENS), as appropriate.

      4. Provide other care depending on manifestations (e.g., urinary incontinence or retention, bowel incontinence or constipation, impaired mobility). Care is similar to that for a client with spinal cord injury (see Section VII.F).

      5. Provide reassurance and emotional support as the client and family cope with the diagnosis and uncertain prognosis (see Chapter 21, Cancer Nursing).

G. Evaluation

      1. The client reports adequate pain control.

      2. The client demonstrates maximum use of remaining abilities in self-care and mobility.

      3. The client maintains skin integrity.

      4. The client verbalizes realistic expectations about the future and expresses feelings about his or her condition and its impact on his or her life.

      5. Family members verbalize understanding of the client's condition and demonstrate the willingness and ability to assist the client in functioning at his or her optimum level.

      6. The client reports satisfaction with sexual expression.

      7. The client exhibits no bowel or bladder problems.

IX. Intervertebral disk herniation

A. Description: a disorder involving impingement of a vertebral disk's nucleus pulposus on spinal nerve roots, causing pain and possible neuromuscular deficit

B. Etiology and incidence

      1. Herniated disk can result from:
         a. Degenerative disorders
         b. Trauma
         c. Congenital predisposition

      2. A common back problem, herniated disk most commonly affects men younger than age 45.

C. **Pathophysiology and management**

1. Rupture of the annulus pulposus (the disk's outer ring) allows part of the nucleus pulposus (the soft, gelatinous inner portion) to protrude and press against spinal nerve roots, producing symptoms.
2. Herniation can occur anywhere along the vertebral column but is most common in the lumbar area.
3. Clinical manifestations vary with the location and degree of herniation and the course of its progression. In lumbar disk herniation, pressure on the sciatic nerve can produce severe—sometimes debilitating—pain and if chronic, possible motor and sensory changes.
4. Therapeutic interventions may include traction, bedrest, and surgery.

D. **Assessment findings**

1. Common signs and symptoms of herniated disk include:
   a. Back pain (in lumbar herniation, often with radiation down the posterior thigh and leg), exacerbated by coughing, sneezing, or straining
   b. Varying degrees of motor and sensory impairment (e.g., muscle weakness, diminished deep tendon reflexes in the lower extremities)
   c. Positive straight-leg raising test or LeSegue's test
2. CT scan, MRI, or myelography may reveal the location of herniation.

E. **Nursing diagnoses**

1. Anxiety
2. Impaired Physical Mobility
3. Pain

F. **Planning and implementation**

1. Assess the site, nature, course, and progress of back pain.
2. Monitor motor and sensory status.
3. Provide conservative management, if indicated, including:
   a. Encouraging bedrest
   b. Positioning with head of bed elevated at 30° and knees slightly flexed
   c. Applying heat
   d. Instructing in appropriate exercises
4. If laminectomy is ordered to remove protruding disk fragments, provide appropriate perioperative care (see Chapter 24, Perioperative Nursing).
5. After surgery:
   a. Assess strength, sensation, and movement of extremities.
   b. Keep the client in proper body alignment when in bed

(provide a firm mattress) and when turning (use log-rolling).

   c. Encourage the client to wear well-fitted, safe walking shoes when ambulating.

   d. Teach proper body mechanics to prevent injury.

   e. Caution the client to avoid slippery surfaces and activities that can involve sudden back movements.

G. Evaluation

   1. The client reports reduced pain; facial expression and body movements reflect increased comfort.

   2. The client walks with a normal gait.

X. Multiple sclerosis (MS)

A. Description: a progressively disabling demyelinating disease affecting nerve fibers of the brain and spinal cord and marked by periodic exacerbations and remissions

B. Etiology and incidence

   1. The cause of MS is unknown; theories include a slow-growing virus, an autoimmune process, and an allergic response to an infectious agent.

   2. Incidence is greater in women than in men and is highest in temperate climates; age of onset is typically between age 20 and 40.

C. Pathophysiology and management

   1. MS produces patches of demyelination throughout the central nervous system, impeding transmission of nerve impulses.

   2. The random pattern of demyelination causes widely varying neurologic effects.

   3. The course of MS is marked by periodic and unpredictable exacerbations and remissions.

   4. Prognosis is variable; MS can cause rapid, sometimes fatal, disability, but about 70% of clients lead active, productive lives with long periods of remission.

   5. Management relies heavily on lifestyle modification and adaptations.

D. Assessment findings

   1. Clinical manifestations of MS vary widely but may include:

     a. Visual problems: diplopia, blurred vision, nystagmus

     b. Motor dysfunction: muscle weakness, paralysis, spasticity, hyperreflexia, tremors, gait ataxia

     c. Fatigue

     d. Bladder or bowel incontinence

     e. Mental changes: mood swings, irritability, depression

   2. No single diagnostic test confirms diagnosis. Lumbar puncture and CSF analysis may reveal elevated CSF gamma globu-

lins; MRI may confirm the presence of demyelinating plaques.

E. **Nursing diagnoses**
1. Anxiety
2. Body Image Disturbance
3. Bowel Incontinence
4. Fatigue
5. Risk for Injury
6. Impaired Physical Mobility
7. Altered Role Performance
8. Functional Incontinence

F. **Planning and implementation**
1. Assess the nature and degree of neuromuscular deficits and their effect on the client's lifestyle.
2. Assess the client's sleep and rest patterns; encourage adequate rest to avoid fatigue.
3. Assist the client in planning lifestyle modifications to decrease stress and fatigue and maximize functional abilities.
4. **Administer adrenocorticotropic hormones such as corticotropin (ACTH) to stimulate release of adrenal cortex hormones, which help to improve nerve conduction. Instruct client to notify physician if serious side effects such as fluid retention, muscle weakness, abdominal pain, or headache occur.**
5. Administer corticosteroids as prescribed (see Section II.D).
6. Provide appropriate care during exacerbations (e.g., help the client establish bladder and bowel control, prevent skin breakdown, prevent and treat muscle spasticity).

G. **Evaluation**
1. The client demonstrates positive adjustment to altered lifestyle.
2. The client exhibits a low anxiety level.

XI. **Parkinson's disease**
A. **Description: a progressive neurologic disorder secondary to degeneration of basal ganglia in the cerebrum**
B. **Etiology and incidence**
1. The etiology of Parkinson's disease is unknown.
2. Suspected causes include viral infection, chemical toxicity, cerebrovascular disease, and effects of such drugs as major tranquilizers and reserpine.
3. The second most common neurologic disorder in the elderly, Parkinson's disease affects about 1 in 100 persons over age 60; incidence is higher in men than in women.

C. Pathophysiology and management
    1. Dopamine, a neurotransmitter secreted by the basal ganglia, is essential to extrapyramidal function; depletion of dopamine diminishes normal neuromuscular inhibiting mechanisms.
    2. Characteristic neurologic deficits associated with Parkinsonism include bradykinesia, muscle rigidity, and resting tremor.
    3. Progressive deterioration continues for about 10 years; death commonly results from pneumonia or another infection.

D. Assessment findings
    1. Common clinical manifestations include:
        a. Tremor, an early sign, commonly affecting the hands and more prominent at rest; also known as resting and "pill rolling" tremor
        b. Bradykinesia (dyskinesia, akinesia): loss of spontaneous movement, slowness in voluntary movement, difficulty initiating movement
        c. Rigidity: decreased muscle tone and stiffness, with jerky movements ("cogwheel rigidity")
        d. Fatigue and muscle weakness
        e. Stooped posture, shuffling gait marked by arm swinging
        f. Impaired ability to turn in bed and rise from chair
        g. Masklike facial expression, increased blinking reflex
        h. Autonomic manifestations, such as oily skin (seborrhea) and excessive perspiration
        i. Dysphagia, drooling
        j. Monotone speech, impaired articulation (dysarthria)
        k. Constipation, due to decreased fluid intake and autonomic dysfunction
        l. Depression, withdrawal
    2. No tests confirm Parkinson's disease; however, urinalysis may reveal increased dopamine levels, to support diagnosis.

E. Nursing diagnoses
    1. Impaired Verbal Communication
    2. Constipation
    3. Risk for Injury
    4. Knowledge Deficit
    5. Impaired Physical Mobility
    6. Altered Nutrition: Less than body requirements
    7. Self Care Deficit
    8. Self Esteem Disturbance
    9. Sleep Pattern Disturbance
   10. Impaired Social Interaction
   11. Altered Role Performance

F. Planning and implementation

    1. Administer antiparkinson, anticholinergic, and antihistamine agents as prescribed (see Section II.D).

    2. If indicated, prepare the client for stereotaxic surgery to reduce tremors and rigidity.

G. Evaluation

    1. The client demonstrates the ability to perform activities of daily living (ADLs).

    2. The client exhibits adequate social interaction.

XII. **Amyotrophic lateral sclerosis (ALS)**

A. Description: a progressively debilitating and eventually fatal disease involving degeneration of motor neurons

B. Etiology and incidence

    1. The cause of ALS is unknown.

    2. ALS affects 2 to 7 of every 100,000 persons—men more than women; onset typically occurs between ages 40 and 70.

C. Pathophysiology and management

    1. ALS is marked by progressive destruction of motor cells in the anterior gray horns and pyramidal tract; both upper and lower motor neurons are affected.

    2. As motor neurons die, the muscle cells that they supply undergo atrophic changes. Progressive paralysis results.

    3. Prognosis varies; most ALS clients die within 3 to 10 years of onset, usually from secondary causes such as pneumonia.

    4. There is no known cure; care is supportive.

D. Assessment findings

    1. Clinical manifestations vary with the location of affected motor neurons and disease stage, and may include:

        a. Progressive weakness, atrophy, spasticity, and tremors of upper extremities, followed by involvement of lower extremities and then respiratory muscles

        b. Fatigue

        c. Impaired speech, chewing, and swallowing

        d. Breathing difficulty

        e. Depression

    2. There are no diagnostic studies specific to ALS; diagnosis is based on history and neurologic findings.

E. Nursing diagnoses

    1. Ineffective Airway Clearance

    2. Risk for Aspiration

    3. Body Image Disturbance

    4. Impaired Verbal Communication

    5. Ineffective Individual and Family Coping

    6. Impaired Gas Exchange

   7. Hopelessness
   8. Powerlessness
   9. Altered Role Performance
  10. Risk for Impaired Skin Integrity
  11. Impaired Swallowing

  F. **Planning and implementation**

    1. Because no treatment currently is available to slow disease progression, provide supportive care, focusing on:

      a. Maximizing functional abilities (e.g., mobility, self-care, communication)

      b. Preventing skin breakdown

      c. Preventing respiratory complications

      d. Ensuring adequate nutrition

      e. Providing intellectually stimulating activities since the client typically experiences no cognitive deficits

    2. Provide emotional support as the client and family deal with the poor prognosis and the grieving process.

  G. **Evaluation**

    1. The client demonstrates the ability to perform ADLs to the maximum of his or her functional capacity.

    2. The client displays no respiratory complications, skin breakdown, or other untoward problems.

    3. The client and family exhibit positive coping with absence of depression.

XIII. **Myasthenia gravis**

  A. **Description: a progressive disorder affecting neuromuscular transmission of impulses in voluntary muscles**

  B. **Etiology and incidence**

    1. Myasthenia gravis is thought to be an autoimmune response.

    2. Incidence is one in 25,000 persons and is higher in women; initial symptoms typically occur between ages 20 and 40.

  C. **Pathophysiology and management**

    1. In myasthenia gravis, acetylcholine receptor (AChR) antibodies interfere with impulse transmission across myoneural junctions.

    2. This causes abnormal weakness and fatigability of skeletal muscle, particularly of the eyes, face, jaw, and neck; also may involve muscles of upper extremities and respiratory muscles.

    3. The disorder follows an unpredictable course of periodic exacerbations and remissions. Drug therapy allows many clients to lead normal lives; however, progressive weakness of respiratory muscles may cause life-threatening respiratory distress or myasthenic crisis.

D. **Assessment findings**
   1. Clinical manifestations typically include:
      a. Abnormal weakness of any striated muscle (particularly of the face, neck, and arms and hands), typically worsening after activity and improving with rest
      b. Severe fatigue
      c. Drooping facial muscles; ptosis
      d. Diplopia
      e. Impaired chewing and swallowing
      f. Breathing difficulty due to weak respiratory muscles
   2. Diagnosis is based on history of weakness of specific muscle groups; positive Tensilon test confirms diagnosis.

E. **Nursing diagnoses**
   1. Ineffective Airway Clearance
   2. Risk for Aspiration
   3. Fatigue
   4. Impaired Gas Exchange
   5. Altered Role Performance

F. **Planning and implementation**
   1. Administer anticholinesterase agents as prescribed (see Section II.D).
   2. If indicated, prepare the client for other treatments, such as plasmapheresis or thymectomy.
   3. Prevent problems associated with swallowing difficulty; provide small, frequent meals, and keep suctioning equipment readily available.
   4. Encourage adjustment in lifestyle to prevent fatigue.

G. **Evaluation**
   1. The client exhibits positive adjustment to lifestyle changes.
   2. The client remains free of respiratory complications.
   3. The client demonstrates adequate ability to perform ADLs.

XIV. **Guillain-Barré syndrome**
   A. **Description: an acute, rapidly progressive form of polyneuritis producing muscle weakness and mild sensory disturbances**
   B. **Etiology and incidence**
      1. Guillain-Barré syndrome is a postinfectious polyneuritis of unknown origin that commonly follows febrile illness.
      2. It can develop at any age but is most common between ages 30 and 50; incidence is about equal in men and women.
   C. **Pathophysiology and management**
      1. Segmental demyelination of peripheral nerves causes inflammation and degeneration in sensory and motor nerve roots.
      2. Most clients experience spontaneous and complete recovery although mild deficits may persist.

D. **Assessment findings**
1. Common signs and symptoms include:
   a. Paresis in the legs (usually the initial manifestation)
   b. Motor weakness progressing to involve the entire peripheral nervous system, including respiratory muscles
   c. Paresthesias
2. Progression may involve total or partial paralysis.
3. Lumbar puncture and CSF analysis may reveal elevated CSF proteins.

E. **Nursing diagnoses**
1. Anxiety
2. Ineffective Gas Exchange
3. Impaired Physical Mobility

F. **Planning and implementation**
1. Explain all procedures and care measures to help reduce the client's anxiety.
2. Monitor respiratory status (if respiratory muscles are involved).
3. Assist with plasmapheresis, if prescribed.

G. **Evaluation**
1. The client exhibits a low level of anxiety.
2. The client remains free of complications.
3. The client experiences a complete return of function.

XV. **Meningitis**
A. **Description: infection or inflammation of the meninges covering the brain and spinal cord**
B. **Etiology and incidence**
1. Bacterial meningitis most often results from previous infection with *Neisseria meningitidis, Streptococcus pneumoniae,* or *Haemophilus influenzae.*
2. Aseptic meningitis may be caused by viral infection or other causes.
3. Children are more prone than adults because of their greater propensity for respiratory infection.

C. **Pathophysiology and management**
1. Infective organisms that enter the brain quickly disseminate through the meninges and into the ventricles.
2. This dissemination may result in:
   a. Meningeal congestion
   b. Cerebral edema
   c. Increased ICP
   d. Generalized inflammation with exudate formation
   e. Hydrocephalus if exudate blocks ventricular passages
3. Prognosis is good with early detection and prompt treatment;

however, untreated meningitis (or delayed treatment) commonly proves fatal, particularly in children and elderly persons.

D. Assessment findings

1. Clinical manifestations may include:
    a. Headache and fever
    b. Altered level of consciousness
    c. Signs of meningeal irritation: nuchal rigidity, positive Brudzinski's and Kernig's signs, exaggerated deep tendon reflexes, opisthotonos
    d. Signs and symptoms of increased ICP (see Section III.D.3)
2. Diagnosis is confirmed by isolation and identification of the causative organism in CSF.

E. Nursing diagnoses

1. Pain
2. Other nursing diagnoses associated with increased ICP (see Section III.E)

F. Planning and implementation

1. **Check for allergies before administering prescribed IV antibiotics, such as penicillin and ampicillin, which cross the blood–brain barrier into the subarachnoid space in concentrations sufficient to inhibit bacterial growth. Assess IV site frequently.**
2. Apply a hypothermia blanket, as prescribed, to relieve hyperthermia.
3. Intervene as appropriate to reduce increased ICP (see Section III.F).

G. Evaluation

1. The client maintains body temperature within normal range.
2. The client reports or exhibits reduced pain.
3. The client exhibits no signs and symptoms of increased ICP.

XVI. Bell's palsy

A. Description: a disorder of the facial nerve (CN VII) producing unilateral facial paresis or paralysis

B. Etiology and incidence

1. Bell's palsy results from facial nerve inflammation, most commonly due to infection, vascular disorders, or local trauma. In some cases, an autoimmune reaction may be involved.
2. It affects all age groups but is most prevalent in persons younger than age 60.

C. **Pathophysiology and management**
   1. The inflamed, edematous facial nerve becomes compressed, causing paresis or paralysis of facial muscles.
   2. In most clients, spontaneous recovery occurs within 3 to 5 weeks. Partial recovery may leave the client with facial contractures.

D. **Assessment findings**
   1. Clinical manifestations include:
      a. Drooping mouth on one side, possibly with drooling
      b. Possible pain
      c. Inability to close the eyelid on the affected side
   2. Diagnosis is based on client history and signs and symptoms.

E. **Nursing diagnoses**
   1. Body Image Disturbance
   2. Risk for Injury
   3. Altered Nutrition: Less than body requirements

F. **Planning and implementation**
   1. Administer prescribed adrenal corticosteroids (prednisone) during exacerbation of Bell's palsy to decrease inflammation and facial nerve edema (see Section II.D).
   2. Provide small, frequent feedings of soft foods.
   3. Provide eye care; teach client to close lids periodically and to use artificial tears.
   4. Apply a facial sling to support facial muscles.
   5. Massage facial muscles gently and apply heat.

G. **Evaluation: Client exhibits complete return of function.**

Bibliography

Bolander, V. R. (1994). *Sorensen & Luckmann's basic nursing: A physiologic approach* (3rd ed.). Philadelphia: W. B. Saunders.

Cochran, I., et al. (1994). Stroke care: Piecing together the long-term picture. *Nursing 94, 24*(6): 34–42.

Clark, J., Queener, S., & Karb, V. (1990). *Pharmacologic basis of nursing practice* (4th ed.). St. Louis: C. V. Mosby.

Karch, A. (1995). *Lippincott's nursing drug guide*. Philadelphia: J. B. Lippincott.

Laskowski-Jones, L. (1993). Acute spinal cord injury: How to minimize the damage. *AJN, 93*(12): 22–32.

Smeltzer, S. C., & Bare, B. G. (1996). *Brunner & Suddarth's textbook of medical-surgical nursing* (8th ed.). Philadelphia: Lippincott-Raven Publishers.

Springhouse Corporation. (1992). *Nursing student's guide to drugs*. Spring House, PA: Springhouse Corp.

STUDY QUESTIONS

1. A client has sustained a severe blow to the head. When monitoring the client for signs of increasing ICP, the nurse should be particularly alert for
   a. pupillary changes
   b. difficulty arousing the client
   c. decreasing blood pressure
   d. elevated temperature

2. Appropriate actions for a client experiencing a tonic–clonic seizure would include which of the following?
   a. placing a tongue blade between the teeth
   b. elevating the head
   c. protecting the head and extremities from contact with other objects
   d. restraining the arms and legs

3. A client has suffered a subarachnoid hemorrhage and complains of pain when moving the head. The nursing diagnosis of Pain would be related to
   a. blood causing irritation of the meninges
   b. lack of oxygen to the parietal lobe
   c. increased production of CSF
   d. decrease in neurotransmitters

4. Which of the following parameters should the nurse use in evaluating the effectiveness of interventions to prevent the complication of bladder infection in a client with a neurologic problem?
   a. Cystogram reveals normal findings.
   b. The client does not complain of pain.
   c. Urine output is 150 mL/day.
   d. Temperature is within normal limits, and urine culture is negative.

5. A client has undergone a craniotomy to remove a glioma-type brain tumor. The client responds minimally to stimuli and respirations sound very moist. These findings would lead the nurse to make the nursing diagnosis of
   a. Decreased Cardiac Output
   b. Ineffective Airway Clearance
   c. Ineffective Breathing Pattern
   d. Anxiety

6. A client has sustained a severe head injury and damaged the prefrontal lobe. The nurse should remain particularly alert for which of the following problems?
   a. visual impairment
   b. swallowing difficulty
   c. impaired judgment
   d. hearing impairment

7. When placing a meal tray in front of a client who has sensory and perceptual problems that affect the right visual field (right homonymous hemianopia), the nurse should
   a. Place all the food on the right side of the tray.
   b. Before leaving the room, remind the client to look over all the tray.
   c. Place food and utensils within the client's left visual field and leave the client alone.
   d. Stay with the client, and periodically draw her attention to the food on the right side of the tray.

8. The nurse should include which of the following in preprocedure teachings for a client scheduled for carotid angiography?
   a. "You will be put to sleep before the needle is inserted."
   b. "The test will take several hours."
   c. "You may feel a burning sensation when the contrast dye is injected."
   d. "There will be no complications."

9. What deficits would the nurse expect in a right-handed person experiencing a stroke affecting the left side of the cortex?
   a. expressive aphasia and paralysis on the right side of the body
   b. expressive aphasia and paralysis on the left side of the body
   c. dysarthria and paralysis on the right side of the body
   d. mixed aphasia and paralysis on the right side of the body

10. Which of the following would be the most important consideration in providing emergency care to a person with a possible cervical spinal injury?
   a. Monitor vital signs every 5 minutes.
   b. Place the neck in a flexed position.
   c. Check to see if the client can move his or her toes.
   d. Immobilize the head and spine, keeping them in alignment.

11. What would be the most appropriate intervention for a client with aphasia who states, "I want a . . ." and then stops?
   a. Wait for the client to complete the sentence.
   b. Immediately begin showing the client various objects in the environment.
   c. Leave the room and come back later.
   d. Begin naming various objects that the client could be referring to.

12. Which of the following statements would be most appropriate when assisting a client who has the nursing diagnoses of Altered Thought Processes with Self Care Deficits?
   a. "What would you like to do first; brush your teeth?"
   b. "Where is your toothbrush?"
   c. "When would you like to have your bath?"
   d. "Would you like to brush your teeth, or do you want me to do it for you? It's good to do things for yourself."

13. Which of the following positions would be most appropriate for a client with right-sided paralysis following a stroke?

   a. on the side with support to the back, with pillows to keep the body in alignment, hips slightly flexed, and hands tightly holding a rolled washcloth
   b. on the side with support to the back, pillows to keep the body in alignment, hips slightly flexed, and a washcloth placed so that fingers are slightly curled
   c. on the back with two large pillows under the head, a pillow under the knees, and a footboard
   d. on the back with no pillows used, with trochanter rolls and a footboard

14. To prevent infection in a client with a subdural intracranial pressure monitoring system in place, the nurse should
   a. Use aseptic technique when cleaning the insertion site and connections.
   b. Use clean technique for cleansing connections and aseptic technique for the insertion site.
   c. Use sterile technique when cleansing the insertion site.
   d. Close any leaks in the tubing with tape.

15. In assisting a client diagnosed with multiple sclerosis, which of the following topics would be important to include in client teaching?
   a. the effects that stress and fatigue have on symptoms
   b. the need for small, frequent meals
   c. the need for vigorous exercise
   d. the positive effects of a high-protein diet

For additional questions, see
***Lippincott's Self-Study Series* Software**
Available at your bookstore

ANSWER KEY

1. **Correct response: b**
   The first sign of pressure on the reticular activating system in the brain stem is a decrease in responsiveness.
   a. Pupillary changes occur later.
   c. Systolic blood pressure increases.
   d. Temperature changes vary and may not be present even with severe decreases in responsiveness.
   Comprehension/Physiologic/Assessment

2. **Correct response: c**
   Protecting the client by moving objects so that the arms and legs do not hit them and placing a soft object under the head are the most important immediate interventions.
   a. Trying to force a tongue blade or other object into the mouth may damage teeth.
   b. Nothing is gained by elevating the client's head since breathing will return to normal after the activity stops.
   d. Restraining movement may result in injury or stiffness following the seizure.
   Application/Safe care/Evaluation

3. **Correct response: a**
   Pain, particularly on movement of the neck, results from blood leakage into the CSF; time will be required for it to be absorbed.
   b and c. Lack of oxygen and increased CSF production usually do not occur.
   d. Neurotransmitters are not involved in the process.
   Knowledge/Physiologic/Analysis (Dx)

4. **Correct response: d**
   Bladder infections result from a variety of causes in many clients with neurologic problems. Elevated temperature occurs in urinary and respiratory infections. A negative urine culture would be another indicator of the absence of infection.

   a. Cystography is done to evaluate bladder function, not detect infection.
   b and c. Pain on urination or oliguria are indicators of infection.
   Comprehension/Physiologic/Evaluation

5. **Correct response: b**
   Clients with decreased arousal frequently have airway problems caused by immobility or by pathology in the brain stem. Attention to respirations and frequent assessment of airway for suctioning are indicated.
   a. Decreased cardiac output would not cause moist sound.
   c. The breathing pattern may be altered, but moist sounds do not indicate a change in pattern.
   d. Anxiety may result from difficulties in breathing, but this client probably is not alert enough to experience anxiety.
   Application/Physiologic/Analysis (Dx)

6. **Correct response: c**
   A number of areas of the brain are involved in cognition and thinking, but damage to the prefrontal area usually results in impaired judgment and insight.
   a. Vision problems may occur with pathology in the occipital lobe or in the pituitary area (optic chiasm).
   b. Swallowing problems result from damage to cranial nerve IX in the brain stem.
   d. Hearing impairment commonly occurs with damage to CN VIII.
   Comprehension/Safe care/Assessment

7. **Correct response: d**
   This client needs to learn to scan the entire visual field.
   a, b, and c. These interventions are not as appropriate as d.
   Analysis/Health promotion/ Implementation

8. *Correct response: c*
Providing a client with information about expected sensations often helps decrease anxiety. The contrast medium commonly causes a burning sensation as it passes through the cerebral arteries.
  a. Clients rarely receive general anesthesia for an angiogram.
  b. The test usually takes less than an hour.
  d. Various complications—such as airway obstruction and vasospasm with sensory and motor deficits—may occur after an angiogram.
Application/Health promotion/Implementation

9. *Correct response: d*
Most aphasias involve both expressive and receptive components, although one may dominate. The speech center is most often found on the nondominant side; the left side of the brain controls the right side of the body.
  a, b, and c. These deficits would not be expected in this client.
Analysis/Physiologic/Assessment

10. *Correct response: d*
Immobilization in alignment will prevent possible fractures or dislocated bone from damaging the spinal cord.
  a. Monitoring the client is important but secondary to immobilization.
  b. Flexing the neck can cause spinal cord damage.
  c. Clients with suspected back injuries should avoid movement until evaluations rules out cord damage.
Application/Safe care/Implementation

11. *Correct response: a*
It often takes time for an aphasic person to select a proper word; the nurse should let the person try to express himself or herself without letting the person become too frustrated.
  b, c, and d. These interventions would not be appropriate in this situation.
Analysis/Psychosocial/Implementation

12. *Correct response: b*
Simple questions and directions are most appropriate; this client probably is not capable of making decisions at this time.
  a, c, and d. Because all of these statements ask the client to make a decision, they would be inappropriate in this situation.
Analysis/Psychosocial/Planning

13. *Correct response: b*
The optimum position is one that approximates normal body functioning.
  a. Curling the fingers tightly can lead to contractures.
  c and d. Placing too many pillows under the head may interfere with breathing and pull the rest of the body out of alignment.
Analysis/Health promotion/Evaluation

14. *Correct response: c*
Utmost care is needed to prevent introducing organisms into the subdural space; therefore, sterile technique is required.
  a and b. Sterile technique is required.
  d. Leaking tubing should be replaced.
Application/Safe care/Planning

15. *Correct response: a*
Studies have shown that stress and fatigue adversely affect the course of the disease. Teaching stress-management techniques and helping the client adjust his or her schedule to ensure adequate rest will be beneficial.
  b. Small, frequent feedings are not a priority in a client with MS.
  c. Vigorous exercise can lead to fatigue.
  d. Increased protein intake is not associated with MS treatment.
Application/Health promotion/Planning

Eye, Ear, Nose, Sinus, and Throat Disorders

I. Eyes

  A. **Structures (Fig. 15-1)**

    1. Anatomically, the eye can be divided into three layers, or coats (outer, middle, and inner), and the refractive media (Fig. 15-1).

    2. The outer, protective layer consists of the:
      a. Sclera: white, opaque, fibrous connective tissue
      b. Cornea: the anterior continuation of the sclera, transparent and avascular

    3. The middle, vascular layer (also known as the uveal tract) includes the:
      a. Choroid: a thin, pigmented membrane containing blood vessels that supply eye tissues
      b. Ciliary body: the anterior continuation of the choroid containing muscles that change the shape of the lens to focus vision
      c. Iris: the central extension of the ciliary body consisting of two muscles and a central opening, the pupil, which constricts and dilates to regulate the amount of light entering the eye's interior (constricts with strong light and near vision, dilates with dim light and far vision)

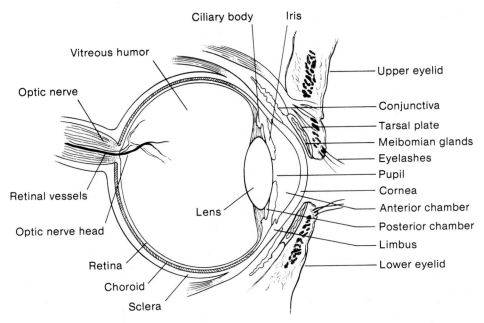

FIGURE 15-1.
Transverse section of the eye. (From Fuller, J., & Schaller-Ayers, J. [1994]. *Health assessment: A nursing approach* [2nd ed.]. Philadelphia: J. B. Lippincott.)

4. The inner, neural layer—the retina—contains layers of nerve cells, including rods and cones, that translate lightwaves into neural impulses for transmission to the brain.

5. Refractive media include the:
   a. Cornea
   b. Aqueous humor: watery fluid filling the eye's anterior chamber that serves as a refracting medium and maintains the hydrostatic intraocular pressure (IOP)
   c. Lens: a biconvex crystalline body located behind the pupil that changes shape for accommodation (focusing)
   d. Vitreous humor: a jellylike substance filling the posterior cavity behind the lens, acting as a refractive medium and maintaining the shape of the eye

B. Function

1. Vision depends on a complex coordination of ocular structures that mediate passage of light rays reflected from an external object to the retina and transmit visual images to the brain for interpretation.

2. Normally, light passes through the refractive media to the retina, where an inverted and reversed image forms.

3.   In the retina, rods and cones convert the projected image into nerve impulses and transmit them to the optic nerve.
4.   Impulses travel along the optic nerve to the brain's optic chiasm and then to the cerebral cortex, where they are interpreted as sight.

II.   Overview of eye disorders
A.   Assessment
1.   The visual fields confrontation test evaluates the peripheral extent of visual fields (other than central reading vision); normal findings include 60 degrees nasally, 50 degrees upward, 90 degrees temporally, 70 degrees downward.
2.   IOP measurement requires a tonometer applied to the cornea. Normal IOP ranges from 12 to 21 mmHg; pressure is increased in glaucoma.

3.   **In vision testing, a Snellen chart is used to evaluate visual acuity and newsprint is used to assess near vision. Normal visual acuity is considered to be $^{20}/_{20}$, in which the numerator represents the distance from the person to chart and the denominator the distance at which a normal eye can read the line; the larger the denominator, the poorer the vision.**
4.   Used to prescribe corrective lenses, the refraction test requires the person to read a Snellen chart through various corrective lenses to measure errors of focus: myopia (nearsightedness), hyperopia (farsightedness), astigmatism (inability to focus horizontal and vertical rays on retina).
5.   Ophthalmoscopic examination evaluates blood vessels and structures of the posterior eye (fundus), detecting retinal changes due to neurologic or vascular conditions.

B.   Psychosocial implications
1.   A client with a visual problem may experience coping difficulties related to:
     a.   Unknown prognosis
     b.   Chronicity or long-term nature of the condition
2.   The client also may experience self-concept changes associated with:
     a.   Altered body image due to blindness or the need to wear eyeglasses
     b.   Potential for loss of independence
3.   The client may have to adjust to lifestyle changes related to potential changes in:
     a.   Role performance
     b.   Occupational performance, with possibility of job loss
     c.   Self-care ability

4. Changes in social interaction patterns related to vision problems may lead to:
   a. Depression
   b. Isolation

III. General nursing interventions in eye care

A. Ophthalmic medication administration

1. **Ensure that all eye medications are sterile.**
2. **Do not use unlabeled, cloudy, or discolored solutions.**
3. **Avoid contact with the eye to prevent contaminating the medication bottle or tube tip.**
4. **Treat each eye separately (i.e., separate medication and equipment); treat the uninfected eye first to avoid cross contamination.**
5. To instill eye drops:
   a. Tilt the client's head back slightly; expose the lower conjunctival sac by pulling down gently on the cheekbone.
   b. Have the client look up.
   c. Resting your hand on the client's forehead for support, to prevent eye injury during administration, instill the prescribed amount of medication onto the lower conjunctiva.
   d. Close the lid gently and press on the nasal-lacrimal canal (inner canthus) to prevent systemic drug absorption and resulting side effects.
   e. Wipe excess secretions with a sterile cotton ball, wiping from the inner to the outer canthus.
6. To instill eye ointment:
   a. Follow the same basic procedure as for instilling eye drops.
   b. Have the client close the lid and roll the eye after instillation.

B. Eye patch application

1. Have the client close both eyes during patch application.
2. Apply the patch and secure it with two strips of tape extending from the midforehead to the lateral cheekbone.
3. **Never apply pressure unless prescribed; if pressure is indicated, use two or three pads and more tape.**
4. Never change an eye patch without a physician's order.

C. Eye shield application

1. Apply an eye shield, alone or over an eye patch, to protect the eye from pressure or irritation.
2. Rest the shield on the bony prominences of the brow, cheek, and nose, and secure it in place with strips of trans-

parent tape in the same manner as for an eye patch (medial top to lateral bottom).

IV. General nursing interventions in eye surgery

A. Preoperative care

1. Explain expected preoperative procedures (e.g., sedation, local or general anesthetic) to reduce anxiety associated with the unfamiliar and unexpected.

2. For the same reason, explain what to expect postoperatively (e.g., eye patch application, prescribed positioning, activity restrictions, ophthalmic medication use, measures to prevent increased IOP, a small amount of serous drainage and subjunctival hemorrhage postoperatively, and eyelid edema for several days).

B. Postoperative care

1. Take precautions to prevent increased IOP, such as:
   a. Instructing the client to lie on the unoperated side
   b. Avoiding constipation (e.g., by administering stool softeners)
   c. Encouraging the client to avoid sneezing or coughing (or to cough with the mouth open, if necessary)
   d. Administering an antiemetic to a nauseous client to prevent vomiting
   e. Washing the client's hair, when allowed, with the neck hyperextended rather than flexed
   f. Instructing the client to avoid excessive exertion, such as lifting and pushing objects

2. Take precautions to prevent injury, such as:
   a. Orienting the client to the hospital environment
   b. Keeping a call bell and other needed items within the client's reach and in a consistent place
   c. Keeping the bed in a low position with the side rails up
   d. Providing adequate room light, or dimming lights if the client experiences photophobia
   e. Assisting the client with ambulation, if indicated
   f. Advising the client not to rub the eyes or touch an eye patch

3. Relieve postoperative discomfort with proper positioning and analgesics as prescribed; avoid opiates, which may cause vomiting or constipation.

4. **Instruct the client to report any sharp pain or feelings of pressure in the eye, which may indicate hemorrhage, increased IOP, or infection. Also instruct the client to report signs and symptoms of additional complications,**

such as coughing, marked restlessness, or any eye pain unrelieved by analgesics.

5. Promote mobility within postoperative restrictions; post any prescribed activity restrictions on the client's bed.
6. Prevent sensory deprivation by:
    a. Rooming the client with another well-oriented, active person if possible
    b. Providing sensory stimulation (e.g., talk to the client often, provide a radio or TV, encourage frequent visitation by family and friends)
    c. Frequently reorienting the client to the environment and the date and time of day
7. Promote adequate nutrition; assist the client with eating and drinking, as necessary, to ensure adequate intake and prevent choking and aspiration.
8. Teach appropriate self-care measures, which may include:
    a. Not removing an eye patch unless specifically ordered
    b. Wearing an eye shield at night or when lying down
    c. Taking sponge baths or showers without getting water on the face
    d. Wearing dark glasses and dimming room lights if experiencing photophobia or using dilating drops
    e. Using medications as prescribed

V. Retinal detachment

A. Description: separation of the retina from the choroid in the posterior eye

B. Etiology and incidence
1. Retinal detachment may result from trauma, age-related degenerative changes, or cataract removal.
2. It most commonly affects persons older than age 40.

C. Pathophysiology and management
1. Retinal layers separate from the choroid, creating a subretinal space.
2. Vitreous fluid seeps between these layers, disrupting choroidal blood supply.
3. Detachment may be partial, causing varying degrees of visual deficits, or total, causing blindness in the affected eye.
4. In most cases, surgery is indicated to reattach the retina.

D. Assessment findings
1. Clinical manifestations typically include:
    a. Recurrent flashes of light and floating spots initially
    b. Progressive blurring of vision in the affected eye, followed by visual field deficits, with the area of visual loss depending on the area of detachment

    2. The client is commonly anxious, confused, and fearful of blindness.

    3. Ophthalmoscopic examination may reveal an area of gray, opaque retina, possibly with fold, holes, or tears.

E. **Nursing diagnoses**

    1. Anxiety

    2. Risk for Injury

    3. Knowledge Deficit

    4. Impaired Physical Mobility

    5. Pain

    6. Sensory/Perceptual Alteration: Visual

F. **Planning and implementation**

    1. Provide information regarding surgical options, which may include:

        a. Creating localized chorioretinal adhesions to reapproximate the retina and choroid through cryotherapy, photocoagulation, laser surgery

        b. Sealing the retina to the choroid with scleral buckling surgery

        c. Injecting an intraocular gas bubble to promote adhesion

    2. Limit mobility by:

        a. Positioning the client in bed preoperatively as prescribed (usually with the detached area dependent), and instructing the client to avoid lying face down, stooping, or bending

        b. Enforcing bedrest for 1 day postoperatively, positioned supine or on the unoperated side unless directed otherwise

    3. Promote adaptation to perceptual impairment:

        a. Preoperatively, patch both eyes if detachment threatens the macula.

        b. Using the correct technique, administer a mydriatic agent to dilate the pupil for intraocular assessment and to accommodate refraction; administer a cycloplegic agent to paralyze the ciliary accommodative muscles before refraction (see Section III.A).

          ▶ *Parasympatholytic (anticholinergic) drugs* with combined mydriatic and cycloplegic effects such as atropine sulfate (Atropisol) and scopolamine hydrobromide (Isopto Hyoscine)

          ▶ *Sympathomimetic (adrenergic) drugs* which do not include cycloplegia but cause vasoconstriction and reduce intraocular pressure such as epinephrine (Glaucon) and phenylephrine HCL (Neo-Synephrine)

        c.   Postoperatively, patch the affected eye for 1 to 4 hours; encourage visitors, socialization, sensory stimulation, and diversional activities.

    4.   Relieve discomfort

        a.   Preoperatively, administer sedation as prescribed, promote comfort and relaxation, and minimize eye strain.

        b.   Postoperatively, administer mild analgesics for discomfort, and apply cool or warm compresses to swollen eyelids.

    5.   Provide postoperative instructions, covering:

        a.   Activities allowed and restricted

        b.   Position prescribed

        c.   Resumption of activity: resuming ADLs gradually and as tolerated, commonly resuming light work in 3 weeks and normal activity in 6 weeks; avoiding heavy lifting, deep bending, or stooping (possibly for life); avoiding bumping or otherwise injuring the head

G. **Evaluation**

    1.   The client adheres to activity and positioning requirements.

    2.   The client displays low anxiety during the period of visual impairment.

    3.   The client reports adequate comfort level following surgery.

    4.   The client follows recommendations for activity resumption.

    5.   The client remains free of eye and other injuries.

VI. **Glaucoma**

  A. **Description**

    1.   Glaucoma refers to a group of disorders characterized by abnormally elevated intraocular pressure (IOP), which can damage the optic nerve.

    2.   Types include:

        a.   Chronic open-angle glaucoma

        b.   Acute closed-angle (or narrow-angle) glaucoma

  B. **Etiology and incidence**

    1.   Glaucoma may be congenital and usually is acquired (hereditary tendency).

    2.   The second most common cause of blindness in the United States, glaucoma affects about 2% of the population older than age 40.

  C. **Pathophysiology and management**

    1.   In chronic open-angle glaucoma, obstruction to outflow of aqueous humor through the trabecular meshwork to canal of Schlemm leads to increased IOP. It usually is bilateral.

2. Increased IOP eventually destroys optic nerve function, causing blindness.

3. Acute closed-angle glaucoma typically involves sudden, complete, unilateral closure with pupil dilation stimulated by dark environment, emotional stress, or mydriatic drugs. It is considered a medical emergency; delay in treatment leads to blindness within several days of onset.

D. Assessment findings

1. Clinical manifestations of chronic open-angle glaucoma typically include:
   a. No early symptoms
   b. Insidious visual impairment, blurring
   c. Diminished accommodation
   d. Gradual loss of peripheral vision (tunnel vision)
   e. Mildly aching eyes
   f. Halos around lights later with elevated IOP

2. Acute closed-angle glaucoma is commonly marked by:
   a. Transitory attacks of diminished visual acuity
   b. Colored halos around lights
   c. Reddened eye with excruciating pain
   d. Headache
   e. Nausea and vomiting

3. Important diagnostic tests for glaucoma include:
   a. Tonometry, which detects elevated IOP
   b. Slit-lamp examination
   c. Gonioscopy to differentiate between chronic open-angle and acute closed-angle glaucoma

E. Nursing diagnoses

1. Anxiety
2. Risk for Injury
3. Knowledge Deficit
4. Sensory/Perceptual Alterations: Visual

F. Planning and implementation

1. **As prescribed, manage chronic open-angle glaucoma with recommended pharmacologic agents. Forewarn client that these medications may cause transient blurring.**
   a. As prescribed, administer *miotics*, which lower IOP by constricting the pupils and by promoting outflow of aqueous humor. Medications include:

   ▸ *Parasympathomimetic (cholinergic) drugs* such as pilocarpine hydrochloride (Pilocar), carbachol (Miostat)
   ▸ *Cholinesterase inhibitors* such as echothiophate (Iodide), demecarium bromide (Humorsol)

      b. Administer *beta-adrenergic blockers*, which decrease the formation of aqueous humor and prevent the sympathetic response of pupil dilation. Medications include timolol (Timoptic), betaxolol (Betoptic).

      c. Administer *carbonic anhydrase inhibitors* such as acetazolamide (Diamox), which reduce the formation of aqueous humor thereby lowering IOP. Urge the client, who is self-administering medication, not to miss doses.

2. **Teach client how to administer eye medications correctly; have the client perform a return demonstration (see Section III.A).**

3. Provide information about laser trabeculoplasty if medication therapy proves ineffective.

4. Provide information regarding management of acute closed-angle glaucoma, including:

      a. Immediate surgical opening of the eye chamber

      b. Carbonic anhydrase inhibitors intravenously (IV) or intramuscularly (IM) to restrict production of aqueous humor

      c. Osmotic agents (mannitol, glycerol)

      d. Surgical or laser peripheral iridectomy after acute episode is relieved

      e. Prophylactic peripheral iridectomy of the unaffected eye before discharge

5. Provide general preoperative and postoperative care and teaching (see Section IV).

6. Teach the client about specific safety precautions, including:

      a. Avoiding mydriatics like atropine, which may precipitate acute glaucoma in a client with closed-angle glaucoma

      b. Carrying prescribed medications at all times

      c. Carrying a medical identification card or wearing a bracelet stating the type of glaucoma and need for medication

      d. Taking extra precautions at night (e.g., use handrails, providing extra lighting to compensate for impaired pupil dilation from miotic use)

G. Evaluation

1. The client verbalizes understanding of prescribed medications and demonstrates appropriate administration technique.

2. The client verbalizes the importance of carrying a medical identification card specifying his or her glaucoma.

3. The client verbalizes understanding of the need to avoid activities that can increase IOP.

4. The client demonstrates compliance with the postoperative regimen.

VII. Cataracts

A. Description: gradually progressive opacity of the lens or lens capsule that leads to visual loss

B. Etiology and incidence

1. The most common cause of cataracts is aging; about 85% of persons older than age 80 experience this problem to some degree.

2. Other possible causes include trauma, drug or chemical toxicity, genetic defects, and secondary effects of other diseases.

C. Pathophysiology and management

1. Altered nutrient metabolism within the lens triggers cataract formation.

2. The lens becomes cloudy and has reduced accommodative power.

3. Light rays cannot pass through the opaque lens to the retina, causing vision loss.

4. Cataracts develop bilaterally, but progression varies in each eye. Treatment involves removal and replacement of the lens.

D. Assessment findings

1. Clinical manifestations include:
   a. Progressively worsening blurred vision
   b. Cloudy-appearing lens
   c. No pain or eye redness

2. Ophthalmoscopic or slit-lamp examination confirms diagnosis.

E. Nursing diagnoses

1. Anxiety
2. Knowledge Deficit
3. Pain
4. Sensory/Perceptual Alteration: Visual

F. Planning and implementation

1. Provide information regarding lens extraction surgery covering:
   a. Preoperative medications:

   ▶ *Sympathomimetic (adrenergic) drugs* such as epinephrine (Glaucon) and phenylephrine (Neo-Synephrine), which cause vasoconstriction and reduce IOP

   ▶ *Hyperosmotic agents,* such as mannitol (Osmitrol) and

glycerol (Osmoglyn), which elevate plasma osmolality and enhance flow of water into the extracellular fluid thereby reducing IOP

m b. **Directions for correct eye medication administration technique (see Section III.A)**

c. What to expect after lens removal: client becomes aphakic (without lens); client may experience hyperopia (farsightedness); with one eye aphakic and the other with lens, client will experience diplopia (double vision)

d. What to expect after lens removed with intraocular lens (IOL) implant: client becomes pseudophakic (has false lens); IOL enables immediate binocular vision if vision is good in other eye; vision will be fine-tuned with glasses

2. Relieve postoperative discomfort with analgesics and atropine eye drops as prescribed. Instruct the client to report severe eye pain immediately; this may indicate increasing IOP or hemorrhage.

3. Provide postoperative teaching, covering:
    a. Discharge, which usually occurs a few hours after surgery
    b. The need for a patch and shield over the operative eye
    c. Patch change by the surgeon the second postoperative day
    d. The need for eye protection: wearing glasses during day (sunglasses at first), using an eye shield at night to prevent rubbing the eye, avoiding straining, lying on back or unaffected side when in bed, reading only in moderation, maintaining sedentary lifestyle for 2 weeks

4. Assist the client with adaptation to altered vision and rehabilitative requirements; explain the need to:
    a. Wear temporary, thick, convex cataract glasses if one eye is aphakic and the other has poor visual acuity.
    b. Wear an eye patch over a glass or phakic eye for binocular vision, if one eye is aphakic and the other phakic (with lens).
    c. Turn the head to the side to scan the entire visual field to compensate for impaired peripheral vision.
    d. Compensate for altered spatial relationships.
    e. Wear permanent glasses prescribed after healing is complete in 2 to 12 months.
    f. Administer steroid-antibiotic eye drops, such as dexamethasone (Maxidex Ophthalmic Solution) and flu-

orometholone (Fluor-Op), which decrease nonpyrogenic inflammation and help prevent infection postoperatively after IOL insertion.

 ▸ **Caution client that medication may initially cause sensitivity to bright light. Suggest wearing sunglasses; instruct client on correct administration technique (see Section III-A).**

g. Administer cycloplegic drops, such as atropine sulfate (Atropisol) or scopolamine hydrobromide (Isopto Hyoscine), to paralyze ciliary accommodative muscles before refraction for 1 to 2 months postoperatively if no IOL was inserted.

 ▸ **Instruct client to notify physician if eye pain occurs after administration (a possible indication of underlying glaucoma).**

G. Evaluation
1. The client verbalizes the need to take precautions and avoid complications.
2. The client exhibits positive adjustment to altered vision and rehabilitative requirements.

VIII. Ears
A. Structures (Fig. 15-2)
1. External ear
    a. Structures of the external ear include the auricle, external auditory canal, and tympanic membrane, also called the eardrum (Fig. 15-2).
    b. The auricle and external auditory canal receive and direct sound waves to the tympanic membrane.
2. Middle ear
    a. Ossicles (consisting of the malleus, incus, and stapes) move and conduct sound waves from the external ear to inner ear.
    b. The eustachian tube equalizes pressure on both sides of the tympanic membrane.
    c. The middle ear communicates with mastoid air cells of the temporal bone.
3. Inner ear (labyrinth)
    a. The vestibule contains receptors that respond to the position of the head as it relates to gravity.
    b. The cochlea contains the organ of Corti (receptor end organ of hearing).
    c. Semicircular canals contain sensory organs of equilibrium.

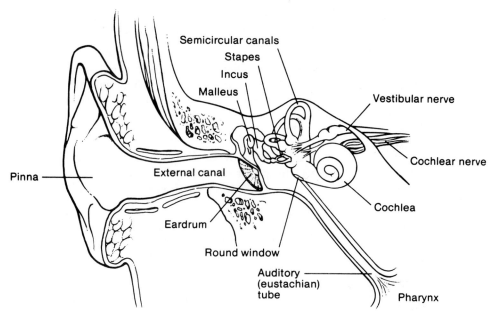

FIGURE 15-2.
Structures of the ear. (From Fuller, J., & Schaller-Ayers, J. [1994]. *Health assessment: A nursing approach*. Philadelphia: J. B. Lippincott.)

4. The acoustic nerve (CN VIII) connects the cochlea, semicircular canals, and vestibular receptors with the brain.

B. Function

1. The ears are involved in both the hearing and position sense (balance and equilibrium).
2. In hearing, sound waves are directed by the external ear through the external auditory meatus where they strike the tympanic membrane, causing it to vibrate.
3. These vibrations trigger movement of the ossicles in the middle ear, whose stapes transmit the vibrations through the fluid in the inner ear to the cochlea and the organ of Corti.
4. Movement in the organ of Corti stimulates the sensory ends of the cochlear branch of the acoustic nerve (CN VIII), which sends impulses to the temporal lobe for interpretation as sound.
5. For position sense, fluid in the semicircular canals of the inner ear responds to body movement by stimulating nerve cells that line the canals. These cells transmit impulses through the vestibular branch of the acoustic nerve to the brain for maintenance of balance and equilibrium.

IX. Overview of ear disorders

A. Assessment

1. Tympanic membrane (eardrum) inspection involves straightening the external auditory canal of an adult by pulling the auricle up and back while tilting the client's head slightly; normal findings include an intact, shiny, pearly gray, concave membrane that moves with swallowing.

 2. Hearing acuity can be screened by having the client identify the point near the ear at which he or she can hear a whispered voice or ticking watch; normally, the client should hear the sound at a distance of 2 feet or so.

3. The Weber test evaluates bone conduction with a tuning fork placed on the midline of the head; normally, the tone is heard equally in both ears by bone conduction.

4. The Rinne test uses a tuning fork to evaluate air conduction and bone conduction; normally, air conduction is greater than bone conduction (positive Rinne).

5. Audiometry should be performed by an audiologist certified by the American Speech and Hearing Association.

6. Assessment of nose and throat should accompany ear assessment because infection in these areas may lead to ear problems.

B. Psychosocial implications

1. A client with a hearing problem may experience coping difficulties related to:
   a. Unknown prognosis
   b. Chronicity or long-term nature of the condition

2. The client also may experience self-concept changes associated with:
   a. Altered body image due to deafness or the need for a hearing aid
   b. Potential for loss of independence

3. The client may have to adjust to lifestyle changes related to potential changes in:
   a. Role performance
   b. Occupational performance, with possibility of job loss
   c. Self-care ability

4. Changes in social interaction patterns related to hearing problems may lead to:
   a. Depression
   b. Isolation

X. Conductive hearing loss

A. Description

1. Conductive hearing loss refers to various problems involving impaired passage of sound from the external ear to the inner ear.
2. Specific conditions include:
   a. Cerumen impaction
   b. External otitis media
   c. Serous otitis media
   d. Suppurative otitis media
   e. Otosclerosis

B. Etiology and incidence

1. Cerumen impaction usually occurs in persons who naturally produce large amounts of cerumen.
2. Causes of external otitis media include infection (bacterial or fungal), excessive moisture in the auditory canal (swimmer's ear), and trauma.
3. Serous otitis media may result from eustachian tube obstruction, sudden changes in atmospheric pressure, allergy, and viral disease.
4. Suppurative otitis media may follow viral disease, tympanic membrane perforation, or prolonged forceful nose blowing. It is most common in infants and young children because of their immature and relatively poorly draining eustachian tubes.
5. Otosclerosis appears to be a hereditary condition; it affects women twice as often as men and typically develops between ages 15 and 30.

C. Pathophysiology and management

1. Impacted cerumen in external ear can block sound from reaching the tympanic membrane.
2. External otitis media involves inflammation of the external ear, with crust formation and edema in the auditory canal.
3. Serous otitis media involves sterile fluid accumulation in the middle ear. It may be acute or chronic; frequent recurrences can threaten hearing.
4. Suppurative otitis media involves pus accumulation in the middle ear and possibly extending into adjacent structures. Chronic recurrence may lead to tympanic membrane perforation.
5. In otosclerosis, spongy bone grows over the normal bony labyrinth, causing the footplate of the stapes to become fixed in the oval window of the otic capsule.

D. **Assessment findings**

1. Cerumen impaction is often visible; the client demonstrates some degree of hearing loss.
2. External otitis media is commonly marked by:
   a. Itching and pain
   b. Watery or purulent discharge
3. Manifestations of serous otitis media include:
   a. Plugged feeling in ear
   b. Reverberation of the client's own voice
   c. Hearing loss
4. Suppurative otitis media typically produces:
   a. Throbbing ear pain
   b. Fever, hearing loss, nausea, and vomiting
   c. Feeling of increased pressure in the ear
   d. Bright red, bulging or retracted tympanic membrane
   e. Possible tympanic membrane rupture with discharge (otorrhea)
5. Otosclerosis may be marked by:
   a. Reduced air conduction compared to bone conduction on Rinne test
   b. Mixed hearing loss or sensorineural hearing loss
   c. Tinnitus

E. **Nursing diagnoses**

1. Knowledge Deficit
2. Risk for Injury
3. Impaired Physical Mobility
4. Pain
5. Sensory/Perceptual Alteration: Auditory
6. Social Isolation

F. **Planning and implementation**

1. Instruct the client in general ear care and hearing protection measures, including:
   a. Protecting the ears from loud noises with plugs, muffs, and so forth
   b. Chewing gum or sucking hard candy when flying to open the eustachian tube and allow air into middle ear
   c. Never inserting any object into the auditory canal beyond the extent of vision
   d. Inserting no object smaller than the finger into the ear
   e. Blowing the nose with the mouth open and both nostrils open to prevent forcing contaminated material into the middle ear

 f. **Instruct client to pull the top of the ear up and**

back when instilling ear drops. (This straightens the ear canal.)

2. If appropriate, teach the client to remove impacted cerumen by first softening it with instilled peroxide or glycerol preparations, such as Debrox, and then irrigating the ear in 2 or 3 days to remove the wax. Instruct the client:
   a. To keep otic solution in ears for 15 minutes by tilting head sideways or by putting cotton in ear
   b. To notify the physician if inflammation or irritation occurs
   c. Not to use the solution for more than 4 consecutive days

3. Provide care to a client with tympanic membrane perforation as follows:
   a. Maintain strict asepsis.
   b. Do not irrigate the ear.
   c. Protect from water contamination by having the client wear ear plugs and a bathing cap.
   d. Recognize a client at risk for labyrinthitis or meningitis.

4. For a client with impaired hearing, enhance communication:
   a. Do not rely on the hospital's intercom system.
   b. Do not exclude the client from conversations in the room.
   c. Avoid startling the client; get the client's attention before speaking to him or her.
   d. Ensure adequate lighting; face the person, speak slowly and distinctly with voice slightly raised (but without shouting), use nonverbal cues.
   e. Use a message board if necessary.
   f. Insert a hearing aid if indicated.

5. Treat external otitis media with topical antibiotics and steroids, gentle debridement, and acid-alcohol solutions to sterilize the auditory canal as prescribed.

6. Prepare a client with serous otitis media for treatment, which may include:
   a. Needle aspiration
   b. Myringotomy (incision into the tympanic membrane to relieve pressure and remove pus)

7. Provide prescribed treatments for a client with suppurative otitis media, which may include:
   a. Systemic antibiotics (for at least 7 days)
   b. Nasal decongestants
   c. Analgesics
   d. Heat and cold applications

8. If indicated, prepare a client with suppurative otitis media for surgery, which may involve:
   a. Mastoidectomy (if the mastoid is involved)
   b. Myringoplasty (repair of perforated tympanic membrane)
   c. Tympanoplasty (replacement or rebuilding of middle ear structures)
9. Prepare a client with otosclerosis for surgery, as indicated, which may include:
   a. Stapedectomy (replacement of diseased ossicles with prostheses)
   b. Fenestration (creation of a new window into the labyrinth to provide a new pathway for sound)
10. Prepare a client undergoing ear surgery for postoperative expectations and requirements:
    a. Inform the client that hearing may not improve noticeably until swelling leaves the operative area and packs are removed.
    b. Explain expected postoperative restrictions on positioning and movement.
    c. Instruct the client not to sneeze, cough, blow his or her nose, or touch the ear or dressing until allowed.
11. Take steps to prevent postoperative injury due to postoperative complications:
    a. Monitor for signs and symptoms of infection (e.g., temperature elevation, headache, drainage).
    b. Do not disturb the inner dressing.
    c. Avoid applying pressure to the ear or ear dressing, which could dislodge a graft or prosthesis.
    d. If the client experiences vertigo, note nystagmus and record the direction of eye movement and effects of position changes.
    e. Observe for signs of facial nerve injury (e.g., inability to frown, wrinkle forehead, close eyes, bare teeth, or pucker lips). (*Note:* Injury may be temporary, due to swelling, or it may be permanent.)
    f. Protect the eye if facial nerve injury occurs.
    g. Instruct the client to report tinnitus, fluctuating hearing, or vertigo.
12. Promote mobility within postoperative restrictions:
    a. Maintain bedrest for up to 48 hours.
    b. Position the client on his or her side with the operative ear up, to prevent displacement of graft; with operative ear down, to enhance drainage; or on the unoperative side, to minimize nausea and vomiting.

13. Relieve postoperative discomfort and guard against injury by:
    a. Maintaining the prescribed position
    b. Keeping the bed rails up and assisting the client with ambulation
    c. Teaching the client to use hand rails (vertigo may threaten safety) and avoid contraindicated or sudden movements
    d. Avoiding jarring the client or the bed
    e. Instructing the client to breathe deeply through an open mouth
    f. Medicating for pain or nausea as indicated
    g. Providing a light or liquid diet to control nausea as necessary
14. Provide the client with self-care instructions, including:
    a. Avoiding getting the ear wet to prevent infection
    b. Avoiding persons with upper respiratory infection
    c. Avoiding bending, straining, and flying until allowed in the postoperative stapedectomy period
    d. Taking the full course of prescribed medications, even after symptoms are relieved
    e. Taking care to prevent burns with a hair dryer if the auricle is numb

G. **Evaluation**
   1. The client demonstrates understanding of effective ear care and hearing protection measures.
   2. The client is free of discomfort and complications postoperatively.
   3. The client verbalizes understanding of self-care and follow-up instructions.

XI. **Menière's disease**
   A. **Description: a chronic disorder of the inner ear involving sensorineural hearing loss, severe vertigo, and tinnitus**
   B. **Etiology and incidence**
      1. The cause of Menière's disease is unknown; it is associated with aging and may follow middle ear infection or head trauma.
      2. It affects men slightly more often than women and most commonly occurs between ages 40 and 50.
   C. **Pathophysiology and management**
      1. Menière's disease appears to involve overproduction or decreased absorption of endolymph, with resultant degeneration of vestibular and cochlear hair cells.
      2. Recurrent attacks result in progressive sensorineural hearing loss (especially low tones), usually unilateral in nature.

D. **Assessment findings**
1. Menière's disease may produce:
    a. Sudden episodes of severe whirling vertigo, with the inability to stand or walk; an episode may last up to several hours
    b. Buzzing tinnitus that worsens before and during an episode
    c. Nausea, vomiting, and diaphoresis
    d. Possibly, brief loss of consciousness with nystagmus
2. Audiometric testing reveals sensorineural hearing loss.

E. **Nursing diagnoses**
1. Anxiety
2. Risk for Injury
3. Knowledge Deficit
4. Pain
5. Sensory/Perceptual Alteration: Auditory
6. Social Isolation

F. **Planning and implementation**

1. **Provide a safe, quiet, dimly lit environment, and enforce bedrest during acute episodes.**
2. Provide emotional support and reassurance to alleviate anxiety.
3. Relieve discomfort with antivertigo agents to decrease sensation of imbalance and dizziness. Different agents are used to determine which is best for the client during an acute attack. Examples include dimenhydrinate (Dramamine), meclizine (Antivert), and diazepam (T-Quil).
4. Provide self-care instructions covering:
    a. The nature of the disorder
    b. The need for a low-salt diet
    c. The importance of avoiding stimulants and vasoconstrictors (e.g., caffeine, decongestants, alcohol)
    d. Self-administration of appropriate medications:
       ▸ *Atropine sulfate* to decrease vertigo during acute attack (Advise client to drink plenty of fluid because the drug causes urinary retention and hesitancy.)
       ▸ *Diuretics,* such as acetazolamide (Diamox) or chlorothiazide (Diuril), which cause diuresis that decreases pressure in the ear and minimizes vertigo (Instruct client to report signs of hypokalemia including muscle cramps, weakness, fatigue; weight gain over 3 lb daily; or excessive diuresis.)
       ▸ *Vasodilators,* such as tolazoline (Priscoline), methantheline (Banthine), niacin (nicotinic acid) which relax vascu-

lar smooth muscle thereby reducing tinnitus (Teach client how to prevent orthostatic hypotension.)

▶ *Antihistamines,* such as dimenhydrinate (Dramamine) or meclizine (Antivert), which suppress vestibular activity thereby decreasing vertigo, nausea, and vomiting (Warn client to avoid hazardous activities, take drug with food to minimize GI distress, rinse mouth with water or chew sugarless gum to relieve dry mouth.)

    5. Discuss potential treatment options:

      a. Conservative management: psychotherapy, allergic hyposensitization, low sodium diet, antihistamines, vasodilators, steroids, antiemetics

      b. Surgery: sac decompression, shunts, ultrasound, labyrinthectomy

G. **Evaluation**

    1. The client reports relief of symptoms due to exacerbation of Menière's disease.

    2. The client remains free from injury during episode.

    3. The client verbalizes understanding of the prescribed self-care regimen and the importance of compliance.

XII. Nose and sinuses

A. **Nose**

    1. The nasal passages, or turbinates, are three bony structures (superior, middle, and inferior) located between the roof of the mouth and the frontal, ethmoid, and sphenoid bones of the skull.

    2. The lining of the nasal turbinates is highly vascular; the nasal vestibule just inside the nares contains cilia—tiny hairs that filter inspired air.

    3. Nasal passages filter, warm, and humidify inspired air.

    4. Enervated by the olfactory nerve (CN I), the nose provides the function of olfaction (smell); the senses of taste and smell are closely related.

B. **Sinuses**

    1. The four paranasal sinuses (frontal, maxillary, ethmoidal, and sphenoidal) are air cavities located around and draining into the nasal turbinates.

    2. The sinuses produce mucus for the nasal cavity and give timbre and resonance to the voice.

XIII. Overview of nose and sinus disorders

A. **Nose and olfactory function assessment**

    1. Assess olfaction by having person identify various odors.

    2. Insert speculum blades ½ inch into nares, resting index finger on side of client's nose.

    3. Inspect for pallor, edema, masses, polyps, redness.

B. Sinus assessment

    1. Inspect the nasal mucosa for redness and discharge.

    2. Palpate the frontal and maxillary sinuses for tenderness.

XIV. **Epistaxis**

  A. Description: severe nosebleed

  B. Etiology and incidence

    1. Epistaxis may be spontaneous or may result from trauma (usually nose picking).

    2. It also may be associated with chemical irritation, acute or chronic infection (such as rhinitis or sinusitis), purpura, leukemia and other blood dyscrasias, hypertension, anticoagulant therapy, or deviated septum.

  C. Pathophysiology and management

    1. In children, epistaxis usually originates in the anterior nose and tends to be mild; in adults, it tends to originate in the posterior nose and be more severe.

    2. Slight to moderate epistaxis usually causes no complications; severe bleeding (persisting longer than 10 minutes after pressure is applied) may cause blood loss up to 1 L/hour.

  D. Assessment findings

    1. Clinical manifestations may include:

      a. Bleeding through the nares, blood trickling into the oropharynx

      b. Blood in the corners of eyes (through the lacrimal ducts)

      c. Blood in the auditory canal if the tympanic membrane is perforated

    2. Nasal inspection with a bright light and speculum may locate the source of bleeding.

  E. Nursing diagnoses

    1. Ineffective Airway Clearance

    2. Risk for Injury

    3. Pain

  F. Planning and implementation

    1. **Intervene to control bleeding, as follows:**

      a. **Have the client sit upright, breathe through the mouth, and refrain from talking.**

      b. **Compress the soft outer portion of the nares against the septum for 5 to 10 minutes.**

      c. **Instruct the client to avoid nose blowing during or after the episode.**

    2. If pressure does not control bleeding, insert anterior packing or posterior packing as appropriate. Keep scissors and a hemostat on hand to cut the strings and remove the packing in the event of airway obstruction.

3. Monitor bleeding: Inspect for blood trickling into the posterior pharynx; observe for hemoptysis, hematemesis, frequent swallowing or belching; instruct the client not to swallow but to spit out any blood.

4. If indicated, provide information regarding electrocautery.

G. **Evaluation**

1. The client remains calm and exhibits no or only minor breathing difficulty.

2. Bleeding is controlled.

3. The client reports adequate pain relief.

XV. Throat

A. **Larynx**

1. Transition between upper and lower airways

2. Permits vocalization

B. **Epiglottis**

1. Part of larynx that protects lower airway

2. Covers larynx during swallowing

XVI. Overview of throat disorders

A. **Assessment**

1. Examine the posterior pharynx with a warmed mirror (to prevent fogging) and tongue depressor, instructing the client to open the mouth wide and take a deep breath to flatten the posterior tongue.

2. Observe color and symmetry; note any exudate, ulcerations, or swelling.

3. Palpate the neck for enlarged lymph nodes.

4. Palpate the neck to assess position and mobility of the trachea; lateral deviation may indicate a mass in the neck or mediastinum.

B. **Psychosocial implications**

1. The client with laryngeal cancer may experience coping difficulties related to:
   a. Unknown progression of symptoms
   b. Chronicity or long-term nature of the disease
   c. Fear of death
   d. Altered communication

2. The client may experience self-concept changes due to:
   a. Body image change after laryngectomy
   b. Potential loss of independence
   c. Altered role performance

3. Disease-related changes in social interaction patterns may result in depression and isolation.

XVII. **Foreign body aspiration**
  A. Description: partial or total occlusion of the larynx or lower airway by an aspirated object
  B. Etiology and incidence
    1. Children may aspirate a variety of objects.
    2. Food is the most common cause of airway obstruction in adults.
  C. Pathophysiology and management
    1. Objects may be aspirated into the upper airway or lower airway (below the larynx).
    2. Aspirated objects can enter the right main bronchus.
    3. Complete airway obstruction may rapidly lead to cardiopulmonary arrest.
  D. Assessment findings
    1. Clinical manifestations of airway obstruction include:
       a. Signs of respiratory distress
       b. Weak, ineffective cough
       c. High-pitched noises on inspiration
       d. Clutching of neck with hands
       e. Inability to speak with complete obstruction
    2. Cyanosis and loss of consciousness may occur with complete obstruction.
  E. Nursing diagnoses
    1. Anxiety
    2. Ineffective Breathing Pattern
  F. Planning and implementation
    1. **If the client can speak (indicating partial airway obstruction):**
       a. **Position for optimal ventilation.**
       b. **Encourage coughing.**
    2. **If the client cannot speak (indicating complete obstruction):**
       a. **Call for help immediately.**
       b. **Perform abdominal thrust (Heimlich) maneuver; use lower sternal thrust for an obese or pregnant victim.**
       c. **Remove an object in the larynx with a finger or forceps via laryngoscopy.**
       d. **Remove an object in the lower airway through bronchoscopy.**
       e. **Prepare to assist with emergency cricothyroidotomy if necessary.**
    3. Help relieve anxiety:
       a. Do not leave the client unattended.

        b.   Encourage the client to resume a normal breathing pattern and to talk about the episode after obstruction is relieved.

  G. **Evaluation**
      1. The client breathes without difficulty.
      2. The client demonstrates anxiety relief after airway clearance and discussion of the episode.

XVIII. Laryngeal cancer

  A. **Description: neoplasm of the larynx; types include:**
      1. Intrinsic: involving the vocal cords
      2. Extrinsic: involving another part of the larynx

  B. **Etiology and incidence**
      1. Predisposing factors to laryngeal cancer include:
          a.   Familial tendency
          b.   Cigarette smoking
          c.   Chronic vocal straining
          d.   Prolonged alcohol ingestion
      2. Laryngeal cancer is the most common cancer of the head and neck; incidence is highest in men (ages 50 to 65).

  C. **Pathophysiology and management**
      1. Most laryngeal tumors are slow-growing, squamous cell carcinomas.
      2. Intrinsic tumors are typically slow growing with little tendency to spread.
      3. More rapid-growing extrinsic tumors may spread to the lymph nodes of the neck or to the thyroid gland.
      4. Prognosis generally is favorable with early detection and treatment.

  D. **Assessment findings**
      1. The earliest and predominant sign of intrinsic laryngeal cancer is persistent hoarseness.
      2. Extrinsic laryngeal cancer commonly is marked by:
          a.   No early hoarseness
          b.   Throat pain and burning when drinking hot or acidic liquids (e.g., orange juice)
          c.   Pain possibly radiating to the ear
          d.   Possibly, enlarged lymph nodes or lump in the neck with metastasis
      3. Late symptoms of both types include:
          a.   Dysphagia and hoarseness
          b.   Dyspnea, cough, hemoptysis, foul-smelling breath
          c.   Weight loss
      4. Studies that aid diagnosis include laryngoscopy, CT scan, laryngography, tissue biopsy, and chest radiograph (to detect metastases).

E. **Nursing diagnoses**
1. Ineffective Airway Clearance
2. Anxiety
3. Ineffective Breathing Pattern
4. Impaired Verbal Communication
5. Risk for Injury
6. Knowledge Deficit
7. Altered Nutrition: Less than body requirements

F. **Planning and implementation**
1. Provide information regarding treatments, which may include:
   a. Radiation therapy (see Chapter 21, Cancer Nursing)
   b. Combination therapy, including chemotherapy (see Chapter 21, Cancer Nursing)
   c. Partial laryngectomy for intrinsic type; retains normal airway and phonation
   d. Radical neck dissection or modified radical neck on involved side
   e. Total laryngectomy: pharyngeal opening closed; speech and breathing altered; all airflow is through permanent tracheostomy
   f. Total laryngectomy with laryngoplasty: dermal tube allows exhalation of air into pharyngeal cavity; client closes permanent tracheostomy opening with finger to speak; speech production is similar to normal
2. Determine the client's understanding of the treatment plan; answer questions, address concerns, and clarify any misconceptions.
3. Encourage the client and family members to ventilate feelings and concerns related to diagnosis, prognosis, treatment, recovery, and altered function.
4. Prepare the client and family for expected postoperative alterations in breathing, speech, and appearance as appropriate.
5. Plan for an alternative means of communication before surgery (e.g., message board, magic slate, use of call bell, hand signals).
6. Initiate a preoperative evaluation by a speech pathologist if indicated.
7. Refer the client and family to support groups, such as the American Cancer Society and laryngectomy groups (e.g., Lost Chord Club, New Voice Club).
8. Promote adequate ventilation postoperatively:
   a. Place the client in Fowler's position after recovery from anesthesia.

b. Turn the client frequently to promote ventilation and drainage.

c. Provide laryngectomy care; suction as needed.

d. Assess diaphragmatic movement on the affected side; nerve damage may occur during surgery.

e. Observe for signs of impaired gas exchange: restlessness, labored breathing, apprehension, increased pulse rate.

f. Administer pain medications as needed; avoid medications that can depress respiration.

g. Encourage early ambulation.

9. Prevent postoperative infection and hemorrhage at the laryngectomy site:

a. Clean the stoma daily with saline or prescribed solution.

b. Monitor wound drainage.

10. Provide an alternative means of communication postoperatively:

a. Keep the call bell readily available at all times.

b. Provide a magic slate or flash cards.

c. Instruct the client in rudiments of lip reading or sign language.

d. Have electronic devices accessible as appropriate.

11. Encourage the client to work with the speech pathologist; esophageal speech training for total laryngectomy typically begins 1 week after surgery.

12. If indicated, prepare the client for tracheoesophageal puncture and prosthesis fitting after laryngectomy heals.

13. Promote adequate nutrition:

a. Provide enteral feeding using nasogastric tube, total parenteral nutrition if nutritionally debilitated, or enteral feeding via cervical pharyngectomy (initial tube placement by surgeon; subsequent placements by nurse) as indicated.

b. Discuss the decreased sense of taste and smell that commonly occurs postoperatively; reassure the client that these senses should improve over time.

c. Provide frequent oral hygiene.

d. Assess for swallowing difficulty due to swelling, alteration of structure, or nerve damage from surgery; assure the client that swallowing will be easier once the laryngectomy tube is removed (3 to 6 weeks postoperatively).

e. After tube removal, begin oral feeding with thick liquids (which are easier to swallow), introducing solid foods as tolerated.

14. Assist the client in adapting to home maintenance management:
   a. Encourage gradual assumption of self-care.
   b. Teach tracheal and stomal care: expect frequent coughing initially with tracheal breathing; maintain clear airway; support neck when changing positions at first; wipe stoma after coughing; cleanse around stoma twice daily (lubricate skin with non–oil-based ointment); provide adequate hydration and humidification of environment; avoid air conditioning.
   c. Teach laryngectomy protection: prevent water from entering the stoma; take tub baths or use a hand-held shower (swimming not recommended); protect stoma from hair sprays, loose hair, and powders; carry an identification card or wear a bracelet informing first-aid providers of special resuscitation requirements.
15. Teach airway care for a client discharged with a laryngectomy tube in place.

G. Evaluation

1. The client demonstrates effective communication method(s).
2. The client expresses a hopeful attitude about recovery.
3. The client exhibits effective ventilation without difficulty or signs of hypoxia or hypercapnia postoperatively.
4. The client exhibits no signs of hemorrhage or infection.
5. The client maintains adequate nutritional status.
6. The client verbalizes understanding of appropriate self-care techniques for airway management and laryngectomy protection.

Bibliography

Bolander, V. R. (1994). *Sorensen & Luckmann's basic nursing: A physiologic approach* (3rd ed.). Philadelphia: W. B. Saunders.

Clark, J., Queener, S., & Karb, V. (1990). *Pharmacologic basis of nursing practice* (4th ed.). St. Louis: C. V. Mosby.

Karch, A. (1995). *Lippincott's nursing drug guide*. Philadelphia: J. B. Lippincott.

Mosby's Patient Teaching Guides. (1994). St. Louis: C. V. Mosby.

Nettina, S. (1996). *The Lippincott manual of nursing practice* (6th ed.). Philadelphia: J. B. Lippincott.

Rankin, S. H., and Stallings, D. (1990). *Patient education: Issues, principles and guidelines*. Philadelphia: J. B. Lippincott.

Smeltzer, S. C., & Bare, B. G. (1996). *Brunner & Suddarth's textbook of medical-surgical nursing* (8th ed.). Philadelphia: Lippincott-Raven Publishers.

Springhouse Corporation. (1992). *Nursing student's guide to drugs*. Spring House, PA: Springhouse Corp.

STUDY QUESTIONS

1. To prevent systemic side effects from drug absorption during eyedrop instillation, the nurse should
   a. Press on the outer canthus of the eye.
   b. Press on the inner canthus of the eye.
   c. Have the client close his or her eyes tightly.
   d. Have the client lie supine a few minutes.

2. Correct preoperative positioning for a client diagnosed with a retinal detachment at the inner aspect of the right eye would be
   a. Fowler's position
   b. supine with a small pillow
   c. right side-lying
   d. left side-lying

3. Which medication would be the most appropriate analgesic for a client who complains of periocular aching after a surgical repair of a detached retina?
   a. Tylenol
   b. codeine
   c. Demerol
   d. morphine

4. A client who has both eyes patched after a surgical repair of a retinal detachment is calling for a dog named Joey and asks the nurse to check the gate to make certain it's locked. An appropriate nursing diagnosis for this behavior would be
   a. Ineffective Coping related to knowledge deficit
   b. Anxiety and Fear related to loss of vision
   c. Sensory/Perceptual Alterations related to loss of vision
   d. Risk for Social Isolation related to vision loss

5. During the nursing history, the nurse would expect a client undergoing surgical correction of glaucoma to state that he or she has
   a. been seeing flashes of light and floaters
   b. recently had a motor vehicle accident while changing lanes
   c. been having headaches, nausea, and redness of the eyes
   d. been having more frequent episodes of double vision

6. The *most* relevant nursing diagnosis for the client admitted for surgical correction of glaucoma would be
   a. Anxiety and Fear related to loss of vision
   b. Pain
   c. Self Care Deficit related to impaired vision
   d. Risk for Injury due to increased intraocular pressure

7. The expected outcome in the evaluation of interventions for the client with acute closed-angle glaucoma is that the client
   a. experiences miosis
   b. experiences mydriasis
   c. reports relief of eye pain
   d. reports relief of nausea and vomiting

8. A nursing history of a client with cataract would most likely include client complaints of
   a. eye pain
   b. floaters
   c. eye redness
   d. blurred vision

9. The *priority* nursing diagnosis for a client admitted to the hospital with an acute episode of Menière's disease should be
   a. Sensory/Perceptual Alteration (kinesthetic)
   b. Pain due to nausea and vomiting
   c. Risk for Fluid Volume Deficit due to vomiting
   d. Risk for Injury due to vertigo

10. The chief complaint of a client who is experiencing an acute exacerbation of Menière's disease would be
    a. vertigo
    b. dizziness
    c. severe ear pain
    d. sudden deafness

11. A client with Menière's disease should receive dietary instruction concerning which type of diet?
  a. high in protein
  b. high in salt
  c. low in protein
  d. low in salt

12. Appropriate hygienic teaching for nose blowing includes having the individual blow with
  a. both nostrils open and mouth open
  b. both nostrils open and mouth closed
  c. alternate nostrils open and mouth closed
  d. alternate nostrils open and mouth open

13. A client has just returned from having nasal surgery with posterior packing in place. The nurse plans interventions focused on control of bleeding by observing that the client
  a. appears to be anxious
  b. has discoloration about the eyes
  c. is frequently swallowing
  d. has a tarry stool

14. The nurse who is admitting a client scheduled for a total laryngectomy determines that the client understands the consequences of the planned surgery by the statement
  a. "I'll be breathing and talking as usual after surgery."
  b. "I'll be breathing as usual but talking differently after surgery."
  c. "I'll be breathing through my neck, but my talking will be the same after surgery."
  d. "I'll be breathing through my neck and will have to talk in a new way after surgery."

15. A 61-year-old client is scheduled for a total laryngectomy. During the preoperative teaching it is most important that the nurse
  a. explain the surgery and obtain informed consent for it
  b. prearrange an alternative communication system with the client
  c. have someone with this type of surgery visit the client
  d. teach the client how to perform suctioning effectively and confidently

16. The nurse knows that the client with a total laryngectomy understands the discharge teaching concerning the tracheal stoma when the client states
  a. "I should stay in my air-conditioned house as much as possible."
  b. "I should not have any episodes of coughing once the swelling goes down."
  c. "I should only take tub baths or use hand-held shower heads."
  d. "I should lubricate the skin around my stoma with petroleum jelly."

For additional questions, see
Lippincott's Self-Study Series Software
Available at your bookstore

ANSWER KEY

1. **Correct response: b**
   Pressing the inner canthus occludes the nasal–lacrimal canal, where absorption takes place.
   a. The outer canthus does not communicate with a duct.
   c. Squeezing the eyes shut might express the medication.
   d. Position would not affect flow into the canal.
   Comprehension/Physiologic/Implementation

2. **Correct response: d**
   The client generally is positioned so that the detached area is dependent.
   a, b, and c. The other positions would not accomplish this goal of management.
   Analysis/Safe care/Planning

3. **Correct response: a**
   Discomfort is usually mild.
   b. Codeine is constipating and may lead to straining and increased IOP.
   c. Demerol often causes nausea and vomiting.
   d. Morphine causes both nausea and vomiting and constipation, which should be avoided after eye surgery.
   Comprehension/Physiologic/Implementation

4. **Correct response: c**
   Sensory deprivation with both eyes patched can lead to perceptual impairment with confusion and memory dysfunction.
   a, b, and d. Although the other diagnoses are also appropriate for the client with eye surgery and loss of vision, the nurse should recognize that the client's behavior reflects disorientation and a disturbance of thought related to sensory deprivation.
   Analysis/Psychosocial/Analysis (Dx)

5. **Correct response: b**
   a. Gradual loss of peripheral vision is characteristic of glaucoma, whereas flashes of light and floaters are characteristic of retinal detachment.
   c. Nausea, headache, and eye redness are seen with an episode of acute (sudden) closed-angle closure.
   d. Double vision occurs when one eye has a lens and the other is aphakic.
   Knowledge/Physiologic/Assessment

6. **Correct response: d**
   The nursing diagnosis reflects the nurse's understanding of the primary pathophysiology of glaucoma (increased IOP).
   a, b, and c. The other diagnoses also should be incorporated into the plan of care.
   Knowledge/Health promotion/Analysis (Dx)

7. **Correct response: a**
   Acute closed-angle glaucoma is a medical emergency; the immediate goal is to open the angle with miotics to prevent blindness.
   b, c, and d. Eye dilation would aggravate the emergency and cause discomfort, nausea, and vomiting.
   Analysis/Physiologic/Evaluation

8. **Correct response: d**
   a and c. Cataracts lead to progressive worsening and blurring of vision and are not associated with eye pain or redness (seen in glaucoma).
   b. Floaters are characteristic of retinal detachment.
   Application/Physiologic/Assessment

9. **Correct response: d**
   Vertigo is the outstanding problem associated with Menière's.
   a. The severe rotational whirling sensation makes the client unable to balance while standing or walk without falling.
   b. Pain and discomfort is usually associated with a feeling of pressure.
   c. Nausea is commonly present and may lead to fluid loss, but the risk of

the client falling is more of a priority nursing concern for client safety.
Analysis/Safe care/Analysis (Dx)

10. **Correct response: a**
Meniäre's is characterized by sudden, severe episodes of vertigo during which the client has a sensation of spinning.
   b. Dizziness should be distinguished from true rotational vertigo.
   c and d. A feeling of pressure but not pain is also characteristic, and hearing loss is progressive, not sudden.
Application/Physiologic/Assessment

11. **Correct response: d**
It is thought that Meniäre's is due to edema of the semicircular canals; a low-salt diet is often prescribed as well as diuretic drugs.
   a, b, and c. High-salt foods should be avoided, but protein intake should have no relation to Menière's (hypoproteinemia might aggravate edema).
Application/Health promotion/ Evaluation

12. **Correct response: a**
Keeping both nostrils and mouth open prevents forcing contaminated material into the middle ear (otitis media).
   b, c, and d. All other responses would increase risk of middle ear infection.
Application/Health promotion/ Implementation

13. **Correct response: c**
Drainage trickling down the posterior pharynx (noted with flashlight) and swallowing, belching, or hematemesis indicate continued bleeding.
   a. Anxiety is common due to the necessity to mouth-breathe.
   b. Black eyes occur with surgical trauma and are expected.
   d. Tarry stools indicate previous, but not current, bleeding.
Analysis/Safe care/Planning

14. **Correct response: d**
All airflow is through a permanent tracheostomy with a total laryngectomy, necessitating esophageal speech or use of an electronic device.
   a. Breathing and talking are unchanged with partial laryngectomy.
   b. All airflow will be through the neck.
   c. Even with laryngoplasty, the tracheostomy is occluded during speech.
Application/Safe care/Analysis (Dx)

15. **Correct response: b**
Since all airflow will be through the neck and the larynx will be removed, some form of communication must be assured before surgery (e.g., magic slate, signals).
   a. It is the surgeon's responsibility to explain surgery.
   c. If possible, psychologic preparation is enhanced with a visit from another laryngectomy client.
   d. Suctioning is easier to teach postoperatively with a tracheostomy present.
Application/Health promotion/Planning

16. **Correct response: c**
Actions should be taken to prevent water from entering the stoma site; for example, the client may take only tub baths, use hand-held shower heads, and avoid swimming.
   a. Adequate hydration and humidification should be provided. Air-conditioning would provide a dry environment.
   b. Initially, frequent coughing is expected with tracheal breathing; this will decrease with time, but the client will always have coughing episodes.
   d. The skin around the stoma site should be lubricated with a non–oil-based ointment.
Application/Health promotion/ Evaluation

Musculoskeletal Disorders

I. Musculoskeletal system

A. Structures

1. The body contains 206 different bones; types include:
   a. Long bones (e.g., femur, humerus, radius)
   b. Short bones (e.g., tarsals, carpals)
   c. Flat bones (e.g., skull, sternum, ribs, ilium)
   d. Irregular bones (e.g., mandible, vertebrae, ear ossicles)
   e. Sesamoid bones (e.g., patella)
2. Articulations (joints) are of various types:
   a. Synarthroses (fixed) (e.g., skull sutures)
   b. Amphiarthroses (slightly movable; e.g., vertebral joints)
   c. Diarthroses (freely movable; e.g., hip, knee, wrist)
3. The skeletal muscle system includes:
   a. Fasciculi: bundles of muscle fibers covered with connective tissue
   b. Muscle sheaths: connective tissue covering groups of muscle bundles
4. Ligaments are strong fibrous connective tissue binding bones.
5. Tendons are strong, fibrous, nonelastic connective tissue extending from muscle sheaths.
6. Cartilage types include:
   a. Hyaline: pearly, blue cartilage covering articular bone surfaces

      b. Fibrocartilage: white, tough, fibrous tissue found in knee

      c. Yellow: elastic, fibrous cartilage found in larynx, external ear

B. **Function**

  1. Bone functions include:

      a. Protection of vital organs

      b. Support for body tissue

      c. Assistance in movement through leverage and attachment for muscles

      d. Hematopoiesis (red blood cell production)

      e. Storage of mineral salts

  2. Functions of freely movable joints include:

      a. Abduction: away from midline

      b. Adduction: toward midline

      c. Circumduction: circle movement

      d. Extension: straightening

      e. Flexion: bending

      f. External rotation: laterally turning on axis

      g. Internal rotation: medially turning on axis

      h. Supination: facing upward

      i. Pronation: facing downward

  3. Skeletal muscle functions include:

      a. Facilitation of voluntary body movement through contraction

      b. Maintenance of body posture

      c. Production of body heat

  4. Ligaments provide joint stability and allow restricted joint movement.

  5. Tendons bind muscles to bones.

  6. Cartilage functions include:

      a. Absorption of weight, shock, stress, and strain

      b. Protection of bones, joints, and joint tissue

II. **Overview of musculoskeletal disorders**

  A. **Assessment**

    1. Health history should cover:

      a. Biographic data (age and sex; socioeconomic status and living conditions, including home layout; conditions that may affect health or rehabilitation; occupation, including physical activity required)

      b. Exercise patterns: type, frequency, energy expended

      c. Hobbies: type, amount of energy required

      d. Diet: type, frequency, and amount of food consumption, including proteins, carbohydrates, calcium, other nutrients

  e. Drug, tobacco, and alcohol intake (include both pre-scribed and over-the-counter drugs)

  f. Family history of musculoskeletal problems

  g. Past history of illnesses, conditions, medication use

2. The nurse also should elicit information on the client's present problem, including:

  a. Onset and course

  b. Symptoms (e.g., pain, swelling, altered movement, color changes, stiffness, deformity, sensory changes)

  c. Treatment received

  d. Perception of problem and expectations of outcome

  e. Lifestyle impacts

  f. Any other concurrent health problems

3. Physical examination involves:

  a. Upright body alignment: posture

  b. Bone discrepancies: contour, length, alignment, symmetry

  c. Bone motion: smoothness

  d. Gait: coordination, rhythm, stride, balance

  e. Joint alignment, symmetry, size, shape, contour, stability, tenderness, heat, swelling

  f. Joint movement: range, smoothness, pain, crepitus, clicks

  g. Muscle mass: shape, size, contour, symmetry, firmness

  h. Muscle strength: symmetry, resistance, contractility

  i. Muscle discrepancies: hypertrophy, atrophy, fasciculation, spasms

B. **Laboratory studies and diagnostic tests**

  1. Roentgenography (radiography, radiograph, photographic images) detects musculoskeletal structure, integrity, texture, or density problems; allows evaluation of disease progression and treatment efficacy.

  2. Bone scans detect skeletal trauma and disease.

  3. Arthrography studies soft tissues and contours of joint cavities.

  4. Arthrocentesis allows analysis of synovial fluid, blood, or pus aspirated from a joint cavity.

  5. Myelography can detect herniation, tumor, and congenital or degenerative conditions of the spinal canal.

  6. Electromyography (EMG) measures muscle electrical impulses for diagnosis of muscle or nerve disease.

  7. Biopsy (aspiration, punch, needle, or incision) studies bone, synovium, or muscle tissue.

  8. Computed tomography (CT) scans study soft tissue, bone,

E. Planning and implementation

1. For a client who sustains a sprain:
   a. Elevate or immobilize the affected joint, and apply ice packs immediately.
   b. Assist with tape, splint, or cast application as necessary.
   c. Instruct the client in use of assistive device (e.g., crutches), if indicated.
   d. Prepare the client with a severe sprain for surgical repair or reattachment, if indicated.
   e. Instruct the client in prescribed weight-bearing activities and activity restrictions.
   f. Teach the client how to take prescribed analgesics, for example:

   m ▸ **Instruct the client to take pain medication as soon as pain starts.**
   ▸ **Caution client that medication may cause drowsiness, and advise client to avoid activities requiring alertness.**

   g. Instruct the client on additional comfort measures:

   ▸ Elevate affected extremity to decrease edema (swelling).
   ▸ Apply cold compresses to constrict blood vessels and warm compresses to dilate vessels and improve circulation.
   ▸ Do no weight-bearing on affected extremity.

2. For a client suffering muscle or tendon strain:
   a. Instruct the client to allow the muscle or tendon to rest and repair itself by avoiding use for approximately 1 week, then progressing activity gradually until healing is complete.
   b. Teach appropriate stretching exercises to be performed after healing to help prevent reinjury.
   c. Prepare the client for surgical repair in severe injury.

F. Evaluation

1. For sprains:
   a. The client reports reduced pain.
   b. The client states appropriate measures to enhance comfort and promote healing.
   c. The client exhibits adequate tissue perfusion in the affected area.
   d. The client demonstrates proper care of cast or use of assistive device.
   e. The client demonstrates proper performance of prescribed rehabilitative exercises.

2. For strains:
   a. The client reports decreased pain and weakness within 3 to 5 days after injury.

> b. The client resumes normal activity without further injury following healing.

VIII. Dislocations

A. **Description: displacement of a bone from its normal articulation with a joint**

B. **Etiology and incidence**

1. A dislocation may be congenital (e.g., congenital hip displacement) or may result from trauma (e.g., abnormal twisting) or disease of surrounding joint tissue (e.g., Paget's disease).

2. Common locations of dislocation include the shoulder, elbow, wrist, digits, hip, knee, ankle, and vertebrae.

C. **Pathophysiology and management**

1. Traumatic dislocation may cause severe stress to associated joint structures, interrupting blood supply and causing nerve damage.

2. If untreated, this may lead to avascular necrosis or nerve palsy in the affected area.

D. **Assessment findings**

1. Common signs and symptoms of dislocation include:
   a. Pain
   b. Visible disruption of joint contour
   c. Swelling
   d. Ecchymoses
   e. Impaired joint mobility
   f. Change in extremity length
   g. Change in axis of dislocated bones (rotation)

2. Severe dislocation may produce circulatory or sensory changes in the affected joint and limb.

3. Radiograph findings may confirm dislocation.

E. **Nursing diagnoses**

1. Risk for Injury
2. Impaired Physical Mobility
3. Pain
4. Altered Tissue Perfusion: Peripheral

F. **Planning and implementation**

1. Immobilize the affected joint during transport to medical care.

2. Assist the physician in reducing displaced parts as necessary.

3. Keep the joint immobilized as prescribed, using bandages, splints, a cast, or traction.

4. **Assess for signs of neurovascular impairment.**

5. After removal of the immobilizing device, instruct the client

to exercise the joint as prescribed to promote return to normal function.

6. Instruct the client in the use of assistive devices (e.g., crutches) as indicated.

G. Evaluation

1. The client reports reduced pain.
2. The client states appropriate measures to enhance comfort and promote healing.
3. The client exhibits adequate tissue perfusion and sensory function in the affected area.
4. The client demonstrates proper care of cast or use of assistive device.
5. The client demonstrates proper performance of prescribed rehabilitative exercises and safety precautions to prevent reinjury.

IX. Fractures

A. Description

1. A fracture is a traumatic injury interrupting bone continuity.
2. Fractures are classified according to type and extent as:
   a. Closed simple, uncomplicated: not causing a break in the skin
   b. Open compound, complicated: involving trauma to surrounding tissue and a break in the skin
   c. Incomplete: partial cross-section break with incomplete bone disruption
   d. Complete: complete cross-section break severing the periosteum
   e. Impact: fracture ends forcibly wedged together
   f. Comminuted: several breaks of bone with splinters, fragments
   g. Displaced: separation of fragments at fracture site
   h. Complicated: involving injury to surrounding tissue
   i. Articular: involving a joint surface
   j. Extracapsular: a break near but not in a joint capsule
   k. Intracapsular: involving a joint capsule
   l. Epiphyseal: break in long bones involving ossification center

B. Etiology and incidence

1. Fractures can result from crushing force or direct blow.
2. Torsion fractures can occur from sudden twisting motion; persons with osteoporosis are at particular risk.
3. Extremely forceful muscle contraction also can cause fractures.

C. **Pathophysiology and management**
  1. Fracture occurs when stress placed on a bone exceeds the bone's ability to absorb it.
  2. Stages of normal fracture healing include:
     a. Inflammation
     b. Cellular proliferation
     c. Callus formation
     d. Callus ossification
     e. Mature bone remodeling
  3. Potential complications of fracture include:
     a. Life-threatening systemic fat embolus, most commonly developing within 24 to 72 hours after fracture (symptoms include personality changes, restlessness, dyspnea, crackles, white sputum)
     b. Nonunion of the fracture site
     c. Arterial damage during treatment
     d. Compartment syndrome
     e. Infection, possibly sepsis
     f. Hemorrhage, possibly leading to shock
  4. Management involves repair of fracture.

D. **Assessment findings**
  1. Clinical manifestations of fracture may include:
     a. Pain
     b. Swelling
     c. Tenderness
     d. Abnormal movement and crepitus
     e. Loss of function
     f. Ecchymoses
     g. Visible deformity
     h. Paresthesias and other sensory abnormalities
  2. Radiograph and other imaging studies may identify the site and type of fracture.

E. **Nursing diagnoses**
  1. Body Image Disturbance
  2. Risk for Infection
  3. Risk for Injury
  4. Impaired Physical Mobility
  5. Pain
  6. Altered Role Performance
  7. Self Care Deficit
  8. Self Esteem Disturbance
  9. Altered Tissue Perfusion: Peripheral

F. **Planning and implementation**
  1. Immobilize a fractured extremity with splints in the position of the deformity before moving the client.

2. Avoid straightening the injured body part if a joint is involved.
3. Cover any breaks in the skin with clean or sterile dressings.
4. Support the affected body part above and below the fracture site when moving the client.
5. Explain all procedures and treatments, emphasizing the importance of the client's participation in the treatment regimen.
6. Provide nonpharmacologic interventions (e.g., relaxation, massage, guided imagery) to help relieve pain.
7. Administer analgesics as appropriate (see Section II.D).
8. Elevate the injured extremity above the level of the client's heart for the first 24 hours or as directed.
9. Apply cold packs as ordered for the first 24 hours.
10. Assist the client with active range-of-motion exercises to unaffected body parts to help maintain function.
11. Promote the client's participation in self-care activities within limitations of the injury and treatment regimen.
12. Explain prescribed activity restrictions and necessary lifestyle modifications due to impaired mobility.
13. Teach the proper use of assistive devices as indicated.
14. Provide appropriate nursing interventions associated with prescribed treatment modalities (see Sections III, IV, and V as appropriate).
15. Monitor closely for signs and symptoms of complications.

G. Evaluation

1. The client participates actively in pain management.
2. The client reports relief of pain and discomfort.
3. The client exhibits adequate tissue perfusion.
4. The client demonstrates normal movement in unaffected body parts.
5. The client participates in muscle-strengthening exercises of affected body parts, if indicated.
6. The client maintains independence in self-care within limits of the injury and treatment plan.
7. The client actively participates in the prescribed medical regimen.
8. The client remains free of potential systemic complications.
9. The client regains maximum use of the affected body part.

X. Compartment syndrome

A. Description: a condition involving increased pressure and constriction of nerves and vessels within an anatomic compartment (e.g., the volar compartment of the forearm and the anterior and deep posterior compartments of the leg)

B. **Etiology and incidence**
1. Compartment syndrome can result from:
   a. Decrease in compartment size
   b. Increase in compartment contents
2. Decrease in compartment size may result from closure of fascial defects or excessively tight bandages, casts, or splints.
3. Increase in compartment contents can result from swelling, bleeding, or muscle hypertrophy.

C. **Pathophysiology and management**
1. The primary problem in compartment syndrome is decreased tissue perfusion due to vessel constriction.
2. Compromised tissue and cellular perfusion persisting longer than 4 to 6 hours can cause nerve and muscle ischemia, resulting in permanent damage (e.g., Volkmann's ischemic contracture).
3. Early detection of compartment syndrome is essential to enable prompt intervention aimed at relieving pressure and preventing tissue and nerve damage.

D. **Assessment findings**
1. Cardiovascular effects: diminished capillary refill, cyanotic nailbeds, pulselessness distal to the involved area
2. Neurologic effects: deep, throbbing, unrelenting pain in the affected area; paresthesias; paralysis distal to the involved area
3. Musculoskeletal effects: hard, swollen muscle, weakness with muscle stretch deterioration

E. **Nursing diagnoses**
1. Risk for Injury
2. Pain
3. Altered Tissue Perfusion: Peripheral

F. **Planning and implementation**
1. Recognize that this condition represents a medical emergency requiring prompt intervention.
2. Elevate the affected extremity to the heart level and apply cold packs to control edema.
3. Release constrictive dressings immediately.
4. If indicated, bivalve a constrictive cast by splitting it along both sides to release pressure; leave the cast in place for support, however.
5. If pressure is not relieved in 1 to 2 hours, prepare the client for fasciotomy, and assist with the procedure as necessary.
6. Promote correction of deformities with physical therapy and exercise as prescribed.

G. **Evaluation**
1. The client exhibits increased tissue perfusion.

2. The client reports decreased pain.
3. The client demonstrates adequate functioning in the affected limb.
4. The client displays no resulting injury after compartment release.

XI. Osteoarthritis

(*Note:* See Chapter 12, Immunologic Disorders, for a discussion of rheumatoid arthritis.)

A. Description: a slowly progressive, degenerative joint disease characterized by variable changes in weight-bearing joints

B. Etiology and incidence

1. Osteoarthritis is associated with obesity, aging, trauma, genetic predisposition, and congenital abnormalities.
2. The most common form of arthritis, osteoarthritis affects both sexes about equally, with onset generally after age 40.

C. Pathophysiology and management

1. Osteoarthritis causes deterioration of the joint cartilage and formation of reactive new bone at joint margins and in subchondral areas.
2. Disability varies from limitation of finger movement to severe hip and knee degeneration.
3. Progression is also variable; joints with minor deterioration may remain stable for years.
4. Management may involve surgery, pain medications, and physical therapy.

D. Assessment findings

1. Clinical manifestations of osteoarthritis include:
   a. Pain and muscle spasm, more pronounced after exercise, at night, and in the early morning
   b. Limited motion in affected joints
   c. Joint "grating" on movement
   d. Flexion contractures, primarily in the hip and knee
   e. Joint tenderness, Heberden's nodes in interphalangeal joints
2. Radiographs may confirm diagnosis.

E. Nursing diagnoses

1. Body Image Disturbance
2. Impaired Physical Mobility
3. Pain
4. Altered Role Performance
5. Self Care Deficit

F. Planning and implementation

1. Apply warm compresses or diathermy to sore joints.
2. Massage surrounding muscles, not overinflamed joints.

3. Promote adequate rest and reduction of stress.
4. Position the client to prevent flexion deformity using foot board, splints, sandbags, wedges, or pillows as needed.
5. Remove splints routinely, if used, to exercise joints.
6. Plan activities that promote optimal function and independence.
7. Consult with a physical therapist for an exercise plan.
8. Teach the client about:

   a. **Prescribed analgesics and their effects (see Section II.D). Advise client to take medication as soon as pain starts, and warn that medication may cause drowsiness.**
   b. NSAIDs (see Section II.D)
   c. Prescribed exercises (only within tolerance level and with modified weight bearing using assistive devices as indicated)
   d. Use of assistive devices, if needed, for ADLs
   e. Correct posture techniques while standing and sitting
9. Prepare the client for surgical treatment as indicated (e.g., osteotomy, arthroplasty, total joint replacement).
10. Caution against resorting to nontraditional, nonmedical treatments, but respect the client's right to choose such a treatment if he or she obtains relief.

G. Evaluation
1. The client reports reduced pain.
2. The client maintains or increases joint movement and muscle strength.
3. The client verbalizes understanding of prescribed medications, exercise, and other aspects of treatment.
4. The client participates in ADLs to the greatest level possible within disease limitations.

XII. Gouty arthritis
A. Description: a metabolic disease marked by urate crystal deposits in joints throughout the body, causing local irritation and inflammatory responses
B. Etiology and incidence
1. Gouty arthritis apparently is linked to a genetic deficit in purine metabolism.
2. For the most part, it affects men older than age 30.
C. Pathophysiology and management
1. Gout is characterized by formation of tophus deposits in soft tissues and urate crystals in joint synovia.
2. It primarily affects joints in the feet (especially the great toe) and legs, but may strike in any joint.

3. The disorder follows a variable course of periodic attacks, often with years-long symptom-free periods between attacks.
4. Eventually, it can lead to chronic disability and, in some cases, severe hypertension and progressive renal failure.
5. Common treatment measures include medication, rest, and dietary changes.

D. Assessment findings
1. The client commonly reports sudden attacks, usually at night, with periodic remissions and exacerbations.
2. Typical manifestations include:
   a. Pain, usually monarticular, acute, crushing, and pulsating
   b. Joint swelling and inflammation
   c. Intolerance to the weight of bed linens over the affected joint
   d. Pruritus or skin ulceration over the affected joint
3. Severe disease may produce signs of renal involvement (e.g., oliguria, low back pain, hypertension).
4. Laboratory findings may include:
   a. Urate crystals in synovial fluid
   b. Hyperuricemia
   c. Elevated serum uric acid level
5. In advanced disease, radiograph may show joint damage.

E. Nursing diagnoses
1. Body Image Disturbance
2. Altered Nutrition: Less than body requirements
3. Pain
4. Altered Role Performance
5. Self Care Deficit
6. Impaired Skin Integrity

F. Planning and implementation
1. Administer such gout-controlling antiinflammatory drugs as colchicine, which suppresses inflammation, and indomethacin (Indocin).

   a. **Explain that colchicine is given for acute attacks and *stopped* when severe side effects, such as abdominal pain, diarrhea, and nausea and vomiting occur.**
   b. **Give indomethacin with food to minimize GI distress.**
2. As prescribed, provide uricosuric drugs, such as probenecid (Benemid), which increase uric acid excretion and reduce serum urate levels.

   a. **Because probenecid is for long-term treatment, be sure to clarify drug order for acute attack.**

        b.   **Urge client to drink 2 to 3 liters of fluid daily and to report any decrease in urine output.**

    3.   Administer uric acid synthesis inhibitors, such as allopurinol (Zyloprim), as prescribed. This medication reduces the amount of uric acid delivered to the kidneys.

        a.   **Tell client that drug will take about 1 week to decrease uric acid level.**

        b.   **Maintain adequate hydration and monitor urine output.**

    4.   Apply ice to affected joints.

    5.   Maintain strict bedrest for 24 hours after an attack.

    6.   Elevate affected limbs.

    7.   Provide a bed cradle to keep bed linen off affected joints.

    8.   Teach the client about:

        a.   The prescribed medication regimen

        b.   The need to increase fluid intake to 3 L/day

        c.   Dietary modifications to limit foods high in purine (e.g., organ meats, anchovies, sardines, shellfish, chocolate, meat extracts)

  G. **Evaluation**

    1.   The client reports reduced pain.

    2.   The client experiences minimal skin irritation over affected joints.

    3.   The client demonstrates minimal side effects to the medication regimen.

    4.   The client verbalizes knowledge of prescribed medications, dietary modifications, and other treatments.

    5.   The client demonstrates reduced frequency and severity of acute attacks.

    6.   The client participates in self-care activities and ADLs as much as possible.

XIII. **Bone tumors**

  A. **Description**

    1.   Bone tumors can be either benign or malignant.

    2.   Types include:

        a.   Osteochondroma: benign tumor usually at the ends of long bones

        b.   Ecchondroma: painful, benign tumor of hyaline cartilage

        c.   Osteogenic sarcoma: highly metastasizing, malignant bone tumor

        d.   Chondrosarcoma: malignant tumor of hyaline cartilage

        e.   Multiple myeloma: malignant tumor arising from bone marrow

B. **Etiology and incidence**
1. The etiology of bone cancer is unclear.
2. Bone cancer is relatively rare; only an estimated 6000 new bone and soft tissue sarcomas occur each year in the United States.
3. Various types predominate in certain age groups:
   a. Osteochondroma: childhood and adolescence
   b. Ecchondroma: childhood and adolescence
   c. Osteogenic sarcoma: younger than age 25
   d. Chondrosarcoma: adult males
   e. Multiple myeloma: between age 50 and 70

C. **Pathophysiology and management**
1. Benign bone tumors usually are slow growing and well circumscribed.
2. Primary malignant bone tumors arise from bone tissue cells or bone marrow components. Cellular characteristics and disease progression vary with type and location.
3. Primary tumors tend to involve contiguous tissues readily and metastasize to the lungs early.
4. Therapy may include surgery, chemotherapy, and other measures.

D. **Assessment findings**
1. Clinical manifestations are highly variable but may include:
   a. Bone pain, possibly severe and persistent or only mild
   b. Varying degrees of movement limitation
   c. Palpable, fixed mass on bone
   d. Sensory disturbance in affected areas secondary to nerve compression
   e. Pathologic fracture in affected bone
   f. Systemic effects (e.g., weight loss, mild fever, malaise)
2. Important laboratory studies and diagnostic tests include:
   a. Chest radiograph to detect lung metastasis
   b. Bone scan to detect extension of bone lesions
   c. Biopsy for tumor identification
   d. Arteriography
   e. Urinalysis and blood chemistries (Elevated alkaline phosphatase is a common finding.)

E. **Nursing diagnoses**
1. Ineffective Family Coping
2. Ineffective Individual Coping
3. Risk for Injury
4. Pain
5. Altered Role Performance
6. Self Care Deficit

F. Planning and implementation

1. Administer analgesics as appropriate (see Section II.D).
2. Assist with position change and ambulation to prevent stress on affected, weakened bones.
3. Provide client or family teaching, covering:
   a. Use of assistive devices as ordered
   b. Action and possible side effects of chemotherapeutic drugs
   c. Medication and treatment regimens for home care
4. Encourage the client and family members to express feelings and concerns; convey an accepting, reassuring demeanor.
5. Prepare the client for surgery and possible limb salvage or amputation as indicated. (Malignant tumors are thoroughly removed with wide excision, resection of the affected part, or amputation of the entire limb to prevent metastasis.)
6. Refer the client and family to appropriate support groups.
7. Encourage the client's maximum independence within limitations of the condition.

G. Evaluation

1. The client reports adequate pain relief.
2. The client experiences no injuries, including pathologic fractures.
3. The client (and family members as appropriate) verbalize understanding of the prescribed treatment regimen.
4. The client and family members demonstrate appropriate coping skills in dealing with the disease and its prognosis.
5. The client maintains independence in ADLs living within limitations imposed by the disease.

XIV. Osteomyelitis

A. Description: severe pyogenic bone infection

B. Etiology and incidence

1. Osteomyelitis can result from trauma or secondary infection (most commonly with *Staphylococcus aureus*).
2. It tends to affect persons with low resistance or with decreased blood flow to a trauma site.
3. Blood-borne osteomyelitis (hematogenic) is more common in children secondary to throat infection.
4. Osteomyelitis secondary to trauma or orthopedic surgical procedures is more common in older persons.

C. Pathophysiology and management

1. Blood stream circulation of infectious microbes to susceptible bone leads to:
   a. Inflammation
   b. Increased vascularity
   c. Edema

    2. The organisms grow and form pus within the bone, and abscess formation may occur.

    3. This deprives the bone of its blood supply, eventually leading to necrosis.

    4. Necrosis stimulates new bone formation (involucrum) by the periosteum; this pushes old bone (sequestrum) out of the abscess or a sinus.

    5. Management measures include comfort measures, antibiotic therapy, and possibly surgery.

D. **Assessment findings**

    1. Osteomyelitis is commonly marked by:
        a. Localized bone pain
        b. Tenderness, heat, and swelling in the affected area
        c. Guarding of the affected area
        d. Restricted movement in affected area
        e. Systemic symptoms (e.g., high fever and chills [acute osteomyelitis], low-grade fever and generalized weakness [chronic osteomyelitis])
        f. Purulent drainage from a skin abscess

    2. Laboratory studies may reveal:
        a. Leukocytosis on WBC count
        b. Elevated erythrocyte sedimentation rate
        c. The causative organism identified on blood culture
        d. Bone involvement in advanced disease demonstrated by radiograph and bone scan

E. **Nursing diagnoses**

    1. Risk for Injury
    2. Impaired Physical Mobility
    3. Pain
    4. Impaired Skin Integrity

F. **Planning and implementation**

    1. Administer analgesics as appropriate (see Section II.D).
    2. Instruct the client on other comfort measures (guided imagery, relaxation techniques, biofeedback).
    3. Support an affected limb above and below the affected area.
    4. Elevate the affected limb to reduce swelling.
    5. Administer antibiotics, such as semisynthetic penicillin and cephalosporins, which will inhibit cell wall synthesis thereby decreasing the infection. Before administering, check client for drug allergy.
    6. Provide local treatments as prescribed (e.g., warm saline soaks).
    7. Provide a diet high in protein and vitamins C and D to promote healing.
    8. Teach the client about:
        a. Activity restrictions

    b. Self-care techniques

    c. Home wound care and IV therapy, if ordered

   9. Prepare the client for surgical debridement, bone grafting, or amputation as appropriate.

G. **Evaluation**

  1. The client reports adequate pain control.

  2. The client performs ADLs within activity restrictions.

  3. The client demonstrates self wound care and IV therapy, if prescribed.

  4. The client states signs and symptoms of further complications to watch for and report.

Bibliography

Bolander, V. R. (1994). *Sorensen & Luckmann's basic nursing: A physiologic approach* (3rd ed.). Philadelphia: W. B. Saunders.

Clark, J., Queener, S., & Karb, V. (1990). *Pharmacologic basis of nursing practice* (4th ed.). St. Louis: C. V. Mosby.

Doenges, M. E. (1993). *Nursing care plans: Guidelines for planning and documenting patient care* (3rd ed.). Philadelphia: F. A. Davis.

Nettina, S. (1996). *The Lippincott manual of nursing practice* (6th ed.). Philadelphia: Lippincott-Raven Publishers.

Pagana, K. D., & Pagana, T. J. (1994). *Diagnostic testing and nursing implications* (4th ed.). St. Louis: C. V. Mosby.

Sahrmann, S. (1995). *Diagnosis and exercise management of musculoskeletal pain syndromes.* St. Louis: C. V. Mosby.

Smeltzer, S. C., & Bare, B. G. (1996). *Brunner & Suddarth's textbook of medical-surgical nursing* (8th ed.). Philadelphia: Lippincott-Raven Publishers.

Springhouse Corporation. (1992). *Nursing student's guide to drugs.* Spring House, PA: Springhouse Corp.

STUDY QUESTIONS

1. Emergency care for a client whose left arm is grossly deformed with ends of the humerus protruding through the skin would include
   a. applying gentle traction to align the fractured bone ends, then splinting the entire extremity in corrected position
   b. covering the broken skin and bone ends with a clean material, then splinting in the position of the deformity
   c. wrapping a tight, clean covering around the broken skin and bone ends, then applying gentle traction to the fracture
   d. leaving the broken skin and bone fragments uncovered and splinting the deformed arm above the elbow at the fracture site

2. During the nursing assessment, the client with a fractured femur and pelvis becomes restless, exhibits dyspnea, and coughs up white sputum. In addition, the nurse auscultates crackles. The nurse would suspect
   a. compartment syndrome
   b. deep vein thrombosis (DVT)
   c. fat embolism
   d. osteomyelitis

3. The nurse evaluates the effectiveness of analgesic medications for osteoarthritis by noting which of the following?
   a. The client has increased motion in joints that have contractures.
   b. The client's Heberden's nodes disappear.
   c. The client reports decreased pain after exercise and at night.
   d. The client demonstrates the ability to perform ADLs.

4. Which client statement would alert the nurse for the potential complication of cast syndrome in a client with a hip spica cast?
   a. "My skin is sensitive in warm, dry environments."
   b. "I become highly emotional when I feel confined in small spaces."
   c. "I had a postoperative infection when I had my appendix removed."
   d. "I felt more pain in my hip yesterday than I do today."

5. The nurse's teaching plan for a client who has gouty arthritis and who is starting a low-purine diet would include instructing the client to avoid which of the following foods?
   a. citrus fruits
   b. green vegetables
   c. organ meats
   d. fresh fish

6. Which of the following nursing diagnoses would be the most important when planning activities for a client receiving chemotherapy for osteogenic sarcoma of the femur?
   a. Altered Role Performance related to discomfort, pain, and impaired mobility
   b. Impaired Skin Integrity related to inflammatory response to chemotherapy
   c. Risk for Injury: pathologic fracture related to effects of tumor and chemotherapy
   d. Ineffective Individual Coping related to diagnosis and treatment regimen

7. If the physician orders Buck's traction until the client with a fractured hip has surgery, the nurse should plan for which of the following traction applications?
   a. continuous, balanced suspension skeletal traction
   b. intermittent, running skeletal traction
   c. continuous, running skin traction
   d. intermittent, balanced suspension skin traction

8. Which priority nursing intervention should be included in the plan of care

following application of Buck's traction for a client who has a fractured hip?
a. turning and repositioning with pillows every hour to prevent deformity
b. cleaning the traction application site every 8 hours to improve circulation
c. checking the traction ropes and pulleys every hour for proper alignment
d. checking neurovascular function every 2 hours in the affected leg

9. A client diagnosed with degenerative joint disease secondary to osteoarthritis is scheduled for a total hip replacement of the right leg. During the preoperative period, the nurse should focus assessment primarily on
a. local and systemic infections
b. self-care ability
c. response to pain medications
d. range of motion in the affected joint

10. After a right total hip replacement, the client's right leg should be maintained in correct position by
a. placing an abductor wedge or pillows between the legs
b. placing sandbags or pillows to keep leg adducted
c. elevating the affected leg on two pillows or supports
d. positioning the client supine and on the operative side

11. When discussing physical activities with the client who has just undergone a right total hip replacement, the nurse should instruct the client to
a. Avoid weight bearing until the hip is completely healed.
b. Intermittently cross and uncross legs several times daily.
c. Maintain hip flexion at 90 degrees when sitting.
d. Limit hip flexion to only 45 to 60 degrees.

12. Discharge planning for a client with a total right hip replacement would include explaining the signs and symptoms of joint dislocation. The nurse would determine that the client understands the instructions by the client's identification of which of the following symptoms?
a. positive Homans' sign and inability to bear weight
b. painless, sudden deformity of the affected hip joint
c. severe hip pain with shortening of the extremity
d. severe pain and swelling of the affected hip joint

13. Which of the following signs and symptoms would indicate the need to decrease or stop the dosage of colchicine for the client experiencing an acute gout attack?
a. bleeding gums and bruising
b. nausea, vomiting, and diarrhea
c. gastric irritation and heartburn
d. blurred vision and nausea

14. Eight hours after a client receives a long-leg cast on the left leg, the client complains of unrelenting pain. The pain remains severe even after the nurse administers pain medication. Additional signs and symptoms that support the suspected diagnosis of compartment syndrome would include
a. diminished capillary refill and cyanotic nailbeds on the left leg
b. warm, tender left calf and increased size of the left calf muscle
c. ability to insert two fingers into the distal and proximal portion of cast
d. a low-grade temperature and bilateral wheezing and crackles heard during lung auscultation

ANSWER KEY

1. **Correct response: b**
   The fracture described is an open, compound fracture. Emergency care for this fracture is to prevent movement until the limb is immobilized. The wound should be covered with a clean (or sterile if available) dressing to prevent further contamination, then splinted with as little movement as possible.
   a, c, and d. No attempts to align or reduce the fracture should be made, and the bone fragments should not be touched or pushed back into place.
   Application/Safe care/Implementation

2. **Correct response: c**
   The presenting features of fat embolism are cerebral disturbances manifested by mental status changes, tachypnea, dyspnea, crackles, wheezes, and large amounts of thick, white sputum.
   a. Some presenting features of compartment syndrome are cyanotic nailbeds; paresthesias and throbbing, unrelenting pain; and hard, swollen muscle.
   b. Swelling, warmth, and tenderness in the affected area are hallmarks of DVT.
   d. Features of osteomyelitis include localized bone pain; tenderness, heat, and swelling; restricted movement; fever and chills.
   Application/Physiologic/Assessment

3. **Correct response: c**
   Clients with osteoarthritis experience increased joint pain after exercise, at night, and early morning. Pain medication should relieve the pain during these times.
   a, b, and d. These observations would not specifically reflect analgesic effectiveness.
   Knowledge/Health promotion/ Evaluation

4. **Correct response: b**
   A client immobilized in a large cast may experience either psychologic or physiologic complications. The psychologic complication is a claustrophobic reaction involving acute anxiety and possible irrational behavior. Physiologic effects may include tachypnea, diaphoresis, dilated pupils, tachycardia, and elevated blood pressure related to the acute anxiety. Clients who report problems with claustrophobia are at risk for this complication.
   a and c. These findings would alert the nurse to possible infection.
   d. This finding is related to progress, not cast syndrome.
   Analysis/Psychosocial/Assessment

5. **Correct response: c**
   Clients with gouty arthritis have a disorder of purine metabolism with abnormal amounts of urates in the body. Urate crystals become deposited in parts of the body causing local irritation and an inflammatory response. Treatment usually consists of lowering the serum urate level to dissolve crystalline deposits through dietary restrictions. Foods high in purine that should be avoided are organ meats, anchovies, sardines, shell fish, chocolate, and meat extracts.
   a, b, and d. The other foods listed are all important to a well-balanced diet.
   Comprehension/Health promotion/ Planning

6. **Correct response: c**
   Osteogenic sarcoma is a primary malignant bone tumor affecting bone cells. The tumor and chemotherapy leaves the bone weakened and makes the client more vulnerable to pathologic fractures. The nurse should prevent stress on the weakened bone by assisting the client with position changes and ambulation.

a, b, and d. Although these diagnoses may be relevant and important to care, they are not the most important.

Comprehension/Safe care/Analysis (Dx)

7. *Correct response: c*

Continuous traction is used to treat fractures, whereas intermittent traction is used to treat muscle spasms or to reduce pain. In this situation, the client has a fractured femur and therefore needs the continuous pull to immobilize the fracture until surgery is performed. The nurse should always assume traction is continuous unless otherwise ordered by the physician. Buck's traction is an extension traction that exerts a straight pull on the leg. The traction is applied to the skin of the lower leg using tape, sponge rubber, or plastic materials.

a, b, and d. These other forms of traction would be inappropriate for this type of injury.

Knowledge/Physiologic/Planning

8. *Correct response: d*

Neurovascular checks should be done every 2 hours for a client in traction to detect complications early.

a. A client receiving traction should be turned and positioned correctly about every 2 hours unless he or she is placed on a special mattress to prevent pressure ulcers.

b. The traction tape should remain in place, but the area should be palpated to determine tenderness caused from pressure, decreased circulation, or nerve pressure.

c. The nurse should check the ropes, pulleys, and weights for proper alignment and traction pull every 8 hours.

Application/Physiologic/Implementation

9. *Correct response: a*

Infection is a major concern for any client undergoing orthopedic surgery. It can be especially harmful for clients with joint replacements because infection may prevent achieving a functional joint postoperatively and necessitate another surgical procedure.

b, c, and d. Although these all may be important factors to assess, infection represents the primary concern.

Application/Safe care/Assessment

10. *Correct response: a*

Following total hip replacement, the client should be kept flat while in a recumbent position with the affected extremity in an abducted position. This is accomplished by placing an abduction wedge or pillows between the client's legs.

b. Adduction of the affected leg could cause dislocation of the hip replacement.

c. Hip flexion should never be beyond 45 to 60 degrees when elevating the leg or while sitting.

d. The client should be turned only 45 degrees on the unoperated side with full support to the operative leg to keep it in the abduction position.

Application/Physiologic/Implementation

11. *Correct response: d*

Following a total hip replacement, the client should be instructed to avoid any activities that cause hip adduction (crossing legs), flexion beyond 90 degrees (sitting in low chairs or on low toilet seats), and rotation (pivoting on affected leg).

a. Progressive weight-bearing exercises are encouraged early depending on physician's orders.

b. Crossing the legs causes hip adduction, which is contraindicated following hip replacement surgery.

c. The client should be taught to limit hip flexion to only 45 to 60 degrees.

Application/Safe care/Implementation

12. *Correct response: c*

Dislocation of the hip prosthesis is a complication from extreme positions of hip adduction or flexion or from infec-

ANSWER KEY

tion of the affected area. Signs and symptoms of hip dislocation include severe hip pain, shortening of the extremity, internal or external rotation of the extremity, and inability to move the hip.

a. A positive Homans' sign indicates thrombophlebitis, an unrelated complication.

b. Hip dislocation invariably produces pain.

d. Swelling may or may not occur with dislocation.

Analysis/Health promotion/Evaluation

13. **Correct response: b**
Antiinflammatory medications (colchicine) are commonly prescribed to control acute attacks. Larger doses and high blood levels are needed. Doses are usually prescribed to the maximum level tolerated, determined by the appearance of symptoms such as nausea, vomiting, and diarrhea.

a, c, and d. These signs and symptoms represent side effects of aspirin and must be addressed separately (e.g., giving enteric-coated tablets to reduce gastric irritation).

Analysis/Physiologic/Evaluation

14. **Correct response: a**
Clinical manifestations of compartment syndrome may include diminished capillary refill, cyanotic nailbeds, pulselessness distal to the involved area; deep, throbbing unrelenting pain in affected area; paresthesias; paralysis distal to the involved area.

b. These are indicative of deep vein thrombosis.

c. The nurse should be able to insert two fingers under proximal and distal end of cast.

d. These are not signs and symptoms of compartment syndrome.

Application/Physiologic/Assessment

Liver, Biliary, and Pancreatic Disorders

17

I. Hepatic system

A. Structures

1. Liver

  a. Located in the right upper abdominal quadrant, the liver is divided into four lobes: the left, right, caudate, and quadrate.

  b. The lobes are further subdivided into smaller units known as lobules.

  c. Blood supply to the liver is from the portal vein (75%), which drains the gastrointestinal (GI) tract, and from the hepatic artery (25%).

  d. The liver contains various cell types, including hepatocytes (liver cells) and Kupffer cells (phagocytic cells that engulf bacteria).

2. Biliary system

  a. Canaliculi, the smallest bile ducts located between liver lobules, receive bile from hepatocytes.

  b. The canaliculi form larger bile ducts, which lead to the hepatic duct.

  c. The hepatic duct from the liver joins the cystic duct

from the gallbladder to form the common bile duct, which empties into the duodenum.

d. Flow of bile into the intestine is controlled by the sphincter of Oddi.

e. The gallbladder is a hollow, pear-shaped organ, 3" to 4" long, attached to the liver under the right lobe.

f. The gallbladder normally holds 30 to 50 mL of bile and can hold up to 70 mL when fully distended.

3. Pancreas

a. A slender, fish-shaped organ, the pancreas lies horizontally in the abdomen behind the stomach and extends roughly from the duodenum to the spleen.

b. The functional pancreatic exocrine unit is the secreting acinus.

c. Pancreatic acini are arranged in lobules with channels that extend to the main lobular duct.

d. The acini normally produce between 1200 and 3000 mL of pancreatic juice daily.

B. Function

1. **Liver functions include:**

a. **Regulating blood glucose level; making glycogen, which is stored in hepatocytes**

b. **Synthesizing glucose from amino acids of lactate through gluconeogenesis**

c. **Converting ammonia produced from gluconeogenetic by-products and bacteria to urea**

d. **Synthesizing plasma proteins such as albumin, globulins, clotting factors, and lipoproteins**

e. **Breaking down fatty acids into ketone bodies**

f. **Storing vitamins and trace metals**

g. **Affecting drug metabolism**

h. **Secreting bile**

2. Continuously formed by hepatocytes (about 1 L/day), bile comprises:

a. Water, electrolytes, lecithin, fatty acids, cholesterol

b. Bilirubin: pigment derived from breakdown of hemoglobin; conjugated with glucuronic acid by hepatocytes, producing direct or conjugated bilirubin that is secreted into bile

c. Bile salts: (made from cholesterol) emulsify fat, reabsorbed in distal ileum and returned to the liver via the portal vein

3. Metabolic functions of the biliary system include:

a. Draining bile from hepatocytes to the gallbladder by way of the biliary tree

b. Storing bile in the gallbladder and releasing it to the duodenum; mediated by the hormone cholecystokinin

4. The pancreas has both endocrine and exocrine functions. (Endocrine functions are discussed in Chapter 10, Endocrine and Metabolic Disorders.) Exocrine functions include:

a. Producing pancreatic juice, which contains three types of digestive enzymes: amylase (hydrolyzes carbohydrate to disaccharides), lipase (hydrolyzes fat to fatty acids and glycerol), trypsin (proteolytic enzymes that split proteins); controlled by the vagus and two hormones, pancreozymin and secretin

b. Secreting water and bicarbonate to neutralize gastric juice

II. Overview of liver, biliary, and pancreatic disorders

A. Assessment

1. Assess liver size by percussing the upper and lower liver borders.
2. Record the level at which the lower border descends below the right costal margin.
3. Palpate the liver, if possible, to assess:
   a. Consistency and firmness
   b. Pain
   c. Shape
   d. Nodules

B. Laboratory studies and diagnostic tests: liver

1. Liver function tests
   a. Alkaline phosphatase level
   b. Serum glutamic-pyruvic transaminase (SGPT)—now more commonly known as ALT—and serum glutamic-oxaloacetic transaminase (SGOT)—now known as AST
   c. Lactic dehydrogenase (LDH)
   d. Serum proteins
   e. Direct and indirect bilirubin
   f. Serum ammonia
   g. Clotting factors
   h. Serum lipids
2. Liver biopsy, sampling of liver tissue by needle aspiration for histologic analysis, is done to establish diagnosis of specific liver disease.
3. Other important liver studies include:
   a. Computed tomography (CT) scan to detect neoplasms, cysts, abscesses, and hematomas
   b. Angiography to visualize hepatic circulation or masses
   c. Splenoportography to determine adequacy of portal blood flow
   d. Liver scan to demonstrate liver size and shape

C. **Laboratory studies and diagnostic tests: biliary system**
  1. Ultrasonography can detect calculi (gallstones) or a dilated common bile duct.
  2. Radionuclide imaging of the biliary tree and gallbladder can aid diagnosis of acute cholecystitis.
  3. Cholecystography detects gallstones and assesses the gallbladder's ability to fill, concentrate, and contract.
  4. Endoscopic retrograde cholangiopancreatography (ERCP) allows direct visualization of the common bile ducts and pancreatic duct.
  5. Percutaneous transhepatic cholangiography (PTC) is useful in distinguishing jaundice caused by liver disease.

D. **Laboratory studies and diagnostic tests: pancreas**
  1. Blood studies
     a. Serum amylase and lipase levels: important aids in diagnosing pancreatitis
     b. White blood cell (WBC) count: usually elevated in pancreatitis
     c. Serum bilirubin levels: possibly elevated in pancreatic dysfunction
  2. Radiographic studies of the abdomen and chest may differentiate pancreatitis from other disorders.
  3. Ultrasonography and CT scanning are used to identify increased pancreas size and to detect pancreatic cysts, pseudocysts, or tumors.
  4. Stool analysis evaluates fat content: normally around 20%, may range from 50% to 90% in pancreatic disease.
  5. ERCP is the most helpful study in the diagnosis of pancreatitis; it also enables tissue biopsy for analysis and differentiates pancreatitis from carcinoma.

E. **Psychosocial implications**
  1. The client with a liver, biliary, or pancreatic disorder may experience coping difficulty related to:
     a. Progressive nature of the disorder
     b. Chronicity of the disorder
     c. Fear of death
     d. Limitations in function
     e. Pain
     f. Guilt associated with the disorder's cause
  2. The client also may express self-concept concerns related to:
     a. Role changes toward increased dependence
     b. Loss of sexuality and sexual function
     c. Body image changes
  3. Lifestyle concerns may be related to potential changes in:
     a. Physical and functional ability

b. Work performance, with possible job loss
c. Self-care ability
4. Disease-related changes in social interactions may result in depression, isolation, rejection, and hopelessness.

III. Jaundice

A. Description: a symptom or syndrome characterized by increased bilirubin concentration in blood; classified as hemolytic, hepatocellular, or obstructive

B. Etiology and incidence
1. Hemolytic jaundice can result from:
   a. Transfusion reaction
   b. Hemolytic anemia
   c. Severe burns
   d. Autoimmune hemolytic anemia
2. Causes of hepatocellular jaundice include hepatitis, yellow fever, and alcoholism.
3. Obstructive jaundice may be:
   a. Extrahepatic, caused by bile duct plugging from gallstones, an inflammatory process, tumor, or pressure from enlarged gland
   b. Intrahepatic, resulting from pressure on channels from inflamed liver tissue or exudate
4. Jaundice also may be hereditary.

C. Pathophysiology and management
1. Hemolytic jaundice, caused by increased destruction of red blood cells, results in the inability to excrete bilirubin as quickly as it forms.
2. Hepatocellular jaundice results from the inability of diseased liver cells to clear normal amounts of bilirubin, due to defective uptake, consumption, or transport mechanisms.
3. Bile deposition in the skin, mucous membranes, and sclera results in characteristic yellow tinging of these structures.
4. Management may require dietary modifications.

D. Assessment findings
1. Clinical manifestations of jaundice include:
   a. Dark, foamy urine due to increased bile in urine
   b. Light or clay-colored stools due to lack of bile in the small bowel
   c. Pruritus due to increased bile acids in skin
   d. Inability to tolerate fatty foods due to absence of bile in the small intestine
2. The client may be mildly or severely ill with other symptoms such as anorexia, fatigue, nausea, weakness, and possible weight loss.

3. Laboratory study findings in jaundice may include:
    a. Conjugated bilirubin (direct): normal or elevated
    b. Unconjugated bilirubin (indirect): normal or elevated
    c. Total bilirubin: elevated
    d. Urine bilirubin: absent or elevated
    e. Urine urobilinogen: decreased or increased
    f. Fecal urobilinogen: elevated, decreased, or absent
    g. AST (or SGOT): normal or elevated
    h. ALT (or SGPT): normal or elevated
    i. Partial thromboplastin time: normal or prolonged

E. Nursing diagnoses
1. Activity Intolerance
2. Anxiety
3. Altered Nutrition: Less than body requirements
4. Risk for Impaired Skin Integrity

F. Planning and implementation
1. Assess the client's level of activity.
2. Intervene to reduce anxiety; reinforce the physician's explanations of the cause and expected outcome of jaundice, and encourage the client to express feelings and concerns.
3. Assess dietary intake and nutritional status; promote a high-carbohydrate intake, with protein intake consistent with that recommended for hepatic encephalopathy.

m   **4. Assess for pruritus, and provide frequent skin care.**

G. Evaluation
1. The client verbalizes understanding of appropriate carbohydrate and protein intake.
2. The client exhibits decreased anxiety.
3. The client exhibits decreased jaundice and pruritus.

IV. Portal hypertension

A. Description: elevated pressure in the portal vein associated with increased resistance to blood flow through the porta hepatis

B. Etiology and incidence
1. Major causes of portal hypertension include:
    a. Cirrhosis
    b. Mechanical obstruction (e.g., thrombosis, tumor)
2. Incidence information is similar to that for cirrhosis.

C. Pathophysiology and management
1. Obstruction of portal venous flow through the liver leads to:
    a. Formation of esophageal, gastric, and hemorrhoidal varicosities due to increased venous pressure
    b. Accumulation of fluid in the abdominal cavity (ascites)
2. The spleen and other organs that empty into the portal system also undergo the effects of congestion.

D. Assessment findings

    1. Signs and symptoms of portal encephalopathy include:

        a. Shifting dullness or fluid wave on abdominal percussion

        b. Dilated abdominal vessels radiating from the umbilicus (caput medusae)

        c. Enlarged, palpable spleen

        d. Bruits detected over the upper abdominal area due to esophageal and gastric varicosities

    2. Important diagnostic tests include portal pressure measurement, liver scans, splenoportography, abdominal angiography, and liver biopsy.

E. Nursing diagnoses

    1. Activity Intolerance

    2. Body Image Disturbance

    3. Decreased Cardiac Output

    4. Fear

    5. Fluid Volume Excess

    6. Risk for Injury

    7. Pain

    8. Risk for Impaired Skin Integrity

    9. Altered Tissue Perfusion: Cardiopulmonary and Renal

F. Planning and implementation

    1. Measure and record abdominal girth and body weight daily.

    2. As prescribed, administer diuretics such as ethacrynic acid (Edecrin) and furosemide (Lasix) to induce diuresis and thereby reduce fluid retention.

        a. Monitor intake and output.

        b. Monitor client for hypovolemia, hypokalemia, and hyponatremia.

        c. Keep in mind that diuretic therapy can precipitate encephalopathy.

    3. Administer a prescribed aldosterone-blocking agent such as spironolactone (Aldactone) which supplements diuretic action and helps prevent potassium loss.

        a. Give drug at mealtime to enhance absorption.

        b. Instruct client to report mental confusion or lethargy at once.

    4. Encourage the client to verbalize feelings about body image and self-concept changes.

    5. Observe the client closely for signs and symptoms of vascular collapse following paracentesis, the removal of fluid from the peritoneal cavity (see Fig. 17-1).

    6. If indicated, prepare the client for peritoneojugular (LeVeen) shunting to shunt ascitic fluid to the venous system.

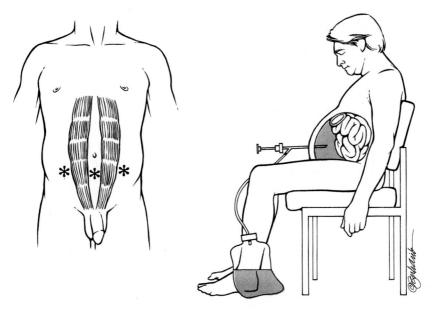

FIGURE 17-1.

When the client with ascites undergoes paracentesis (aspiration of fluid for testing or drainage), the trocar is inserted to avoid the musculature (see stars at left). To prevent hypotension, oliguria, hyponatremia, and possible shock, no more than 2 to 3 L of fluid should be aspirated. (From Smeltzer, S. C., & Bare, B. G. [1992]. *Brunner and Suddarth's Textbook of medical-surgical nursing* [7th ed.]. Philadelphia: J. B. Lippincott.)

G. Evaluation

1. The client exhibits reduced abdominal girth and body weight.
2. The client maintains adequate electrolyte balance.
3. The client verbalizes feelings about body image and self-concept.
4. The client exhibits no evidence of vascular collapse.

V. Hepatic encephalopathy

A. Description: a neurologic syndrome developing as a complication of liver disease; may be acute and self-limiting or chronic and progressive

B. Etiology and incidence

1. Possible causes of hepatic encephalopathy include:
   a. Severe liver injury
   b. Hepatocellular failure
   c. Portal shunting directly from the portal system to systemic venous circulation
   d. Increased serum ammonia levels secondary to GI bleeding, high-protein diet, or bacterial growth in the intestine and uremia
2. Incidence information is similar to that for cirrhosis.

C. **Pathophysiology and management**
1. Hepatic encephalopathy results from accumulation of ammonia and other identified toxic metabolites in blood due to the liver cells' inability to convert ammonia to urea.
2. Increased blood ammonia concentration leads to neurologic dysfunction and possible brain damage.

D. **Assessment findings**
1. Clinical manifestations include:
   a. Neurologic dysfunction progressing from minor mental aberrations and motor disturbances to coma
   b. Asterixis or flapping tremor of hands (also called liver flap)
2. Laboratory tests may reveal:
   a. Elevated serum ammonia level
   b. Elevated serum bilirubin level
   c. Prolonged prothrombin time

E. **Nursing diagnoses**
1. Ineffective Airway Clearance
2. Risk for Injury
3. Sensory/Perceptual Alterations
4. Impaired Skin Integrity

F. **Planning and implementation**

 1. **Closely monitor neurologic status for any changes.**
2. Measure and record daily weight, fluid intake, and output.
3. Take vital signs every 4 hours; watch for changes from baseline.
4. Assess for signs and symptoms of infection.
5. Evaluate serum ammonia values daily.
6. Reduce or eliminate the client's dietary protein intake if you detect evidence of impending coma.
7. Administer a high cleansing enema to reduce ammonia absorption.

 8. **Assess the client's history for drug allergies before administering prescribed antibiotics, such as neomycin (Miciguent). Provided orally or as a retention enema, this agent inhibits ammonia-forming bacteria in the GI tract, thereby reducing ammonia and improving neurologic status.**
9. Monitor electrolyte status and intervene as indicated to correct any imbalances.

 10. **Monitor client closely and administer a conservative dose of prescribed sedative or analgesic medication because liver damage will alter drug metabolism.**
11. Administer lactulose (Cephulac) as prescribed to reduce serum

ammonia levels by inducing catharsis which decreases colonic pH and inhibits fecal flora from producing ammonia from urea.

a. Advise client to expect two or three soft stools daily (ammonia is removed along with the stool), and explain that watery diarrhea indicates overdose.

b. **Dilute medication with fruit juice to modify sweetness.**

G. Evaluation

1. The client exhibits increased level of consciousness.
2. The client maintains adequate intake and output.
3. The client maintains vital signs within normal ranges.
4. The client exhibits normal serum ammonia level.
5. The client displays no evidence of infection or injury.

VI. Bleeding esophageal varices

A. Description: a hemorrhagic process involving dilated, tortuous veins in the submucosa of the lower esophagus

B. Etiology and incidence

1. The most common cause is portal hypertension resulting from obstructed portal venous circulation.
2. Incidence information is similar to that for cirrhosis.

C. Pathophysiology and management

1. In portal hypertension, collateral circulation develops in the lower esophagus as venous blood diverted from the GI tract and spleen due to portal obstruction seeks an outlet.
2. Due to excessive intraluminal pressure these collateral veins become tortuous, dilated, and fragile. They are particularly prone to ulceration and hemorrhage.
3. Ruptured esophageal varices are the most common cause of death in clients with hepatic cirrhosis.

D. Assessment findings

1. Present with hematemesis and melena, if ulcerated massive hemorrhage occurs
2. Signs of hepatic encephalopathy
3. Dilated abdominal veins
4. Ascites
5. Endoscopy confirms diagnosis

E. Nursing diagnoses

1. Activity Intolerance
2. Decreased Cardiac Output
3. Fear
4. Risk for Injury
5. Pain
6. Risk for Impaired Skin Integrity
7. Altered Thought Processes

F. Planning and implementation

    1. Monitor vital signs and urinary output to evaluate fluid balance.

    2. Assess level of consciousness.

    3. **Infuse vasopressin (Pitressin) intravenously or intraarterially as prescribed to constrict the splanchnic arterial bed and reduce portal pressure. Closely monitor client for such vasoconstrictive effects as angina or bowel ischemia.**

    4. If the physician performs balloon tamponade to control bleeding, explain the procedure to the client to reduce fear and enhance his or her cooperation with insertion and maintenance of the esophageal tamponade tube, and monitor closely to prevent accidental removal or displacement of the tube with resultant airway obstruction (see Fig. 17-2).

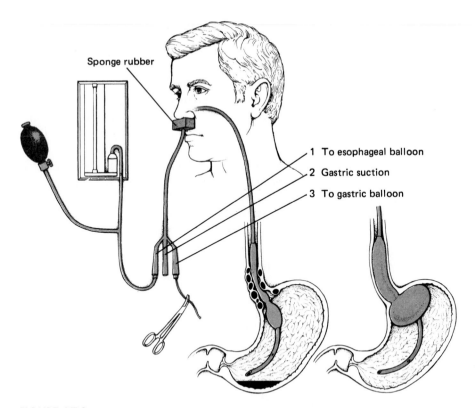

Sponge rubber

1 To esophageal balloon

2 Gastric suction

3 To gastric balloon

FIGURE 17-2.

To stop variceal bleeding, an esophageal tamponade tube (also called a compression balloon tube) may be advanced and secured so that the compression balloon can be inflated against the bleeding site (at right). The various lumens permit inflation, deflation, suction, and other procedures. (From *The Lippincott manual of nursing practice* [2nd ed., 1991]. Philadelphia: J. B. Lippincott.)

5. If the physician orders iced saline lavage, focus nursing interventions on:
   a. Ensuring nasogastric tube patency to prevent aspiration
   b. Observing gastric aspirate for evidence of bleeding
   c. Protecting the client from chilling
6. After injection sclerotherapy, if performed, assess for:
   a. Aspiration
   b. Esophageal perforation
   c. Rebleeding
7. After portal-systemic surgical intervention, if done, monitor for such complications as:
   a. Development of systemic encephalopathy
   b. Liver failure
   c. Rebleeding

G. Evaluation
1. The client verbalizes understanding of the disorder and procedures used.
2. The client communicates needs and fears.
3. The client reports reduced fear related to potential hemorrhage.
4. The client maintains a patent airway with no aspiration.
5. The client maintains intact skin integrity.
6. The client remains free of massive hemorrhage.
7. The client reports increased comfort resulting from treatment.

VII. Hepatitis
A. Description: an inflammatory disorder of the liver parenchyma occurring in hepatitis A, hepatitis B, hepatitis C, and toxic or drug-induced hepatitis
B. Etiology and incidence
1. Hepatitis usually results from viral infection; however, it also can result from toxicity or certain drugs.
2. The hepatitis A virus (an RNA virus) may be transmitted via the fecal–oral route or from contaminated food or water. This virus is endemic in some parts of the world; children younger than 15 years are at greatest risk.
3. The hepatitis B virus (a DNA virus) may be transmitted parenterally or by intimate contact with carriers; persons with acute disease; or contaminated instruments, syringes, or needles. Incidence is greatest in areas with high population densities and poor hygienic conditions.
4. Hepatitis (linked to an unidentifiable virus) can result from transfusion of contaminated blood products, exposure to infected persons in renal transplant and dialysis units, or parenteral drug abuse.
5. Toxic or drug-induced hepatitis results from chemicals or

medications that damage the parenchyma (e.g., carbon tetra-chloride, halothane, acetaminophen).

C. Pathophysiology and management

1. After exposure to a hepatitis virus, incubation period varies: typically about 30 days for hepatitis A, 90 days for hepatitis B, and 50 days for hepatitis C.

2. Hepatocellular damage results from the body's immune response to the virus or toxin and is characterized by diffuse inflammatory infiltration with local necrosis.

3. Bile flow is interrupted, antigen–antibody complexes activate the complement system, bilirubin diffuses into tissues, bile salts accumulate, and hepatomegaly and splenomegaly occur.

4. In uncomplicated cases, hepatocellular repair usually is completed within 3 to 4 months of onset.

5. Possible complications include fulminating hepatitis (a rare but life-threatening condition), chronic hepatitis, a chronic carrier state for hepatitis B surface antigen, cholestatic hepatitis, aplastic anemia, and pancreatitis.

6. Management relies first on prevention and immunization and on administration of immune globulins.

D. Assessment findings

1. Hepatitis A is commonly marked by:
   a. Initially, headache, malaise, fatigue, anorexia, lethargy, fever, flulike respiratory symptoms
   b. In the icteric phase, dark urine, scleral icterus, jaundice, liver tenderness and perhaps enlargement
   c. Elevated serum transaminase levels, presence of hepatitis virus antibodies

2. Hepatitis B resembles hepatitis A clinically but usually with more severe manifestations. Fever and respiratory symptoms are rare; arthralgias and rash may occur.

3. Hepatitis C and toxic or drug-induced hepatitis typically resemble viral hepatitis in onset and symptoms; may progress to hepatic failure.

E. Nursing diagnoses

1. Activity Intolerance
2. Fatigue
3. Knowledge Deficit
4. Altered Nutrition: Less than body requirements
5. Altered Sexuality Patterns
6. Social Isolation

F. Planning and implementation

1. Ensure that the client receives adequate fluid intake, sufficient rest, and proper nutrition.

2. Intervene to provide symptomatic relief as appropriate.
3. Administer blood transfusions or electrolyte supplements as ordered.
4. Teach the client health maintenance measures related to the type of hepatitis, which may include:
   a. Hepatitis A: good sanitation and personal hygiene practices, effective sterilization procedures, administration of immune globulin
   b. Hepatitis B: administration of specific hepatitis B immune globulin, hepatitis B vaccine for preexposure, immunization of high-risk persons
   c. Hepatitis C: mandatory screening of blood donors, avoidance of certain medications and alcohol
   d. Toxic or drug-induced hepatitis: avoidance of the causative agent

G. **Evaluation**
1. The client maintains adequate fluid and nutrient intake.
2. The client reports decreased fatigue.
3. The client verbalizes understanding of preventive measures and self-care to maintain health status.

VIII. Cirrhosis

A. **Description: a chronic, degenerative liver disease marked by diffuse destruction and fibrotic regeneration of hepatic cells; classified as Laennec's, posthepatic, and biliary cirrhosis**

B. **Etiology and incidence**
1. Major causes of cirrhosis include:
   a. Alcoholism and chronic nutritional deficiencies (Laennec's cirrhosis)
   b. Bile duct disorders that suppress bile flow (biliary cirrhosis)
   c. Various types of hepatitis (posthepatic cirrhosis)
2. Incidence is twice as high in men as in women; peak incidence occurs between ages 40 and 60.

C. **Pathophysiology and management**
1. In cirrhosis, liver cells are injured or destroyed and replaced with scar tissue. Regeneration of liver tissue is patchy, resulting in a characteristic "hobnail" appearance.
2. Fibrosis and other changes in hepatocytes and reticular cells, as well as vascular and bile duct changes, lead to decreased blood and bile flow. Obstructed blood flow results in portal hypertension and esophageal varices.
3. Impaired hepatic functions include gluconeogenesis, detoxification of drugs and alcohol, bilirubin metabolism, vitamin absorption, and hormonal metabolism.

D. **Assessment findings**

1. Clinical manifestations include:
   a. Enlarged, firm liver
   b. Chronic dyspepsia
   c. Constipation or diarrhea
   d. Gradual weight loss
   e. Ascites
   f. Splenomegaly
   g. Spider telangiectases
   h. Dilated abdominal blood vessels
   i. Signs and symptoms of portal hypertension (late)
2. Laboratory study results may include:
   a. Destruction and fibrosis of liver tissue seen on biopsy
   b. Abnormal thickening and masses revealed on liver scan
   c. Elevated ALT, AST, and LDH levels
   d. Hypoalbuminemia
   e. Elevated prothrombin time
   f. Reduced bromsulphalein dye excretion

E. **Nursing diagnoses**

1. Activity Intolerance
2. Risk for Injury
3. Altered Nutrition: Less than body requirements
4. Risk for Impaired Skin Integrity
5. Altered Thought Processes

F. **Planning and implementation**

1. Promote adequate rest and relaxation.
2. Ensure good nutritional intake.
3. Prevent threats to skin integrity.
4. Minimize the risk of bleeding.
5. Minimize metabolic derangements that can cause further deterioration of mental status.

G. **Evaluation**

1. The client demonstrates independence in activities.
2. The client exhibits improved nutritional status.
3. The client exhibits improved skin integrity.
4. The client demonstrates reduced risk of bleeding.
5. The client demonstrates improved mental status.

IX. **Liver cancer**

A. **Description: a rare form of cancer with a high mortality rate; may be primary (benign or malignant) or metastatic**

B. **Etiology and incidence**

1. Adenoma, a benign primary tumor, is associated with use of oral contraceptives or androgens; incidence is increasing, primarily in women.

    2. Occurring most frequently in men, hepatoma (or hepatocellular carcinoma)—the most common malignant primary tumor—has been linked to various factors, including hepatitis B, chronic liver disease, anabolic steroid use, and long-term androgen therapy.

    3. Metastatic liver cancer is associated with approximately one half of all late cancer cases. In the United States, it is up to 20 times more prevalent than primary liver tumors.

C. **Pathophysiology and management**

    1. Primary liver tumors originate in hepatocytes, connective tissue, or blood vessels (hepatomas) or in intrahepatic bile ducts (cholangiomas).

    2. Metastatic cancer can spread from virtually any body area but is mostly associated with breast, lung, and colon cancer.

    3. Processes of liver metastasis include:

        a. Extension from adjacent organs

        b. Migration by way of the hepatic arterial system or the portal venous system

        c. Seeding from peritoneal migration

    4. Although benign, adenomas carry a high risk of rupture due to their high vascularity.

    5. Malignant liver cancer is almost always fatal, with death occurring an average of 6 months after diagnosis.

    6. Treatment may include chemotherapy, surgery, or transplantation.

D. **Assessment findings**

    1. Possible clinical manifestations of hepatoma include:

        a. Recent weight loss, weakness, and fatigue

        b. Hepatomegaly, jaundice, ascites

        c. Liver mass detected on palpation

    2. Pertinent laboratory studies may reveal:

        a. Anemia

        b. Elevated alkaline phosphatase

        c. Hypoproteinemia

        d. Decreased activity on liver function studies

        e. Filling defects revealed on liver scans

    3. Positive tissue biopsy confirms diagnosis.

E. **Nursing diagnoses**

    1. Ineffective Breathing Pattern

    2. Fear

    3. Risk for Infection

    4. Altered Nutrition: Less than body requirements

    5. Pain

    6. Altered Role Performance

    7. Risk for Impaired Skin Integrity

F. **Planning and implementation**
1. Provide emotional support for the client and family, and help them cope with the diagnosis of cancer and its poor prognosis.
2. Teach the client and family about the prescribed treatment plan, which may include radiation therapy, chemotherapy, or surgery (resection or liver transplantation).
3. If the physician institutes percutaneous biliary drainage to bypass obstructed biliary ducts, teach the client catheter care and signs of infection to watch for and report.
4. If liver transplantation was performed, provide postoperative care, including:
    a. Administering prescribed immunosuppressive drugs to prevent tissue rejection (See Chapter 21, Cancer Nursing)
    b. Monitoring for and reporting signs of rejection
5. Arrange for home health care follow-up after discharge.

G. **Evaluation**
1. The client reports minimal discomfort and adequate pain control.
2. The client displays minimal respiratory compromise.
3. The client maintains adequate nutritional status.
4. The client exhibits improved skin and tissue integrity.
5. The client remains free of infection.
6. The client and family members communicate fears and receive adequate emotional support.

X. **Cholelithiasis and cholecystitis**

A. **Description**
1. Cholelithiasis refers to calculi formation in the gallbladder.
2. Cholecystitis is acute or chronic inflammation of the gallbladder.

B. **Etiology and incidence**
1. Gallstone formation results from changes in bile components or bile stasis, which may be associated with such factors as infection, cirrhosis, pancreatitis, celiac disease, diabetes mellitus, pregnancy, and oral contraceptive use.
2. Cholelithiasis is extremely common, affecting approximately 20% of the population in the United States. It is the fifth leading cause of hospitalization in adults and is associated with about 90% of all gallbladder disease in the United States.
3. Incidence is greater in women than in men before age 50 and approximately equal in both sexes after age 50.
4. Acute cholecystitis may be calculous (with gallstones) or acalculous (without gallstones) and can result from:
    a. Obstruction of the cystic duct with an impacted gallstone (90% to 95% of cases)

    b.   Tissue damage due to trauma, massive burns, or surgery

    c.   Gram-negative septicemia

    d.   Multiple blood transfusions

    e.   Prolonged fasting

    f.   Hypertension

    g.   Overuse of narcotic analgesics

5. Although chronic cholecystitis may follow acute cholecystitis, it often occurs independently; it is almost always associated with gallstone formation.

6. Acute cholecystitis is most common in middle-aged persons; the chronic form usually affects the elderly. Incidence of either type is greater in women than in men (about 3:1).

C. Pathophysiology and management

    1. Calculi usually form from solid constituents of bile; the three major types are:

        a.   Cholesterol gallstones, the most common type, thought to form in supersaturated bile

        b.   Pigment gallstones, formed mainly of unconjugated pigments in bile precipitate

        c.   Mixed types, with characteristics of pigment and cholesterol stones

    2. Up to one half of persons with gallstones are asymptomatic and require no intervention.

    3. In some cases, however, gallstones can obstruct the cystic duct, causing cholecystitis, or the common bile duct, where they are termed choledocholithiasis.

    4. In cholecystitis, inflammation causes the gallbladder wall to become thickened and edematous and the cystic lumen to increase in diameter.

    5. Submucosal hemorrhage, mucosal ulceration, and polymorphonuclear infiltration follow.

    6. If inflammation spreads to the common bile duct, obstruction of bile drainage can lead to jaundice.

    7. Other possible complications include:

        a.   Empyema (pus-filled gallbladder)

        b.   Perforation

        c.   Emphysematous cholecystitis

    8. Treatment for cholelithiasis and cholecystitis may involve:

        a.   Chenodeoxycholic acid to dissolve gallstones (effective in dissolving about 60% of radiolucent gallstones)

        b.   Nonsurgical removal (e.g., lithotripsy or extracorporeal shock wave therapy)

        c.   Surgical treatment (e.g., cholecystectomy [gallbladder removed after ligation of cystic duct and artery], choledochostomy [incision into the common bile duct for calculi removal], cholecystomy [gallbladder opened; stones, bile, or pus removed; drainage tube placed])

9. Pigment gallstones cannot be dissolved and must be excised.

D. Assessment findings

1. Many clients with cholelithiasis are asymptomatic.
2. Possible clinical manifestations include:
   a. Episodic (commonly following a high-fat meal), cramping pain in the right upper abdominal quadrant or the epigastrium, possibly radiating to the back near the right scapular tip (biliary colic)
   b. Nausea and vomiting
   c. Fat intolerance
   d. Fever and leukocytosis
   e. Signs and symptoms of jaundice
3. Biliary ultrasonography (cholecystosonography) can detect gallstones in most cases.
4. Acute cholecystitis is commonly marked by:
   a. Biliary colic
   b. Tenderness and rigidity in the right upper quadrant elicited on palpation (Murphy's sign)
   c. Fever
   d. Nausea and vomiting
   e. Fat intolerance
   f. Signs and symptoms of jaundice
5. Manifestations of chronic cholecystitis commonly include:
   a. Pain, less severe than in the acute form
   b. Fever, also less severe than in the acute form
   c. Fat intolerance
   d. Heartburn
   e. Flatulence
6. Laboratory and diagnostic study findings in acute or chronic cholecystitis may include:
   a. Leukocytosis
   b. Elevated alkaline phosphatase
   c. Detection of gallstones on ultrasonography
   d. Inability to visualize the gallbladder on HIDA scanning or oral cholecystography

E. Nursing diagnoses

1. Risk for Fluid Volume Deficit
2. Risk for Infection
3. Altered Nutrition: Less than body requirements
4. Pain
5. Risk for Impaired Skin Integrity

F. Planning and implementation

1. Intervene to relieve pain; give prescribed analgesics.

    2. Promote adequate rest.

    3. Administer antacids, such as Maalox, Amphojel, or Mylanta, to neutralize gastric acid and decrease acid irritation.

      a. **Shake medication in suspension form well.**

      b. **Instruct client to take other medications 1 or 2 hours before or after taking antacid to prevent altered absorption.**

    4. Assess nutritional status, and promote a high-protein, high-carbohydrate, low-fat diet.

    5. Monitor fluid balance, and administer IV fluids as prescribed.

    6. Monitor for signs and symptoms of possible complications.

    7. Teach the client about planned treatments; prepare him or her for scheduled procedures as appropriate.

G. Evaluation

    1. The client reports only minimal discomfort.

    2. The client remains free of infection.

    3. The client maintains adequate fluid volume.

    4. The client exhibits intact, uncompromised skin integrity with no evidence of jaundice.

    5. The client maintains adequate nutritional status and verbalizes understanding of dietary recommendations to help control symptoms.

XI. Acute pancreatitis

A. Description: inflammation of the pancreas ranging from a relatively mild, self-limiting disorder to rapidly fatal, acute hemorrhagic pancreatitis

B. Etiology and incidence

    1. The major causes of acute pancreatitis are:

      a. Alcoholism

      b. Cholecystitis

      c. Surgery involving or near the pancreas

    2. Other possible predisposing factors include:

      a. Viral hepatitis, mumps, peptic ulcer disease, periarteritis, hyperlipidemia, hypercalcemia, anorexia nervosa, shock with ischemia, trauma to the pancreas, ERCP

      b. Use of medications such as thiazide diuretics, furosemide, valproic acid, estrogens, tetracycline, azathioprine, mercaptopurine, sulfonamides, and glucocorticoids

    3. Men most commonly develop pancreatitis related to alcoholism, trauma, or peptic ulcer; in women, pancreatitis is most commonly associated with cholecystitis.

C. Pathophysiology and management

    1. Acute pancreatitis involves various pathologic changes, ranging from edema and inflammation to necrosis and hemorrhage.

2. Due to abnormal pancreatic enzyme activation in the pancreas (instead of in the GI tract), the pancreas begins to digest itself.

3. Kinin activation alters cell membrane permeability, causing a loss of protein-rich fluid into the tissues and peritoneal cavity and producing hypovolemia.

D. Assessment findings

1. Clinical manifestations of acute pancreatitis include:
   a. Abdominal tenderness with back pain
   b. GI problems: nausea, vomiting, diarrhea, steatorrhea
   c. Fever
   d. Jaundice
   e. Mental confusion
   f. Flank or umbilical bruising
   g. Hypotension
   h. Signs of hypovolemia
   i. Possibly, respiratory distress

2. Laboratory studies may reveal elevated amylase, lipase, and WBC levels.

E. Nursing diagnoses

1. Ineffective Breathing Pattern
2. Fluid Volume Deficit
3. Altered Nutrition: Less than body requirements
4. Pain

F. Planning and implementation

1. Administer analgesics, such as acetaminophen with codeine (Tylenol 3) for mild pain; propoxyphene (Darvon) for moderate pain; or meperidine (Demerol) and morphine (Duramorph) for severe pain. These drugs alter perception of and response to pain while depressing the CNS.

   a. **Assess pain on scale of 1 (least pain) to 10 (worst pain) and rule out complications or new condition requiring physician's attention.**
   b. **Administer appropriate medication and implement safety precautions.**
   c. **Evaluate effectiveness of medication within 30 minutes of delivery.**

2. Perform nasogastric suction as needed.
3. Assess fluid and electrolyte status, and provide replacement therapy as indicated.
4. Administer blood transfusions and parenteral nutrition as prescribed.
5. Maintain optimal respiratory status; place the client in semi-

Fowler's position to decrease pressure on the diaphragm, and teach the client coughing and deep breathing techniques.

n   6.   **Administer histamine (H$_2$) receptor antagonists, such as cimetidine (Tagamet), ranitidine (Zantac), or famotidine (Pepsid), to suppress gastric acid. Instruct client to continue taking medication even after pain subsides.**

G.   Evaluation
1.   The client reports decreased pain.
2.   The client exhibits improved fluid and nutritional status.
3.   The client demonstrates adequate respiratory function.

XII.   Chronic pancreatitis

A.   Description: progressive pancreatic inflammation resulting in permanent structural damage to pancreatic tissue

B.   Etiology and incidence
1.   Chronic pancreatitis typically results from repeated episodes of acute pancreatitis.
2.   More than half of all cases of chronic pancreatitis are associated with alcoholism.

C.   Pathophysiology and management
1.   With repeated attacks of pancreatitis, pancreatic cells are progressively replaced with fibrous tissue, causing increased pressure within the pancreas.
2.   Eventually, this results in mechanical obstruction of the pancreatic duct, common bile duct, and duodenum.
3.   Other effects include atrophy of the ductal epithelium, inflammation, and destruction of pancreatic cells.
4.   Management measures include drug and diet therapies, and possibly surgery.

D.   Assessment findings
1.   Chronic pancreatitis is commonly marked by pain, weight loss, steatorrhea, and anorexia.
2.   Laboratory study findings typically reveal:
      a.   Pancreatic calcification detected on ERCP
      b.   Abnormal glucose tolerance test

E.   Nursing diagnoses
1.   Diarrhea
2.   Altered Nutrition: Less than body requirements
3.   Pain

F.   Planning and implementation
1.   Provide symptomatic treatment, focusing on relieving pain, promoting comfort, and treating new attacks.
2.   Manage any endocrine insufficiency, such as diabetes mellitus, by initiating dietary and insulin therapy.

3. Administer pancreatic enzymes such as pancrelipase (Pancreatin), which replaces the enzymes necessary to digest protein, starches, and fats.

𝍄 a. **Administer dose just before or during the meal.**
   b. **Do not crush (or chew) the medication, which has an enteric coating to protect it from gastric juices.**

4. Help the client reduce pancreatic secretions by:
   a. Promoting a low-fat diet
   b. Encouraging avoidance of caffeine and alcohol
   c. Providing instruction on the use of antacids (see Section X.F.3).
   d. Offering instruction on the use of histamine (H_2) receptor antagonists such as cimetidine (see Section XI.F.6).

5. Prepare the client for surgery to relieve pain and drain cysts, if indicated.

G. Evaluation

1. The client reports only minimal discomfort.
2. The client maintains adequate nutritional status.
3. The client reports reduced frequency of diarrhea and steatorrhea.

XIII. Pancreatic cancer

A. Description: tumors, most commonly adenocarcinomas, of the pancreas

B. Etiology and incidence

1. Pancreatic cancer is linked to such factors as:
   a. Exposure to chemicals
   b. High-fat diet
   c. Cigarette smoking
   d. Chronic pancreatitis

2. Pancreatic cancer is second only to colon cancer as a cause of GI cancer-related death. Incidence is greater in men than in women; peak incidence occurs between age 55 to 65.

C. Pathophysiology and management

1. Carcinoma may arise in any portion of the pancreas (head, body, or tail), producing clinical manifestations that vary, depending on the location.

2. The overall 5-year survival rate for all clients with pancreatic cancer is less than 5%.

3. Treatment may involve:
   a. Surgery, aimed at either cure or symptom palliation
   b. Chemotherapy
   c. Radiation therapy for palliation

D. Assessment findings

1. The following may be initial manifestations or may develop

only when cancer is in an advanced stage: anorexia, weight loss, abdominal pain, jaundice, diarrhea or steatorrhea, palpable epigastric mass.

    2. Laboratory and diagnostic studies may reveal:

        a. Elevated serum APT level (in 80% of clients)

        b. Elevated carcinoembryonic antigen (CEA), LDH, AST, and serum amylase levels

        c. Hyperglycemia

        d. Structural abnormalities detected on upper GI series

        e. Mass demonstrated by ultrasonography or CT scan

        f. Pancreatic duct stricture seen on ERCP

        g. Tissue biopsy positive for malignancy

E. Nursing diagnoses

    1. Ineffective Breathing Pattern

    2. Altered Nutrition: Less than body requirements

    3. Pain

    4. Impaired Tissue Integrity

F. Planning and implementation

    1. Assess the client's level of pain frequently, and administer pain medications (see Section XI.F.1).

    2. Assess for and report any changes affecting nutritional needs. Administer parenteral nutrition as prescribed.

    3. Monitor serum glucose level, and observe for signs of hyperglycemia.

    4. As prescribed, administer pancreatic enzymes (see Section XII.F.3).

    5. Prepare the client for pancreatoduodenectomy (removal of most of the pancreas to excise a resectable tumor), if indicated.

    6. After surgery, provide postoperative care:

        a. Assess respiratory status: Encourage and assist the client to cough and deep-breathe every hour, and help him or her change position often.

        b. Avoid placing pressure on anastomoses and sutures.

        c. Irrigate the nasogastric tube and other tubes gently and only if prescribed. Withhold oral intake until GI function returns.

        d. Inspect surgical incisions for inflammation, infection, and abscess formation.

        e. Maintain aseptic technique when handling wound dressings.

G. Evaluation

    1. The client reports only minimal discomfort.

    2. The client exhibits minimal or no respiratory compromise.

    3. The client maintains adequate nutritional status.

    4. The client exhibits improved skin and tissue integrity.

Bibliography

Bolander, V. R. (1994). *Sorensen & Luckmann's basic nursing: A physiologic approach* (3rd ed.). Philadelphia: W. B. Saunders.

Bouchier, I. A. D., et al. (1993). *Gastroenterology: Clinical science and practice* (2nd ed.). Philadelphia: W. B. Saunders.

Carpenito, L. J. (1995). *Nursing diagnosis: Application to clinical practice* (6th ed.). Philadelphia: J. B. Lippincott.

Clark, J., Queener, S., & Karb, V. (1990). *Pharmacologic basis of nursing practice* (4th ed.). St. Louis: C. V. Mosby.

Gitnick, G., LaBreque, D. R., & Moody, F. G., Jr. (1992). *Diseases of the liver and biliary tract*. St. Louis: C. V. Mosby.

Nettina, S. (1996). *The Lippincott manual of nursing practice* (6th ed.). Philadelphia: J. B. Lippincott.

Scherer, J. C., & Timby, B. K. (1995). *Introductory medical-surgical nursing* (6th ed.). Philadelphia: J. B. Lippincott.

Schiff, L., & Schiff, E. R. (1993). *Diseases of the liver* (7th ed.). Philadelphia: J. B. Lippincott.

Smeltzer, S. C., & Bare, B. G. (1996). *Brunner & Suddarth's textbook of medical-surgical nursing* (8th ed.). Philadelphia: J. B. Lippincott.

Society of Gastroenterology Nurses and Associates. (1993). *SGNA gastroenterology nursing: A core curriculum*. St. Louis: C. V. Mosby.

Springhouse Corporation. (1992). *Nursing student's guide to drugs*. Spring House, PA: Springhouse Corp.

Surawicz, C. S., & Owen, R. (1995). *Gastrointestinal and hepatic infections*. Philadelphia: W. B. Saunders.

STUDY QUESTIONS

1. Bile is synthesized by which type of cell?
   a. enterocyte
   b. hepatocyte
   c. Kupffer cell
   d. Acinar cell

2. For which of the following reasons would a client with jaundice develop the nursing diagnosis of Risk for Impaired Skin Integrity?
   a. Jaundice is associated with decubitus formation.
   b. Jaundice impairs urea production, which produces pruritus.
   c. Jaundice produces pruritus due to impaired bile acid excretion.
   d. Jaundice leads to decreased tissue perfusion.

3. For which of the following reasons would the nurse explain placement of an esophageal-tamponade tube to a bleeding client?
   a. to obtain cooperation and reduce fear
   b. to begin teaching for home care
   c. to have client assist with tube insertion
   d. to maintain client's level of anxiety

4. Which of the following nursing plans would be *most* helpful with a client with chronic pancreatitis?
   a. Teach client to modify protein in diet.
   b. Encourage client to exercise daily.
   c. Allow client to liberalize fluid intake.
   d. Counsel client to stop alcohol consumption.

5. Which of these pancreatic fluids are secreted from the acinar exocrine cell?
   a. insulin
   b. glucagon
   c. trypsin
   d. pancreozymin

6. A client with acute cholecystitis will usually demonstrate which of the following nutritional alterations?
   a. Altered Nutrition: Less than body requirements related to poor oral intake due to anorexia
   b. Altered Nutrition: More than body requirements related to decreased gastrointestinal losses
   c. Altered Nutrition: More than body requirements related to decreased nutrient requirements
   d. Altered Nutrition: Less than body requirements related to long-term malnutrition

7. Evaluation of the resolution of elevated direct or conjugated serum bilirubin generally indicates correction of which of the following?
   a. hepatocellular damage
   b. impaired bile excretion
   c. Kupffer cell damage
   d. hemolysis

8. Pancreatic lipase performs which of the following functions?
   a. breaks down fat into fatty acids and glycerol
   b. transports fatty acids into the brush border
   c. triggers cholecystokinin to contract the gallbladder
   d. breaks down protein into dipeptides and amino acids

9. After administering diuretic therapy to a client with ascites, which of the following nursing actions most helps ensure safe care?
   a. Measure serum potassium for hyperkalemia.
   b. Assess the client for hypervolemia.
   c. Measure body weight weekly.
   d. Document precise intake and output.

10. Which evaluation criteria would the nurse establish for a client in hepatic coma?
    a. Client is oriented to time, place, and person.
    b. Client exhibits no ecchymotic areas.

c. Client increases oral intake to 2000 calories/day.

d. Client exhibits increased serum albumin.

11. For a client with a LeVeen or peritoneojugular shunt, the nurse should note presence of ascites because the shunt

a. was placed to reduce portal hypertension

b. was placed to reduce ascites

c. diverts blood to the inferior vena cava

d. reduces bacterial ammonia production in the GI tract

12. When planning pain management for a client following a pancreatoduodenectomy, the *best* plan for nursing care would be to

a. Hold pain medication because this operative procedure is minor.

b. Give pain medication regularly regardless of respiratory status.

c. Bypass assessment since the client is unable to express pain with this procedure.

d. Administer pain medication frequently as prescribed.

13. With the nursing diagnosis Knowledge Deficit about self-care activities at home following cholecystitis, the nurse would use which of the following criteria to evaluate the client's understanding of an appropriate diet?

a. The client selects low-carbohydrate food divided into six small meals.

b. The client selects high-fat, high-carbohydrate meals.

c. The client selects low-fat, high-carbohydrate meals.

d. The client selects high-fat, low-protein meals.

14. When caring for a client following percutaneous transhepatic cholangiography, the nurse's evaluation of the client would be that the client demonstrates absence of

a. fever and chills

b. hypertension

c. bradycardia

d. nausea and diarrhea

15. In planning for home care of a client with hepatitis A, which of the following preventive measures should the nurse emphasize to protect the client's family?

a. Keep the client in complete isolation.

b. Use good sanitation with dishes and shared bathroom.

c. Avoid contact with blood-soiled clothing or dressings.

d. Forbid sharing of needles or syringes.

16. Which of the following is the *most* important intervention for Risk for Injury secondary to altered clotting mechanisms in a client with hepatic cirrhosis?

a. Allow the client complete independence of mobility.

b. Apply pressure to injection sites.

c. Administer antibiotics as prescribed.

d. Increase nutritional intake.

For additional questions, see
Lippincott's Self-Study Series Software
Available at your bookstore

ANSWER KEY

1. **Correct response: b**
   Hepatocytes (liver cells) synthesize and secrete bile into the canaliculi.
   a. Enterocytes are cells within the small intestine.
   c. Kupffer cells are the phagocytic cells of the liver.
   d. Acinar cells are the exocrine cells of the pancreas.
   Knowledge/Physiologic/Assessment

2. **Correct response: c**
   Pruritus occurs secondary to decreased bile acid excretion.
   a. Jaundice is not associated with decubitus formation; edema and hypoalbuminemia are.
   b and d. Jaundice itself does not impair urea production or lead to decreased tissue perfusion.
   Comprehension/Safe care/Analysis (Dx)

3. **Correct response: a**
   This tube is placed in critical situations; thus, the client will be fearful.
   b. This tube is used only short term and is not indicated for home use.
   c. The tube is large and uncomfortable and would not be inserted by the client.
   d. A client's anxiety should be decreased, not maintained.
   Application/Psychosocial/Implementation

4. **Correct response: d**
   Continued alcohol consumption may cause recurrent attacks.
   a. Protein modification in the diet is not necessary for this client.
   b. Exercise is helpful for health promotion but not most helpful for this client.
   c. Liberalizing fluid intake may be helpful but not most helpful in this client.
   Analysis/Health promotion/Planning

5. **Correct response: c**
   Trypsin is the proteolytic enzyme in pancreatic fluid.
   a and b. Insulin and glucagon are pancreatic hormones secreted by the beta and alpha endocrine cells.
   d. Pancreozymin is released from the intestine and acts on the pancreas.
   Knowledge/Physiologic/Assessment

6. **Correct response: a**
   Anorexia, nausea, vomiting, or pain will lead to decreased oral intake.
   b. The client may have increased GI losses with vomiting.
   c. As with an acute inflammatory process, nutrient requirements may increase.
   d. Cholecystitis generally is not associated with long-term malnutrition.
   Comprehension/Physiologic/ Analysis (Dx)

7. **Correct response: b**
   Elevated direct bilirubin level indicates impaired bile excretion.
   a and c. Hepatocyte or Kupffer cell damage generally does not cause elevated bilirubin.
   d. Hemolysis leads to elevated indirect or unconjugated bilirubin levels.
   Application/Physiologic/Evaluation

8. **Correct response: a**
   Lipase hydrolyzes fat into fatty acids and glycerol.
   b. Lipase does not perform this transport function.
   c. Fat itself triggers cholecystokinin release.
   d. This is the function of trypsin, not lipase.
   Comprehension/Physiologic/Assessment

9. **Correct response: d**
   Careful intake and output measurement is essential for safe diuretic therapy.
   a. Hypokalemia, not hyperkalemia, commonly occurs with diuretic therapy.
   b. A client should be assessed for hypovolemia after increased urine output.
   c. This client should be weighed daily.
   Analysis/Self care/Implementation

10. *Correct response: a*

With resolving hepatic coma, the client should be able to express orientation to time, place, and person.

b. Ecchymotic areas are related not to hepatic coma but to decreased synthesis of clotting factors.

c. Although oral intake may be related to level of consciousness, oral intake or lack of it is more closely related to anorexia.

d. Serum albumin does not indicate level of consciousness, but rather reflects hepatic synthetic ability.

Application/Self care/Evaluation

11. *Correct response: b*

This shunt diverts peritoneal ascites back into the venous system.

a and c. The shunt does not reduce portal hypertension or divert blood.

d. This shunt has no effect on bacterial growth or ammonia production.

Application/Self care/Implementation

12. *Correct response: d*

This is a major operative procedure generally done for a painful disorder; therefore, pain medication should be administered frequently.

a. This is a long, major, extensive procedure.

b. With analgesia administration, respiratory status should always be assessed.

c. Because this procedure should not impair a client's ability to express pain, pain should be assessed.

Application/Health promotion/Planning

13. *Correct response: c*

The client should reduce fat intake and substitute fat calories with carbohydrates.

a. Reducing carbohydrate intake would be contraindicated.

b and d. A high-fat diet may lead to another attack of cholecystitis.

Application/Health promotion/ Analysis (Dx)

14. *Correct response: a*

Fever and chills may indicate septicemia, a common postprocedure complication.

b. Hypotension, not hypertension, is associated with septicemia.

c. Tachycardia, not bradycardia, is most likely to occur.

d. Nausea and diarrhea may occur but are not classic signs of sepsis.

Analysis/Physiologic/Evaluation

15. *Correct response: b*

Hepatitis A is transmitted through the fecal–oral route.

a. Complete isolation is not required.

c and d. These precautions are for hepatitis B, not hepatitis A.

Analysis/Health promotion/Planning

16. *Correct response: b*

With altered clotting mechanisms, prolonged application of pressure to injection or bleeding sites is important.

a. Complete independence may increase potential for injury, because an unsupervised client may injure himself or herself and bleed excessively.

c and d. Antibiotics and good nutrition are important to promote liver regeneration; however, they are not most important for a client with increased bleeding potential.

Analysis/Health promotion/ Implementation

Renal and Urinary
Disorders

18

I. **Renal and urinary system**
   A. Structures
   B. Function

II. **Renal and urinary system overview**
   A. Assessment
   B. Laboratory studies and diagnostic tests
   C. Psychosocial implications

III. **Urinary retention**
   A. Description
   B. Etiology and incidence
   C. Pathophysiology and management
   D. Assessment findings
   E. Nursing diagnoses
   F. Planning and implementation
   G. Evaluation

IV. **Urinary incontinence**
   A. Description
   B. Etiology and incidence
   C. Pathophysiology and management
   D. Assessment findings
   E. Nursing diagnoses
   F. Planning and implementation
   G. Evaluation

V. **Neurogenic bladder dysfunction**
   A. Description
   B. Etiology and incidence
   C. Pathophysiology and management
   D. Assessment findings
   E. Nursing diagnoses
   F. Planning and implementation
   G. Evaluation

VI. **Urinary tract infection (UTI)**
   A. Description
   B. Etiology and incidence
   C. Pathophysiology and management
   D. Assessment findings
   E. Nursing diagnoses
   F. Planning and implementation
   G. Evaluation

VII. **Urolithiasis (renal calculi)**
   A. Description
   B. Etiology and incidence
   C. Pathophysiology and management
   D. Assessment findings
   E. Nursing diagnoses
   F. Planning and implementation
   G. Evaluation

VIII. **Urinary tract cancer**
   A. Description
   B. Etiology and incidence
   C. Pathophysiology and management
   D. Assessment findings
   E. Nursing diagnoses
   F. Planning and implementation
   G. Evaluation

IX. **Acute renal failure**
   A. Description
   B. Etiology and incidence
   C. Pathophysiology and management
   D. Assessment findings
   E. Nursing diagnoses
   F. Planning and implementation
   G. Evaluation

I. Renal and urinary system

A. Structures

1. The kidneys are paired organs located on either side of the vertebral column between the 12th thoracic and 3rd lumbar vertebrae in the posterior abdomen behind the peritoneum.

2. Kidney components include (Fig. 18-1):

    a. Cortex: outer portion containing the glomerules, tubules, and part of the loop of Henle

    b. Medulla: middle portion containing part of the loop of Henle and the collecting ducts

    c. Pelvis: inner portion where urine is collected; the narrowed portion becomes the proximal aspect of the ureter as it approaches the hilum

    d. Hilum: area where nerves, blood vessels, and the ureter enter the kidney

    e. Minor and major calyces: recesses of the pelvis that receive urine from papillae of collecting ducts

    f. Renal column: cortical tissue between pyramids in the cortex

    g. Pyramids: collecting ducts with bases on the border between the cortex and medulla; apices form papillae as they extend toward the pelvis

    h. Papillae: apices of pyramids through which urine travels to the renal pelvis

    i. Fibrous capsule: outer covering that adheres to the renal parenchyma

3. The functional unit of the kidney, the nephron contains the glomerulus and tubules; specific components include:

    a. Glomerulus: beginning of the nephron; a tuft of capillaries supplied by afferent arterioles and drained by efferent arterioles within Bowman's capsule

    b. Proximal tubule: convoluted portion with border of microvilli lining the lumen

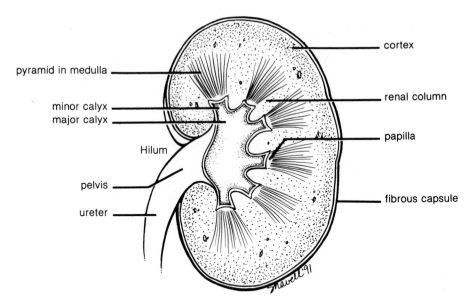

pyramid in medulla

minor calyx

major calyx

Hilum

pelvis

ureter

cortex

renal column

papilla

fibrous capsule

FIGURE 18-1.
Gross structure of a bisected kidney.

    c.   Loop of Henle: narrows as it moves from the cortex to the medulla

    d.   Distal tubule: passes between afferent and efferent arterioles of glomerulus as it moves back into the cortex

    e.   Collecting duct: passes through the cortex and medulla receiving the terminal end of several nephrons

4.   Renal circulation involves (Fig. 18-2):

    a.   Renal artery, branching from the abdominal aorta

    b.   Interlobar arteries, whose subdivisions carry blood into the corticomedullary zone

    c.   Arcuate arteries, forming arches around bases of pyramids

    d.   Interlobular arteries, subdivisions of the arcuate arteries supplying the renal capsule

5.   Renal innervation is supplied through both sympathetic and parasympathetic nerves. Adrenergic fibers also are in proximity to juxtaglomerular apparatus.

6.   Urinary system components include:

    a.   Ureters, extending from the renal pelvis to the urinary bladder

    b.   Bladder, which serves as a reservoir for urine until it is excreted from the body

    c.   Urethras, extending from the base of the bladder to the urinary meatus; approximately 4 cm long in men, 20 cm long in women

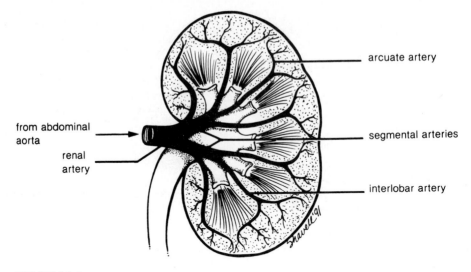

FIGURE 18-2.
Blood supply to the kidney. The renal artery branches from the abdominal aorta.

B. Function

 1. Table 18-1 gives a summary of major nephron component functions. Additional functions include:

  a. Blood pressure regulation by renin secretion

  b. Red blood cell production regulation by erythropoietin secretion

  c. Metabolism of vitamin D

 2. Ureters transport urine to the bladder via peristaltic waves of smooth muscle; the ureterovesical junction prevents backflow of urine (reflux).

 3. Micturition (voiding) is under voluntary and involuntary control. The urge to void normally occurs when 150 to 300 cc urine has accumulated; the bladder normally contains no urine after voiding (residual urine).

II. Overview of renal and urinary function

 A. Assessment

  1. The health history should focus on obtaining information about:

   a. Usual voiding pattern

   b. Changes in this pattern

   c. Artificial orifice

   d. Difficulty in starting or maintaining a urine stream

   e. Feeling of urgency

   f. Urine characteristics: odor, color, cloudy, or clear

   g. Incontinence

   h. Pain, burning

TABLE 18-1.
Major Functions of Nephron Components

NEPHRON COMPONENT	MAJOR FUNCTIONS
Glomerulus	Filtration
Proximal tubule	65% Na^+ and H_2O reabsorbed (antidiuretic hormone [ADH] not required) Glucose, K^+, amino acids reabsorbed HCO_3^- reabsorbed H^+ secreted Urea reabsorbed Filtrate leaves isotonic
Loop of Henle	Countercurrent multiplying and exchange mechanisms established between long, thin loops of Henle of juxtamedullary nephrons and adjacent vasa recta Filtrate leaves hypotonic
Distal tubule	Na^+ reabsorbed and K^+ secreted in presence of aldosterone; opposite occurs in absence of aldosterone Water reabsorbed with Na^+; ADH also influences water reabsorption Filtrate leaves hypotonic or isotonic
Collecting duct	Na^+ and K^+ regulated by aldosterone Acid–base regulation; H^+ secretion, HCO_3 reabsorption, NH_3 secretion, NH_4 excretion ADH determines final urine volume

        i.   History of disease process, surgical procedures, or trauma affecting the urinary system

        j.   Pertinent medication use (e.g., diuretics, antibiotics, narcotics, nephrotoxins, cholinergics, phenacetin)

        k.   Allergies

  2. Important physical examination steps include:

        a.   Inspecting the masses in the upper abdomen and flank area

        b.   Inspecting the external meatus for signs of discharge, cleanliness, location, and size

        c.   Palpating for the lower poles of the right and left kidney; note enlargement

        d.   Percussing above the symphysis pubis for a distended bladder

        e.   Auscultating for bruits over the renal arteries

B. **Laboratory studies and diagnostic tests**

  1. Urinalysis involves assessment of:

        a.   Color: normally yellow to amber

        b.   Opacity: normally clear

        c.   Odor: normally faintly aromatic

        d.   Specific gravity: normally 1.005 to 1.025

       e.   Osmolality: normally 300 to 900 mOsm/kg

       f.   pH: normally 4 to 8

       g.   Glucose, ketones, protein: normally negative

       h.   Red blood cells and white blood cells: normally none to trace amounts

       i.   Sediment (crystals or casts): normally none

       j.   Bacteria: normally none

       k.   Amount: normally 1500 to 2000 mL/24 hours

  2. Blood analysis includes:

       a.   Plasma creatinine: excellent indicator of renal function; normally 0.3 to 1 mg/dL, rises with renal failure

       b.   Blood urea nitrogen (BUN): normally 10 to 20 mg/dL; rises with renal failure and influenced by protein intake, catabolism, and bleeding

  3. Culture and sensitivity testing detects infective microorganisms; requires a midstream clean-catch urine specimen.

  4. Creatinine clearance evaluates glomerular filtration rate (GFR); increases as renal function diminishes.

  5. Vascular studies include:

       a.   Radionuclide tests: renal scan (provides anatomic information); renogram (provides information about renal blood flow, GFR, and tubular secretion)

       b.   Renal arteriography: outlines renal vasculature

       c.   Renal venography: outlines renal veins

  6. Plain roentgenogram of kidneys, ureters, and bladder (KUB) visualizes size, shape, and position of urinary structures.

  7. Ultrasound studies identify gross renal anatomy.

  8. Computed tomography scan detects renal masses, vascular disorders, and filling defects of the collecting system.

  9. Intravenous and retrograde pyelography (IVP) and cystourethrography provide information about the size, shape, and position of urinary tract structures and evaluate renal excretory function.

  10. Hemodynamic studies evaluate motor and sensory function of the bladder and micturition process.

  11. Cystoscopic examination allows direct endoscopic visualization of the entire urinary tract.

  12. Bladder and kidney biopsy determines the nature and extent of disease.

C. **Psychosocial implications**

  1. A client with a renal or urinary disorder may experience coping difficulty related to:

       a.   Chronic nature of the disorder

       b.   Progressive nature of symptoms

       c.   Fatigue

   d. Fear of dying

   e. Embarrassment (at incontinence)

  2. The client also may have self-concept concerns related to:

   a. Body image changes (with urinary diversion)

   b. Altered sexual function

   c. Role changes toward increased dependence

  3. Lifestyle concerns may be related to potential changes in:

   a. Physical activity

   b. Work performance, with the possibility of job loss

   c. Self-care ability

  4. Disease-related changes in social interactions may lead to isolation, hopelessness, and depression.

III. Urinary retention

 A. **Description: retention of urine in the bladder in the presence of normal urine production, with the inability to release it even when the micturition reflex is activated**

 B. **Etiology and incidence**

  1. Common causes of retention in males include:

   a. Benign prostatic hypertrophy

   b. Urethral stricture

   c. Calculi or foreign body in the urethra

   d. Urethritis

   e. Tumor

   f. Phimosis

  2. In females, possible causes include:

   a. Urethral obstruction secondary to stricture, calculi, vaginal cysts, tumor, edema

   b. Retroverted gravid uterus

  3. Causes in both sexes include:

   a. Reflex spasm of sphincters following surgery of invasive procedures

   b. Trauma

   c. Neurogenic bladder dysfunction

   d. Medications (e.g., anticholinergics, antihistamines)

   e. Fecal impaction

   f. Psychogenic retention

 C. **Pathophysiology and management**

  1. Bladder catheterization commonly reveals residual urine.

  2. Retention may be acute or chronic. Management aims to increase urine flow naturally or by catheterization.

  3. Chronic retention can lead to overflow incontinence or residual urine.

  4. Other possible complications include urinary tract infection, bladder distention and damage, and hydronephrosis.

D. Assessment Findings

    1. Common clinical manifestations include:

        a. Reports of inability to void, urgency, hesitancy, dribbling

        b. Lower abdominal pain or discomfort

        c. Restlessness, diaphoresis

        d. Visible or palpable bladder distention

        e. Dullness on bladder percussion

        f. Possibly, signs and symptoms of lower urinary tract infection

E. Nursing diagnoses

    1. Risk for Infection

    2. Pain

    3. Urinary Retention

F. Planning and implementation

    1. Facilitate bladder emptying through such actions as providing privacy, running water, having the client assume a normal voiding position, and providing pain relief.

    2. If the client cannot void, perform intermittent catheterization to prevent overdistention of the bladder.

    3. Administer alpha adrenergic blockers such as phenoxybenzamine (Dibenzyline), which decreases the urinary sphincter's resistance to outflow, causing urination and reducing pain.

        a. **Caution client that orthostatic hypotension may occur.**

        b. **Administer with food to decrease GI distress.**

    4. If indicated, prepare the client for surgical intervention (e.g., dilation of urethra, cystoplasty).

G. Evaluation

    1. The client demonstrates a normal voiding pattern.

    2. The client displays no evidence of urinary tract infection.

    3. The client reports relief of pain related to urinary retention.

IV. Urinary incontinence

A. Description

    1. Incontinence refers to the inability of the urinary sphincters to control release of urine.

    2. Types include:

        a. Enuresis (bedwetting): usually a childhood problem

        b. Stress incontinence: dribbling resulting from any kind of physical stress (e.g., coughing, sneezing, laughing; most commonly affects women)

        c. Urgency incontinence: inability to hold back urine flow when feeling the urge to void

        d. Paradoxical incontinence: urine retention with overflow, marked by involuntary voiding of small amounts

      e.   Continuous incontinence: completely uninhibited micturition reflex, with an unpredictable voiding pattern

B. **Etiology and incidence**

    1.   Temporary episodes of incontinence can result from:

        a.   Inflammation

        b.   Stress

        c.   Certain medications (e.g., narcotics, tranquilizers, sedatives, diuretics, antihistamines, antihypertensive drugs, atropinelike drugs)

    2.   Persistent or permanent incontinence may result from neuromuscular dysfunction due to such disorders as:

        a.   Bladder lesions

        b.   Spinal cord injury

        c.   Multiple sclerosis

        d.   Spinal cord tumor

        e.   Complications of pelvic surgery

        f.   Cerebrovascular accident

        g.   Large bowel disease (e.g., spastic colon, diverticular disease)

    3.   Anatomic causes of incontinence include:

        a.   Weak abdominal and perineal muscle tone due to obesity, sedentary lifestyle

        b.   Sphincter weakness or damage from obstetric trauma, surgery, or congenital conditions

        c.   Urethral deformity due to recurrent urinary tract infections, trauma, surgery, or estrogen-deficiency vulvitis

        d.   Altered urethrovesical angle in women linked to previous pregnancies and perineal muscle weakness

    4.   In some persons, incontinence stems from psychosocial factors (e.g., rebellion, dependence, regression, anxiety, attention-getting behavior).

    5.   Incidence increases with age.

C. **Pathophysiology and management**

    1.   **The embarrassment associated with incontinence often damages a person's self-esteem and can become an overwhelming negative factor in the person's life.**

    2.   Incontinence is commonly viewed as an infantile behavior and may provoke feelings of helplessness, hopelessness, and frustration.

D. **Assessment findings**

    1.   Clinical manifestations of incontinence may include:

        a.   Clothing or bedding wet with urine

        b.   Reports of dribbling, urgency, hesitancy, or inability to get to the bathroom before voiding starts

      2.   The client may exhibit or express anxiety, frustration, depression, poor self-esteem, or other psychologic distress.

E. **Nursing diagnoses**
1. Anxiety
2. Body Image Disturbance
3. Knowledge Deficit
4. Powerlessness
5. Self Esteem Disturbance
6. Impaired Skin Integrity
7. Incontinence: Functional, Reflex, Stress, Total, Urge

F. **Planning and implementation**
1. Protect the client's skin by keeping him or her dry; change clothing and bed linens as necessary.
2. Provide bladder training if indicated.
3. Encourage fluid intake of 2 to 2.5 L/day, if not contraindicated.
4. If indicated, teach the client to do perineal and Kegel exercises to help improve muscular control. The exercises can be done lying, sitting, or standing as follows:
   a. Contract the perineal muscles as though stopping urination.
   b. Sustain contraction for 5 to 10 seconds and release.
   c. Repeat 10 times, 3 or 4 times a day.
5. Check the client's medication regimen for any drugs that could cause or contribute to incontinence.
6. Refer the client for psychologic evaluation as appropriate.

G. **Evaluation**
1. The client reports fewer episodes of incontinence.
2. The client demonstrates skill at Kegel exercises by an ability to stop voiding in midstream.
3. The client demonstrates application of bladder control training by a normal voiding pattern.
4. The client verbalizes the need to drink at least 2 L of fluid daily.

V. **Neurogenic bladder dysfunction**

A. **Description: dysfunction of the bladder due to impaired neurologic control secondary to central or peripheral nervous system lesions**

B. **Etiology and incidence**
1. Major causes of neurogenic bladder include:
   a. Spinal cord injury or tumor
   b. Herniated intervertebral disk
   c. Cerebrovascular accident and other cerebral disorders
   d. Neurologic disorders such as multiple sclerosis, diabetes mellitus, syphilis

       e.   Congenital anomalies (e.g., spina bifida, myelomeningo-cele)

       f.   Infection

  2. An upper motor neuron lesion causes spastic neurogenic bladder; a lower motor neuron lesion, flaccid neurogenic bladder.

C. **Pathophysiology and management**

  1. Spastic (reflex or autonomic) neurogenic bladder, the most common type, involves:

       a.   Loss of conscious sensations and cerebral motor control

       b.   Reduced bladder capacity and marked bladder wall hypertrophy

       c.   A pattern of spontaneous, uncontrolled voidings

  2. In flaccid (atonic, nonreflex, areflexic, or autonomous) neurogenic bladder, the following sequence occurs:

       a.   Inability of bladder musculature to contract allows the bladder to fill until it becomes grossly distended.

       b.   When intrabladder pressure reaches a certain point, small amounts of urine dribble from the urethra.

       c.   Sensory loss may make the client unaware of incontinence.

       d.   Extreme, prolonged bladder distention can result in damage to bladder musculature, urinary stasis and infection, and renal infection.

  3. Mixed neurogenic bladder—usually associated with lesions at the conus–cauda equina junctions—involves a combination of spastic and flaccid dysfunction.

  4. Possible long-term complications of neurogenic bladder include urinary tract infection, hydronephrosis, urolithiasis, and renal failure.

  5. Bladder retraining and catheterization are management measures.

D. **Assessment findings**

  1. Clinical manifestations of neurogenic bladder vary widely depending on type and degree of neurologic damage; common signs and symptoms include:

       a.   Residual urine detected on bladder catheterization

       b.   Some degree of incontinence

       c.   Bladder distention

       d.   Restlessness

  2. Pertinent laboratory and diagnostic studies include:

       a.   BUN, creatinine clearance, and serum creatinine to evaluate renal function

       b.   Cystography to detect vesicoureteral reflux

       c.   Urethrography to detect urethral complications

       d.   Urine pressure and flow studies

        e.   Cystoscopy to assess muscle fiber status and perform tissue biopsy

E. Nursing diagnoses
1. Anxiety
2. Body Image Disturbance
3. Knowledge Deficit
4. Powerlessness
5. Self Esteem Disturbance
6. Impaired Skin Integrity
7. Altered Urinary Elimination

F. Planning and implementation
1. Intervene as appropriate depending on the type and underlying cause of neurogenic bladder.
2. Provide bladder retraining, if indicated.
3. Perform bladder catheterization (continuous or intermittent) as appropriate.
4. If indicated, teach the client self-catheterization techniques.
5. Encourage adequate fluid intake (2 to 2.5 L/day).

G. Evaluation
1. The client demonstrates proper application of the bladder retraining program.
2. The client demonstrates proper self-catheterization technique, if appropriate.
3. The client verbalizes the need to drink at least 2 L of fluid daily.

VI. Urinary tract infection (UTI)

A. Description
1. Inflammation and infection of urinary tract structures is classified as upper UTI or lower UTI.
2. Upper UTIs include pyelonephritis (inflammation of the kidney).
3. Lower UTIs include:
    a.   Ureteritis (inflammation of the ureter)
    b.   Cystitis (inflammation of the bladder wall), the most common type
    c.   Urethritis (inflammation of the urethra)

B. Etiology and incidence
1. UTIs result from pathogenic microorganisms in the urinary tract (e.g., *Escherichia coli*, *Proteus*, *Klebsiella*, *Enterobacter*).
2. Predisposing factors include:
    a.   Loss of resistance to invading microorganisms
    b.   Sexual intercourse
    c.   Indwelling catheterization
    d.   Urine stasis

      e.   Urinary tract instrumentation
      f.   Residual urine
      g.   Urinary reflux
      h.   Bladder overdistention
      i.   Loss of intact mucosal lining
      j.   Metabolic disorders
   3.   Women develop UTI more frequently than men because of their shorter urethras; approximately 25% of all women experience UTI at some time. Incidence in women increases with aging; incidence in men peaks after age 50.

C. **Pathophysiology and management**
   1.   Pyelonephritis commonly occurs secondary to urine reflux into the kidney.
   2.   In lower UTI, infection typically ascends from the urethra to the bladder and, possibly, to the ureter.
   3.   Other pathways of infection include blood and lymph.
   4.   Management includes treating the infection.

D. **Assessment findings**
   1.   Common manifestations of acute pyelonephritis include:
      a.   Flank pain
      b.   Costovertebral angle tenderness
      c.   Fever, chills
      d.   Dysuria
      e.   Frequency and urgency
      f.   Malaise
      g.   Possibly bloody or cloudy urine
      h.   Urinalysis findings: elevated WBC count, white cell casts, bacteria
   2.   Lower UTI may be marked by:
      a.   Frequency and urgency
      b.   Burning on urination
      c.   Nocturia
      d.   Inflamed, swollen meatus in urethritis
      e.   Bacteriuria and RBCs in urine
      f.   Urine culture identifying the causative microorganism

E. **Nursing diagnoses**
   1.   Risk for Fluid Volume Deficit
   2.   Knowledge Deficit
   3.   Pain
   4.   Altered Urinary Elimination

F. **Planning and implementation**
   1.   As prescribed, administer broad-spectrum antibiotics, such as co-trimoxazole (Bactrim), sulfasoxazole (Gantrisin), nitrofurantoin (Furan), cephadrine (Velosef), and cefaclor (Ceclor), which fight the organism causing the UTI.

n a. **Assess the client for drug allergies before administering medication. Monitor client carefully after administration.**

b. **Instruct the client to take all medication exactly as prescribed even if signs and symptoms subside.**

c. **Advise taking drug with meals to minimize possible GI distress.**

2. Apply heat to the perineum to decrease discomfort.
3. Provide instruction, covering:
   a. The need to increase fluid intake to 3 to 4 L/day
   b. The need to frequently and completely empty bladder
   c. Hygienic measures (e.g., wearing cotton underwear, wiping from front to back, avoiding tub baths)
   d. The importance of acidifying urine through an acid–ash diet (high in meats, cranberry juice)
   e. The need for follow-up care

G. **Evaluation**
1. The client verbalizes understanding of the prescribed medication regimen.
2. The client verbalizes understanding of the need to drink 3 to 4 L of fluid daily.
3. The client demonstrates normal voiding pattern without residual urine.
4. The client reports decreased pain and discomfort.
5. The client states proper hygiene measures to adopt.
6. The client states foods that can help acidify urine.
7. The client schedules a follow-up appointment.

VII. Urolithiasis (renal calculi)

A. **Description: calculi in the urinary tract—bladder, ureters, and, most commonly, kidneys**

B. **Etiology and incidence**
1. Predisposing factors in calculi formation include:
   a. Immobility
   b. Hypercalcemia
   c. Urinary tract infection
   d. Urine stasis
   e. High urine specific gravity
   f. Genetic predisposition
2. Incidence peaks between ages 30 and 50 and is higher in men than in women.

C. **Pathophysiology and management**
1. Calculi are formed by deposition of crystalline substances, including calcium oxalate, calcium phosphate, and uric acid.

    2. Most calculi contain calcium or magnesium in combination with phosphorus or oxalate.

    3. Calculi may pass through the urinary tract or they may lodge, causing obstruction leading to infection and possibly hydronephrosis.

D. **Assessment findings**

    1. Clinical manifestations vary with the location, size, and cause of calculi and may include:

        a. Acute, sharp, intermittent pain (ureteral colic)

        b. Dull, tender, ache in the flank (renal colic)

        c. Nausea and vomiting accompanying severe pain

        d. Fever and chills

        e. Hematuria

        f. Abdominal distention

        g. Pyuria

        h. Rarely, oliguria or anuria

    2. Laboratory and diagnostic studies may reveal:

        a. Visible calculi seen on KUB radiograph

        b. Mineral content of calculi detected on stone analysis

        c. Determination of calculi size and location using IVP

        d. Obstructive changes, such as hydronephrosis, detected on renal ultrasonography

E. **Nursing diagnoses**

    1. Risk for Infection

    2. Knowledge Deficit

    3. Pain

    4. Altered Urinary Elimination

F. **Planning and implementation**

    1. Assess the client's level of pain frequently and provide pain control because shock or syncope may result from excruciating pain.

        a. As prescribed, administer IV pain medications, such as meperidine (Demerol), which elevates the pain threshold and thereby alters the client's response to pain.

        ▶ Assess the client's pain level on a standard pain scale; rule out any complications that may require medical attention; implement safety precautions; evaluate effectiveness of pain medication within 30 minutes of administration.

        b. Encourage bedrest.

        c. Teach relaxation techniques.

        d. Provide hot baths or moist heat to the flank areas.

        e. Encourage around-the-clock, high-fluid intake if client is not nauseated or vomiting.

2. Administer antiemetics, such as promethazine (Phenergan) or hydroxyzine (Vistaril), which inhibit the medullary chemoreceptor trigger zone, thereby alleviating nausea and vomiting.

𝍩 a. **Administer IV or deep IM.**
   b. **Institute safety precautions because drug may cause drowsiness.**

3. Prepare the client who cannot pass the calculus spontaneously for one of the following nonsurgical procedures:
   a. Extracorporeal shock wave lithotripsy (ESWL)—used to break up calculus so that client can pass the particles during urination
   b. Ureteroscopy—insertion of instruments through a cystoscope to visualize and access the calculus and then remove or fragment it with laser energy or ultrasound
   c. Stone dissolution—infusion of chemolytic solutions (alkylating or acidifying agents) through a percutaneous nephrostomy tube; used for clients who are poor risks for other treatments
   d. Endourologic procedures—which integrate the skills of the radiologist and urologist, to extract renal calculi without major surgery: an endoscopic instrument is introduced through a percutaneous nephrostomy and calculus is extracted by forceps or a basketlike device on the instrument.

4. Prepare the client for nephrolithotomy (incision into the kidney for removal of the calculus) if nonsurgical methods fail.
   a. Monitor for signs and symptoms of dehydration resulting from postobstructive diuresis.
   b. Intervene as necessary to restore fluid balance.

5. Inform the client that chemical analysis of the calculus is performed to determine stone's composition (calcium oxalate, calcium phosphate, urate); the composition guides further diet therapy.

6. Institute measures to help prevent stone recurrence, such as:
   a. Encouraging dietary modifications based on the stone's composition
   b. Increasing fluid intake to 3 to 4 L/day
   c. Promoting increased physical activity
   d. Monitoring urine pH
   e. Administering drugs such as aluminum hydroxide (Amphojel), sodium cellulose phosphate (Calcibind), cholestyramine (Questran), allopurinol (Lopurin).

   𝍩 ▸ **Explain that diet therapy should continue while client is taking these medications.**

G. Evaluation
1. The client reports relief of pain.
2. The client exhibits a normal voiding pattern without pain.
3. The client states appropriate foods in the prescribed diet to help prevent calculi formation.
4. The client verbalizes the need to drink 3 to 4 L of fluid daily.
5. The client expresses the intention to increase activity as tolerated.

VIII. Urinary tract cancer

A. Description: neoplasms of the kidney, bladder, or elsewhere in the urinary system

B. Etiology and incidence
1. The etiology of urinary tract cancer is unclear; known risk factors include:
   a. Long-term cigarette smoking
   b. Exposure to carcinogens (e.g., pesticides and various industrial chemicals)
   c. Familial predisposition
2. Renal cancer affects men more often than women. Incidence of bladder cancer is two to three times greater in men than in women; peak incidence occurs between ages 50 and 70.

C. Pathophysiology and management
1. Kidney tumors include:
   a. Adenocarcinomas, accounting for about 90% of all renal tumors
   b. Renal cell carcinomas of the parenchyma
   c. Sarcomas of connective tissue
2. Kidney cancer may metastasize readily to the other kidney and to the lung, bone, brain, and liver.
3. Primary bladder tumors are papillomatous growths within the bladder lumen and possibly infiltrating the bladder wall.
4. Bladder cancer tends to metastasize to the liver, bone, and lung.
5. Malignant urethral neoplasms are uncommon but include squamous cell carcinomas and adenocarcinomas.
6. Management may call for chemotherapy, radiation therapy, and surgery, among other treatments.

D. Assessment findings
1. Clinical manifestations vary with the site and type of cancer but may include:
   a. Gross, painless hematuria
   b. Dysuria
   c. Palpable mass in kidney or bladder
   d. Lower abdominal or flank pain (a late symptom)

          e.   Fever

          f.   Cachexia

          g.   Fatigue

          h.   Hypertension

   2.   Laboratory studies may reveal:

          a.   Hypercalcemia

          b.   Erythrocytosis

          c.   Elevated ESR

          d.   Abnormal liver function studies

   3.   Pertinent diagnostic procedures include:

          a.   Urine cytology

          b.   Excretory urography

          c.   Cystoscopy

          d.   Ultrasonography of the urinary tract

E.   **Nursing diagnoses**

   1.   Anxiety

   2.   Fatigue

   3.   Knowledge Deficit

   4.   Pain

   5.   Self Esteem Disturbance

   6.   Altered Urinary Elimination

F.   **Planning and implementation**

   1.   Administer antineoplastic agents, such as vinblastine; metho-trexate, vinblastine, cisplatin (MVC); cisplatin cyclophospha-mide, doxorubicin. These agents used alone or in combina-tion exert cytotoxic activity on the cancer cells. (See Chapter 21 for nursing interventions for chemotherapy.)

   2.   Prepare the client for radiation therapy or surgery (e.g., cys-tectomy, nephrectomy) as ordered.

   3.   Teach the client about self-care measures (e.g., catheter, stoma, drainage appliance, and skin care; nutritional and fluid intake; sexual activity).

   4.   Promote positive coping strategies, and encourage reliance on available support systems.

   5.   Help the client and family work through the grieving process.

G.   **Evaluation**

   1.   The client verbalizes increased knowledge related to self-care.

   2.   The client states possible side effects of chemotherapy or radi-ation therapy.

   3.   The client demonstrates a willingness to seek support or help as appropriate.

   4.   The client can express feelings and fears about the diagnosis, treatment, and prognosis.

IX. Acute renal failure

A. Description

1. Acute renal failure is defined as sudden, rapid, potentially reversible deterioration of renal function.
2. It can be classified according to underlying cause as:
   a. Prerenal azotemia, stemming from decreased blood flow to kidneys
   b. Postrenal obstruction, involving obstruction to urine outflow
   c. Renal parenchymal failure, involving intrinsic damage to renal structures

B. Etiology and incidence

1. Causes of prerenal azotemia include factors that interfere with renal perfusion, such as:
   a. Hypovolemia (e.g., from hemorrhage, shock, burns)
   b. Increased intravascular capacity (e.g., due to sepsis, neurogenic shock)
   c. Cardiac disorders (e.g., myocardial infarction, arrhythmias)
   d. Renal artery obstruction
   e. Hepatorenal syndrome
2. Possible causes of postrenal obstruction include:
   a. Ureteral obstruction due to calculi, strictures, trauma, or pregnancy
   b. Bladder obstruction (e.g., cancer, prostatic hypertrophy)
3. Renal parenchymal failure can result from:
   a. Acute tubular necrosis (ATN), which accounts for about 75% of all cases of acute renal failure
   b. Acute glomerulonephritis
   c. Acute pyelonephritis

C. Pathophysiology and management

1. Acute renal failure typically occurs in four phases:
   a. Onset phase: extending from the time of the precipitating event to the beginning of the oliguric–anuric phase
   b. Oliguric–anuric phase: marked by urine output <400 mL/day, volume overload, elevated BUN and creatinine, electrolyte abnormalities, metabolic acidosis, uremia
   c. Diuretic phase: extending from the time output becomes >400 mL/day to the time BUN stops rising and stabilizes in normal range; electrolyte and acid–base problems begin to normalize
   d. Convalescent phase: extending from the time BUN stabilizes until the client returns to normal activity; may

take up to 2 years to regain 70% to 80% of normal function

2. Management includes drug therapy and dialysis.
3. Systemic effects of acute renal failure are widespread and may include:
   a. Fluid and electrolyte imbalances
   b. Acidosis
   c. Increased susceptibility to infection
   d. Anemia
   e. Platelet dysfunctions
   f. GI disturbances (e.g., anorexia, nausea, vomiting, diarrhea or constipation, stomatitis)
   g. Pericarditis
   h. Uremic encephalopathy

D. Assessment findings
1. Clinical manifestations depend on the underlying condition. Some of the most common include:
   a. Altered urine output; may be oliguria, anuria, or (rarely) polyuria
   b. Hypertension or hypotension
   c. Tachypnea
   d. Signs of fluid overload or extracellular fluid depletion
2. Laboratory studies may reveal the following:
   a. Urine osmolality: in prerenal azotemia, >900 mOsm/kg; in postrenal obstruction, may be normal; in renal parenchymal failure, <250 mOsm/kg
   b. Urine sodium: in prerenal azotemia, <20 mEq/L; in postrenal obstruction, may be normal; in renal parenchymal failure, >27 mEq/L
   c. Elevated BUN, serum creatinine, and potassium levels
   d. Decreased blood pH, bicarbonate, hemoglobin, and hematocrit

E. Nursing diagnoses
1. Fatigue
2. Risk for Fluid Volume Deficit
3. Risk for Fluid Volume Excess
4. Risk for Infection
5. Knowledge Deficit
6. Impaired Physical Mobility
7. Altered Thought Processes
8. Altered Tissue Perfusion: Renal
9. Altered Urinary Elimination

F. Planning and implementation
1. Provide prompt, aggressive interventions to manage the underlying problem.

2. During the oliguric–anuric phase:

   a. Assess fluid balance; restrict intake to urine output plus 500 mL/day.

   b. Monitor serum potassium level and assess for effects of hyperkalemia; restrict potassium in diet as necessary; administer sodium polystyrene sulfonate (Kayexalate), which removes potassium from the intestines.

   ⁿ ▸ **Administer orally, by nasogastric tube, or by retention enema (retained for 30 to 45 minutes).**
   ▸ **Monitor serum potassium level.**

   c. Monitor for acidosis. As prescribed, administer an alkalinizing agent, such as sodium bicarbonate, which will elevate the plasma pH thereby causing potassium to move into the cells and lower the serum potassium levels.

   ⁿ ▸ **Monitor arterial blood gas values for signs of metabolic acidosis or alkalosis.**

   d. Assess for infection, especially of the respiratory and urinary tracts.

   ⁿ ▸ **Do not leave urinary catheter in place.**
   ▸ **Assess for allergies before administering prescribed antibiotics.**

   e. Monitor for hyperphosphatemia. As prescribed, administer phosphate-binding agents, such as aluminum hydroxide, which decrease absorption of phosphate from the intestines thereby decreasing serum phosphate levels.

   ⁿ ▸ **Instruct client to restrict sodium intake, drink plenty of fluids, and follow a low-phosphate diet.**

   f. Monitor for hypocalcemia. As prescribed, administer calcium supplements.

   ⁿ ▸ **Assess for hypercalcemia by checking for Chvostek's and Trousseau's signs.**

   g. Prevent GI bleeding. As prescribed, administer H_2 receptor antagonists, such as cimetidine (Tagamet), which decreases gastric acid production.

   ⁿ ▸ **If administered intravenously, watch site for infiltration.**

   h. Promote comfort. As prescribed, administer short-acting barbiturates to control pain, and assess for CNS complications such as drowsiness, confusion, delirium, coma, convulsions.

    i.   As prescribed, administer steroids, such as prednisone or methylprednisolone, to decrease inflammation.

    ▶ **Do not discontinue steroidal drug abruptly (doing so may lead to adrenal insufficiency); rather, decrease dosage slowly.**

    j.   Provide a high-calorie and low-protein diet, with hyperalimentation if the client cannot eat.

    k.   If indicated, prepare the client for dialysis to correct hyperkalemia, fluid overload, acidosis, or severe uremia.

    l.   Adjust dosages of drugs secreted by the kidney as necessary.

G.   **Evaluation**

    1.   The client exhibits normal renal function, as evidenced by stabilized:

        a.   Urine output

        b.   Urine osmolality

        c.   Urine sodium levels

        d.   Blood pressure

        e.   Fluid balance

    2.   The client demonstrates the ability to perform ADLs without undue fatigue.

    3.   The client verbalizes knowledge about the course of illness and required follow-up care.

X.   **Chronic renal failure**

    A.   **Description: the end result of progressive, irreversible loss of functioning renal tissue**

    B.   **Etiology and incidence**

        1.   Chronic renal failure usually develops gradually (may take up to several years); in some cases, it may occur rapidly because of an acute disorder (e.g., unresolved acute renal failure).

        2.   Major causes include:

            a.   Hypertensive nephropathy

            b.   Diabetic nephropathy

            c.   Chronic glomerulonephritis

            d.   Chronic pyelonephritis

            e.   Lupus nephritis

            f.   Polycystic kidney disease

            g.   Chronic hydronephrosis

    C.   **Pathophysiology and management**

        1.   Three basic stages of chronic renal failure have been identified:

            a.   Decreased renal reserve: renal function 40% to 50% of normal; homeostasis maintained

            b.   Renal insufficiency: renal function 20% to 40% of nor-

mal; GFR, clearance, and urine concentration decreased; homeostasis altered
  c. End-stage renal disease: renal function less than 10% to 15% of normal; all renal functions severely decreased; homeostasis significantly altered
2. In chronic renal failure, end products of metabolism accumulate in blood instead of being excreted in urine. Retention of sodium and water leads to edema, congestive heart failure, and hypertension. Conversely, episodes of diarrhea and vomiting may lead to sodium and water depletion, exacerbating uremia and producing hypotension and hypovolemia.
3. Metabolic acidosis occurs, interfering with the kidney's ability to excrete hydrogen ions, produce ammonia, and conserve bicarbonate.
4. Decreased GFR results in:
  a. Increased serum phosphate
  b. Decreased serum calcium
  c. Increased parathormone but depleted bone calcium, leading to bone changes (e.g., uremic bone disease, osteomalacia)
  d. Increased serum magnesium
5. Erythropoietin production decreases, resulting in anemia.
6. Neurologic complications develop, such as:
  a. Altered mental function
  b. Personality and behavioral changes
  c. Convulsions
  d. Coma
7. Table 18-2 gives more information on the widespread pathologic effects of chronic renal failure.
8. During the final stages of chronic renal failure, dialysis or kidney transplant is necessary to sustain life.

D. **Assessment findings**
1. Major clinical manifestations of chronic renal failure depend on the stage of the disorder:
  a. Decreased renal reserve: client asymptomatic as long as he or she is not exposed to severe physiologic or psychologic stress
  b. Renal insufficiency: polyuria and nocturia, signs and symptoms of mild anemia
  c. End-stage renal disease: widespread systemic manifestations (see Table 18-2)
2. Characteristic laboratory findings include:
  a. Anemia
  b. Elevated BUN, serum creatinine

(text continues on page 557)

TABLE 18-2.
Systemic Manifestations of Chronic Renal Failure and Management

SYSTEM	MANIFESTATIONS	PATHOPHYSIOLOGIC BASIS	MANAGEMENT
Cardiovascular	Fluid overload; edema	Decreased excretion of water	Dietary fluid restriction
	Congestive heart failure	Fluid overload	Dietary sodium restriction
		Hypertension	Dietary potassium restriction
	Electrolyte imbalances	Decreased excretion of electrolytes	Alkaline medications (e.g., Shohl's solution, Bicitra, sodium bicarbonate)
	Metabolic acidosis	Decreased hydrogen ion secretion	Antihypertensive medications
		Decreased bicarbonate ion reabsorption and generation	Correction of electrolyte imbalance
		Retention of acid end products of metabolism	Dialysis
	Hypertension	Decreased ammonia synthesis and ammonium excretion	
		Fluid overload	
		Increased sodium retention	
	Arrhythmias	Inappropriate activation of the renin angiotension system	
		Electrolyte imbalances, especially hyperkalemia, hypocalcemia, and variations in sodium levels	
	Pericarditis, effusion, and tamponade	Uremic toxins	
		Increased pericardial membrane permeability	
Hematopoietic	Anemia	Decreased erythropoietin secretion by kidneys	Iron supplements
		Loss of red blood cells through the GI tract, mucous membranes, or dialysis	Folic acid supplements
			Androgens
			Blood transfusions
		Decreased red blood cell survival time due to uremic toxins	Dialysis
		Uremic toxins interfering with folic acid action	Epogen
	Alterations in coagulation	Platelet dysfunction due to uremic toxins	
	Increased susceptibility to infection	Decreased neutrophil phagocytosis and chemotaxis due to uremic toxins	
Integumentary	Pallor	Uremic anemia	Bath oils and lotions
	Yellowness	Retained urochrome pigment excreted through the skin	Dialysis
	Dryness	Decreased secretions from oil and sweat glands due to uremic toxins	Correct hyperphosphatemia
			Self-care instruction

(continued)

TABLE 18-2.
Systemic Manifestations of Chronic Renal Failure and Management (Continued)

SYSTEM	MANIFESTATIONS	PATHOPHYSIOLOGIC BASIS	MANAGEMENT
Integumentary (*cont.*)	Pruritus	Dry skin Calcium or phosphate deposits in the skin Uremic toxins effect on nerve endings	
	Purpura and ecchymosis	Increased capillary fragility Platelet dysfunction	
	Uremic frost (seen only in terminal or severely critically ill clients)	Urea or urate crystals excreted through the skin	
Psychosocial	Decreased mentation, decreased concentration, and altered perceptions (even to the point of frank psychoses)	Uremic toxins producing uremic encephalopathy Electrolyte imbalances Metabolic acidosis Tendency to develop cerebral edema	Dialysis Psychosocial counseling Client and family education
Skeletal	Hypocalcemia and hyperphosphatemia	Hyperphosphatemia due to decreased renal excretion Decreased GI absorption of calcium due to decreased renal conversion of vitamin D	Dialysis Calcium supplements Vitamin D supplements Self-care instruction
	Osteodystrophy	Increased osteoclastic activity in response to an increased secretion of parathyroid hormone	Phosphate-binding medications given with meals—Amphojel, Basaljel
	Metastatic calcifications	Deposition of calcium phosphate crystals in soft tissue and other structures	
Respiratory	Pulmonary edema	Fluid overload Increased pulmonary capillary permeability Left ventricular dysfunction	Fluid restriction Dialysis Cardiovascular treatments
	Pneumonia or pneumonitis	Thick tenacious oral secretions due to decreased fluid intake	Antibiotics Pulmonary hygiene (coughing and deep-breathing exercises, oral care) Acidosis treatment
	Kussmaul respirations	A weak, lethargic client with a depressed cough reflex due to uremia Decreased pulmonary macrophage activity Fluid overload An increase in the rate and depth of respirations to decrease the amount of carbon dioxide in the body to compensate for the metabolic acidosis.	

(*continued*)

TABLE 18-2.
Systemic Manifestations of Chronic Renal Failure and Management (Continued)

SYSTEM	MANIFESTATIONS	PATHOPHYSIOLOGIC BASIS	MANAGEMENT
Neuromuscular	Drowsiness, confusion, coma, and irritability Tremors, twitching, and convulsions Peripheral neuropathy Stage 1: restless leg syndrome and paresthesias Stage 2: motor involvement leading to footdrop Stage 3: paraplegia	Uremic toxins producing a uremic encephalopathy Metabolic acidosis Electrolyte imbalances Uremic toxins producing a uremic encephalopathy Decreased nerve conduction, both motor and sensory, due to uremic toxins	Dialysis Seizure precautions Safety precautions during ambulation, exercise, and ADLs
Gastrointestinal	Anorexia, nausea, and emesis Stomatitis and uremic halitosis Gastritis and bleeding Bowel problems: diarrhea Constipation	Uremic toxins Decomposition of urea in the GI tract releasing ammonia, and irritating the mucosa Uremic toxins Decomposition of the urea in the oral cavity releasing ammonia Uremic toxins Decomposition of urea in the GI tract releasing ammonia, which irritates the GI mucosa producing small ulcerations Increased capillary fragility Uremic toxins Hypermotility due to electrolyte imbalances, especially hyperkalemia Hypomotility due to electrolyte imbalances, decreased fluid intake, decreased activity, and decreased bulk in the diet	Dialysis Oral hygiene Oral assessment Hemoglobin and hematocrit monitoring Diarrhea or constipation control Increased dietary bulk Exercise regimen Self-care instruction

     c.   Elevated serum phosphorus
     d.   Decreased serum calcium
     e.   Decreased serum proteins (particularly albumin)
     f.   Low blood pH

E. Nursing diagnoses
1. Activity Intolerance
2. Anxiety
3. Ineffective Individual Coping
4. Risk for Fluid Volume Deficit
5. Risk for Fluid Volume Excess
6. Knowledge Deficit
7. Altered Nutrition: Less than body requirements
8. Impaired Skin Integrity
9. Altered Urinary Elimination

F. Planning and implementation
1. Provide conservative therapy, as indicated, which may include:
   a. Fluid control; daily fluid intake equaling 500 mL (insensible loss) plus the amount of the previous 24 hours' urinary output
   b. Dietary modifications: decreased protein intake (approximately 1 g/kg ideal body weight; of this amount 85% to 90% should be high biologic value protein—containing complete essential amino acids [e.g., fish, poultry, eggs]—and 10% to 15% low biologic value protein—containing incomplete amino acids [e.g., nuts, cereals, breads]); decreased sodium; decreased potassium; high-calorie foods of simple sugars and carbohydrates (e.g., candy and butter balls)
   c. Medication administration (see Table 18-2)
   d. Symptomatic treatment (see Table 18-2)
2. Prepare the client for peritoneal dialysis, if indicated. Assist with the procedure as instructed, maintaining septic technique and monitoring for signs and symptoms of peritonitis (e.g., rigid, boardlike abdomen; fever; cloudy peritoneal fluid).
3. Prepare the client for and assist with hemodialysis, if indicated. Provide proper shunt care, and assess for possible complications (e.g., bleeding due to heparinization, hypovolemia and hypotension due to excessive water removal, dialysis disequilibrium syndrome [headache, confusion, seizures] due to rapid removal of urea from plasma).
4. Prepare the client for kidney transplantation, if indicated. Provide postoperative care for any client who has undergone major surgery (see Chapter 24, Perioperative Nursing), with special attention to catheter patency and adequacy, intake and output, fluid replacement, and protection from infection.

Monitor for signs and symptoms of complications such as graft rejection (fever, elevated WBC, electrolyte abnormalities, abnormal renogram) and infection stemming from immunosuppressive therapy (sepsis pneumonia, wound infection, urinary tract infection).

G. Evaluation

1. The client limits fluid intake to 500 cc plus amount equal to previous 24 hours' output.
2. The client states foods allowed and prohibited in the prescribed diet.
3. The client demonstrates reduced anxiety.
4. The client exhibits the ability and desire to mobilize or identify resources to help with lifestyle adjustments.
5. The client demonstrates the ability to participate in dialysis if it is to be done in the home setting.
6. The client verbalizes ways to reduce the risk of infection.
7. The client states the intention to adjust his or her activity level to reduce fatigue.

Bibliography

Bolander, V. R. (1994). *Sorensen & Luckmann's basic nursing: A physiologic approach* (3rd ed.). Philadelphia: W. B. Saunders.

Clark, J., Queener, S., & Karb, V. (1990). *Pharmacologic basis of nursing practice* (4th ed.). St. Louis: C. V. Mosby.

Nettina, S. (1996). *The Lippincott manual of nursing practice* (6th ed.). Philadelphia: Lippincott-Raven Publishers.

Porth, C. M. (1992). *Pathophysiology: Concepts of altered health states* (4th ed.). Philadelphia: J. B. Lippincott.

Smeltzer, S. C., & Bare, B. G. (1996). *Brunner & Suddarth's textbook of medical-surgical nursing* (8th ed.). Philadelphia: Lippincott-Raven Publishers.

Springhouse Corporation. (1992). *Nursing student's guide to drugs.* Spring House, PA: Springhouse Corp.

STUDY QUESTIONS

1. The nurse monitors for significant changes by focusing on which of the following laboratory tests in a client whose renal function is deteriorating?
   a. blood urea nitrogen (increase)
   b. serum creatinine (decrease)
   c. creatinine clearance (increase)
   d. serum potassium (decrease)

2. Acute tubular necrosis (ATN) is characterized by which of the following?
   a. oliguria (usually)
   b. gradual onset
   c. irreversibility
   d. glucosuria

3. A client with chronic renal failure should manage fluid intake at home by
   a. subtracting the previous day's urine output from 500 mL and limiting intake to milk
   b. adding 500 mL to the previous day's urine output and dividing that amount over the next 24 hours
   c. consuming all of the fluid allowance during the day to prevent nighttime bladder distention
   d. weighing himself or herself before each meal and drinking 500 mL of fluid four times a day

4. After the physician orders a culture and sensitivity test, why would the nurse instruct the client to obtain a clean-catch midstream urine specimen?
   a. The urinary tract normally harbors some microorganisms.
   b. Microorganisms on the client's external genitalia may contaminate the specimen.
   c. The nurse does not want to catheterize the client.
   d. A midstream specimen obtains the largest number of microorganisms in the lower urinary tract.

5. Evaluation of normal kidney response to acidosis would be based on which of the following criteria?
   a. The kidneys secrete excess bicarbonate.
   b. The kidneys absorb hydrogen ions.
   c. The kidneys decrease ammonia production and ammonium excretion.
   d. The kidneys increase urine excretion.

6. Which of following interventions is important for the nurse to implement following kidney biopsy?
   a. Decrease fluid intake to less than 100 mL/day.
   b. Instruct the client to ambulate as soon as possible after the procedure.
   c. Monitor vital signs closely.
   d. Perform neuro checks every 3 to 4 hours for the first 24 hours.

7. ATN may be caused by
   a. prolonged ischemia
   b. Goodpasture's syndrome
   c. ureteral calculi
   d. prostatic hypertrophy

8. The nursing diagnosis Knowledge Deficit related to the need for teaching to prevent pyelonephritis would *least* likely apply to which of following clients?
   a. a 25-year-old sexually active man
   b. a bedridden elderly client with an indwelling (Foley) catheter
   c. an 18-month-old toddler with a history of vesicoureteral reflux
   d. a 55-year-old woman who has been treated for urinary retention

9. Why should the nurse plan to address malnutrition for a client with renal failure?
   a. Anemia causes increased absorption of water-soluble vitamins.
   b. The client requires increased carbohydrate intake.
   c. Increased anabolism occurs in renal failure.
   d. Anemia often causes anorexia, nausea, and vomiting.

10. After dietary instruction, evaluation of effective learning for a client with chronic renal failure would reveal the client's understanding of which fact

about high biologic value (HBV) proteins?

a. They contain the five essential amino acids in each food.

b. They are found in fish, poultry, and eggs.

c. They should compose only a small portion of a dialysis client's total protein intake.

d. They are found in legumes, breads, and cereals.

11. A client with chronic renal failure often experiences pruritus. To intervene effectively, the nurse should teach the client to perform which of these self-care measures at home?

a. increasing dietary intake of phosphate

b. increasing dietary intake of protein

c. applying glycerin to the skin

d. using superfatted soaps and lotions

12. Clinical manifestations and assessment findings that would support a diagnosis of acute pyelonephritis would include:

a. urinary stress incontinence and abdominal pain

b. flank pain, fever, and dysuria

c. burning upon urination and inflamed urinary meatus

d. acute, sharp, intermittent pain and anuria

13. Causes of hypertension associated with chronic renal failure include

a. hypoaldosteronism

b. increased sodium and water retention

c. decreased renin production

d. decreased antidiuretic hormone production

14. On auscultating over the precordium of a client with chronic renal failure, the nurse hears a pericardial friction rub. The nurse should promptly notify the physician because this finding is indicative of

a. pleural effusion

b. cardiac tamponade

c. ventricular arrhythmias

d. anemic pericarditis

15. An 18-year-old renal transplant client has expressed frustration about feeling alone in the hospital room. "I wish I could be out in the waiting room visiting with my friends." Which of the following diagnoses is demonstrated by this client?

a. Ineffective Individual Coping

b. Self Esteem Disturbance

c. Social Isolation

d. Hopelessness

For additional questions, see
Lippincott's Self-Study Series Software
Available at your bookstore

ANSWER KEY

1. **Correct response: a**
   Decreased amounts of urea nitrogen are filtered in renal failure so plasma level increases.
   b, c, and d. Serum creatinine increases, creatinine clearance decreases, and serum potassium increases in renal failure.
   Comprehension/Physiologic/ Implementation

2. **Correct response: a**
   Urine output is usually decreased in ATN.
   b and c. ATN has sudden onset and is usually reversible with treatment.
   d. Glucosuria is not commonly associated with ATN.
   Knowledge/Physiologic/Assessment

3. **Correct response: b**
   Insensible losses (500 mL) plus urine output determine intake in renal failure.
   a. This is an incorrect formulation.
   c. Fluid intake should be divided over a 24-hour period.
   d. This amount of fluid far exceeds the recommended allotment.
   Analysis/Health promotion/Planning

4. **Correct response: b**
   External genitalia normally harbor microorganisms.
   a. The urinary tract is considered sterile.
   c. Catheterization is not necessary for a culture and sensitivity specimen.
   d. This is an incorrect statement.
   Comprehension/Safe care/ Implementation

5. **Correct response: c**
   Ammonia is produced in the renal tubule, and ammonium is excreted in response to acidosis.
   a and b. Bicarbonate is absorbed and hydrogen ions secreted in acidosis.
   d. Urine volume is not affected.
   Comprehension/Physiologic/Evaluation

6. **Correct response: c**
   Vital sign monitoring detects bleeding and shock.
   a. Fluid intake may be increased.
   b. The client remains on bedrest for 6 to 8 hours.
   d. Neuro checks are unnecessary.
   Application/Safe care/Implementation

7. **Correct response: a**
   Ischemia is a common cause of ATN.
   b. Goodpasture's syndrome is glomerular disorder.
   c and d. Calculi and prostatic hypertrophy may cause hydronephrosis.
   Knowledge/Physiologic/Assessment

8. **Correct response: a**
   Kidney infections are caused by immobility, reflux, stasis, and debilitation. Women are more prone to UTI than men.
   b, c, and d. These clients all would be more prone to UTI than a young adult man.
   Analysis/Safe care/Analysis (Dx)

9. **Correct response: d**
   Anorexia, nausea, and vomiting may lead to decreased intake and poor absorption of nutrients.
   a. Anemia may lead to decreased absorption of vitamins.
   b. Increased carbohydrate intake is important to provide energy.
   c. Catabolism commonly occurs in renal failure.
   Analysis/Health promotion/Planning

10. **Correct response: b**
    Fish, poultry, and eggs are good sources of HBV protein.
    a and c. HBV protein contains all essential amino acids and should compose the largest percentage of the total protein intake.
    d. Legumes, breads, and cereals contain low biologic value proteins.
    Analysis/Health promotion/Evaluation

11. *Correct response: d*

Superfatted soaps and lotion help keep skin moist and relieve pruritus.

a. Excess phosphate in chronic renal failure contributes to skin problems.

b. Dietary protein is decreased to help control the level of uremic toxins.

c. Glycerin has a long-term drying effect.

Application/Health promotion/Planning

12. *Correct response: b*

Common clinical manifestations of acute pyelonephritis include: flank pain, fever, chills, dysuria, also costovertebral angle tenderness, frequency and urgency, malaise, possibly bloody or cloudy urine.

a, c, and d. These signs and symptoms do not support the diagnosis of acute pyelonephritis.

Application/Physiologic/Assessment

13. *Correct response: b*

The kidneys' inability to excrete sodium and water leads to increased vascular volume and increased blood pressure.

a and c. Renal failure may involve increased aldosterone and renin production.

d. ADH is not commonly affected by renal failure.

Application/Physiologic/Assessment

14. *Correct response: d*

Pericardial layers rub together due to inflammation from uremic toxins.

a. Pleural effusion may lead to pleural friction rub.

b. Pericardial friction rub would disappear with tamponade.

c. Arrhythmias are unrelated to pericardial friction rub.

Application/Safe care/Implementation

15. *Correct response: c*

An immunosuppressed post-transplant client is placed on mask isolation in a single room and protected from anyone with infection. The client is reflecting social isolation.

a, b, and d. This scenario offers no evidence that the client has disturbed self esteem, nor is there evidence of ineffective coping or hopelessness.

Application/Psychosocial/Analysis (Dx)

Hematologic Disorders

I. **Hematologic system**
   A. Structures
   B. Function

II. **Hematologic system overview**
   A. Assessment
   B. Laboratory studies
   C. Psychosocial implications
   D. Blood transfusion therapy

III. **Complications of blood transfusion**
   A. Overview
   B. Assessment findings
   C. Nursing diagnoses
   D. Planning and implementation
   E. Evaluation

IV. **Anemias: general considerations**
   A. Description
   B. Etiology and pathophysiology
   C. Assessment findings
   D. Nursing diagnoses
   E. Planning and implementation
   F. Evaluation

V. **Iron deficiency anemia**
   A. Description
   B. Etiology and incidence
   C. Pathophysiology and management
   D. Assessment findings
   E. Nursing diagnoses
   F. Planning and implementation
   G. Evaluation

VI. **Megaloblastic anemia**
   A. Description
   B. Etiology and incidence
   C. Pathophysiology and management
   D. Assessment findings
   E. Nursing diagnoses

F. Planning and implementation
G. Evaluation

VII. **Sickle cell anemia**
   A. Description
   B. Etiology and incidence
   C. Pathophysiology and management
   D. Assessment findings
   E. Nursing diagnoses
   F. Planning and implementation
   G. Evaluation

VIII. **Leukemias**
   A. Description
   B. Etiology and incidence
   C. Pathophysiology and management
   D. Assessment findings
   E. Nursing diagnoses
   F. Planning and implementation
   G. Evaluation

IX. **Lymphomas**
   A. Description
   B. Etiology and incidence
   C. Pathophysiology and management
   D. Assessment findings
   E. Nursing diagnoses
   F. Planning and implementation
   G. Evaluation

X. **Multiple myeloma**
   A. Description
   B. Etiology and incidence
   C. Pathophysiology and management
   D. Assessment findings
   E. Nursing diagnoses
   F. Planning and implementation
   G. Evaluation

I. Hematologic system

A. Structures

1. Whole blood consists of formed elements (blood cells) suspended in liquid component (plasma).
2. In an adult, total blood volume is approximately 5 L, constituting 7% to 8% of total body weight.
3. Whole blood contains three types of blood cells:
   a. Erythrocytes (red blood cells—RBCs); average number: 5 million/cubic mL of blood
   b. Leukocytes (white blood cells—WBCs); average total WBC count: 5000 to 10,000 cells per cubic mL of blood
   c. Thombocytes (platelets); normal platelet count: 150,000 to 450,000/cubic mL of blood
4. Erythrocytes, the major cellular element of circulating blood, are biconcave disks normally about 7 μm in diameter containing hemoglobin confined in a plasma membrane.
5. Reticulocytes, immature erythrocytes, may be released prematurely from marrow into circulation under conditions necessitating rapid blood cell production (compensatory mechanism).
6. Leukocytes are divided into two major types based on cell structure:
   a. Granular leukocytes, also called granulocytes or polymorphonuclear leukocytes
   b. Nongranular leukocytes, or mononuclear leukocytes
7. Produced in bone marrow, granulocytes normally comprise 70% of all WBCs. They are subdivided into three types based on staining properties: neutrophils, eosinophils, and basophils.
8. Mononuclear leukocytes are subdivided into:
   a. Lymphocytes, which are produced in bone marrow and undergo differentiation in lymph tissue; comprise 30% of total leukocytes

      b.   Monocytes, which are produced in bone marrow and transform into mature forms called macrophages on release into tissues; comprise 5% of total leukocytes

9.   Thrombocytes are formed from fragments of membrane and cytoplasm from very large cells in bone marrow, lung, and spleen called megakaryocytes; normal life span is 7 to 14 days.

10.   Hematocrit refers to the percentage of total blood volume comprised by cells; normal value is approximately 45%.

11.   Hemoglobin, a protein, comprises about 95% of erythrocyte mass. Hemoglobin has the ability to bind oxygen loosely and reversibly; when combined with oxygen, it's called oxyhemoglobin. Whole blood normally contains about 15 g of hemoglobin per 100 mL of blood.

12.   Plasma, the liquid portion of whole blood remaining after blood cells are removed, constitutes 55% of blood volume and contains large quantities of organic and inorganic substances.

13.   Serum is the fluid remaining when plasma is allowed to clot (i.e., plasma minus fibrinogen and several clotting factors).

14.   Plasma proteins consist primarily of:
      a.   Albumin, the largest of plasma proteins, produced in the liver
      b.   Globulins

15.   Globulins are subdivided into:
      a.   Gamma globulins, consisting mainly of antibodies known as immunoglobulins
      b.   Alpha and beta fractions, including transport proteins and clotting factors, produced in the liver (Table 19-1)

B.   **Function**

    1.   General blood functions include:
      a.   Transporting oxygen absorbed from lungs and nutrients absorbed from gastrointestinal (GI) tract to body cells for cellular metabolism
      b.   Transporting waste products from tissues to excretory organs
      c.   Aiding in chemical, acid–base, and thermal regulation of body
      d.   Transporting hormones and other substances internally secreted to their tissue sites of action
      e.   Aiding in defense against infection through action of antibodies and phagocytes
      f.   Aiding in regulation of extracellular fluid volume
      g.   Promoting hemostasis: arrest of bleeding by blood clot formation, followed by clot dissolution

    2.   All blood cells originate from stem cells. Certain blood cells

TABLE 19-1.
Blood Coagulation Proteins

FACTOR	SYNONYMS	NORMAL PLASMA CONCENTRATIONS (mg/dL)
I	Fibrinogen	200–400
II	Prothrombin	10
III	Tissue thromboplastin, tissue factor	0
IV	Calcium ion	4–5
V	Proaccelerin, labile factor	1
VII	Serum prothrombin conversion accelerator (SPCA), stable factor	0.05
VIII	Antihemophilic factor	1–2
IX	Christmas factor	0.3
X	Stuart-Power factor	1
XI	Plasma thromboplastin antecedent (PTA)	0.5
XII	Hageman factor	3
XIII	Fibrin stabilizing factor (FSF)	1–2
Prekallikrein	Fletcher factor	5
High molecular weight kininogen	Fitzgerald, Flaujeac, Williams factor; contact activation cofactor	6

From Saito, H. (1984). Disorders of hemostasis. Ratnoff, O. D. and Forbes, C. D. (Eds.). Orlando, FL: Grune and Stratton.

derive from bone marrow but undergo differentiation and maturation in various tissues (e.g., lymphocytes, monocytes).

3. Normal erythrocyte production (erythropoiesis), occurring in the bone marrow, is stimulated by erythropoietin (a substance produced primarily by the kidneys) and requires several nutrients, notably iron, vitamin B, folic acid, pyridoxine (vitamin B), and ascorbic acid (vitamin C).

4. Erythrocytes transport oxygen from lungs to tissues. In active tissues, oxygen readily dissociates from hemoglobin; in venous blood, hemoglobin combines with hydrogen ions produced by cellular metabolism, buffering excess acid.

5. The average life span of a circulating erythrocyte is 120 days. Erythrocytes are removed by phagocytosis in the reticuloendothelial system, particularly the liver and spleen. Reticuloendothelial cells produce bilirubin, a pigment from hemoglobin released from destroyed erythrocytes excreted in bile.

6. Leukocytes defend the body against invasion by infectious and parasitic organisms through processes of phagocytosis (ingestion and destruction of invading organisms and foreign particles) and antibody production.

7. Neutrophils are phagocytic cells that arrive early at the site of inflammatory reaction but have a relatively short life span of only several days. Increased numbers (neutrophilia) occur with onset of infection, especially with pyogenic bacteria that augment the body's resistance. Infection also may produce a "shift to the left" (appearance of more immature forms of neutrophils in circulation, such as bands and metamyelocytes).

8. Eosinophils and basophils contain and release potent biologic materials (such as histamine, serotonin, and heparin), which alter blood supply to tissues and help mobilize the body's defense mechanisms.

9. Monocytes, the largest nongranular leukocytes, can phagocytize large foreign particles, cell fragments, and necrotic tissue.

10. Lymphocytes produce substances that aid in attacking foreign cells and substances. B lymphocytes produce antibodies; T lymphocytes kill foreign cells directly or release lymphokines, substances that enhance activity of phagocytic cells.

11. Platelets help control bleeding by:
    a. Physically aggregating and adhering to sites of vascular injury, forming a patch or plug that temporarily stops bleeding
    b. Releasing biochemical substances that activate coagulation factors in plasma to form a stable fibrin clot

12. Approximately 10% to 15% of circulating platelets are continually being consumed in normal, ongoing, intravascular clot formation in repair of small vascular injuries.

13. Plasma provides a medium for circulation of blood cells. Various constituent substances contribute to acid–base balance, blood clot formation and clot lysis, fluid balance, transport of nutritional and hormonal substances, and immunologic defense and surveillance.

14. Capillary walls are impermeable to albumin, creating an osmotic force that maintains fluid volume within the vascular system. Albumin has the ability to bind several plasma substances for transport, such as fatty acids, drugs, metals, and bilirubin.

15. Coagulation or fibrin clot formation results from a complex series of reactions wherein inert plasma proteins are "activated" or transformed into enzymes in sequential manner, ending with thrombin-induced conversion of fibrinogen to fibrin (cascade theory).

16. Initial interactions of coagulation factors may be grouped into three separate pathways (intrinsic, extrinsic, common); clot formation can occur by way of:
    a. Intrinsic and common pathways, where triggering stim-

ulus occurs within circulation (i.e., blood comes in contact with abnormal surface)

    b. Extrinsic and common pathways, when tissue injury releases thromboplastin into circulation

17. The fibrinolytic system is a plasma enzyme system responsible for blood clot removal after blood vessel integrity is restored.

18. Inert plasma protein—plasminogen—is activated into the enzyme plasmin, which digests fibrinogen and fibrin in a process called fibrinolysis.

19. Fibrinolysis produces fibrin split products (FSP), also known as fibrin degradation products, which are removed from circulation by the reticuloendothelial system and liver and spleen; FSP normally is not present in circulation.

II. Hematologic system overview

A. Assessment

1. Inspection of skin and mucous membranes may reveal such color changes as:

    a. Pallor (paleness), occurring with decreased hemoglobin or decreased blood flow

    b. Cyanosis (bluish discoloration), occurring with increased circulating unoxygenated hemoglobin secondary to hypoxia (buccal, peripheral)

    c. Rubor (redness), occurring with increased visibility of normal oxyhemoglobin due to dilation of superficial blood vessels (e.g., fever) or with increased blood flow (e.g., inflammation)

    d. Jaundice (yellowish discoloration), resulting from increased bilirubin levels secondary to RBC hemolysis; appearing first in sclera, then mucous membranes, then generalized

2. Color changes are best assessed where capillary beds are superficial and pigmentation minimal (e.g., nailbeds, hard palate, lips, palms, soles, conjunctivae).

3. Skin and mucous membrane inspection also may reveal:

    a. Petechiae—small, pinpoint hemorrhages on skin or mucous membranes—which most commonly occur with quantitative or qualitative platelet disorders; generally more numerous over bony prominences (increased trauma) or dependent areas (increased venous pressure)

    b. Ecchymoses—bluish-black macula—resulting from seepage of blood into skin or mucous membranes, often secondary to trauma

    c. Pruritus and malignant infiltrative skin lesions, occurring with certain hematologic malignancies (e.g., leukemias and lymphomas)

    d.   Glossitis (inflammation of the tongue) and ulcerative lesions of oral cavity, which occur with certain anemias

    e.   Gingival hypertrophy (enlargement of gums), common in monocytic leukemia due to leukemic cell infiltration

  4. Palpation of the thorax and abdomen can detect:

    a.   Splenomegaly (enlarged spleen), which occurs in various hematologic disorders, including several anemias and hematologic malignancies

    b.   Hepatomegaly (enlarged liver), possibly indicating inflammation (as in hepatitis), venous congestion, or a hematologic malignancy

  5. Lymphadenopathy (enlarged lymph nodes) may point to regional or systemic infection or a hematologic malignancy.

B. **Laboratory studies**

  1. In bone marrow aspiration and biopsy, specimens of bone marrow and bone are obtained by introducing a needle with stylet into the iliac crest (the sternum may be used for aspiration in adults); purposes include:

    a.   Diagnosing hematologic disorders through evaluating precursors of peripheral blood cells or iron content

    b.   Evaluating effectiveness of treatment

    c.   Diagnosing nonhematologic diseases (e.g., infectious diseases, certain granulomas) or staging solid tumor malignancies

  2. Complete blood count includes:

    a.   Enumeration of the number of RBCs, WBCs, and platelets per cubic millimeter of venous blood

    b.   Differential WBC count, or respective percentages of neutrophils, eosinophils, basophils, lymphocytes, and monocytes contributing to the total WBC count

  3. Reticulocyte count detects the percentage of young (1- to 2-day-old) nonnucleated erythrocytes in peripheral blood.

  4. Red blood cell indices involve three calculated measurements of average RBC size and hematocrit and hemoglobin content; helpful in diagnosing and evaluating the severity of anemic disorders. Specific indices include:

    a.   Mean corpuscular hemoglobin: average amount of hemoglobin contained within RBCs

    b.   Mean corpuscular hemoglobin concentration: percentage representing the ratio of the weight of hemoglobin to the volume of an average RBC

    c.   Mean corpuscular volume: value for average RBC size

  5. Hemoglobin electrophoresis provides a means for identifying different hemoglobins (e.g., A, A2, F, S), based on the speed at which they travel when exposed to electrical current.

6. The sickling test detects characteristic sickling of RBCs occurring with sickle cell trait or disease by exposing blood to a reducing agent, thus depriving cells of oxygen.

7. Coombs' test detects immune globulin plasma (indirect Coombs'); used in diagnosing various hemolytic anemias.

8. Leukocyte alkaline phosphatase testing estimates the amount of this enzyme (normally present in high concentrations in neutrophils) through a special stain of peripheral blood.

9. Bleeding time involves measuring in minutes the time it takes for bleeding to stop after a standardized skin puncture, usually on the forearm; helps detect disorders of platelet function.

10. Platelet aggregation measures the time and completeness of platelet aggregate formation in a plasma sample after addition of a triggering agent.

11. Prothrombin time (PT) measures coagulation through extrinsic and common pathways; purposes include:
    a. Monitoring coumarin therapy
    b. Providing a screening test for liver disease and coagulation factor deficiencies

12. Partial thromboplastin time (PTT) evaluates coagulation through intrinsic and common pathways; purposes include:
    a. Monitoring heparin therapy
    b. Screening for coagulation factor deficiencies

13. Thrombin clotting time measures thrombin-induced conversion of fibrinogen to fibrin in the coagulation cascade; used to monitor heparin therapy.

14. Coagulation factor assay provides the definitive test for quantitative deficiency of coagulation factor. In this test, a sample of the client's plasma is added to a sample of factor-deficient plasma, then the amount of correction in PT and PTT is compared with correction by normal plasma (arbitrarily defined as 100% activity).

C. **Psychosocial implications**

1. The client with a hematologic disorder may experience coping difficulty related to:
   a. Progressive nature of disease
   b. Disease chronicity
   c. Limitations imposed by treatments
   d. Fear of dying
   e. The need to learn much self-care information
   f. Ongoing follow-up care or lifelong preventive and therapeutic regimens

2. The client also may have self-concept concerns related to:
   a. Loss of self-esteem

    b.   Body image changes related to the disorder and treatments

    c.   Role changes toward increasing dependence

3.   Disease-related lifestyle concerns may involve changes in:

    a.   Physical ability

    b.   Work performance, with potential for job loss

    c.   Economic stability

    d.   Family dynamics

4.   The disease may lead to changes in social interaction patterns, possibly resulting in isolation, depression, helplessness, and hopelessness.

D. **Blood transfusion therapy**

    1.   Treatment involves instilling whole blood or blood components (specific portion or fraction of blood lacking in client).

    2.   One unit of whole blood consists of 450 mL of blood collected into 60 to 70 mL of preservative or anticoagulant. Whole blood stored for more than 6 hours does not provide therapeutic platelet transfusion, nor does it contain therapeutic amounts of labile coagulation factors (factors V and VIII).

    3.   Blood components include:

        a.   Packed RBCs (100% of erythrocyte, 100% of leukocytes, and 20% of plasma originally present in one unit of whole blood), indicated to increase the oxygen-carrying capacity of blood with minimal expansion of blood volume

        b.   Leukocyte-poor, packed RBCs, indicated for clients who have experienced previous febrile nonhemolytic transfusion reactions

        c.   Platelets, either HLA (human leukocyte antigen) matched or unmatched

        d.   Granulocytes (basophils, eosinophils, and neutrophils)

        e.   Fresh frozen plasma, containing all coagulation factors, including factors V and VIII (the labile factors)

        f.   Single donor plasma, containing all stable coagulation factors but reduced levels of factors V and VIII; preferred for reversing warfarin-induced anticoagulation

        g.   Albumin, a plasma protein

        h.   Cryoprecipitate, a plasma derivative rich in factor VIII, fibrinogen, factor XIII, and fibronectin

        i.   Factor IX concentrate, a concentrated form of factor IX prepared by pooling, fractionating, and freeze-drying large volumes of plasma

        j.   Factor VIII concentrate, a concentrated form of factor VIII, prepared by pooling, fractionating, and freeze-drying large volumes of plasma

    k. Prothrombin complex, containing prothrombin and factors VII, IX, X, and some factor XI

 4. Blood component therapy has the following advantages:

  a. Avoids the risk of sensitizing the client to other blood components

  b. Provides optimal therapeutic benefit while reducing risk of volume overload

  c. Increases availability of needed blood products to larger population

 5. Principles of blood transfusion therapy:

  a. **Whole blood transfusion: Generally indicated *only* for clients who need increased oxygen-carrying capacity and restored blood volume when there is no time to prepare or obtain needed, specific blood components.**

  b. Packed RBCs: Should be transfused over 2 to 3 hours; if client cannot tolerate volume over a maximum of 4 hours, it may be necessary to divide a unit into smaller volumes, properly refrigerating remaining blood until needed. One unit of packed RBCs should raise hemoglobin approximately 1%, hematocrit 3%.

  c. Platelets: Administer as rapidly as tolerated (usually 4 units every 30 to 60 minutes). Each unit of platelets should raise the recipient's platelet count by 6000 to 10,000/mm^3; however, poor incremental increases occur with alloimmunization from previous transfusions, bleeding, fever, infection, autoimmune destruction, and hypertension.

  d. Granulocytes: May be beneficial in selected population of infected, severely granulocytopenic clients (less than 500/mm^3) not responding to antibiotic therapy and expected to experience prolonged, suppressed granulocyte production.

  e. Plasma: Plasma carries a risk of hepatitis equal to that of whole blood. Therefore, if only volume expansion is required, other colloids (e.g., albumin) or electrolyte solutions (e.g., lactated Ringer's) are preferred. Give fresh-frozen plasma as rapidly as tolerated because coagulation factors become unstable after thawing.

  f. Albumin: Indicated to expand blood volume of clients in hypovolemic shock and to elevate level of circulating albumin in clients with hypoalbuminemia. The large protein molecule is a major contributor to plasma oncotic pressure.

  g. Cryoprecipitate: Indicated for treating hemophilia A,

von Willebrand's disease, disseminated intravascular coagulation (DIC), and uremic bleeding.

h. Factor IX concentrate: Indicated for treating hemophilia B; carries a high risk of hepatitis because it requires pooling from many donors.

i. Factor VIII concentrate: Indicated for treating hemophilia A; heat-treated product decreases the risk of hepatitis and HIV transmission.

j. Prothrombin complex: Indicated in congenital or acquired deficiencies of these factors.

III. Complications of blood transfusion

A. Overview

1. *Hemolytic transfusion reaction* **is a life-threatening complication occurring from transfusion of donor blood that is incompatible with the recipient's blood.**

2. In hemolytic transfusion reaction, antibodies in the recipient's plasma combine with antigens on donor erythrocytes, causing agglutination and hemolysis in circulation or in the reticuloendothelial system. Similarly, antibodies in donor plasma combine with antigen on the recipient's erythrocytes; however, complications from infusion of incompatible plasma are less severe than those associated with infusion of incompatible erythrocytes. The most rapid hemolysis occurs in ABO incompatibility; Rh incompatibility is usually less severe.

3. *Delayed hemolytic transfusion reaction* occurs 1 to 2 weeks after transfusion; erythrocytes hemolyzed by antibody are not detectable during crossmatch but are formed rapidly after transfusion. It generally is not dangerous, but subsequent transfusions may be associated with acute hemolytic reaction.

4. In hemolytic reaction, the severity of complications correlates with the amount of incompatible blood transfused; chances of fatal reaction decrease if less than 100 mL of incompatible blood is infused.

5. *Febrile, nonhemolytic transfusion reaction,* the most common type of reaction, is generally caused by sensitivity to leukocyte or platelet antigens.

6. *Septic reaction* is a serious complication resulting from transfusion of a blood product contaminated with bacteria.

7. *Allergic reactions* may result from sensitivity to plasma protein or donor antibody, which reacts with recipient antigen.

8. *Circulatory overload* results from administration at a rate or volume greater than can be accommodated by the circulatory system, precipitating congestive heart failure or pulmonary edema.

9. **Rarely, several *infectious diseases* can be transmitted through blood transfusion.**
    a. Hepatitis B and hepatitis C
    b. Malaria
    c. Syphilis
    d. Acquired immunodeficiency syndrome (AIDS)
10. *Graft-versus-host (GVH) disease* results from engraftment of immunocompetent lymphocytes in bone marrow of immuno-suppressed recipients, which triggers an immune response of the graft against the host.
11. *Reactions associated with massive transfusions* (>10 units of packed RBCs in 1 to 6 hours) include:
    a. Hypocalcemia, resulting from binding of recipient's circulating calcium to anticoagulant (citrate) in packed RBCs
    b. Citrate intoxication due to accumulation of citrate
    c. Hyperkalemia, in which stored RBCs progressively increase extracellular potassium concentration
    d. Exacerbation of liver disease due to increased ammonia levels in stored blood
    e. Hypothermia, in which transfusion of cold blood (below 37°C) at rates > 100 mL/min may produce arrhythmias and cardiac arrest
    f. Aggregates of leukocytes and platelets in the lungs, resulting from accumulation of the aggregates during blood storage
    g. Hemorrhage, resulting from excessive dilution of the recipient's platelets and clotting factors

B. Assessment findings
1. Clinical manifestations of transfusion complications vary depending on the precipitating factor (Table 19-2).
2. Reactions associated with massive transfusion produce varying manifestations (see the appropriate chapter in this text for information on a specific condition).

C. Nursing diagnoses
1. Ineffective Breathing Pattern
2. Decreased Cardiac Output
3. Fluid Volume Deficit
4. Fluid Volume Excess
5. Impaired Gas Exchange
6. Hyperthermia
7. Hypothermia
8. Risk for Infection
9. Risk for Injury

TABLE 19-2.
Assessment Findings in Transfusion Complications

COMPLICATION	ASSESSMENT FINDINGS
Hemolytic transfusion reaction	Fever, chills, low back pain, flank pain, headache, nausea, flushing, tachycardia, tachypnea, hypotension, hemoglobinuria (cola-colored urine)
Delayed hemolytic reaction	Fever, mild jaundice, gradual drop in hemoglobin level, positive Coombs' test result
Febrile nonhemolytic reaction	Temperature rise during or soon after transfusion, chills, headache, flushing, anxiety
Allergic reaction	Hives, generalized pruritus, wheezing, anaphylaxis (rare)
Circulatory overload	Dyspnea, cough, crackles, jugular vein distention
Infectious disease transmission	Rapid or insidious onset of symptoms, depending on specific disease
Graft-versus-host disease	Skin changes (reddening, ulcerations), edema, hair loss, hemolytic anemia, positive Coombs' test result

10. Pain
11. Impaired Skin Integrity
12. Altered Tissue Perfusion
- **D. Planning and implementation**
  - 1. Help prevent transfusion reaction by:
    - a. Meticulously verifying client identification beginning with type and crossmatch sample collection and labeling to double-check blood product and client identification before transfusion; verify with licensed personnel
    - b. Inspecting the blood product for gas bubbles, clotting, or abnormal color before administration
    - c. Beginning transfusion slowly (1 to 2 mL/min) and observing the client closely, particularly during the first 15 minutes (severe reactions usually manifest within 15 minutes after the start of transfusion); take vital signs every 5 minutes
    - d. Transfusing blood within 4 hours, and changing blood tubing every 4 hours to minimize the risk of bacterial growth at warm room temperatures
    - e. Preventing infectious disease transmission through careful donor screening or performing pretests available to identify selected infectious agents
    - f. Preventing GVH disease by ensuring irradiation of blood products containing viable WBCs (i.e., whole blood, platelets, packed RBCs, and granulocytes) before

transfusion; irradiation alters ability of donor lymphocytes to engraft and divide

    g.   Preventing hypothermia by warming blood unit to 37°C before transfusion

    h.   Removing leukocyte and platelet aggregates from donor blood by installing a microaggregate filter (20- or 40-μm size) in the blood line to remove these aggregates during transfusion

2.   Actions to take on detecting any signs or symptoms of reaction include:

    a.   Stopping the transfusion immediately, and notifying the physician

    b.   Disconnecting the transfusion set—but keeping the IV line open with 0.9% saline solution to provide access for possible IV drug infusion

    c.   Sending the blood bag and tubing to the blood bank for repeat typing and culture

    d.   Drawing another blood sample for plasma hemoglobin, culture, and retyping

    e.   Collecting a urine sample as soon as possible for hemoglobin determination

3.   Interventions to address symptoms of the specific reaction include:

    a.   Managing hemolytic reaction by correcting hypotension, DIC, and renal failure associated with RBC hemolysis and hemoglobinuria

    b.   Treating febrile, nonhemolytic transfusion reactions symptomatically with prescribed antipyretics; providing leukocyte-poor blood products for subsequent transfusions

    c.   Managing septic reaction with antibiotics, increased hydration, steroids, and vasopressors as prescribed.

    d.   Administering antihistamines, steroids, and epinephrine for allergic reaction as indicated by the severity of the reaction. (If hives are the only manifestation, transfusion can sometimes continue but at a slower rate.)

    e.   Managing circulatory overload initially by positioning the client upright with feet dependent and providing prescribed diuretics, oxygen, and aminophylline

E.   **Evaluation**

    1.   The client maintains normal breathing pattern.

    2.   The client demonstrates adequate cardiac output.

    3.   The client reports minimal or no discomfort.

    4.   The client maintains adequate fluid balance.

    5.   The client remains normothermic.

    6.   The client remains free of infection.

    7.   The client's skin remains intact with no lesions or pruritus.

    8.   The client has normal electrolyte and blood chemistry values.

IV. Anemias: general considerations

A. **Description: a clinical condition (not a laboratory result) defined as decrease in hemoglobin content or red cell mass that impairs oxygen transport**

B. **Etiology and pathophysiology**

    1.   Anemia is one of the most common problems in clinical practice; it may be a primary pathology or secondary to an underlying condition.

    2.   Anemia is classified according to either morphologic characteristics of erythrocytes or etiologic mechanisms resulting in decreased hemoglobin or RBC mass.

    3.   Morphologic characteristics refer to average RBC size and hemoglobin content. Average RBC size may be normal (normocytic), smaller than normal (microcytic), or larger than normal (hypochromic).

    4.   Physiologic mechanisms include:

        a.   Decreased or ineffective RBC or hemoglobin production (bone marrow failure)

        b.   Decreased or premature RBC destruction (hemolysis)

        c.   Increased RBC loss (hemorrhage)

    5.   Bone marrow failure (i.e., reduced erythropoiesis) may result from nutritional deficiency, toxic exposure, invasion or replacement of marrow by tumor or fibrous tissue, or unknown causes.

    6.   Hemolysis may result from an intrinsic RBC defect incompatible with normal cell survival or from an extrinsic factor that promotes cell destruction.

C. **Assessment findings**

    1.   Clinical manifestations reflect deficient oxygenation of tissues and compensatory cardiopulmonary mechanisms regardless of the cause of anemia, and include:

        a.   Pallor

        b.   Susceptibility to fatigue

        c.   Central nervous system manifestations: headache, dizziness, lightheadedness, slowing of thought processes, irritability, restlessness, and depression

        d.   Effects of increased cardiac workload: tachycardia, palpitations, and angina pectoris or congestive heart failure in susceptible persons

        e.   Tachycardia and dyspnea progressing from exertional to at rest

f.   Complaints of feeling cold due to blood being shunted to areas of greater need

2.   Severity of symptoms depends on:
   a.   Whether anemia is of rapid or gradual onset (Generally, the more rapidly anemia develops, the more severe the symptoms.)
   b.   Cardiopulmonary reserve
   c.   Metabolic requirements
   d.   Other medical disorders
   e.   Specific complications and features associated with the cause of anemia

3.   Clinical and laboratory indices provide information regarding the site and nature of RBC hemolysis. Hemolysis generally occurs within phagocytic cells of the reticuloendothelial system, especially liver and spleen.

4.   Bilirubin is formed within phagocyte by metabolism of hemoglobin, and released into the blood stream, increasing plasma bilirubin concentration. (Levels above 1.5 mg/dL produce visible jaundice of sclera.)

5.   Hemolysis may occur directly in the blood stream in some disorders, releasing hemoglobin into plasma (hemoglobinemia); initially hemoglobin binds to plasma protein—haptoglobin—but when haptoglobin is saturated, hemoglobin diffuses through renal glomeruli and into urine (hemoglobinuria), giving the urine a cola color.

6.   Diagnostic evaluation to determine cause and type of anemia includes:
   a.   Hemoglobin and hematocrit
   b.   RBC indices
   c.   Examination of stained blood capacity
   d.   Reticulocyte count
   e.   Serum iron level
   f.   Total iron binding capacity
   g.   Serum ferritin
   h.   Serum folate level
   i.   Vitamin B_{12} level
   j.   Hemoglobin electrophoresis
   k.   Coombs' test
   l.   White blood cell (WBC) studies—may include bone marrow aspiration and biopsy or studies to determine the source of any chronic blood loss

D.   Nursing diagnoses
1.   Activity Intolerance
2.   Decreased Cardiac Output
3.   Altered Nutrition: Less than body requirements

E. **Planning and implementation**
1. Direct general management toward addressing the cause of anemia and replacing blood loss as needed to sustain adequate oxygenation.
2. Promote optimal activity and protect from injury:
   a. Encourage ambulation and participation in activities of daily living (ADLs) as tolerated; emphasize hazards of immobility (e.g., hypotension, muscle wasting).
   b. Assess the client's subjective response to activity (e.g., complaints of fatigue, weakness, lightheadedness, breathlessness).
   c. Observe for dizziness or unsteady gait, and provide support as necessary.
   d. Provide for adequate rest periods, and defer or replan activities causing undue fatigue.
   e. **Teach the client to avoid sudden movement (e.g., rising from lying to standing or bending position) because the hypotensive effect may cause falling.**
3. Reduce activities and stimuli that cause tachycardia and increased cardiac output:
   a. Monitor vital signs at rest and with activity.
   b. **Encourage the client to report palpitations, chest pain, or dyspnea experienced with activity or psychological stress.**
   c. Provide for a quiet environment and calm activity.
   d. For a client experiencing dyspnea, elevate the head of the bed; avoid gas-forming foods (abdominal distention may aggravate dyspnea); oxygen therapy may be necessary.
   e. Observe and report signs of fluid retention (peripheral edema, neck vein distention, decreased urinary output).
4. Provide for nutritional needs:
   a. Provide high-protein and high-calorie foods and sufficient fruits and vegetables to assure essential nutrients for erythropoiesis.
   b. Discuss necessary dietary alterations with the client and family.
   c. Administer any prescribed nutritional supplements (e.g., iron, vitamin B_{12}, folic acid). See specific anemias for nursing interventions.
   d. Promote small, frequent meals to help cope with problems of fatigue and anorexia.

F. **Evaluation**
1. The client demonstrates normal activity tolerance.

2. The client remains free from injury.
3. The client follows a progressive schedule of rest, activity, and exercise.
4. The client maintains normal cardiac output, as evidenced by:
   a. Vital signs within normal ranges
   b. No signs of fluid retention
5. The client maintains adequate nutritional status.

V. Iron deficiency anemia

A. Description: a type of anemia marked by below-normal total body iron and inadequate hemoglobin production for body requirements

B. Etiology and incidence
1. Iron deficiency anemia can result from:
   a. Chronic blood loss secondary to GI bleeding (e.g., from ulceration, tumor, hemorrhoids, hookworm infestation), excessive menstrual bleeding, multiple pregnancies
   b. Insufficient dietary iron intake
   c. Impaired GI absorption of iron secondary to gastrectomy or prolonged, severe diarrhea
   d. Increased iron requirements during periods of rapid body growth, pregnancy, or menstruation
2. It is the most common type of anemia in all age groups, affecting 10% to 30% of the adult population in the United States.

C. Pathophysiology and management
1. In iron deficiency anemia, body stores of iron decrease, as do stores of transferrin (which binds with and transports iron).
2. This leads to depletion of RBC mass, resulting in decreased hemoglobin concentration and decreased oxygen-carrying capacity of the blood.
3. Treatment involves correcting iron deficiency.

D. Assessment findings
1. Iron deficiency anemia presents primarily with general manifestations of anemia (see Section IV.C).
2. Skin and mucous membrane manifestations may include fissuring at angles of mouth; smooth, sore tongue; and spoon-shaped, brittle nails.
3. Some clients may exhibit pica (craving to eat unusual substances such as clay and laundry starch) or extreme craving for ice.
4. Laboratory studies commonly reveal:
   a. Microcytic hypochromia: RBCs small and relatively devoid of pigment
   b. Hemoglobin proportionally lower than hematocrit and RBC count

       c.   Serum iron concentration low, total iron binding capacity high, serum ferritin low (measure of iron stores)

E. Nursing diagnoses

    1. Activity Intolerance

    2. Decreased Cardiac Output

    3. Altered Nutrition: Less than body requirements

F. Planning and implementation

    1. Direct therapeutic goals at treating the underlying cause of anemia (e.g., GI bleeding) and correcting iron deficit through diet and supplemental iron preparations.

    2. Administer iron, which is used mainly for the synthesis of heme, the essential protein of hemoglobin. Clients should be told to:

       a. **Expect dark stool.**

       b. **Notify physician if side effects, such as diarrhea, constipation, GI upset, or nausea and vomiting become severe or intolerable.**

       c. **Store iron safely out of reach of children (in whom iron poisoning may be fatal).**

    3. Advise client that iron preparations include:

       a. Parenteral: dextran (Imferon)

          ▶ **Administer using Z-track technique to avoid leakage into subcutaneous tissues.**

          ▶ **Caution client that preparation may discolor skin and cause local pain.**

          ▶ **Be alert for possible anaphylactic reaction.**

       b. Oral: ferrous sulfate (Feosol), which should be taken whole, not crushed

       c. Liquid iron

          ▶ **Forewarn client that liquid iron may stain teeth.**

          ▶ **Suggest diluting iron and administering through a straw or dropper placed at back of tongue.**

    4. Provide information on preventive measures including:

       a. Counseling and instruction to high-risk clients (e.g., menstruating and pregnant women)

       b. Reviewing foods high in iron (e.g., organ and other meats, cooked white beans, leafy vegetables, raisins, molasses)

       c. Encouraging taking a source of vitamin C with iron-rich foods to enhance absorption

       d. Advising that tannates (in tea) and carbonates hinder iron absorption

5. Additional nursing interventions include those common to all anemias (see Section IV.F).

G. Evaluation

1. The client demonstrates normal activity tolerance.
2. The client remains free from injury.
3. The client follows a progressive schedule of rest, activity, and exercise.
4. The client maintains normal cardiac output, as evidenced by:
   a. Vital signs within normal ranges
   b. No signs of fluid retention
5. The client maintains adequate nutritional status.

VI. Megaloblastic anemia

A. Description

1. Megaloblastic anemias are hematologic disorders characterized by the production and peripheral proliferation of large, immature, and dysfunctional RBCs.
2. Types include:
   a. Vitamin B_{12} deficiency anemia (pernicious anemia)
   b. Folic acid deficiency anemia

B. Etiology and incidence

1. Vitamin B_{12} deficiency can result from:
   a. Inadequate dietary intake (rare, except in strict vegetarians)
   b. Faulty absorption from the GI tract due to lack of secretion of intrinsic factor, normally produced by gastric mucosal cells
   c. Certain small intestine disorders that impair absorption
2. Causes of folic acid deficiency anemia include:
   a. Inadequate dietary intake, especially of uncooked vegetables and fruits; may occur in clients on prolonged IV hyperalimentation
   b. Impaired absorption in the upper jejunum
   c. Increased requirements, common in alcoholism, pregnancy, chronic hemolytic anemias
   d. Impaired use from administration of drugs that act as folic acid antagonists (e.g., methotrexate)

C. Pathophysiology and management

1. Vitamin B_{12} and folic acid are essential for normal DNA synthesis and hematopoiesis; in deficiency, RBCs cannot produce DNA, so normal nuclear maturation is arrested.
2. Cytoplasmic maturation proceeds, however, resulting in abnormally large cells with increased membrane surface area.
3. Because DNA metabolism is essential to formation of all cellular elements in bone marrow, WBCs and platelets are diminished.

4. Treatment includes vitamin therapy.

D. **Assessment findings**

    1. Both types of megaloblastic anemia present with common general signs and symptoms of anemia (see Section IV.C).

    2. Other manifestations may include:

        a. Smooth, sore tongue

        b. Diarrhea

        c. Paresthesias

        d. Impaired coordination and position sense

        e. Confusion, behavioral changes

    3. Diagnostic tests may reveal:

        a. Low serum and red cell folate levels and serum vitamin B_{12} level

        b. Blood smear showing marked variation in size and shape of cell and a variable number of abnormally large cells with normal hemoglobin concentration

        c. Impaired vitamin B_{12} absorption seen on Schilling test

E. **Nursing diagnoses**

    1. Activity Intolerance

    2. Decreased Cardiac Output

    3. Altered Nutrition: Less than body requirements

F. **Planning and implementation**

    1. **Instruct client about lifelong vitamin B_{12} (cyanocobalamin) replacement therapy for pernicious anemia. Never administer parenteral dose intravenously.**

    2. Discuss folic acid replacement therapy by oral route (possibly IM route if malabsorption is a problem).

        a. Reassure the client that therapy can cease when hemoglobin level returns to normal.

        b. Inform client that chronic alcohol ingestion, anticonvulsant medications, and oral contraceptives will alter folic acid absorption.

    3. Institute general interventions common to all anemias (see Section IV.E).

G. **Evaluation: those common to all anemias (see Section IV.F)**

VII. **Sickle cell anemia**

A. **Description: a severe, chronic, incurable hemolytic anemia resulting from an inherited defective hemoglobin molecule (hemoglobin S) and marked by episodic painful crises**

B. **Etiology and incidence**

    1. Sickle cell anemia results from homozygous inheritance of the hemoglobin S-producing gene.

    2. Incidence is highest in persons of tropical African descent; about 10% of African-Americans carry the abnormal gene (sickle cell trait), and 1 in 600 African-American infants are born with the disease.

3. Significant incidence of sickle cell anemia is also found in the Middle East, the Mediterranean area, India, South America, and the Caribbean islands.

C. Pathophysiology and management

1. The hemoglobin S molecule acquires its characteristic sickle shape when exposed to low oxygen tension.

2. Hemoglobin S is significantly less soluble than normal hemoglobin when it gives up its oxygen; deoxygenated hemoglobin S turns into a firm gel, deforming RBC shape.

3. Hemoglobin S-containing RBCs have a decreased survival time and adhere to vascular endothelium, causing anemia and vascular occlusion.

4. A high concentration of misshaped cells during sickling crises makes blood abnormally viscous, resulting in sluggish circulation and sludging of sickled cells, especially within microcirculation.

5. Occlusion in microcirculation increases hypoxia, which in turn triggers sickling in other RBCs, perpetuating the cycle.

6. The organs most vulnerable to infarction and necrosis include brain, kidneys, bone marrow, and spleen.

7. **If ischemia or infarction occurs, the client experiences severe pain, possibly with swelling and fever—known as painful crisis. Precipitating factors for painful crises include:**
    a. **Dehydration**
    b. **Infection**
    c. **Fatigue**
    d. **Menstruation**
    e. **Alcohol use**
    f. **Emotional stress**
    g. **Acidosis**

8. *Aplastic crises* associated with infection and decreased RBC can cause a precipitous, life-threatening drop in hemoglobin.

9. Increased hemolysis (*hyperhemolytic crises*) can occur with infection, with increased bilirubin levels predisposing to gallstone formation (bilirubin stones).

10. *Sequestration crises* (most common in infants) are characterized by rapid onset of splenomegaly (from blood pooling) and a precipitous drop in hemoglobin.

11. The various types of crises often occur in combination rather than as isolated events.

12. Crises typically become less frequent and severe with aging; risk of death from crisis is greatest in children under age 5 years.

13. In persons with sickle cell anemia, premature death commonly results from the infection or from the effects of recurrent occlusion of microcirculation (e.g., cerebrovascular accident).

14. Management aims to prevent crises and control symptoms.

D. Assessment findings

1. Chronic manifestations of sickle cell anemia include:
   a. Jaundice
   b. Progressively impaired kidney function
   c. Signs and symptoms secondary to hemolysis and thrombosis
   d. Enlarged facial and skull bones
   e. Susceptibility to infections, especially osteomyelitis and pneumonia
   f. Leg ulcers, usually secondary to trauma
   g. Gallstones
   h. Splenomegaly
   i. Cardiomegaly
   j. Tachycardia, flow murmurs
   k. Growth retardation
   l. Delayed puberty
   m. In adulthood, characteristic "spiderlike" body habitus (elongated extremities, narrow shoulders and hips, barrel chest, curved spine, elongated skull)

2. Painful crisis may be marked by:
   a. Severe abdominal, chest, back, muscle, or bone pain
   b. Increased jaundice
   c. Dark urine
   d. Low-grade fever

3. Aplastic crisis may produce:
   a. Pallor
   b. Dyspnea
   c. Lethargy, stupor, possibly coma

4. Acute sequestration crisis is characterized by:
   a. Pallor
   b. Lethargy
   c. If untreated, signs and symptoms of hypovolemic shock

5. Diagnosis of sickle cell anemia is confirmed by:
   a. A stained blood smear exhibiting sickle cells
   b. Serum electrophoresis showing hemoglobin S

E. Nursing diagnoses

1. Risk for Infection
2. Knowledge Deficit
3. Pain

F. **Planning and implementation**
   1. Provide pain relief:
       a. Have the client rest and support affected joints as indicated.

       b. **Administer analgesics for acute, severe pain, which may necessitate oral or parenteral narcotics, such as meperidine (Demerol) or morphine (Duramorph) as follows: Assess the client's pain level; rule out complications; implement safety precautions; administer around-the-clock medication; monitor closely to avoid impaired respiration and decreased oxygenation; evaluate effectiveness of pain medication within 30 minutes of administration.**
       c. Encourage client-controlled analgesia, when appropriate, which may decrease the client's anxiety concerning timely administration of pain medication and provide excellent pain relief using lower total narcotic doses.
       d. Administer fluids (to dilute blood and reverse sludging of cells), and monitor hydration.
   2. Provide information to assist client and family adjustment to disease, its treatment, and prevention of crises:

       a. **Instruct in measures to prevent crises: avoid infections, dehydration, strenuous physical activity, emotional stress, tight or restrictive clothing, high altitudes.**
       b. Folic acid replacement may be indicated to support erythropoiesis.
       c. Simple RBC or exchange transfusion may be indicated for aplastic crisis; for severe, painful crisis unresponsive to other therapies; preoperatively, to dilute the amount of sickled blood; during the final trimester of pregnancy to prevent crisis; or to treat leg ulcers unresponsive to therapy.
       d. Review genetic implications, and refer for counseling as necessary.
       e. Encourage participation in support groups.
   3. Institute infection prevention measures:
       a. Encourage appropriate dental care and prompt treatment for breaks in skin integrity.
       b. Review immunization schedule with client and family.
       c. Instruct the client and family to observe for fever; cough; tachypnea; urinary symptoms; and any reddened, painful, or open areas, and to seek prompt medical attention if they develop.

G. Evaluation
>   1. The client reports minimal or no pain.
>   2. The client and family verbalize understanding of sickle cell disorder, its causes, and signs and symptoms of crisis.
>   3. The client demonstrates appropriated self-care measures to prevent or manage infection.

VIII. Leukemias

A. Description
>   1. Leukemias are malignant disorders of blood-forming tissues characterized by uncontrolled proliferation of WBCs in bone marrow, replacing normal marrow elements, and in the liver, spleen, lymph nodes, and nonhematologic organ systems (skin, kidney, GI tract, and central nervous system).
>   2. Leukemias are classified according to:
>   a. Specific cell line(s) involved: lymphocytic, myelocytic, monocytic
>   b. Maturity of malignant cells: acute (immature cells) and chronic (differentiated cells)
>   3. Types include:
>   a. Acute nonlymphocytic leukemia (ANLL)
>   b. Acute lymphocytic leukemia (ALL)
>   c. Chronic myelogenous leukemia (CML)
>   d. Chronic lymphocytic leukemia (CLL)

B. Etiology and incidence
>   1. Etiology is unknown, but certain factors are associated with increased incidence, including:
>   a. Exposure to radiation
>   b. Chemical agents (e.g., benzene, alkylating chemotherapeutic agents)
>   c. Infectious agents (viruses implicated in animal models)
>   d. Genetic variables (increased incidence reported in clients with Down's syndrome; some reports of increased familial incidence)
>   2. Incidence varies with type:
>   a. ANLL: most common in adults; incidence increases with age
>   b. ALL: most common in children (85% of all cases); accounts for 90% of leukemias in children
>   c. CML: uncommon before age 20; incidence rises with age
>   d. CLL: the most common type of leukemia in persons age 50 and older

C. Pathophysiology and management
>   1. Acute leukemias are rapidly progressive diseases usually char-

acterized by uncontrolled proliferation of very immature cells (blasts) in bone marrow and peripheral tissue.

2. Leukemic blast cells in marrow suppress differentiation and proliferation of normal hemopoietic cells, predisposing to severe anemia, thrombocytopenia (hemorrhage), and granulocytopenia (infection). Acute leukemias typically prove rapidly fatal if untreated.

3. ANLL affects cells committed to granulocytic, monocytic, megakaryocytic, and erythrocytic stem cell lines; typically, aberration in growth of one cell type predominates. The most common types of ANLL involve maturational arrest and proliferation of cells in myeloblastic and monoblastic stages of development.

4. ALL affects lymphoid-committed stem cell lines and is characterized by proliferation of immature lymphoid cells (lymphoblasts) in bone marrow.

5. CML involves malignancy of myeloid stem cells, with more mature cells present than in acute forms and symptoms generally not as severe as in acute forms (i.e., terminal phase of disease involves progression to less differentiated, or blastic, phase). Onset typically is gradual and insidious.

6. CLL is characterized by marked increase in mature lymphocytes in circulation and lymphoid tissue. The disease may be relatively asymptomatic over many years; progressive anemia and thrombocytopenia may result from bone marrow infiltration, immune destruction, or hypersplenism.

D. Assessment findings

1. Clinical manifestations may include:
   a. Petechiae, ecchymoses, epistaxis, gingival bleeding, retinal hemorrhages, or frank bleeding from any body orifice secondary to thrombocytopenia
   b. Gingival hypertrophy (most commonly in AML)
   c. Pallor, fatigue, dyspnea secondary to anemia
   d. Fever, signs and symptoms of infection due to neutropenia
   e. Lymphadenopathy, splenomegaly, hepatomegaly due to tissue invasion
   f. Bone pain, arthralgias secondary to pressure from rapidly proliferating cells in marrow
   g. Neurologic effects secondary to leukemic infiltration of central nervous system

2. Laboratory studies typically reveal:
   a. Peripheral WBC count varying widely (1000 to >100,000/mm^3) but always including immature cells (ANLL/ALL)
   b. Elevated leukocyte count (CML)

      c.   Low leukocyte alkaline phosphatase (CML)

      d.   Elevated leukocyte count, possibly exceeding 100,000/ mm^3 (CLL)

      e.   Decreased erythrocytes, granulocytes, and platelets (CLL)

      f.   A large percentage (60% to 90%) of bone marrow's nucleated cells identified as blasts (which normally comprise up to only 5% of normal marrow elements), with reduced erythroid precursors, mature cells, and megakaryocytes (ANLL/ALL)

      g.   Philadelphia chromosome present in bone marrow cells in over 90% of clients (CML)

E. Nursing diagnoses

    1.   Activity Intolerance

    2.   Ineffective Individual Coping

    3.   Fluid Volume Deficit

    4.   Risk for Infection

    5.   Altered Nutrition: Less than body requirements

    6.   Pain

F. Planning and implementation

    1.   Monitor temperature, and report elevation.

    2.   Assess for and report other signs and symptoms of infection.

    3.   **Recognize that the client is at high risk for infection when absolute neutrophil count falls below 1000/mm^3 and at grave risk when count is 500/mm^3 or less.**

    4.   Obtain cultures and initiate empiric IV antibiotic therapy as prescribed.

    5.   Be aware that classic signs of infection may not be apparent in a client with leukemia.

    6.   Maintain a protective environment as indicated.

    7.   Maintain integrity of skin and mucous membranes.

    8.   Teach the client and family signs and symptoms of infection and preventive techniques.

    9.   Institute measures to prevent bleeding, and monitor for bleeding.

    10.   Provide information on scheduled treatments (see Chapter 21, Cancer Nursing).

        a.   For ANLL and ALL: initial combination chemotherapy, allogenic bone marrow transplantation, consolidation therapy, and intermittent long-term maintenance chemotherapy for several years

        b.   For CML: initial single-agent chemotherapy, followed by long-term, low-dose maintenance therapy; in acute exacerbation phase (blast crisis), possibly bone marrow transplantation

        c.   For CLL: possibly no treatment for asymptomatic clients; for symptomatic clients, initially single-agent chemotherapy, followed by combination chemotherapy and possibly splenectomy for refractory thrombocytopenia

    11.   Promote positive coping mechanisms to help the client and family deal with stressors related to the disease and its treatment.

    12.   Provide pain relief as needed and as prescribed.

    13.   Promote activity in accordance with the client's strength and tolerance. Alternate periods of rest and activity as needed.

    14.   Teach the client safety measures (see Section IV.E).

    15.   Ensure adequate nutrition and hydration.

G.   **Evaluation**

    1.   The client remains free of infection, or infection is minimized.

    2.   The client exhibits minimal or no bleeding.

    3.   The client demonstrates positive coping skills.

    4.   The client reports minimal or no discomfort.

    5.   The client maintains an activity level compatible with blood value changes.

    6.   The client maintains adequate nutritional intake.

    7.   The client exhibits adequate fluid balance.

IX.   Lymphomas

A.   **Description**

    1.   Lymphomas are neoplastic diseases of cells of the lymphoreticular system; lymphocytes and histiocytes (fixed, nonmotile macrophages).

    2.   Classification of lymphomas is based on:

        a.   Predominant malignant cell type (i.e., lymphocytic lymphomas, histiocytic lymphomas, or Hodgkin's disease)

        b.   Degree of malignant cell differentiation (i.e., well-differentiated, poorly differentiated, or undifferentiated)

    3.   Lymphomas usually are divided into two large subgroups based on morphologic appearance of involved lymph nodes:

        a.   Hodgkin's disease

        b.   Non-Hodgkin's lymphomas

    4.   Mycosis fungoides is a rare, chronic, cutaneous T-cell lymphoma producing skin lesions closely resembling those of Hodgkin's disease in lymph nodes and viscera.

B.   **Etiology and incidence**

    1.   The etiology of lymphomas is unknown.

    2.   Hodgkin's disease most commonly affects young adults; incidence is higher in males than in females and peaks in two age groups: age 15 to 38 and after age 50.

    3.   Non-Hodgkin's lymphomas are two to three times more

common in men than in women and affect all age groups, with incidence increasing with age.

4. Mycosis fungoides is rare; peak incidence is between age 40 and 60.

C. Pathophysiology and management

1. Lymphomas usually originate in lymph nodes and may originate in or involve lymphoid tissue throughout body (e.g., spleen, tonsils, stomach wall, liver, bone marrow). They commonly spread to extralymphatic tissue (e.g., lungs, kidneys).

2. The key cell of Hodgkin's disease is the Reed-Sternberg cell, a gigantic, atypical tumor cell of unique morphology and uncertain origin.

3. Different histopathologic subtypes are associated with varying prognoses:
   a. Lymphocyte predominant: most favorable prognosis
   b. Nodular sclerosing: next best prognosis
   c. Mixed cellularity: characteristically more aggressive than either nodular sclerosing or lymphocyte-predominant subtypes
   d. Lymphocyte depleted: most unfavorable prognosis

4. Hodgkin's disease usually shows a highly predictable pattern of spread through lymphatic channels to contiguous nodes. It also may spread via a hematogenous route to extranodal sites (e.g., GI tract, bone marrow, skin, and other organs).

5. The clinical pattern at presentation determines the all-important stage (extent) of disease (Table 19-3) and strongly correlates with histologic subtype.

TABLE 19-3.
Ann Arbor Staging System for Hodgkin's Lymphoma

STAGE*	DESCRIPTION
I	Involvement of a single lymph node region (I) or of a single extralymphatic organ or site (IE)
II	Involvement of two or more lymph node regions on the same side of the diaphragm (II) or localized involvement of extralymphatic organ or site and of one or more lymph node regions on the same side of the diaphragm (IIE)
III	Involvement of lymph node regions on both sides of the diaphragm (III), which may also be accompanied by localized involvement of extralymphatic organ or site (IIIE), the spleen (IIIS), or both (IIISE)
IV	Diffuse or disseminated involvement of one or more extralymphatic organs or tissues, with or without associated lymph node enlargement. The reason for stage IV classification should be identified further by site-defining symbols.

*Systemic symptoms: Each stage is subdivided into A and B categories. A is for clients without defined symptoms; B is for those with. The B classification applies to a client with unexplained weight loss of more than 10% body weight in the 6 months before diagnosis, unexplained fever exceeding 38°C, and night sweats.

6. In non-Hodgkin's lymphomas, the major determinants of clinical patterns of disease and of prognosis are:
    a. Cell type of origin (state of differentiation)
    b. Pattern of growth within involved lymph nodes (follicular or diffuse)
7. Diagnostic terminology has been clarified in a major comparative study. According to the working formulation, three broad groups may be defined:
    a. Low-grade or favorable group: has less aggressive cell types or possesses follicular (also called nodular) growth pattern
    b. Intermediate-grade group: has either aggressive cell types in follicular patterns or diffuse patterns of cells, many or all of which appear aggressive
    c. High-grade or unfavorable group: pattern of growth diffuse and cell type appears highly malignant
8. Non-Hodgkin's lymphomas are more likely than Hodgkin's to involve generalized lymph node disease or extranodal disease at time of diagnosis. Bone marrow invasion, with associated anemia and thrombocytopenia, and immune dysfunction, with associated infections, are evident with these lymphomas.
9. Mycosis fungoides commonly begins in skin as pruritic, red rash, and months or years later manifests with mushroomlike growths (lymphoma) varying in size from 1 to 5 cm. Disease eventually spreads to lymph nodes, spleen, liver, and lungs.

D. Assessment findings

1. Common clinical manifestations of lymphomas include:
    a. Palpable lymph nodes, especially cervical, axillae, or groin
    b. Fatigue
    c. Weight loss
    d. Mild to high fever, often exhibiting Pel-Ebstein fever pattern
    e. Chills, night sweats
    f. Pruritus
2. The disease also may produce signs and symptoms secondary to encroachment of enlarged mediastinal and retroperitoneal lymph nodes, including:
    a. Dyspnea secondary to pressure against trachea
    b. Dysphagia secondary to pressure against esophagus
    c. Laryngeal paralysis and brachial, lumbar, or sacral neuralgias secondary to pressure on nerves
    d. Edema in extremities or effusions into pleura or peritoneum due to pressure on veins
    e. Signs of obstructive jaundice from pressure on the common bile duct

       f.   Splenomegaly

       g.   Hepatomegaly

  3.   Diagnosis and staging of Hodgkin's disease involves:

       a.   Lymph node biopsy to identify histologic features

       b.   Chest radiograph to identify any mediastinal, hilar, or intrapulmonary disease

       c.   CT scan to evaluate lymph node involvement

       d.   Bone marrow biopsy

       e.   Liver function tests and liver scan

       f.   Lymphangiography to detect abdominal lymph node involvement, which may not be seen on CT scan

       g.   Surgical staging laparotomy with splenectomy, liver and multiple lymph node biopsies to identify disease in spleen and lymph nodes below the diaphragm

  4.   Procedures involved in diagnosis and staging of non-Hodgkin's lymphomas include:

       a.   Lymph node biopsy

       b.   Bone marrow aspirate and biopsy

       c.   Liver and renal function tests

       d.   CT scan

       e.   Laparotomy

  5.   Diagnosis of mycosis fungoides involves:

       a.   Biopsy of skin lesions

       b.   Biopsies of lymph nodes, bone marrow, liver

E. **Nursing diagnoses**

  1.   Ineffective Individual Coping

  2.   Risk for Infection

  3.   Altered Nutrition: Less than body requirements

  4.   Pain

F. **Planning and implementation**

  1.   Maintain optimal skin hydration and protection to decrease pruritus.

  2.   Care for skin reactions in radiation treatment fields as prescribed by radiation oncology center.

  3.   Treat fever symptomatically with antipyretics once infection is ruled out.

  4.   Administer analgesics as needed to relieve painful encroachment of enlarged lymph nodes.

  5.   Ensure adequate nutrition and hydration.

  6.   Protect the client from infection.

  7.   Instruct the client and family about treatment protocols (see Chapter 21, Cancer Nursing).

       a.   For Hodgkin's disease: depending on stage, symptoms, and cell type, radiation therapy and combination chemotherapy; in disease resistant to conventional chemotherapy or in relapse, possibly intensive therapy with autologous bone marrow transplant rescue

b. For non-Hodgkin's lymphomas: depending on staging and histopathologic classification, radiation therapy (possibly curative with localized disease) or combination chemotherapy (for widespread disease); in clients with relapsed or refractory disease after initial intensive therapy, possibly autologous (or less commonly, allogeneic) bone marrow transplantation

c. For mycosis fungoides: based on clinical staging, topical chemotherapy (nitrogen mustard) or corticosteroids for skin manifestations, radiation therapy, systemic chemotherapy, or a combination of topical chemotherapy, radiation therapy, and systemic chemotherapy

8. Provide emotional and psychological support during extensive diagnostic testing and treatments.

G. Evaluation

1. The client reports decreased discomfort.
2. The client maintains adequate nutritional intake.
3. The client remains free of infection or exhibits only minor infection.
4. The client demonstrates effective coping with diagnosis and effects of treatment.

X. Multiple myeloma

A. Description: a malignant disease of plasma cells that infiltrates bone, soft tissues, lymph nodes, liver, spleen, and kidneys

B. Etiology and incidence

1. The etiology of multiple myeloma is unclear.
2. Incidence is highest in men older than age 40.

C. Pathophysiology and management

1. Widespread proliferation of immature plasma cells takes place mainly in bone marrow throughout the skeletal system.
2. Plasma cells derived from B lymphocytes normally produce immunoglobulins. Malignant plasma cells produce large quantities of abnormal immunoglobulin or fragments of immunoglobulin protein (Bence Jones protein) that can usually be detected in serum and urine by immunoelectrophoresis.
3. Plasma cell tumors can infiltrate extraskeletal sites such as the skin, mouth, kidneys, and pleura.
4. Osteolytic bone lesions often are associated with hypercalcemia; pathologic fractures are common, especially in vertebrae and ribs.
5. Management usually includes combination chemotherapy or radiation therapy.

D. Assessment findings
1. Characteristic clinical manifestations include:
   a. Severe bone pain
   b. Signs and symptoms of anemia secondary to marrow replacement with plasma cells
   c. Weight loss
   d. Signs and symptoms of renal failure due to precipitation of immunoglobulin in tubules, hypercalciuria, increased uric acid, or infiltration of kidney with plasma cells
   e. Signs and symptoms of infection secondary to impaired antibody production
2. Diagnostic studies include:
   a. Bone marrow aspiration or biopsy demonstrating increased numbers of plasma cells
   b. Serum electrophoresis showing abnormal globulins appearing as monoclonal "spikes"; fragments of these globulins excreted in urine as Bence Jones protein
   c. Radiographs and bone scans revealing numerous osteolytic bone lesions; generalized demineralization of skeleton (osteoporosis) is common

E. Nursing diagnoses
1. Ineffective Individual Coping
2. Risk for Infection
3. Risk for Trauma
4. Pain

F. Planning and implementation
1. Provide pain relief as indicated (e.g., analgesics, back brace).
2. Assess for focal sites of pain that may be palliated with radiation therapy.
3. As indicated, prepare the client for combination chemotherapy to decrease malignant cell mass and relieve pain (see Chapter 21, Cancer nursing).
4. As indicated, prepare the client for radiation therapy to palliate bone pain and reduce the size of extraskeletal plasma cell tumors (see Chapter 21, Cancer Nursing).
5. **Protect the client from injury: Teach measures to prevent pathologic fractures, avoid immobilization (unless ambulation is contradicted due to risk of cord compression with spinal lesion), monitor for and report signs and symptoms of spinal cord compression (e.g., motor weakness or dysfunction, paresthesias or sensory loss, bladder or bowel dysfunction).**
6. Ensure adequate hydration; avoid dehydration, which can precipitate acute renal failure.

7. Monitor serum calcium levels, and assess for signs and symptoms of hypercalcemia:
   a. Restlessness
   b. Confusion
   c. Lethargy
   d. Decreased muscle tone
   e. Cardiac arrhythmias
8. Protect the client from infection.
9. Provide psychosocial and emotional support.

G. Evaluation
1. The client reports relief of bone pain.
2. The client exhibits increased ambulation.
3. The client participates in the planned regimen to prevent injury.
4. The client remains free of infection, or infection is minimized.
5. The client exhibits positive coping skills to deal with the diagnosis and effects of treatment.

XI. Bleeding disorders

A. Description
1. This term refers to various disorders of impaired hemostasis—the physiologic process involved in terminating abnormal bleeding.
2. Specific disorders include:
   a. Thrombocytopenia, a quantitative platelet disorder
   b. Idiopathic thrombocytopenic purpura (ITP), a group of bleeding disorders of unknown etiology
   c. Clotting factor defects (hemophilia A and B)
   d. von Willebrand's disease
   e. Disseminated intravascular coagulation (DIC)

B. Etiology and incidence
1. Thrombocytopenia, the most common cause of generalized bleeding, can result from:
   a. Decreased production of platelets by marrow (e.g., infiltrative diseases of marrow such as leukemia; myelosuppressive therapy; myelofibrosis; drug effects)
   b. Increased platelet destruction (e.g., infection, immune disorders)
   c. Abnormal distribution or sequestration (e.g., hypersplenism)
   d. Loss of platelets from blood stream (e.g., excessive bleeding without replacement, extracorporeal circulation)
2. The etiology of ITP is unknown.

3. Clotting factor defects result from inherited (sex-linked recessive) deficiency of individual coagulation factors.
   a. Hemophilia A involves deficiency of factor VIII (antihemophilic factor); it is the most common inherited disorder of coagulation, affecting approximately 1 in 10,000 of the male population.
   b. Hemophilia B involves deficiency of factor IX (Christmas factor); incidence is 5 to 10 times lower than for hemophilia A.
4. Von Willebrand's disease is a common bleeding disorder of either autosomal dominant or recessive inheritance.
5. DIC always occurs secondary to an underlying disease or condition, including:
   a. Septicemia
   b. Obstetrical complications
   c. Disseminated malignancies
   d. Massive tissue injury (burns and trauma)
   e. Hemolytic transfusion reaction
   f. Shock
   g. Anaphylaxis
6. Other acquired coagulation defects include:
   a. Coumarin drug toxicity, which interferes with synthesis of vitamin-K-dependent coagulation factors by the liver; excessive doses or administration with other drugs that interfere with metabolism can produce prothrombin deficiency
   b. Heparin administration, which interferes with thrombin-induced conversion of fibrinogen to fibrin
   c. Clotting factor deficiencies resulting from impaired synthesis by the liver
   d. Massive transfusion creating a dilutional clotting factor deficiency, unless all coagulation factors included in blood components are transfused

C. Pathophysiology and management
1. Hemostasis (arrest of bleeding) involves three sequential events:
   a. Vascular reaction: immediate vasoconstriction of injured vessels
   b. Formation of platelet plug (normally within 5 minutes of vessel injury), which effectively stops bleeding in small vessels and provides temporary protection in larger injuries
   c. Activation of the clotting cascade, resulting in formation of more permanent, stable fibrin clot

2. Other mechanisms can contribute to hemostasis, including:
   a. Hemorrhage from large wound slowed by abrupt lowering of arterial blood pressure (shock), reducing rate of blood flow throughout body
   b. Hematoma formation or tissue swelling at site of injury, which may slow bleeding by compressing affected vessel
3. A fibrin clot eventually will be lysed by another plasma protein system—the fibrinolytic system—once tissue repair of the vascular endothelium has occurred.
4. Bleeding disorders can result from defects in vessels, platelets, coagulation factors, or the fibrinolytic system.
5. Vascular disorders involve spontaneous rupture of small vessels that are defective or injured; they may be localized or widespread, and result from:
   a. Vascular injury secondary to drug reactions, allergic disorders, collagen-vascular diseases, bacterial infections
   b. Alteration in the connective tissue framework supporting blood vessels due to vitamin C deficiency, adrenocortical hormone excess, senile purpura
6. Thrombocytopenia is marked by a deficient number of circulating platelets. Because platelets play a vital role in coagulation, thrombocytopenia poses a serious threat to hemostasis.
7. ITP involves immune destruction of platelets and production of antiplatelet antibodies, which markedly shorten platelet life span.
8. Bleeding associated with clotting factor defects, which may be very severe, characteristically manifests with large, spreading bruises and bleeding into muscles and joints with even minor trauma. Recurrent joint hemorrhages can result in such severe damage that chronic pain or ankylosis (fixation) of joint occurs.
9. The risk of bleeding correlates with coagulation factor assay results:
   a. Severe bleeding diathesis (high risk of spontaneous bleeding), with 5% or less of circulating factor VIII or IX
   b. Moderate bleeding diathesis (minimal to moderate risk of spontaneous bleeding but high risk of profuse bleeding with surgery or trauma), with 5% to 25% circulating factor VIII or IX
   c. Mild bleeding diathesis (rare spontaneous bleeding, abnormal bleeding with surgery or trauma), with 25% to 40% circulating factor VIII or IX
10. von Willebrand's disease is characterized by mild deficiency of factor VIII (15% to 50% of normal) with impaired platelet function. This results in such manifestations as nosebleeds,

menorrhagia, prolonged bleeding from cuts, and postoperative bleeding; massive soft tissue and joint hemorrhages are absent.

11. DIC is characterized by widespread clotting in microcirculation, leading to consumption of coagulation factors and platelets and ultimately resulting in bleeding. Bleeding can range from minimal occult internal bleeding to profuse hemorrhaging from all orifices. The clinical picture is a complex combination of thrombosis and bleeding; acute renal failure may result from fibrin deposition in renal microcirculation.

D. Assessment findings

1. Signs and symptoms of bleeding disorders vary with the particular defect (Table 19-4).

2. Vascular abnormalities usually manifest as local bleeding into the skin; the term *purpura* refers to extravasation of blood into skin and mucous membranes.

3. Platelet defects, either quantitative or qualitative, usually produce:
   a. Petechiae
   b. Easy bruising
   c. Bleeding that generally stops with local pressure and does not recur when pressure is released

4. Coagulation factor defects usually present with:
   a. Deep tissue bleeding after minor trauma, such as intramuscular hematomas and hemarthroses (bleeding into joint spaces)

TABLE 19-4.
Clinical Distinction Among Blood Vessel, Platelet, and Coagulation Disorders

FINDINGS	DISORDERS OF COAGULATION	DISORDERS OF PLATELETS OR VESSELS ("PURPURIC DISORDERS")
Petechiae	Rare	Characteristic
Deep dissecting hematomas	Characteristic	Rare
Superficial ecchymoses	Common; usually large and solitary	Characteristic; usually small and multiple
Hemarthrosis	Characteristic	Rare
Delayed bleeding	Common	Rare
Bleeding from superficial cuts and scratches	Minimal	Persistent; often profuse
Sex of patient	80%–90% of hereditary forms occur only in males	Relatively more common in females
Positive family history	Common	Rare

        b.   Usually, no petechiae or superficial hemorrhages

        c.   Recurrence of external bleeding several hours after pressure is removed

5. Abdominal, flank, or joint pain may indicate internal bleeding.
6. Hypotension; tachycardia; chest pain; pallor; cool, clammy skin; tachypnea; or altered responsiveness may indicate internal bleeding associated with hypovolemia.
7. Headache and altered neurologic signs and symptoms may indicate cerebral hemorrhage.
8. Vision changes may indicate retinal hemorrhage.
9. Dyspnea, respiratory distress, hemoptysis, cyanosis, or rales may indicate interstitial hemorrhage in lungs.
10. Laboratory findings in thrombocytopenia may include:
    a. Platelet deficiency secondary to underlying disease, generally diagnosed by bone marrow aspiration and biopsy
    b. Platelet deficiency due to increased destruction, as evidenced by marrow showing increased megakaryocytes and normal platelet production
11. In ITP, laboratory studies may indicate:
    a. Abnormalities in platelet size or morphologic appearance
    b. Increased levels of immunoglobulins (IgG) or complement components identified on platelet surface
12. Findings in hemophilia A and B commonly include:
    a. Abnormal coagulation factor assay
    b. Prolonged PTT
13. von Willebrand's disease may be marked by:
    a. Abnormal coagulation factor assay
    b. Normal platelet count
    c. Prolonged bleeding time
    d. Slightly prolonged PTT
14. Laboratory studies in DIC may reveal:
    a. Decreased platelet count
    b. Decreased fibrinogen
    c. Prolonged PT and PTT
    d. Increased FSP
    e. Schistocytes (red cell fragments) on peripheral smear

E. **Nursing diagnoses**
1. Fear
2. Risk for Injury
3. Knowledge Deficit
4. Pain

F. **Planning and implementation**
1. Observe location of petechiae and ecchymoses (e.g., pe-

techiae in the conjunctiva of the eye may be a clinical indication of spontaneous bleeding, as opposed to petechiae over bony prominences or areas subjected to trauma).

2. Note color of ecchymoses to distinguish between old and new bleeding (purple or purplish blue, fading to green, yellow, and brown with time).

3. Observe for frank bleeding from any orifice: mouth (gums), nose, vagina, rectum, urethra. Also look for bleeding from suture lines and venous access sites.

4. Test all drainage and excreta for occult blood (feces, urine, emesis, gastric drainage).

5. Assess joints for swelling, mobility limitation, and pain.

6. **Assess color and temperature of skin (e.g., pale, cool, clammy); note tachypnea, hypotension, tachycardia, palpitations, altered responsiveness, or decreased urine output; these findings may indicate inadequate tissue oxygenation or decreased blood volume.**

7. Measure blood loss; weigh linens, bandages, and the like.

8. Monitor for orthostatic changes in blood pressure and pulse.

9. **Minimize invasive procedures; avoid injections or, if injection is essential, use small-gauge needles with Z-track technique, and apply firm pressure up to 5 minutes.**

10. Avoid increasing intracranial pressure with Valsalva's maneuver in a client with a platelet count <20,000/mm^3, which poses risk of cerebral bleeding. Symptomatically treat cough, constipation, chills, nausea, and vomiting; instruct the client to avoid strenuous activity, forceful nose blowing, and like actions.

11. Warn the client to avoid alcohol and medication containing aspirin, which interfere with platelet function.

12. Instruct the client in general preventive measures, including:
    a. Using an electric shaver instead of a razor
    b. Using a soft or sponge-tipped toothbrush
    c. Maintaining rigorous dental prophylaxis
    d. Avoiding contact sports
    e. Avoiding use of rectal thermometers, suppositories, enemas, and vaginal tampons

13. Intervene to control bleeding, as indicated, which may include:
    a. In thrombocytopenia, prophylactic platelet transfusions, steroids or other immune modulation, hormonal control of menstrual periods
    b. In ITP, corticosteroids, gamma globulin, preparation for splenectomy, immunosuppression therapy (e.g., vincristine, cyclophosphamide, azathioprine)

    c.   In hemophilia A or B, appropriate replacement therapy (factor VIII or IX concentrates) to prevent or treat bleeding

    d.   In von Willebrand's disease, cryoprecipitate, which contains factor VIII, fibrinogen, and factor XIII

    e.   In DIC, transfusion of red cells, platelets, or cryoprecipitate; IV heparin to slow coagulation process

    f.   In coumarin toxicity, oral or parenteral vitamin K to correct prothrombin deficiency; if urgent replacement needed, transfusion of single donor plasma or prothrombin complex concentrates

    g.   To correct excess heparin dosage, protamine sulfate administration

    h.   For factor deficiencies from liver disease, transfusion of fresh frozen plasma, fresh whole blood, or factor IX concentrate

14.   Promote comfort with analgesics, orthopedic devices, and a bed cradle as indicated.

15.   Provide psychological support to the client and family members. Assess their anxiety level and understanding of the disorder and its treatment; encourage verbalization of questions and fears.

16.   Provide information to facilitate the client's participation and control in the preventive and therapeutic regimens; emphasize safe physical activities along with realistic restrictions.

17.   Provide information to assist the client and family members with adjustment to the disease process, including:

    a.   Signs and symptoms in relation to disease pathophysiology

    b.   Rationale for interventions

    c.   Measures to prevent and control bleeding

    d.   Rehabilitative measures (e.g., mobilization and physiotherapy subsequent to hemarthrosis)

    e.   Genetic implications of the bleeding disorder as appropriate

18.   Refer the client and family members to counseling or support groups as indicated.

G.   Evaluation

1.   The client reports minimal or no pain and an acceptable comfort level.

2.   The client regains or maintains adequate tissue perfusion.

3.   The client verbalizes understanding of the cause and treatment of the blood disorder.

4.   The client demonstrates positive coping with the diagnosis and therapeutic regimen.

Bibliography

Bolander, V. R. (1994). *Sorensen & Luckmann's basic nursing: A physiologic approach* (3rd ed.). Philadelphia: W. B. Saunders.

Carpenito, L. J. (1995). *Nursing diagnosis: Application to clinical practice* (6th ed.). Philadelphia: J. B. Lippincott.

Clark, J., Queener, S., & Karb, V. (1990). *Pharmacologic basis of nursing practice* (4th ed.). St. Louis: C. V. Mosby.

Deglin, J. H., & Vallerand, A. H. (1995). *Davis's drug guide for nurses* (4th ed.). Philadelphia: F. A. Davis.

DeVita, V. T., Jr., Hellman, S., & Rosenberg, S. A. (Eds.). (1995). *Important advances in oncology 1995.* Philadelphia: J. B. Lippincott.

Doenges, M. E., Moorhouse, M. F., & Geissler, A. C. (1993). *Nursing care plans: Guidelines for planning and documenting patient care* (3rd ed.). Philadelphia: F. A. Davis.

Leavell, B. S., & Thorp, O. A., Jr. (1987). *Leavell and Thorp's fundamentals of clinical hematology* (5th ed.). Philadelphia: W. B. Saunders.

Nettina, S. (1996). *The Lippincott manual of nursing practice* (6th ed.). Philadelphia: Lippincott-Raven Publishers.

Porth, C. M. (1992). *Pathophysiology: Concepts of altered health states* (4th ed.). Philadelphia: J. B. Lippincott.

Powers, L. W. (1989). *Diagnostic hematology: Clinical and technical principles.* St. Louis: C. V. Mosby.

Smeltzer, S. C., & Bare, B. G. (1996). *Brunner & Suddarth's textbook of medical-surgical nursing* (8th ed.). Philadelphia: Lippincott-Raven Publishers.

STUDY QUESTIONS

1. The most common sign of thrombocytopenia is
   a. petechiae
   b. hemostasis
   c. melena
   d. hemarthrosis

2. Transfusion of which of the following
   blood components would therapeutically provide all of the coagulation factors?
   a. cryoprecipitate
   b. random donor platelets
   c. fresh frozen plasma
   d. stored whole blood

3. Which of the following clinical signs
   and symptoms would suggest an anemia
   secondary to vitamin deficiency rather
   than folic acid deficiency?
   a. smooth, sore tongue
   b. palpitations
   c. paresthesias
   d. dizziness

4. Which of the following nursing interventions should be implemented in caring for a client whose CBC reveals a
   WBC 5000/mm^3, Hgb 12.9 g/dL,
   and platelet count 7000/mm^3?
   a. cough and deep breathe every 4
      hours to prevent infection
   b. platelet transfusions to maintain
      platelet count above 20,000/mm^3
   c. aspirin as needed to control temper-
      ature or chills
   d. stool softeners as needed to prevent
      constipation

5. Client teaching about self-management
   of the fatigue associated with anemia
   should include instructions to
   a. Continue bedrest to conserve en-
      ergy.
   b. Participate in all usual ADLs.
   c. Follow a progressive ambulatory
      program.
   d. Exercise to increase heart rate and
      respiratory rate to build greater en-
      durance.

6. Which of the following would most
   likely be a contributing factor in the development of infection in a client with
   acute leukemia?
   a. myelosuppressive effects of chemo-
      therapy
   b. granulocytopenia
   c. immature WBCs
   d. neutrophilia

7. The nurse would know the client needs
   more instruction concerning prescribed
   ferrous sulfate when the client states
   a. "I take my iron supplements with
      food to enhance their absorption."
   b. "I know that the gastrointestinal
      side effects that I'm experiencing
      are common with ferrous sulfate."
   c. "I eat organ meats weekly because
      they are a good dietary source of
      iron."
   d. "I take vitamin C tablets to enhance
      iron absorption."

8. The client receiving a unit of packed
   RBCs has baseline vital signs of temperature 98°F, BP 136/72 mmHg, pulse
   rate 100, respiratory rate 22; 15 minutes later the temperature is 101°F, BP
   140/76, pulse 104, and respiratory rate
   24. The nurse should:
   a. Continue the transfusion, and mon-
      itor every 15 minutes for develop-
      ment of further signs and symp-
      toms.
   b. Stop the transfusion immediately,
      and notify the physician.
   c. Continue infusion, and administer
      aspirin for fever.
   d. Slow the rate of transfusion, and
      continue monitoring.

9. Which of the following parental actions
   would indicate their ineffective adjustment to their infant son's diagnosis of
   hemophilia?
   a. They request counseling regarding
      family planning.
   b. They request teaching on the pro-

cedure for IV administration of factor VIII.
c. They verbalize feelings of guilt.
d. They discourage their child's participation in sports.

10. A client diagnosed with multiple myeloma would demonstrate a knowledge deficit of the disease process if which of the following occurs?
   a. The client decreases ambulation with bone pain.
   b. The client increases fluid intake.
   c. The client avoids heavy lifting.
   d. The client monitors serum calcium levels.

11. Laboratory findings for a client, aged 57, include WBC, $10,800/mm^3$; Hgb, 11.2 g/dL; platelet count, 100,000/uL; and differential showing neutrophils 4%, bands 0, lymphocytes 94%, monocytes 1%, and eosinophils 1%. Based on these data, the priority nursing diagnosis for the client would be
   a. Risk for Fluid Volume Deficit related to bleeding with thrombocytopenia
   b. Risk for Infection related to neutropenia
   c. Risk for Injury related to anemia
   d. Risk for Injury related to leukocytosis

12. Nursing interventions for the client experiencing a sickle cell crisis would include
   a. administering vitamin B_{12} intravenously and applying cold compresses to joints

b. encouraging passive and active range of motion exercises and turning every hour
c. administering around-the-clock analgesics and increasing fluid intake
d. decreasing fluid intake and applying thromboembolism stockings.

13. Which of the following assessment findings would indicate a positive response to heparin therapy in the client diagnosed with DIC?
   a. increased platelet count
   b. increased fibrinogen
   c. decreased fibrin split products
   d. decreased bleeding

14. Nursing interventions for the client diagnosed with a bleeding disorder would include
   a. administering enteric-coated aspirin
   b. observing for petechiae and ecchymoses
   c. assessing for jugular vein distention
   d. administering ferrous sulfate daily

15. Which of the following would be an inappropriate item to include in planning care for a severely neutropenic client?
   a. Transfuse neutrophils (granulocytes) to prevent infection.
   b. Exclude raw vegetables from the diet.
   c. Avoid administering rectal suppositories.
   d. Prohibit vases of fresh flowers and plants in the client's room.

For additional questions, see
Lippincott's Self-Study Series Software
Available at your bookstore

ANSWER KEY

1. **Correct response: a**
   Petechiae are characteristic of quantitative or qualitative platelet defects since platelets are primarily responsible for cessation of bleeding in small vessels.
   b and c. Although these findings may occur with thrombocytopenia, they are not characteristic.
   d. Hemarthrosis is characteristic of coagulation factor deficiencies.
   Knowledge/Physiologic/Assessment

2. **Correct response: c**
   Fresh frozen plasma contains all the coagulation factors, including the labile factors (V and VIII).
   a. Cryoprecipitate contains factor VIII, fibrinogen, and factor XIII.
   b. Random donor platelets contain large amounts of platelets in a minimum (nontherapeutic) amount of plasma.
   d. Stored whole blood does not include the labile coagulation factors.
   Application/Physiologic/Implementation

3. **Correct response: c**
   Vitamin B_{12} is essential for nervous system function, and the neurologic manifestations of B_{12} deficiency are not seen in folic acid deficiency.
   a. A smooth, sore tongue may be seen with either B_{12} or folic acid deficiency.
   b and d. Palpitations and dizziness are general manifestations of anemia and can be observed in either deficiency.
   Application/Physiologic/Assessment

4. **Correct response: d**
   This client is at risk of spontaneous bleeding. Preventing constipation decreases the risk of intracerebral bleeding secondary to increased intracranial pressure with Valsalva maneuver.
   a. Coughing increases intracranial pressure.
   b. Platelets are not transfused prophylactically in clients with ITP (cells

are destroyed and produce little therapeutic benefit).
   c. Aspirin is contraindicated in bleeding disorders since it interferes with platelet function. Nonaspirin antipyretics should be used instead.
   Analysis/Safe care/Implementation

5. **Correct response: c**
   The client should gradually increase activity and endurance, alternating periods of rest with periods of activity.
   a. Immobility is associated with muscle wasting and hypotension.
   b. Participation in the usual ADLs should be as tolerated, with activities causing undue fatigue replanned or deferred.
   d. Care should be directed toward decreasing activities that necessitate increased cardiac output—like exercise—until the anemia improves.
   Application/Health promotion/Implementation

6. **Correct response: d**
   Neutrophilia, an increase in circulating mature neutrophils, occurs in healthy persons as a compensatory response to the onset of bacterial infection.
   a. Suppression of marrow production of WBCs due to chemotherapy puts the client at profound risk of "nadir" sepsis.
   b. Decreased production of mature granulocytes due to chemotherapy and the disease process places the client at risk of infection.
   c. Immature WBCs, although perhaps present in large numbers, are not functional.
   Comprehension/Health promotion/Evaluation

7. **Correct response: a**
   Adequate iron absorption requires an acid environment; therefore, supplements should be taken between meals.
   b. Various GI side effects are common

(e.g., nausea, heartburn, abdominal cramping).

   c. Organ meats are one of the best food sources of iron.

   d. Vitamin C enhances iron absorption and is included in several iron preparations.

Application/Health promotion/ Analysis (Dx)

8. *Correct response: b*

Temperature elevation may indicate a hemolytic transfusion reaction; therefore, the transfusion must be stopped and the physician and blood bank notified.

   a. If hemolytic transfusion reaction is suspected, the transfusion must be stopped immediately.

   c. Antipyretics may be administered subsequent to physician's order only if the medical diagnosis is febrile, nonhemolytic transfusion reaction.

   d. This is incorrect because the transfusion must be stopped to enable the physician to rule out hemolytic versus nonhemolytic transfusion reaction (due to leukocyte or platelet antigens).

Analysis/Safe care/Implementation

9. *Correct response: d*

Contact sports should be avoided, but noncontact sports (e.g., swimming) are acceptable activities and can contribute to the child's independence and self-esteem. Preventing the child from engaging in safe physical activity may indicate overprotective behavior.

   a. Seeking this knowledge is a positive coping strategy and indicates an understanding of the genetic implications of the disease.

   b. This request indicates an interest in participating in the therapeutic regimen, which is essential in adjusting to illness.

   c. Guilt is a common parental reaction to genetically based illnesses; identifying feelings facilitates coping.

Analysis/Psychosocial/Evaluation

10. *Correct response: a*

Immobilization should be avoided because ambulation prevents further bone resorption and hypercalcemia. Analgesics should be administered to relieve pain and help maintain mobility.

   b. This action indicates knowledge that adequate hydration prevents renal failure.

   c. This precaution is appropriate to protect against pathologic fracture.

   d. This action reflects the client's understanding regarding predisposition to hypercalcemia due to lytic bone lesions.

Comprehension/Health promotion/ Evaluation

11. *Correct response: b*

Although the client's total WBC count is 10,800, only 4% of these cells are neutrophils, placing the client at grave risk of infection (i.e., absolute neutrophil count less than $500/mm^3$).

   a. Although the platelet count is below normal, generally there is no significant risk of bleeding until the count falls to $50,000/mm^3$ or below.

   c. The client's Hgb is near normal.

   d. The WBC count is only slightly above normal; it is the interpretation of the differential that is important.

Analysis/Safe care/Analysis (Dx)

12. *Correct response: c*

The client will be in severe pain and around-the-clock medications will help keep pain at a tolerable level and decrease anxiety about receiving pain medication. Increasing fluid will dilute the blood and reverse sludging of cells.

   a. Vitamin B_{12} is administered in megaloblastic anemia and cold compresses will cause vasoconstriction which will increase pain.

   b. During the crisis have the client rest and support affected joints; exercise will increase pain.

   d. Decreasing fluid will further concentrate blood and increase sludging of cells, causing more pain.

Application/Physiologic/Implementation

13. *Correct response: b*

Effective heparin therapy should stop the process of intravascular coagulation, which should result in increased fibrinogen.

a. Platelet count would increase in effective therapy, due to decreased thrombus formation.

c. Lysis of thrombi should decrease.

d. Bleeding should cease due to the increased availability of platelets and coagulation factors.

Analysis/Physiologic/Evaluation

14. *Correct response: b*

Petechiae are small pinpoint hemorrhages on the skin or mucous membranes which occur with quantitative or qualitative platelet disorders; ecchymoses are bluish-black macula resulting from seepage of blood into skin or mucous membranes, usually secondary to trauma.

a. Aspirin is contraindicated in clients with bleeding disorders.

c. Jugular vein distention is a sign of fluid volume overload and not a bleeding disorder.

d. Iron (ferrous sulfate) is used for anemias, not bleeding disorders.

Application/Physiologic/Implementation

15. *Correct response: a*

Granulocyte transfusion is not indicated to prevent infection.

b. Raw vegetables should be avoided to provide a low-bacterial diet.

c. Rectal temperatures, suppositories, and enemas are contraindicated in order to maintain integrity of mucous membranes.

d. Flower vases and plants should be avoided since stagnant water provides a favorable medium for bacterial growth.

Application/Safe care/Planning

Infectious Disorders

I.   Structures and functions

    A. Infectious process and chain of infection

        1. Infectious agents are organisms capable of causing disease.

        2. Organisms that normally inhibit homeostasis (normal flora) can cause opportunistic diseases.

        3. Not all infections (presence of organisms within a host) cause a pathologic process or disease.

        4. Types of infectious organisms include:

            a. Bacteria
            b. Viruses
            c. Rickettsiae
            d. Protozoa
            e. Fungi
            f. Helminths

5. Virulence refers to an organism's degree of pathogenicity (ability to cause disease).

6. Sources and reservoirs of infection include:
   a. Communicable disease: infectious disease that can be transmitted from an infected person, animal, or object to an uninfected person
   b. Nosocomial infection: infection acquired within a health care facility
   c. Opportunistic infection: infection that occurs in immunocompromised hosts (e.g., elderly persons, organ transplant recipients) caused by microbes that rarely cause infection in hosts with normal immune systems
   d. Reservoirs: commonly moist, warm environments (e.g., sewage, stagnant water)

7. Factors that increase a host's susceptibility to infection include:
   a. Damaged or inadequate defense mechanisms
   b. Debilitation and stress (as in hospitalized clients)
   c. Invasive procedures that provide a route of access for microorganisms (e.g., urinary catheterization)
   d. Therapies that cause immunosuppression (e.g., corticosteroids, chemotherapy)

8. The most common sites of infection are:
   a. Urinary tract
   b. Surgical wounds
   c. Respiratory tract

9. Four modes of transmission to host exist:
   a. Contact (e.g., sexually transmitted diseases [STDs])
   b. Common source of transmission (e.g., shared foods or drinks)
   c. Airborne (e.g., droplet nuclei resulting in tuberculosis, histoplasmosis)
   d. Vector borne (e.g., mosquitoes carrying malaria)

10. Portals of entry—the points at which infectious agents enter the host's body—include:
    a. Skin: by organisms burrowing into skin (e.g., hookworm larvae); through injection by insect bite (e.g., malaria); break in skin integrity (e.g., surgical wound or pressure sore)
    b. Gastrointestinal (GI) tract: typically via contaminated foods and drinks (e.g., cholera)
    c. Respiratory tract: via airborne droplet nuclei (e.g., tuberculosis, influenza)
    d. Genitourinary tract: sometimes via contamination from GI tract, route for STDs

        e.   Placenta: rare, although syphilis spirochete passes through this portal

        f.   Blood: through invasive procedures (e.g., venipuncture) or via insect bites

11. Portals of exit from the host—routes by which infectious agents leave the host body—also include the skin, GI tract, respiratory tract, genitourinary (GU) tract, placenta, and blood.

12. Identifying the portal of exit for a specific microorganism guides interventions to prevent disease transmission (e.g., wearing gown and gloves when bathing and changing bed linen for a client with hepatitis A because the virus leaves the host by way of the feces).

13. The severity of infection and infectious disease depends on both host factors (e.g., susceptibility, amount of exposure) and organism factors (e.g., virulence).

14. Exposure can result in one of four conditions:

    a.   Exposure with no infection

    b.   Subclinical infection

    c.   Disease limited by host responses (resolves without treatment)

    d.   Severe disease requiring treatment

B. **Trends in infectious diseases**

    1. Deaths from infectious diseases have declined greatly in industrialized nations.

    2. Infectious diseases continue to be a major cause of death in developing countries.

    3. Infectious diseases—such as acquired immunodeficiency syndrome (AIDS)—plague both industrialized and developing nations.

II. Overview of infectious disorders

    A. Assessment

        1. Nursing health history should focus on information about:

            a.   Recent exposure to infectious disease from contact with a person who has a known or suspected infection or may be a carrier of infectious disease, or from travel to places where certain infections are endemic

            b.   Current immunization status

            c.   Other medical problems that may compromise defenses (e.g., cancer, diabetes mellitus)

            d.   Systemic symptoms such as fever and chills, dysuria, arthralgias, myalgias, generalized weakness, anorexia

            e.   Signs and symptoms of local infection: redness, swelling, pain, warmth

            f.   Medication use, particularly corticosteroids, antibiotics, cancer chemotherapy

g.   Exposure to insect or animal bites
h.   Sexual practices
i.   Sensitivities, allergies

2.   Significant physical assessment findings include:
a.   Lesions of skin or mucous membranes
b.   Skin rashes
c.   Abnormal drainage from open lesions or body orifices
d.   Lymph node enlargement
e.   Altered nutritional status
f.   Altered vital signs (e.g., elevated temperature, tachycardia, blood pressure changes)
g.   Respiratory abnormalities (e.g., cough, breathing difficulties, changes in lung sounds)

3.   Important laboratory studies and diagnostic tests may include:
a.   Microbiologic specimens: urine, blood, sputum, wound exudate, feces, mucous membrane secretions
b.   White blood cell count: elevated in infection
c.   Serology: presence of antigens or antibodies to specific diseases

B.   Psychosocial implications

1.   The client with an infectious disease may experience coping difficulties related to:
a.   Fear of rejection based on the perceived cause of infection (e.g., unconventional sexual practices)
b.   Uncertainty about recovery and long-term manifestations or complications
c.   Concern about contagion

2.   The client also may have self-concept concerns related to:
a.   Body image changes
b.   Rejection as a sexual partner

3.   Disease-related lifestyle concerns may be associated with potential changes in:
a.   Physical ability
b.   Activity level
c.   Work performance, with potential for job loss

4.   Infectious disease can result in social isolation, possibly leading to isolation and depression.

III.   General nursing interventions for persons with infectious disorders

A.   Treat and prevent further infection (see Sections IV and V).

B.   Promote comfort.

1.   Administer analgesics as prescribed for the client's comfort.

   a.   Assess pain level on pain scale
   b.   Assess client's condition and rule out complications requiring medical attention.

      c. **Implement safety precautions, as appropriate, and evaluate drug effectiveness about 30 minutes after administration.**

2. Reposition the client as needed.
3. Use nonpharmacologic pain control methods when appropriate, such as:
   a. Guided imagery, distraction
   b. Relaxation techniques
   c. Hypnosis
   d. Massage
4. Provide prompt treatment for infection.

C. **Resolve any fluid volume deficit.**

m 1. **Assess for signs and symptoms including:**
   a. **Postural hypotension**
   b. **Tented skin turgor**
   c. **Tachycardia**
   d. **Weight loss**
   e. **Oliguria**
   f. **Weakness**
   g. **Decreased urine specific gravity**
   h. **Flat neck veins**

2. Encourage oral fluid intake.
3. Administer IV fluids if indicated.
4. Monitor intake and output, vital signs.

D. **Improve gas exchange.**

m 1. **Assess for signs and symptoms of impaired gas exchange:**
   a. **Dyspnea**
   b. **Increased respiratory rate and depth**
   c. **Signs of hypoxia, hypercapnia**
   d. **Restlessness, confusion, somnolence**
   e. **Decreased lung sounds, rales, rhonchi, expiratory wheezes**

2. Administer oxygen therapy for hypoxia.
3. Reposition the client to increase lung expansion, perfusion, and ventilation.
4. Encourage good pulmonary hygiene, including:
   a. Coughing and deep breathing exercises
   b. Diaphragmatic breathing
   c. Cessation of smoking and a smoke-free environment
5. Facilitate mobilization of secretions through:
   a. Ensuring adequate hydration
   b. Promoting rest and comfort
   c. Splinting the client's chest during coughing to minimize discomfort

  d. Administering prescribed aerosol treatments

  e. Encouraging ambulation as tolerated

E. **Provide information regarding causes, prevention, and treatment of infection.**

 1. **Assess what the client and family already know.**

 2. Give brief explanations; clarify when necessary.

 3. Use audiovisual aids when available.

 4. Teach:

  a. Methods of preventing infectious disease (e.g., prophylaxis, good personal health)

  b. Ways to prevent disease transmission

  c. Sources of infectious diseases

  d. Treatment for specific infectious disease

  e. Possible complications and reportable symptoms

F. **Reduce elevated body temperature.**

 1. Assess vital signs frequently to monitor the pattern and severity of febrile episodes.

 2. Keep in mind that not every infection is accompanied by fever, and conversely, fever does not always indicate infection. In some clients, fever may be an adaptive response; thus, antipyretic measures are not always indicated.

 3. In cases where antipyretic measures are indicated, provide appropriate interventions, which may include:

  a. Administering antipyretics, such as aspirin or acetaminophen (Tylenol), which act on the thermoregulatory center of the brain to produce diaphoresis and vasodilation.

    ▸ **Do not give aspirin to children because of its association with Reye's syndrome.**

    ▸ **Watch for GI distress and possible bleeding from aspirin.**

  b. Removing heavy or restrictive garments and excess bed linens

  c. Sponging the client's body with tepid water—avoid cold water or direct application of ice

  d. Applying cool compresses to areas of increased blood supply—axilla, groin, face

  e. Using a hypothermia blanket if indicated

 4. Encourage increased fluid intake to replace losses from sweating.

 5. Promote rest and comfort.

 6. Administer antimicrobial therapy to eliminate the cause of fever (see specific disease for medication).

G. **Resolve impairment in tissue integrity.**
1. Monitor for:
   a. Changes in skin color (e.g., blanched or reddened)
   b. Changes in turgor suggesting dehydration or edema
   c. Open lesions
2. Maintain optimal nutrition.
3. Maintain appropriate personal hygiene.
4. Culture any draining lesions.
5. Administer appropriate topical agents.
6. Change dressings as appropriate.

H. **Minimize social isolation.**
1. Explain the rationale for isolation procedures to the client and support persons.
2. Encourage the maximum social contact possible while under isolation.
3. Schedule regular periods to talk with the client.
4. Interact with the client in a caring, nonjudgmental manner.
5. Encourage the client to express anxieties and emotions.
6. Discontinue isolation as soon as possible.
7. Work with the client to devise means of reducing boredom.
8. Teach the client stress-reduction techniques.

IV. **General nursing interventions to prevent infectious disorders in health care facilities**
A. **Reduce host susceptibility.**
1. Improve host nutritional and fluid status.
2. Administer prescribed medical therapy to treat immunodeficiencies.
3. Teach the client about the importance of immunizations and about immunization methods.
4. Prevent damage to host defenses (e.g., avoid invasive procedures when possible).

B. **Prevent nosocomial infections.**
1. To prevent urinary tract infections (UTIs):
   a. Avoid urinary catheterization whenever possible.
   b. Use aseptic technique during catheterization.
   c. Maintain asepsis of urinary drainage systems.
   d. Remove urinary catheters as soon as possible.
   e. Avoid irrigating catheters.
2. To prevent surgical wound infections:
   a. Maintain asepsis intraoperatively.
   b. Use aseptic technique during dressing changes.
   c. Avoid preoperative hair removal when possible; if hair removal is necessary, use clippers or depilatories instead of razors, and remove hair immediately before surgery.

      d.   Limit personnel movement into and out of the operating room (OR) during surgical procedures.

      e.   Change dressings over closed wounds only when wet or if signs and symptoms of infection develop.

  3.   To prevent respiratory tract infections:

      a.   Use only properly disinfected and sterilized respiratory equipment.

      b.   Perform respiratory therapies (e.g., tracheal suctioning) using aseptic technique.

      c.   Assist the client in maintaining respiratory hygiene through deep-breathing and coughing exercises.

  4.   To prevent bacteremias (bacterial infections of blood):

      a.   **Limit invasive procedures whenever possible.**

      b.   **Maintain aseptic technique during invasive procedures.**

      c.   Change IV and intra-arterial fluids and tubing at recommended intervals.

      d.   Assess IV catheter sites for signs of infection.

      e.   Alternate IV catheter sites at recommended intervals.

      f.   Prevent and treat infections at other body sites; microbes from other sites can gain access to vasculature.

C.   **Practice proper handwashing procedures.** *(Thorough handwashing is the most important nursing action to decrease spread of infection.)*

  1.   To wash hands:

      a.   Remove jewelry.

      b.   Use regular soap for routine client care.

      c.   Wash for 10 to 15 seconds under briskly running water for routine client care.

      d.   Keep nails short, and always scrub around and under them.

      e.   Use an antimicrobial product to kill organisms when working with immunocompromised clients or before invasive procedures.

  2.   Be sure to wash your hands:

      a.   Following intense, prolonged client contact

      b.   Before any invasive procedure

      c.   Before and after caring for susceptible clients (e.g., newborns, elderly persons)

      d.   Before and after touching mucous membranes, body fluids, secretions, or excretions—even if gloves were worn

      e.   After contact with objects that likely are contaminated (e.g., urine measuring devices)

      f.   Before entering high-risk units (e.g., intensive care nursery)

      g.   Between direct contacts with different clients

D.   **Institute CDC-recommended precautions in accordance with institution policies.**

    1.   **Wear gloves and other barriers (mask, face shield, impermeable gown) when in contact with, or at risk of contact with, blood or other body fluids and substances.**

    2.   Ensure a private room for:

      a.   Clients with highly communicable or virulent infections

      b.   Clients with poor personal hygiene who are likely to contaminate the environment

    3.   Wear barrier garments to prevent transmitting infection to a client (e.g., an immunosuppressed client at risk for infection)

V.   **General nursing interventions to prevent spread of infectious disease in communities**

  A.   **Perform case finding and reporting.**

  B.   **Provide individual and community teaching.**

    1.   Teach about methods to improve host defenses, including:

      a.   Maintaining adequate nutrition

      b.   Keeping immunizations current

    2.   Teach the importance of chemoprophylaxis (e.g., taking chloroquine when traveling in malaria-infested regions).

    3.   Teach ways to maintain:

      a.   Good hygiene

      b.   Proper sanitation

      c.   Safe meal preparation

      d.   Proper food storage

    4.   Teach guidelines for "safe sex" to prevent STDs.

  C.   **Participate in community immunization programs as possible.**

VI.   **Septicemia and septic shock**

  A.   **Description**

    1.   Septicemia, or sepsis, is a systemic infection of the blood stream producing clinically apparent manifestations.

    2.   **Septic shock is a life-threatening form of shock resulting from uncontrolled septicemia.**

  B.   **Etiology and incidence**

    1.   Septicemia most commonly results from gram-negative bacteria, including *Escherichia coli, Klebsiella, Enterobacter, Pseudomonas aeruginosa, Proteus, Neisseria meningitidis,* and *Bacteroides fragilis.* Gram-positive bacteria—*Staphylococcus aureus* and *Streptococcus pneumoniae*—have been implicated in some cases.

    2. Septicemia can produce septic shock in persons with compromised defenses; approximately 40% of cases of septic shock lead to septicemia.

    3. Risk factors include:
- a. Hospitalization
- b. Invasive procedures
- c. Immunodeficiency
- d. Advanced age
- e. Trauma
- f. Burns
- g. Disorders that result in debilitation

C. **Pathophysiology and management**

    1. The pathophysiology of septic shock is incompletely understood.

    2. It is thought that shock results in reaction to an endotoxin that triggers release of chemical mediators and hormones.

    3. These mediators and hormones cause cardiovascular changes and cellular injury.

    4. Arteriolar and venous spasms cause pooling of blood in pulmonary, renal, splanchnic, and peripheral tissues, leading to tissue anoxia and acidosis.

    5. Intense vasoconstriction increases peripheral resistance, decreases cardiac output, and diminishes blood flow to major organs.

    6. Activation of factor XII of the intrinsic coagulation system can produce intravascular coagulation and fibrinolysis.

    7. Death may occur from vascular collapse.

    8. Septic shock typically occurs in two phases: hyperdynamic and hypodynamic. The sooner the disorder is detected and treated the better the outcome.

D. **Assessment findings**

    1. Septicemia commonly produces fever, chills, prostration, pain, headache, nausea, and diarrhea.

    2. Clinical manifestations of septic shock depend on the stage of shock, causative organism, and client's condition.

    3. Common findings in the hyperdynamic phase include:
- a. Warm, flushed skin
- b. Normal or high urine output
- c. Mild hypotension
- d. Tachycardia
- e. Edema (due to capillary leakage)

    4. Manifestations of the hypodynamic phase include:
- a. Marked hypotension
- b. Cold, dry skin
- c. Oliguria or anuria

    d.   Edema
    e.   Respiratory abnormalities (e.g., apnea, tachypnea)
    f.   Restlessness, confusion secondary to hypoxia
    g.   Altered level of consciousness

  5. Laboratory studies may reveal:
    a.   Causative organism identified on blood cultures
    b.   Metabolic acidosis, indicated by decreased PCO_2, PO_2, HCO_3, and pH
    c.   Clotting abnormalities
    d.   Anemia

E. **Nursing diagnoses**
  1. Decreased Cardiac Output
  2. Impaired Verbal Communication
  3. Ineffective Individual Coping
  4. Fluid Volume Excess
  5. Impaired Gas Exchange
  6. Risk for Infection
  7. Sleep Pattern Disturbance
  8. Altered Tissue Perfusion: Cardiopulmonary

F. **Planning and implementation**
  1. Administer medications and fluids as prescribed to improve cardiac output and tissue perfusion; therapy may include:
    a.   IV fluid replacement
    b.   Inotropic agents which increase myocardial contractility, and vasopressor agents, such as norepinephrine (Levophed), which increases blood pressure

      ▶ Monitor blood pressure and intake and output.
      ▶ Perform essential hemodynamic monitoring.

    c.   Antiinfective agents, such as nafcillin (Unipen), cefazolin (Kefsol), carbenicillin (Geocillin), chloramphenicol (Spectro-Chlor), and gentamicin (Garamycin)

      ▶ Assess for allergies.
      ▶ As appropriate, assess site before and after IV administration.
      ▶ Administer medication around the clock.

    d.   Packed red blood cells, platelets
  2. Take steps to improve gas exchange (see Section III.D).
  3. Explain all procedures to the client to help relieve anxiety.
  4. Encourage the client and family members to communicate feelings and concerns regarding the disorder, its treatment, and possible outcome.
  5. Intervene as indicated to limit blood loss due to clotting abnormalities, including:

a. Protecting the client from trauma that could cause hemorrhage (e.g., bumps, falls)

b. Avoiding venipuncture and other invasive procedures whenever possible

c. Using small-gauge needles when injections and venipuncture are unavoidable

d. Applying firm pressure to venipuncture sites for 3 to 7 minutes; for prolonged bleeding, applying sandbags

e. Preventing the client from coughing, vomiting, or straining with bowel movements

f. Providing assistance with activities of daily living or teaching the client to avoid shaving, brushing with a hard-bristled toothbrush, and flossing

6. Assist an intubated client with communications as needed.

7. Help the client maintain as normal a sleep pattern as possible; keep the room quiet and dimly lit; promote rest and relaxation; cluster necessary procedures to minimize disturbances.

8. Treat and prevent further infection (see Sections III and IV).

G. Evaluation

1. The client exhibits adequate cardiac output and tissue perfusion, as evidenced by:
   a. Normal blood pressure
   b. Warm skin, normal skin color
   c. Normal mentation
   d. Adequate urinary output

2. The client maintains normal fluid balance, as evidenced by:
   a. Elastic skin turgor
   b. Normal blood pressure and heart rate
   c. Absence of venous distention and edema

3. The client maintains adequate gas exchange, as indicated by:
   a. Normal respiratory rate and depth
   b. Normal arterial blood gas values
   c. No dyspnea

4. The client demonstrates the ability to communicate needs, feelings, and concerns.

5. The client is able to sleep uninterrupted for prolonged periods.

6. The client exhibits minimal blood loss.

7. The client remains free from infection.

VII. Gonorrhea: Sexually transmitted disease (STD)

A. Description: a common infection of the genitourinary tract

B. Etiology and incidence

1. The infectious agent is the *Neisseria gonorrhoeae* bacterium.

2. Transmission may occur through:
   a. Sexual intercourse

b. Oral–genital contact

c. Anal–genital contact

3. A newborn may be infected during vaginal delivery.

4. Gonorrhea is a commonly reported communicable disease; incidence is highest in persons aged 15 to 24.

C. **Pathophysiology and management**

1. Short incubation period permits rapid spread.

2. Many disease carriers are asymptomatic.

3. The bacterium generally affects selected epithelial mucous membranes, causing inflammation:

a. Urethritis

b. Cervicitis

c. Proctitis

4. Coinfection with other STDs commonly occurs:

a. AIDS

b. Chlamydia

c. Genital herpes

d. Syphilis

D. **Assessment findings**

1. Common genitourinary manifestations include:

a. In men: dysuria, urethral discharge, prostatitis, urethritis

b. In women: urinary frequency, dysuria, vaginal discharge, pelvic inflammatory disease

2. GI manifestations (most common in homosexual males) may include:

a. Anal itching and irritation

b. Rectal bleeding

c. Diarrhea

d. Painful defecation

3. Oral involvement may produce:

a. Sore throat

b. Lip ulcers

c. Inflamed gingivae

d. Oropharyngeal vesicles

4. Systemic effects (in disseminated gonorrhea) may include:

a. Bacteremia

b. Hemorrhagic skin rash

c. Arthritis

d. Fever

5. Diagnostic tests include:

a. In men: urethral, pharyngeal, anal cultures; gram stain of urethral smears

b. In women: endocervical, anal, pharyngeal cultures

E. **Nursing diagnoses**

1. Risk for Infection

    2. Noncompliance with Treatment and Follow-Up Regimen

    3. Pain

    4. Altered Sexuality Patterns

    5. Social Isolation

    6. Impaired Tissue Integrity

    7. Altered Urinary Elimination

F. **Planning and implementation**

    1. Obtain a complete sexual history, ensuring the client's privacy and covering:

        a. Types of sexual activity engaged in

        b. Number of sexual partners

        c. Previous STDs or exposure to STDs

    2. Minimize social isolation (see Section III.H).

    3. Minimize discomfort through prompt treatment measures which may include:

        a. Administering antiinfective penicillins, such as amoxicillin (Amoxil) and ampicillin (Omnipen), which disturb formation of critical proteins in the bacterial cell wall

        ▶ Assess for drug allergy.

        ▶ **Administer with food to minimize GI upset.**

        ▶ **Instruct client to take all medication exactly as prescribed.**

        b. Administering probenecid (Probalan), which increases serum levels of penicillins and related agents

        ▶ **Instruct client to take food with medication to decrease GI distress.**

        ▶ **Instruct client to drink 8 to 10 glasses of water daily.**

        c. Administering tetracycline, which has bacteriostatic action

        ▶ **Assess for drug allergy.**

        ▶ **Give oral medication on an empty stomach 1 hour before meals with glass of water.**

        ▶ **Do not take within 1–2 hours of having milk products.**

    4. Treat oral or rectal lesions, pharyngitis by:

        a. Instituting prompt antibiotic therapy, as prescribed, with proper follow-up monitoring

        b. Teaching the client to keep affected areas clean

    5. Manage dysuria by instituting prompt antimicrobial therapy and proper follow-up care.

    6. Assist the client in maintaining intimacy with sexual partners through "safe sex" methods such as:

        a. Mutual masturbation

b. Body massage, hugging
c. Using condoms (not 100% effective)
7. Help minimize noncompliance by:
a. Teaching the client reasons for strictly adhering to the treatment and follow-up regimens
b. Treating the client with respect and dignity
c. Ensuring privacy
d. Arranging follow-up appointments at convenient times for the client
8. Teach the client how to prevent spread of disease through:
a. Using forms of safe sex
b. Limiting the number of sex partners and learning the sexual history of potential partners before engaging in sexual contact
c. Referring sex partners for evaluation and treatment
d. Being aware of the high incidence of coinfection with other STDs
e. Seeking follow-up assessment after treatment to prevent recurrence
f. Having periodic check-ups, if sexually active, to identify STDs early
g. Being aware that pregnant women can pass the disease to infants during delivery

G. Evaluation
1. The client maintains social ties without transmitting disease.
2. The client exhibits prompt and complete elimination of symptoms through proper treatment and follow-up.
3. The client complies with the treatment regimen.
4. The client avoids recurrence and other STDs.

VIII. **Staphylococcal infections: specific bacterial infection**
A. **Description: infections caused by pathogenic species of *Staphylococcus*, a gram-positive bacteria; types include bacteremia, pneumonia, enterocolitis, osteomyelitis, food poisoning, and skin infections**
B. **Etiology and incidence**
1. The most common causative bacteria are *Staphylococcus aureus* and *S. epidermis*.
2. Modes of transmission include direct contact, common source, and animal.
3. Persons at greatest risk include those with impaired skin integrity, newborns, and prosthetic heart valves or joints.
C. **Pathophysiology and management**
1. Staphylococci are part of normal flora of the skin and mucous membranes.
2. Staphylococci are widely distributed in air, dust, and fomites.

3. Local involvement may cause skin infections such as boils and abscesses.
4. Systemic involvement may produce:
   a. Bacteremias
   b. Toxic shock syndrome (TSS), associated with menstruation and tampon use
   c. Endocarditis
5. Staphylococci are a common cause of nosocomial infections.
6. *S. epidermidis* is a common cause of infection in clients with intravascular devices.
7. Management involves eradicating the cause.

D. Assessment findings
   1. Skin infection may be manifested by:
      a. Cellulitis
      b. Painful abscesses
      c. Boils
      d. Other skin lesions
   2. Signs and symptoms of food poisoning may include:
      a. Nausea and vomiting
      b. Abdominal cramps
      c. Diarrhea
      d. Anorexia
   3. Invasive infection may produce signs and symptoms of systemic infections such as:
      a. Endocarditis
      b. Meningitis
      c. Arthritis
      d. UTIs
   4. TSS is commonly marked by:
      a. High fever
      b. Diarrhea
      c. Peripheral edema, hypotension, renal failure
      d. Desquamation of skin, especially on soles and palms
      e. Myalgias
   5. Diagnosis is based on culture and gram stain results.

E. Nursing diagnoses
   1. Risk for Altered Body Temperature
   2. Diarrhea
   3. Risk for Infection
   4. Risk for Injury
   5. Pain
   6. Altered Skin Integrity
   7. Altered Tissue Perfusion: Cerebral, Cardiopulmonary, Renal
   8. Altered Urinary Elimination

F.   Planning and implementation
  1.   Intervene to treat fever as indicated (see Section III.F).
  2.   Intervene as appropriate to manage effects of systemic infection (see information on specific infectious disorders in other chapters of this book).
  3.   Intervene as appropriate to minimize pain (see Section III.B).
  4.   Minimize damage to tissue integrity (see Section III.G).
  5.   Intervene as necessary to maintain adequate tissue perfusion (see Section III.D).
  6.   Help minimize transmission of nosocomial infections (see Section IV.B).
  7.   Intervene as necessary to prevent dehydration (see Section III.C)

G.   Evaluation
  1.   The client maintains temperature within normal range without complications.
  2.   The client maintains a normal elimination pattern.
  3.   The client reports no or minimal pain.
  4.   The client maintains or regains integrity of skin and mucous membranes.
  5.   The client maintains adequate tissue perfusion, shown by:
       a.   Adequate blood pressure, urine output
       b.   Normal mentation
       c.   Warm, dry skin of normal color
  6.   The client exhibits minimal blood loss.
  7.   The client demonstrates decreased incidence of nosocomial infections.

IX.   Tuberculosis (TB): specific bacterial infection
  A.   Description: a chronic granulomatous infection that usually affects the pulmonary system but also may invade other organs and tissues
  B.   Etiology and incidence
  1.   Infectious agents include:
       a.   *Mycobacterium tuberculosis*
       b.   *Mycobacterium bovis* (rarely)
  2.   Transmission occurs through inhalation or ingestion of infected droplets from a person with active disease.
  3.   Incidence is highest in crowded, poverty-stricken settings.
  4.   Those at greatest risk include immunocompromised or debilitated persons and persons with a history of previous infection.
  C.   Pathophysiology and management
  1.   Inhaled infected droplets travel to the pulmonary alveoli.
  2.   Here, the bacilli form lesions known as tubercles.

3. Tubercles may heal, leaving scar tissue, or may continue as granuloma, which may heal and may be reactivated later.
4. Granulomas may produce necrosis, liquefaction, sloughing, and cavitation of lung tissue.
5. The initial lesion may disseminate bacilli to other tissues (e.g., kidneys, bones, lymph nodes).
6. Treatment includes medication.

D. Assessment findings

1. In early stages, TB often is without symptoms.
2. Manifestations of advancing TB include:
   a. Fatigue, weight loss
   b. Cough, initially dry, later productive of mucopurulent sputum
   c. Hemoptysis
   d. Fever and chills
3. Diagnostic tests include:
   a. Tuberculin skin test to detect infection
   b. Chest radiograph, sputum sample analysis to identify active disease
   c. Follow-up sputum cultures every 2 to 4 weeks

E. Nursing diagnoses

1. Risk for Altered Body Temperature
2. Ineffective Breathing Pattern
3. Risk for Infection
4. Knowledge Deficit
5. Noncompliance with Treatment Regimen

F. Planning and implementation

1. Take steps to prevent disease transmission, including:
   a. Teaching the client to cover his or her mouth and nose with thick tissue when coughing or sneezing
   b. Ensuring proper disposal of soiled tissues
   c. Emphasizing the importance of handwashing
   d. Instituting TB precautions if the client is hospitalized
2. Provide client and family teaching, covering:
   a. The prescribed medication regimen (typically a 9- to 18-month course); will include one or a combination of the following:

   ▸ **Isoniazid (INH), which inhibits mycobacterial cell wall synthesis; should be administered on an empty stomach and continued as prescribed**
   ▸ **Rifampin (Rifadin), which inhibits RNA synthesis and which is always administered with other antitubercular agents; colors urine, feces, sputum, tears, and sweat red-orange**
   ▸ **Ethambutol (Myambutol), which is usually added as a**

> third agent in resistant disease; may cause changes in visual acuity, perception, and color interpretation, requiring medical attention
>
> ▶ Streptomycin, the initial treatment for suspected resistant or very severe TB; administered by IM injection two to three times a week (check for allergy initially and in follow-up)

    b. The importance of long-term treatment and follow-up care

    c. Possible complications and reportable symptoms (e.g., hemorrhage, pleurisy)

    d. The need to avoid factors that may exacerbate symptoms (e.g., smoking, asbestos, silicone exposure)

    e. The importance of skin testing for family members to identify disease in household contacts

3. Encourage compliance with the prescribed treatment regimen:

    a. Adapt the medication schedule to fit the client's routine as possible.

    b. Be sensitive to the client's situation.

    c. Consult social services to investigate insurance coverage and proper follow-up care.

    d. Help the client minimize medication side effects.

    e. Schedule follow-up appointments at convenient times and places.

    f. Treat the client with dignity and respect.

4. Treat fever as indicated (see Section III.F).

5. Intervene to maintain an effective breathing pattern (see Section III.D).

G. **Evaluation**

  1. The client and family members verbalize measures to help prevent disease transmission.

  2. The client and family members verbalize knowledge of:

    a. Medication regimen

    b. Prevention of disease spread

    c. Recognition of possible complications (e.g., hemorrhage, pleurisy)

  3. The client demonstrates compliance with the medication regimen and follow-up care schedule.

  4. The client maintains normal body temperature.

  5. The client maintains an effective breathing pattern, as evidenced by:

    a. Normal respiratory rate

    b. Regular, nonlabored breathing pattern

    c. Arterial blood gas values within normal ranges

X. Influenza: specific viral infection

   A. **Description: an acute, highly contagious respiratory tract infection**

   B. **Etiology and incidence**

   1. Influenza results from one of three different types of *Myxovirus influenzae,* an RNA myxovirus: Type A, Type B, or Type C.

   2. It usually occurs seasonally in epidemics.

   3. Persons at high risk include young children, elderly persons, persons with chronic diseases, and health care workers.

   C. **Pathophysiology and management**

   1. Infection occurs via droplet transmission from an infected person or by indirect contact (e.g., sharing a contaminated cup).

   2. The infection invades the respiratory tract epithelium, causing inflammation and desquamation; symptoms typically appear after an incubation period of 24 to 72 hours.

   3. Usually a self-limiting disorder, influenza can cause life-threatening complications (e.g., pneumonia) in high-risk persons. Treatment is supportive.

   D. **Assessment findings**

   1. Respiratory manifestations of influenza may include:
      a. Sinusitis
      b. Dyspnea
      c. Sore throat
      d. Nasal stuffiness
      e. Nasal discharge
      f. Dry cough

   2. Other common signs and symptoms include fever, chills, malaise, headache, and myalgias.

   E. **Nursing diagnoses**

   1. Activity Intolerance
   2. Risk for Altered Body Temperature
   3. Ineffective Breathing Pattern
   4. Risk for Infection

   F. **Planning and implementation**

   1. Provide client and family teaching, covering:
      a. Infection prevention measures (see Sections III, IV, and V)

      b. **The importance of annual vaccination for persons at high risk**

   2. Intervene to treat fever when indicated (see Section III.F).

   3. Administer amantadine (Symmtral) to high-risk persons as prophylaxis for influenza A

      a.   **Instruct client how to prevent orthostatic hypotension.**

      b.   **Instruct client to take as directed and not to discontinue abruptly.**

    4.   Take steps to improve breathing patterns, which may include:

      a.   Helping the client relax and positioning him or her properly to ease breathing

      b.   Providing room vaporization and administering antitussive agents for cough and decongestants for nasal stuffiness and secretions

      c.   Encouraging increased fluid intake to liquefy secretions (and to replace fluid losses from fever)

    5.   Encourage adequate rest periods.

G. **Evaluation**

    1.   The client avoids infection.

    2.   The client maintains normal body temperature.

    3.   The client exhibits normal breathing pattern.

    4.   The client regains normal activity tolerance.

XI. **Rocky Mountain spotted fever: specific rickettsial infection**

  A. **Description: a potentially fatal, tick-borne infectious disease marked by fever and skin rash and possibly leading to shock and renal failure**

  B. **Etiology and incidence**

    1.   The infectious agent—*Rickettsia rickettsii*—is transmitted by the dog tick (*Dermacentor variabilis*), wood tick (*Dermacentor andersoni*), and other tick species in the United States.

    2.   Common reservoirs include dogs, rodents, and wild animals.

    3.   Incidence is highest in the south-central and south Atlantic regions of the United States and peaks in early summer.

  C. **Pathophysiology and management**

    1.   The infectious agent reproduces in the endothelium of small and medium-sized blood vessels, causing widespread swelling and degeneration.

    2.   This generalized vasculitis produces disease symptoms, which may involve multiple body organs and systems.

  D. **Assessment findings**

    1.   Clinical manifestations include:

      a.   Malaise, lethargy, stupor

      b.   Severe headache

      c.   Photophobia

      d.   Anorexia

      e.   High, continuous fever with chills

      f.   Rash on extremities, spreading medially (usually occurring on the third to fifth day after onset)

g.   Possible skin necrosis, especially of the ear lobes, scrotum, toes, and fingers
h.   Generalized edema
i.   Myalgia, arthralgia, abdominal pain
j.   Splenomegaly
2.   Laboratory findings may include:
a.   Thrombocytopenia
b.   Coagulation defects
c.   Serologic confirmation of infection

E.   Nursing diagnoses
1.   Risk for Altered Body Temperature
2.   Risk for Infection
3.   Pain
4.   Impaired Skin Integrity

F.   Planning and implementation
1.   Teach preventive measures, including:
a.   Inspecting the skin frequently for ticks when in high-risk areas
b.   Tick removal (flicking an unattached tick off the skin; removing an attached tick with tweezers, grasping it close to the attachment point)
c.   Washing hands and the attachment site immediately after tick removal
2.   Administer medications as prescribed, which may include:
a.   Tetracycline, which has bacteriostatic action and inhibits bacterial protein synthesis and which should be given on an empty stomach 1 hour before meals (assess for drug allergy initially and at follow-up) and 1–2 hours after having milk products
b.   Chloramphenicol (Chloromycetin), a synthetic antiinfective which may produce serious toxic side effects (limiting its use to severe infections)

> ► Instruct client to take drug on empty stomach.
> ► Question prescription that calls for therapy exceeding 14 days.
> ► Teach client to recognize signs of bone marrow depression (bleeding, sore throat, oral mucosal lesions, pallor) and to report them to physician at once.

3.   Intervene to reduce fever as indicated (see Section III.F).
4.   Intervene as appropriate to minimize pain (see Section III.B).
5.   Intervene to minimize damage to skin (see Section III.G).

G.   Evaluation
1.   The client verbalizes knowledge of appropriate preventive measures.
2.   The client maintains body temperature within normal range.

      3.   The client reports minimal or no discomfort.

      4.   The client exhibits resolution of rash without complications.

XII. Candidiasis: specific fungal infection

A. Description: a variable fungal infection producing superficial mucocutaneous and, less commonly, serious systemic manifestations

B. Etiology and incidence

1. Infectious agents are those of the *Candida* genus (e.g., *Candida albicans*, *Candida tropicalis*).
2. These organisms commonly are part of the normal flora of the GI tract, vagina, mouth, and skin.
3. They can cause infection when some change in the body triggers proliferation or systemic invasion; such factors may include:
   a. Immunosuppression
   b. Invasive procedures
   c. Use of broad-spectrum antibiotics
   d. Hyperglycemia
   e. Debilitation
4. A mother with vaginal candidiasis can pass the infection on to her infant during vaginal delivery.

C. Pathophysiology and management

1. Candidiasis usually is a mild, superficial infection affecting the skin, mucous membranes, or nails.
2. Rarely, organisms enter the blood stream and invade deep organs (e.g., meninges, lungs, endocardium), causing serious infection that possibly can lead to shock and death.

D. Assessment findings

1. Manifestations of oral candidiasis (thrush) include:
   a. Creamy, white, curdlike patches on tongue, oral mucosa
   b. Painful, bleeding lesions, especially if patches are scraped
2. Candida esophagitis is marked by:
   a. Painful swallowing, feeling of obstruction with swallowing
   b. Substernal chest discomfort
   c. Nausea and vomiting
3. Signs and symptoms of Candida vaginitis include:
   a. Discharge: scanty to moderate amount, thick, white, curdlike
   b. Severe vulvar pruritus
   c. Vaginal and labial erythema
   d. Symptoms of secondary urethral infection
4. Manifestations of disseminated candidiasis commonly include high fever, chills, hypotension, prostration, and possibly rash; other signs and symptoms depend on the site of infection:

      a.   Pulmonary: hemoptysis, cough

      b.   Renal: flank pain, dysuria, hematuria, pyuria

      c.   Brain: headache, nuchal rigidity, seizures, focal neurologic deficits

      d.   Endocardium: heart murmur, chest pain

      e.   Eye: blurred vision, pain, scotoma, exudate

  5. Diagnosis is based on:

      a.   Tissue culture

      b.   Histologic examination of biopsy specimen

E. **Nursing diagnoses**

  1. Decreased Cardiac Output

  2. Risk for Infection

  3. Altered Nutrition: Less Than Body Requirements

  4. Altered Oral Mucous Membrane

  5. Pain

  6. Impaired Tissue Integrity

  7. Altered Tissue Perfusion

F. **Planning and implementation**

  1. Alleviate pain as indicated (see Section III.B).

  2. Relieve pruritus, as necessary, by:

      a.   **Administering antipruritic medication, such as diphenhydramine (Benadryl), which prevents initiation and transmission of nerve impulses thereby decreasing itching (Advise client that drowsiness may occur initially but usually subsides with continued use.)**

      b.   Applying cool compresses to affected areas

      c.   Keeping affected areas clean, dry, and open to air (if possible)

  3. Institute measures to prevent infection: oral, esophageal, disseminated (see Section IV).

  4. Teach client to prevent vaginal candidiasis by:

      a.   Encouraging her to have sex partners checked for infection and to use condoms to prevent transmission

      b.   Avoiding tight-fitting underwear and pants

      c.   Avoiding synthetic underwear; wear cotton ones instead

      d.   Practicing good perineal hygiene

  5. Promote good nutrition by:

      a.   Assessing for signs and symptoms of undernutrition: malaise, fatigue, nausea, vomiting (risk factors); physical and biochemical indices of malnourishment

      b.   Observing for decrease in intake or loss of interest in food

      c.   Encouraging a high-calorie, high-protein diet

      d.   Monitoring weight

       e.   Encouraging small, frequent meals, especially if the client is fatigued or nauseated

       f.   Administering antiemetics as necessary

       g.   Administering total parenteral nutrition or tube feedings, if indicated

6. Help the client maintain oral mucosal integrity by:

       a.   Promoting frequent, thorough mouth care

       b.   Instructing the client to avoid alcohol-containing mouthwashes, which dry the mucosa and can cause pain

       c.   Administering topical antifungal agents as needed

       d.   Observing for signs of disseminated infection

7. Promote good skin integrity by:

       a.   Applying topical antifungal agents as prescribed

       b.   Keeping affected areas clean, dry, and open to air

       c.   Observing for signs of disseminated infection

8. Intervene as necessary to maintain adequate cardiac output and tissue perfusion.

9. Administer prescribed medications, which may include:

       a.   Nystatin (Nystex), miconazole (Monistat), or ketoconazole (Nizoral) for mucocutaneous candidiasis

         ▶ **Teach client who is taking oral medication to clean mouth before taking drug, then swish and swallow.**

         ▶ **Instruct client to wash hands before and after applying vaginal medication.**

         ▶ **Tell client to continue drug as prescribed to prevent reinfection (usually for 1 to 2 weeks after symptoms subside).**

       b.   Amphotericin B (Fungizone) for disseminated or deep organ candidiasis

         ▶ **Monitor IV administration closely.**

         ▶ **Be alert for signs and symptoms of renal damage.**

         ▶ **Monitor client's potassium, calcium, magnesium, and liver enzyme levels regularly.**

G. **Evaluation**

  1. The client reports minor or no discomfort.

  2. The client reports reduced pruritus.

  3. The client avoids infection or reinfection and doesn't spread infection to others.

  4. The client maintains adequate nutritional status.

  5. The client displays intact oral mucosa that returns to normal state without complications.

  6. The client maintains intact skin that returns to normal state without complications.

7. The client maintains adequate tissue perfusion and cardiac output.

XIII. Malaria: specific protozoal infection

A. Description: a serious infectious disease caused by protozoa transmitted to the blood stream through mosquito vectors

B. Etiology and incidence

1. Malaria is caused by protozoa of the genus *Plasmodium;* species include *Plasmodium falciparum, P. vivax, P. malariae,* and *P. ovale.*

2. The organism usually is transmitted to humans through the bite of the female *Anopheles* mosquito.

3. Other modes of transmission include:
   a. Transfusion of infected blood
   b. Parenteral inoculation (e.g., sharing contaminated needles)
   c. Placental leak during delivery

4. Malaria affects over 300 million people worldwide; it is endemic in tropical and subtropical climates.

C. Pathophysiology and management

1. After injection, *Plasmodium* sporozoites migrate through the blood stream to parenchymal liver cells.

2. Cystlike structures are formed; these contain merozoites, which invade erythrocytes, engulf hemoglobin, and eventually cause cell rupture.

3. Erythrocyte rupture releases heme (malaria pigment), cell debris, and more merozoites that, unless destroyed by phagocytosis, enter other erythrocytes.

4. An infected person then becomes a reservoir of malaria whose blood can transmit the disease to others through mosquito vectors.

5. Hepatic parasites may persist for years, producing a chronic carrier state.

6. Prognosis is good with treatment; if untreated, however, malaria can prove fatal—most commonly from disseminated intravascular coagulation or other serious complications.

D. Assessment findings

1. Common clinical manifestations include:
   a. Fever and chills, usually following a characteristic pattern of recurrence every 48 to 72 hours (depending on protozoan species)
   b. Diaphoresis
   c. Effects of pancytopenia

2. Uncomplicated malaria also may produce such signs and symptoms as nausea, fatigue, malaise, dizziness, headache, and myalgias accompanying recurrent fever.

3. Severe infections (usually associated with *P. falciparum*) may be marked by:
   a. Anemia
   b. Jaundice
   c. Renal insufficiency
   d. Adult respiratory distress syndrome (ARDS)
   e. Hemoglobinuria
   f. Diarrhea
   g. Coma
4. Relapses are common and may recur for several years.
5. Diagnosis is confirmed by identification of *Plasmodium* parasites in peripheral blood.

E. Nursing diagnoses
   1. Risk for Altered Body Temperature
   2. Risk for Infection
   3. Knowledge Deficit
   4. Pain

F. Planning and implementation
   1. Teach prevention techniques to persons traveling to areas where malaria is endemic, including:
      a. Remaining in screened areas whenever possible and using mosquito nets when outdoors
      b. Using insect repellent
      c. Staying indoors during mosquitoes' most active feeding period (dusk until dawn)
      d. **Taking a prophylactic antimalarial agent, such as chloroquine (Aralen), with meals to decrease GI distress, reporting any visual or hearing changes to physician, and avoiding prolonged sun exposure**
      e. Wearing clothing that covers most of the body
   2. Teach strategies for prevention of disease spread, such as:
      a. Urging travelers to high-risk areas to seek prompt medical advice for flulike symptoms
      b. Instructing travelers to malaria-ridden areas to refrain from donating blood for up to 3 years following exposure
   3. Teach about prescribed drug therapy, including the agent, dosage schedule, duration (usually 3 to 14 days depending on the agent), and possible side effects.
   4. Provide other nursing interventions to reduce fever, minimize discomfort, and address other symptoms (see Section III).

G. Evaluation
   1. The client states appropriate measures to prevent exposure to or infection with the malaria parasite.

2. The client verbalizes understanding of early signs and symp-
    toms and treatment of malaria.
3. The client maintains normal body temperature.
4. The client reports minimal or no discomfort.
5. The client verbalizes understanding of measures to prevent
    transmission of infectious disease to other persons.

XIV. Ascariasis: specific helminthic infection

**A. Description: a parasitic infection caused by roundworm infesta-
    tion**

B. Etiology and incidence

1. The infectious organism is *Ascaris lumbricoides,* a large
    roundworm (15 to 35 cm long).
2. Infection is transmitted by ingesting ova contained in conta-
    minated food, water, or soil. Direct person-to-person trans-
    mission does not occur.
3. Ascariasis occurs worldwide but is most common in tropical
    regions with poor sanitation and in Asia, where many farmers
    use human feces for crop fertilization.

C. Pathophysiology and management

1. After ingestion, *A. lumbricoides* ova hatch and release larvae,
    which penetrate the intestinal wall and travel through the
    blood stream to the lungs and heart.
2. In the lungs, larvae penetrate alveoli and move up the respira-
    tory tree to the pharynx.
3. From the pharynx, larvae are swallowed; they then travel
    through the GI tract back to the small intestine, where they
    mature into worms. This entire process takes about 3
    months.
4. The life span of *A. lumbricoides* is approximately $1\frac{1}{2}$ years.
5. Heavy infestation can cause obstruction of the trachea, intes-
    tine, bile duct, pancreatic duct, or appendix, producing severe
    pain and other symptoms.
6. Management focuses on prevention and drug therapy.

D. Assessment findings

1. Some infections are asymptomatic.
2. Large numbers of worms in the intestine may produce severe
    cramping pain and nausea and vomiting.
3. Invasion of the lungs is commonly marked by dyspnea, fever
    and chills, cough, pneumonia.
4. Eosinophilia commonly occurs during the larval stage.
5. Ascariasis is confirmed by ova or adult worms in stool.

E. Nursing diagnoses

1. Impaired Gas Exchange
2. Risk for Infection

        3.   Altered Nutrition: Less than body requirements

        4.   Pain

F.   **Planning and implementation**

        1.   Teach preventive measures to people traveling to high-risk areas, including:

            a.   Practicing good personal hygiene

            b.   Avoiding ingestion of contaminated food or water

        2.   Intervene to minimize discomfort, improve gas exchange, and improve nutrition (see Section III).

        3.   Administer prescribed medications, which may include:

            a.   Piperazine citrate (Antepar), which paralyzes the parasite

      ▶ **Advise client that laxatives, enemas, or dietary restrictions are unnecessary.**

      ▶ **Instruct client to notify physician if muscular weakness, tremors, nausea or vomiting, or abdominal cramps occur.**

            b.   Mebendazole (Vermox), which depletes the glycogen that the parasites need for survival (the tablet form may be chewed, swallowed whole, or crushed and mixed with food)

            c.   Pyrantel pamoate, which paralyzes the worms, may be given with milk, fruit juice, or food; laxatives, enemas, or dietary restrictions are unnecessary.

G.   **Evaluation**

        1.   The client avoids or exhibits resolution of roundworm infection.

        2.   The client states the importance of early identification and prompt treatment of infection.

        3.   The client reports minor or no discomfort.

        4.   The client demonstrates adequate gas exchange.

        5.   The client maintains adequate nutrition.

Bibliography

Bolander, V. R. (1994). *Sorensen and Luckmann's basic nursing: A physiologic approach* (3rd ed.). Philadelphia: W. B. Saunders.

Clark, J., Queener, S., & Karb, V. (1990). *Pharmacologic basis of nursing practice* (4th ed.). St. Louis: C. V. Mosby.

Gorbach, S. L., Bartlett, J. G., & Blacklow, N. R. (1992). *Infectious diseases.* Philadelphia: W. B. Saunders.

Hoeprich, P. D., Jordan, M. C., & Ronald, A. R. (1994). *Infectious diseases* (5th ed.). Philadelphia: J. B. Lippincott.

Nettina, S. (1996). *The Lippincott manual of nursing practice* (6th ed.). Philadelphia: Lippincott-Raven Publishers.

Porth, C. M. (1992). *Pathophysiology: Concepts of altered health states* (4th ed.). Philadelphia: J. B. Lippincott.

Smeltzer, S. C., & Bare, B. G. (1996). *Brunner and Suddarth's textbook of medical-surgical nursing* (8th ed.). Philadelphia: Lippincott-Raven Publishers.

Springhouse Corporation. (1992). *Nursing student's guide to drugs.* Spring House, PA: Springhouse Corp.

STUDY QUESTIONS

1. The nurse discovers a sputum sample at a client's bedside. The sample is dated with today's date, along with the client's name and identification number, but there is no time marked on it. What should the nurse do in this situation?
   a. Send the sample to the clinical laboratory immediately.
   b. Discard the sample, and collect another one as soon as possible.
   c. Send the sample to the clinical laboratory immediately, but call the laboratory to tell them that the collection time is unknown.
   d. Refrigerate the sample, and call the clinical laboratory to pick up the specimen as soon as possible.

2. The nurse would assess which of the following signs and symptoms of the male client with suspected gonorrhea?
   a. dysuria, urethral discharge, and urethritis
   b. warm flushed skin, chills, and prostration
   c. painful abscesses, skin lesions, and cellulitis
   d. malaise, headache, and myalgias

3. When planning care for a client in a health care facility, the nurse must be aware that a nosocomial infection
   a. occurs only in immunocompromised hosts
   b. occurs in at least 30% of clients in a given hospital
   c. usually is present within a community but is not always clinically apparent
   d. is acquired in a health care facility

4. Nursing interventions for the client with elevated body temperature secondary to an infectious process would include
   a. sponging the client's body with ice water
   b. encouraging decreased fluid intake

   c. administering antipyretic medications
   d. applying heavy and restrictive garments

5. Which of the following interventions are recommended to prevent nosocomial wound infections?
   a. Shave hair 24 hours before surgical procedure.
   b. Change dressings on closed wounds every 6 hours.
   c. Do not change IV and intra-arterial fluids and tubing unless the client exhibits signs of infection.
   d. Maintain asepsis during surgery by limiting personnel movement in and out of the OR.

6. In a neonatal intensive care unit, which of the following actions should the nurse perform before caring for clients?
   a. Wash hands using a new bar of soap.
   b. Soak all rings in isopropyl alcohol for 5 minutes.
   c. Don sterile gloves instead of washing hands.
   d. Scrub around and under nails.

7. Which of the following would most likely be a major nursing diagnosis for a person in the hypodynamic phase of septic shock and would require prompt intervention?
   a. Ineffective Individual Coping
   b. Altered Urinary Elimination
   c. Decreased Cardiac Output
   d. Risk for Infection

8. A client with septicemia is at risk for coagulation defects. Specific indicators of minimal blood loss would include
   a. blood pressure of 102/64 mmHg
   b. hematocrit of 42
   c. tented skin turgor
   d. heart rate of 135 beats per minute

9. Which of the following behaviors show that a client understands measures that may prevent him or her from acquiring influenza?

a. The client covers nose and mouth with a handkerchief when sneezing or coughing.

b. The client takes prophylactic antibiotics.

c. The client receives the appropriate flu vaccine each year.

d. The client asks to have a throat culture done to detect infection.

10. Which of the following instructions should the nurse give to a person planning a backpacking trip in an area known to have ticks that carry organisms causing Rocky Mountain spotted fever?

a. Inspect the face and hands frequently for ticks.

b. When an unattached tick is found on the skin, flick it off.

c. When an attached tick is found, remove it by crushing it between your fingernails.

d. When an attached tick is found, remove it by rubbing soap on it.

11. Which of the following statements would indicate that a client does not have the knowledge necessary to prevent recurrent vaginal candidiasis?

a. "I douche regularly with a vinegar preparation."

b. "I now wear only cotton underwear."

c. "I have stopped using oral contraceptives."

d. "My boyfriend now wears a condom when we have vaginal intercourse."

12. While on a trip to a tropical region, the nurse determines that a traveling companion is at risk for malaria because the friend

a. takes prophylactic chloroquine

b. wears long-sleeved shirts and pants

c. seems to nap often

d. takes frequent evening walks

13. A 68-year-old client has just been admitted with uncontrolled diabetes and congestive heart failure. What actions should the nurse take to minimize this client's risk of nosocomial infection?

a. Insert a urinary catheter as soon as possible.

b. Monitor PO_2 and other arterial blood gas values every 30 minutes.

c. Change IV catheter sites only when they become infected.

d. Teach and assist the client to perform coughing and deep-breathing exercises frequently.

14. The client asks the nurse, "How does someone get tuberculosis?" The nurse's best response would be

a. "Tuberculosis is transmitted by breathing air containing droplets from another person infected with TB."

b. "You can only get tuberculosis through blood transfusions."

c. "Tuberculosis can be transmitted through sexual intercourse."

d. "Frequent handwashing can prevent the spread of tuberculosis."

15. When assessing a person with suspected ascariasis, which of the following findings would the nurse expect to find?

a. severe headache and photophobia

b. creamy, white, curdlike patches on tongue

c. history of exposure to animal bites

d. abdominal cramping, nausea and vomiting

ANSWER KEY

1. **Correct response: b**
   Prompt delivery and analysis of microbiologic specimens is essential. Because the specimen had set for an unknown period, it must be discarded.
   a, c, and d. These actions would be inappropriate; another sample must be obtained.
   Application/Safe care/Planning

2. **Correct response: a**
   Common genitourinary manifestations of gonorrhea in men include dysuria, urethral discharge, prostatitis, and urethritis.
   b. These are signs and symptoms of septicemia or septic shock.
   c. These are signs and symptoms of a bacterial infection.
   d. These are signs and symptoms of a viral infection.
   Knowledge/Physiologic/Assessment

3. **Correct response: d**
   Nosocomial infections are those that are acquired during hospitalization.
   a. Nosocomial infections can occur in immunocompromised persons as well as in persons with normal immune systems.
   b. Although there can be multiple cases of nosocomial infections within an institution, they can also occur in a single client.
   c. An endemic infection is one that is usually present within a community but is not always clinically apparent.
   Knowledge/Physiologic/Planning

4. **Correct response: c**
   Antipyretic agents will affect the thermoregulatory center of the brain, resulting in diaphoresis and vasodilation, thereby decreasing temperature.
   a, b, and d. The body should be sponged with tepid water, fluid intake should be increased, and heavy or restrictive clothing should be removed.
   Application/Physiologic/Implementation

5. **Correct response: d**
   Maintaining asepsis during surgery by limiting personnel movement in and out of the OR helps to prevent surgical wound infection.
   a. Preoperative hair removal should be avoided when possible but, if necessary, should be done immediately before surgery using clippers or depilatories.
   b. Dressings over closed wounds should be changed only when wet or if signs and symptoms of infection develop.
   c. IV and intra-arterial fluids and tubing should be changed at recommended intervals and not after infection has occurred.
   Knowledge/Health promotion/Planning

6. **Correct response: d**
   Proper handwashing includes scrubbing the nails thoroughly.
   a. In special care units, an antimicrobial cleanser should be used instead of plain soap.
   b. Jewelry should be removed before washing hands.
   c. Wearing gloves is not a substitute for handwashing.
   Application/Safe care/Planning

7. **Correct response: c**
   Although ineffective coping may occur, especially in earlier stages of septicemia, the hypodynamic phase represents a grave situation in which the client may be obtunded or comatose. Septicemia may have begun as a UTI, but at the hypodynamic stage, the UTI is not likely to be a major problem. Oliguria is the probable alteration in urinary elimination. Although the client with sepsis is at risk for potential, additional infections, the major problem is complications of existing infection.
   a, b, and d. These diagnoses, although possibly pertinent, would most likely be lower in priority than

Decreased Cardiac Output for this client.

Comprehension/Physiologic/ Analysis (Dx)

8. **Correct response: b**
   Hematocrit indicates the percentage of total blood volume comprised by cells; normal value is approximately 45%.
   a, c, and d. These answers represent abnormal values. The blood pressure should be above 110/70, the skin turgor should be elastic, and heart rate should be between 80 and 100 beats per minute.

Application/Physiologic/Evaluation

9. **Correct response: c**
   Vaccination is the best method of protecting against infection.
   a. Covering the nose and mouth when sneezing or coughing will protect others but will not protect the client from getting the flu.
   b. Antibiotics, which work against bacteria, will not be effective against the influenza virus.
   d. Submitting to diagnostic procedures will not prevent the client from contracting influenza.

Application/Health promotion/ Evaluation

10. **Correct response: b**
    Unattached ticks should be removed by flicking them off the skin.
    a. Ticks are most likely to burrow into skin in warm, moist areas of the body, including the scalp. The face and hands are less likely areas of burrowing.
    c. Attached ticks should never be crushed because crushing may expose broken skin to contaminated tick secretions. Rather, they should be removed with tweezers.
    d. Rubbing soap on an attached tick will not help remove it.

Comprehension/Health promotion/ Implementation

11. **Correct response: a**
    Douches have not been shown to be effective against recurrent vaginitis.
    b. Cotton underwear is recommended because cotton is more absorbent than synthetic fabrics and thus keeps the perineal area drier.
    c. Since oral contraceptive use is associated with increased incidence of recurrent candidiasis, many practitioners recommend alternative birth control.
    d. Condom use lessens the chance of transmitting the fungus between sexual partners.

Application/Health promotion/ Evaluation

12. **Correct response: d**
    Because mosquitoes feed at night, being out after dusk increases the risk of acquiring the disease.
    a. Prophylactic chloroquine is an appropriate intervention to prevent infection.
    b. Wearing clothes that cover most of the body helps prevent infection.
    c. Fatigue is a symptom of infection but does not indicate increased risk for infection.

Analysis/Health promotion/Assessment

13. **Correct response: d**
    This intervention prevents nosocomial pneumonias.
    a. For this client, urinary catheterization should be avoided whenever possible.
    b. Frequent invasive procedures increase risk of nosocomial bacteremias.
    c. IV sites should be changed at regular intervals and when signs of infection occur.

Application/Physiologic/Implementation

14. **Correct response: a**
    Transmission of tuberculosis occurs through inhalation or ingestion of infected droplets from a person with active disease.

b and c. These are not routes of transmission for TB.

d. Handwashing will not prevent the spread of TB.

Comprehension/Health Promotion/ Implementation

15. Correct response: d

Although some ascariasis infections are asymptomatic, worms in the intestines usually cause severe abdominal cramping and nausea and vomiting. Invasion of the lungs results in dyspnea, fever, chills, and cough.

a. These are signs and symptoms of Rocky Mountain spotted fever.

b. These are signs oral candidiasis (thrush).

c. Ascariasis is not transmitted through animal bites.

Analysis/Physiologic/Assessment

Cancer Nursing

I. Overview of cancer

A. Description

1. Cancer is the general name given to a large group of diseases characterized by:
   a. Uncontrolled growth and spread of abnormal cells
   b. Proliferation: rapid reproduction by cell division
   c. Invasion: growth of primary tumor into surrounding tissue
   d. Metastasis: spread or transfer of cancer cells from one organ or part to another not directly connected
2. Many cancers are now theorized to be multifocal or systemic (e.g., breast cancer); however, no one theory is proven.
3. The metastatic process may be divided into three stages:
   a. Invasion of neoplastic cells from primary tumor into surrounding tissue with penetration of blood or lymph; occurs because cells are not encapsulated
   b. Spread of tumor cells through lymph or circulation or by direct expansion
   c. Establishment and growth of tumor cells at secondary site; either in lymph filter (lymph nodes) or in organs from venous circulation

B. Theory of pathogenesis

1. Healthy cells are transformed by unknown mechanisms on exposure to certain etiologic agents, including:
   a. Viruses (e.g., Epstein-Barr, herpes simplex type II, cytomegalovirus, papillomavirus, hepatitis B)
   b. Chemical carcinogens (e.g., chromium, cobalt, tar, soot, asphalt, nitrogen mustards, certain plastics, aniline dyes, hydrocarbons in cigarette smoke, air pollutants from industry, crude paraffin oil, fuel oils, nickel, asbestos, and arsenicals)
   c. Physical stressors (e.g., excessive exposure to sunlight or radiation, chronic irritation)
   d. Hormonal factors (e.g., imbalance of endogenous or exogenous hormones, such as estrogen or diethylstilbestrol [DES])
   e. Genetic factors (e.g., abnormal chromosome patterns, such as Burkitt's lymphoma, chronic myelogenous or acute leukemia, and skin cancers; or familial predisposition, such as in breast, endometrial, colorectal, stomach, and lung cancer)
2. Cancer development is closely linked to immune system failure, as evidenced by:
   a. Increased incidence of malignancy in organ transplant recipients who receive immunosuppressive therapy

b. Increased risk for developing secondary cancers in clients receiving long-term chemotherapy to treat a primary malignancy

3. Cancer occurrence typically reflects a combination of genetic inheritance, host mechanisms, and environmental influences.

II. Neoplasms

A. Proliferative patterns

1. Benign and malignant cells display different characteristics of cellular growth; the degree of differentiation (anaplasia) determines cells' malignant potential.

2. *Hyperplasia* involves an increase in the number of cells in a tissue; may be a normal or an abnormal cellular response.

3. *Metaplasia* refers to the conversion of one type of cell in a tissue to another type not normal for that tissue. It results from an outside stimulus affecting parent stem cells and may be reversible or progress to dysplasia.

4. *Dysplasia* refers to a change in size, shape, or arrangement of normal cells into bizarre cells; may precede an irreversible neoplastic change.

5. *Anaplasia* involves a change in the structure of cells and in their orientation to one another, characterized by a loss of differentiation and a return to a more primitive form. The resulting poorly differentiated, irregularly shaped cells are nearly always malignant.

6. *Neoplasia* refers to abnormal benign or malignant cell growth.
   a. Benign neoplasm: usually harmless, does not infiltrate other tissues
   b. Malignant neoplasm: always harmful; may spread or metastasize to tissues far from the original site

B. Characteristics of normal cells

1. The replicative cell cycle is divided into the following intervals:
   a. G0: resting phase
   b. G1: cellular production of RNA and protein in preparation for DNA synthesis; length of phase dependent on cell type
   c. S: synthesis of DNA and proteins; phase length typically 6 to 8 hours
   d. G2: RNA synthesis in preparation for mitosis; lasts only a few hours
   e. M: mitosis (cell division), resulting in two daughter cells; duration ranges from 1 to several hours

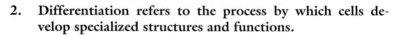

2. **Differentiation refers to the process by which cells develop specialized structures and functions.**

3. Normal cells spread until they make contact with other cells, at which point growth stops (contact inhibition).

4. Normal cells contribute in some way to homeostasis.

C. **Characteristics of neoplastic cells**

1. Neoplastic cells typically appear larger than normal cells, with bigger nuclei. They may bear little resemblance to the normal tissue cells.

2. These cells exhibit uncontrolled proliferation with no contact inhibition.

3. Neoplastic cells serve no homeostatic function.

D. **Characteristics of neoplastic tumors**

1. Neoplastic tumors are disorganized, irregular nests or sheets of neoplastic cells.

2. They tend to flourish in antagonistic physical, chemical, hormonal, and viral environments.

3. Tumors contain a high percentage of proliferating cells.

4. Approximately 20 doublings of tumor cells must occur to produce a 1-mm tumor—the smallest mass clinically detectable.

5. Some tumors have the ability to metastasize—spread from the original site to distant organs. Certain types of tumors are more likely to metastasize to certain sites.

III. **Epidemiology**

A. **Incidence**

1. The number of reported cancer cases has increased steadily since 1900; factors contributing to this rise include:
   a. Increasingly precise diagnostic methods
   b. Better gathering, analysis, and publication of statistics
   c. Increased life span (Older persons are more vulnerable to cancer because of accumulated years of exposure to carcinogens.)

2. Currently in the United States, more than 1 million new cases of cancer are diagnosed annually.

3. Cancer affects every age group, but more than 50% of cancers occur in persons older than age 65.

4. Men experience a higher overall incidence than women.

5. Cancer incidence is higher in industrialized nations of the world and in industrial sectors of more developed countries.

B. **Mortality**

1. **Cancers are second only to cardiovascular diseases as the leading cause of death in the United States.**

2. In order of frequency, leading causes of cancer deaths include:
   a. In men: cancers of the lung, colon or rectum, and prostate
   b. In woman: cancers of the lung, breast, and colon or rectum

C. **Survival**

1. **A person exhibiting no evidence of disease for at least 5 years after diagnosis usually is considered cured; however, some cancers may require longer periods of scrutiny.**
2. Generally, 5-year survival rates have increased since the 1940s.
3. Current statistics reveal encouraging survival trends in certain cancers, including:
   a. Acute lymphocytic leukemia in children
   b. Hodgkin's disease
   c. Burkitt's lymphoma
   d. Ewing's sarcoma
   e. Wilms' tumor
   f. Rhabdomyosarcoma
   g. Choriocarcinoma
   h. Testicular cancer
   i. Ovarian cancer
   j. Osteogenic sarcoma
4. Unfortunately, survival rates have not improved significantly for some major cancers (e.g., lung and colon).

IV. Prevention and detection

A. **Early detection**

1. **Recognizing early signs and symptoms and seeking prompt treatment can significantly reduce morbidity and mortality of several types of cancer.**
2. Cancer's seven early warning signals include:
   a. Change in bowel or bladder habits
   b. A sore that does not heal
   c. Unusual bleeding or discharge
   d. Thickening of lump in breast or elsewhere
   e. Indigestion or difficulty in swallowing
   f. Obvious change in wart or mole
   g. Nagging cough or hoarseness

B. **Primary prevention**

1. **Cancer prevention focuses on reducing risk factors—factors in the external and internal environment that increase a persons' susceptibility to cancer development.**
2. General factors that influence cancer incidence and mortality include:
   a. Sex
   b. Age
   c. Geographic location
   d. Socioeconomic status
   e. Ethnic or cultural background

   f.   Personal habits
   g.   Occupation
   h.   Personal and family health histories
3. Specific risk factors vary with the type of cancer and include:
   a.   Breast cancer: age, familial history in mother or sisters, precancerous condition on breast biopsy, obesity, first pregnancy after age 30, nulliparous status
   b.   Colorectal cancer: colorectal polyps, family history of colorectal cancer, inflammatory bowel disease, high-fat and low-fiber diet
   c.   Lung cancer: cigarette smoking, involuntary smoke inhalation, occupational exposures such as asbestos
   d.   Cervical cancer: early age at first intercourse, multiple sexual partners, human papilloma virus (HPV) infection (condyloma or warts), smoking
   e.   Endometrial cancer: obesity, prolonged use of unopposed postmenopausal estrogens, hypertension, diabetes
   f.   Urinary tract or bladder cancer: smoking, exposure to chemical carcinogen, family history of bladder cancer
   g.   Oral cancer: smoking and alcohol use, use of smokeless tobacco
   h.   Prostate cancer: no known risk factors
   i.   Skin cancer: fair skin, sun exposure, severe sunburn in childhood, and familial conditions such as dysplastic nevus syndrome
4. Risk reduction involves specific actions aimed at decreasing (but not eliminating) the risk of cancer development.
5. The American Cancer Society (ACS) has issued the following nutritional guidelines to reduce the risk of many types of cancer:
   a.   Avoid obesity.
   b.   Decrease total dietary fat intake.
   c.   Eat more high-fiber foods, such as whole grain cereals, fruits, and vegetables.
   d.   Include foods rich in vitamins A and C in the daily diet.
   e.   Include cruciferous vegetables (e.g., cabbage, broccoli, brussels sprouts, kohlrabi, cauliflower) in the diet.
   f.   Consume alcoholic beverages only in moderation.
   g.   Consume salt-cured, smoked, and nitrite-cured foods only in moderation.
6. Other accepted risk-reduction measures include:
   a.   Avoid tobacco use. (Cigarette smoking accounts for approximately 83% of lung cancer cases and 30% of all cancer deaths; use of smokeless tobacco increases the risk of mouth, laryngeal, throat, and esophageal cancers.)

    b.   Avoid excessive sun exposure, particularly between 10 A.M. and 3 P.M. (Almost all cases of nonmelanoma skin cancers are considered sun related; sun exposure also is a major factor in melanomas).

    c.   Avoid exposure to industrial agents known to increase cancer risk (e.g., nickel, chromate, asbestos, vinyl chloride).

C.   Secondary prevention

    1.   Secondary prevention involves detection and case-finding efforts to achieve early diagnosis (Table 21-1).

TABLE 21-1.
Summary of American Cancer Society Recommendations for the Early Detection of Cancer in Asymptomatic People

TEST OR PROCEDURE	SEX	AGE	FREQUENCY
Sigmoidoscopy, preferably flexible	M&F	50 and over	Every 3–5 years
Fecal occult blood test	M&F	50 and over	Every year
Digital rectal examination	M&F	40 and over	Every year
Prostate exam*	M	50 and over	Every year
Pap test [to detect cervical cancer]	F	All women who are, or who have been, sexually active, or have reached age 18, should have an annual Pap test and pelvic examination. After a woman has had three or more consecutive satisfactory normal annual examinations, the Pap test may be performed less frequently at the discretion of her physician.	
Pelvic examination	F	18–40 Over 40	Every 1–3 years with Pap test Every year
Endometrial tissue sample	F	At menopause, if at high risk†	At menopause and thereafter at the discretion of the physician
Breast self-examination	F	20 and over	Every month
Breast clinical examination	F	20–40 Over 40	Every 3 years Every year
Mammography‡	F	40–49 50 and over	Every 1–2 years Every year
Health counseling and cancer check-up§	M&F M&F	Over 20 Over 40	Every 3 years Every year

*Annual digital rectal examination and prostate-specific antigen should be performed on men 50 years and older. If either is abnormal further evaluation should be considered.
†History of infertility, obesity, failure to ovulate, abnormal uterine bleeding, or unopposed estrogen or tamoxifen therapy.
‡Screening mammography should begin by age 40.
§To include examination for cancers of the thyroid, testicles, ovaries, lymph nodes, oral region, and skin.
Revised November 1992, Guidelines for the cancer related checkup: An update. Atlanta, GA: American Cancer Society.

2. After early detection, prompt intervention may halt the cancerous process in some cases.

V. Cancer diagnosis

A. Early detection

1. **Early detection commonly hinges on thorough, accurate:**
   a. **Familial and environmental history**
   b. **Physical examination**
   c. **Evaluation of laboratory data and test findings**
2. ACS guidelines for early detection of breast cancer appear in Table 21-1.

B. Tumor staging

1. Cancer staging is based on:
   a. Characteristics of primary tumor (both clinical and histologic)
   b. Involvement of lymph nodes
   c. Evidence of metastasis
2. The TNM system (T = tumor, N = node, M = metastasis) is the most commonly used staging method; designations include:
   a. TO = no evidence of primary tumor
   b. TS = carcinoma in situ (neoplasm that remains confined to site of origin, potentially invasive if not surgically removed)
   c. T1, T2, T3, T4 = progressive increase in tumor size and involvement
   d. NO = regional lymph nodes not demonstrably abnormal
   e. N1, N2, N3 = increasing degrees of demonstrable abnormality of regional lymph nodes
   f. MO = no evidence of distant metastasis
   g. M1, M2, M3 = ascending degrees of distant metastasis, including metastasis to distant lymph nodes
3. Other staging systems in widespread use include:
   a. Duke's for colon cancer
   b. Clark's for malignant melanoma

C. Tumor grading

1. Performed by a pathologist, grading involves evaluating the extent to which tumor cells differ from their normal precursors, then assigning a corresponding numerical value to reflect this differentiation.
2. Low numerical grades reflect well-differentiated tumors that deviate minimally from normal cells.
3. High numerical grades reflect poorly differentiated tumors that deviate substantially from normal cells; the highest grades are assigned to the most aberrant tumors.

D. Classification of malignant neoplasms: see Table 21-2

TABLE 21-2.
Classification of Neoplasms

PARENT TISSUE	BENIGN TUMOR	MALIGNANT TUMOR
Epithelium		
Skin and mucous membrane	Papilloma Polyp	Squamous cell carcinoma Basal cell carcinoma Transitional cell carcinoma
Glands	Adenoma Cystadenoma	Adenocarcinoma
Endothelium		
Blood vessels	Hemangioma	Hemangioendothelioma Angiosarcoma
Lymph vessels	Lymphangioma	Lymphangiosarcoma
Bone marrow		Multiple myeloma Ewing's sarcoma Leukemia Lymphosarcoma Lymphangioendothelioma
Lymphoid tissue		Reticular cell sarcoma (difficult to classify because of cell embryology) Lymphatic leukemia
Connective tissues		
Embryonic fibrous tissue	Myxoma	Myxosarcoma
Fibrous tissue	Fibroma	Fibrosarcoma
Adipose tissue	Lipoma	Liposarcoma
Cartilage	Chondroma	Chondrosarcoma
Bone	Osteoma	Osteogenic sarcoma
Synovial membrane	Synovioma	Synovial sarcoma
Muscle tissue		
Smooth muscle	Leiomyoma	Leiomyosarcoma
Striated muscle	Rhabdomyoma	Rhabdomyosarcoma
Nerve tissue		
Nerve fibers and sheaths	Neuroma Neurinoma (neurilemmoma) Neurofibroma	Neurogenic sarcoma Neurofibrosarcoma
Ganglion cells	Ganglioneuroma	Neuroblastoma
Glial cells	Glioma	Glioblastoma Spongioblastoma
Meninges	Meningioma	

(continued)

TABLE 21-2.
Classification of Neoplasms (Continued)

PARENT TISSUE	BENIGN TUMOR	MALIGNANT TUMOR
Pigmented neoplasms		
Melanoblasts	Pigmented nevus	Malignant melanoma Melanocarcinoma
Miscellaneous		
Placenta	Hydatidiform mole Dermoid cyst	Choriocarcinoma Embryonal carcinoma Embryonal sarcoma Teratocarcinoma

E. **Cancer management**
   1. Major treatment modalities for cancer include:
       a. Surgery
       b. Radiation therapy
       c. Chemotherapy
   2. Other treatments that may be useful in certain cancers include:
       a. Immunotherapy
       b. Biologic response modifiers
       c. Bone marrow transplantation
   3. Selection of recommended treatment depends on such factors as:
       a. Cancer type and stage
       b. Site
       c. Sensitivity to anticancer drugs
       d. Previous treatments
       e. Concurrent organ system dysfunction

VI. **Cancer management: surgery**
   A. **Description: surgical removal of tumors, the most commonly used treatment modality for cancer**
   B. **Objectives**
       1. Preventive or prophylactic surgery involves removing precancerous lesions (e.g., unusual skin growth, colorectal polyps, cervical cancer in situ).
       2. Diagnostic surgery is done to confirm or rule out malignancy from analysis of tissue samples obtained from incisional, excisional, or needle biopsies.

   3. **Curative surgery, the most widely used cancer treatment, is a localized intervention aimed at removing all tumor tissue while limiting structural and functional impairment.**

4. Reconstructive surgery aims to improve the client's quality of life by restoring maximal function and appearance; best outcomes depend on the cancer site and extent of surgery.
5. Palliative surgery is done to:
   a. Retard tumor growth
   b. Decrease tumor size
   c. Relieve distressing manifestations of cancer when cure is no longer possible

C. **Nursing diagnoses: Basic nursing diagnoses applying to general preoperative and postoperative client care also apply to care of clients undergoing cancer surgery (see Chapter 24, Perioperative Nursing).**

D. **Planning and implementation: Basic principles of preoperative and postoperative nursing care also apply to cancer surgery (see Chapter 24, Perioperative Nursing).**

E. **Evaluation: Evaluation criteria for clients undergoing cancer surgery are similar to those for all surgical clients (see Chapter 24, Perioperative Nursing).**

VII. Cancer management: radiation therapy (RT)

A. **Description and overview**
   1. RT involves directing high-energy ionizing radiation to destroy malignant tumor cells without harming surrounding tissues.
   2. Types of ionizing radiation include:
      a. Radiographs
      b. Gamma rays
      c. Electrons
      d. Beta particles
   3. Generally, RT is used as localized treatment for solid tumors; approximately 50% of cancer clients receive RT at some point during the course of disease.
   4. RT interrupts cellular growth by damaging cellular DNA. The degree of cellular DNA damage from RT depends on such factors as:
      a. Cell division rate (Rapidly dividing cells are more radiosensitive.)
      b. Phase of the cell cycle (Cells undergoing DNA synthesis and mitosis are most sensitive.)
      c. Cell oxygenation level (Well-oxygenated cells are more sensitive.)
      d. Degree of cell differentiation (Poorly differentiated cells may be more sensitive than well-differentiated cells.)
   5. Damage may occur at time of treatment or later, when cells attempt to divide.

6. **Each body organ can receive only a specific, limited amount of radiation before irreparable damage to normal tissue occurs.** Tissue damage can be minimized through:
    a. Fractionation: dividing total radiation dose into small, frequent doses; tumor cells less able to repair than normal cells
    b. Alternating sites of entry (ports) of radiation so that normal tissue receives only a portion of the total dose
    c. Using customized blocks and shields, whenever possible, to protect normal tissues

B. **Objectives**
    1. Curative therapy aims to eradicate all disease and give the client the same life expectancy as a person who never had cancer. RT is often curative for such cancers as:
        a. Hodgkin's disease
        b. Testicular seminomas
        c. Localized cancers of the head and neck
        d. Cervical cancers
    2. RT also may be used as a control or an adjunct to other therapy, with the goal of prolonged and improved survival without disease eradication; examples include:
        a. Preoperative RT to shrink a tumor
        b. Postoperative RT to eradicate microscopic disease
        c. RT in conjunction with chemotherapy to prevent leukemic infiltration to the brain and spinal cord
    3. RT may be used as palliative therapy in advanced cancer to relieve symptoms of metastatic disease (e.g., pain, obstruction, bleeding, pathologic fractures).

C. **Sources of radiation therapy**
    1. External RT (teletherapy) usually is applied by high-energy radiograph machines (e.g., betatron, linear accelerator) or machines containing a radioisotope (e.g., cobalt 60). Clients receiving external RT do not retain radioactivity after therapy.
    2. Internal radiation therapy (brachytherapy) involves placing specially prepared radioisotopes directly into or near the tumor itself or into systemic circulation. Sources include:
        a. Sealed source: isotopes placed in applicators, needles, seeds, ribbons, or catheters before placement into malignant tumor or cavities; removed when exposure time is adequate or may be left in tumor permanently (depends on half-life of source)
        b. Unsealed source: used in systemic therapy and administered intravenously or orally (e.g., phosphorus 32, iodine 131)

D. **Principles of radiation protection**
1. Close contact with persons receiving internal radiation therapy provides exposure to small amounts of radiation.
2. The nurse should follow calculated safe time and distance parameters specified by the radiation physicist.

3. **Protection from exposure to excessive radiation depends on time, distance, and shielding.**
   a. Time: The less time spent close to a radiation source, the lower the exposure.
   b. Distance: The greater the distance from the source, the lower the exposure.
   c. Shielding: Using lead or other materials to absorb energy helps reduce exposure in some cases; the type of rays emitted determines the radioactive precautions specified by the radiation safety officer.

E. **Radiation therapy side effects**
1. Side effects are directly related to the body site being irradiated.
2. The severity of side effects depends on:
   a. Radiation dosage (daily or fractionated dose and total dose)
   b. Type of radiation
   c. Proximity of tumor to skin surface
   d. Size of treatment field
3. When counseling a client about possible side effects, be sure to emphasize the benefits of therapy.

F. **Nursing diagnoses**
1. Diarrhea
2. Fatigue
3. Risk for Infection
4. Risk for Injury
5. Altered Nutrition: Less than body requirements
6. Pain
7. Risk for Impaired Skin Integrity
8. Social Isolation
9. Impaired Tissue Integrity

G. **Planning and implementation**
1. Never refer to radiation skin reactions as burns.
2. Supplement teaching about skin care as necessary, covering:
   a. Keeping the treatment area dry
   b. Washing with water only, patting skin dry

   c. **Never applying ointment, powder, lotion, heat, ice, or other substances to the treatment field unless prescribed by the radiotherapist**

    d.   **Avoiding washing off target marks made by the radiation therapist**

    e.   Shaving with an electric razor only in the treatment area

    f.   Avoiding clothes that rub or bind

    g.   Avoiding sun exposure to the treatment site

3. Monitor WBC count, and notify the therapist if it drops below 2000/μL.

4. Teach the client with depressed WBC count the signs and symptoms of infection to watch for and report.

5. Monitor platelet count, and notify the therapist if it drops below 100,000/mm^3.

6. Teach the client with depressed platelet count to:
   a. Avoid physical trauma and aspirin products.
   b. Recognize and report signs of hemorrhage.
   c. Avoid parenteral injections.

7. Reassure the client that fatigue commonly results from RT and is not an indicator of worsening disease.

8. Teach the client how to conserve energy for priority activities; encourage adequate rest.

9. Promote a high-protein, high-calorie diet (if the client is not diabetic).

10. Provide a bland diet as indicated.

11. Monitor the oral cavity daily for signs of stomatitis.

12. Urge the client to avoid smoking and alcohol ingestion.

13. Monitor fluid and electrolyte balance, and record daily weights.

14. Promote increased fluid intake—up to 3000 mL/day, if not contraindicated.

15. Encourage oral hygiene only as prescribed by the radiation therapist; warn the client to avoid commercial mouthwashes.

16. Offer artificial saliva or sugarless candy to increase salivation if xerostomia (dryness due to salivary changes) occurs.

17. Monitor stools for diarrhea; if indicated, reinforce a low-residue diet and high fluid intake, and administer antidiarrheal medication as prescribed.

18. If the client complains of nausea, administer antiemetics as prescribed, and plan rest periods before and after meals.

19. Assess for central nervous system (CNS) changes; report any significant findings.

20. Assess the client's compliance with the prescribed medication regimen (e.g., steroids).

21. Encourage the client to express feelings and concerns related to potential hair loss secondary to RT.

22. Suggest covering the head with a wig, scarf, or hat to reduce embarrassment.

23. Promote gentle hair care to minimize loss (see Section VIII.J.40–41 for more information).
24. Monitor for urinary system complications (e.g., hematuria, dysuria, frequency).
25. Reinforce radiation safety precautions.
26. Promote measures to reduce social isolation, such as:
    a. Frequent telephone calls to friends and relatives
    b. Television, radio, puzzles, hobbies depending on mobility
    c. Frequent staff checks on the client with time to talk with him or her whenever possible

H. Evaluation

1. The client shows no evidence of altered skin integrity secondary to RT.
2. The client demonstrates proper skin care techniques.
3. The client displays no evidence of infection related to RT.
4. The client exhibits no evidence of bleeding related to platelet depression.
5. The client verbalizes understanding of the need to alter activities to adjust to weakness and fatigue.
6. The client maintains a normal bowel elimination pattern.
7. The client maintains dietary intake sufficient to meet nutritional needs.
8. The client reports no pain related to complications from RT.
9. The client interacts with others appropriately to reduce social isolation.

VIII. Cancer management: chemotherapy

A. Description and overview

1. Chemotherapy involves administering antineoplastic drugs to promote tumor cell death by interfering with cellular functions and reproduction.
2. It is a systemic cancer intervention for widespread disease or when the risk of undetectable disease is high.
3. Chemotherapy is administered to eradicate neoplastic cells, allowing the body's immune system to destroy remaining tumor cells.
4. Each exposure to chemotherapy destroys a percentage of tumor cells (20% to 90%), depending on dosage (cell-kill theory).
5. Repeated doses over a prolonged period are necessary to achieve tumor regression.

B. Objectives

1. *Curative therapy* involves early, aggressive treatment aimed at eradicating disease. Cure is considered to be achieved when the client exhibits no evidence of disease; reference points of

5- and 10-year survival rates are used. After cure, the client would have the same expected life span as age- and sex-matched persons without cancer.

2. A second attempt at curative intervention when disease recurs is known as *salvage therapy.*

3. *Control therapy* aims to cause or sustain tumor regression and diminish symptoms to extend and improve the client's quality of life when cure is no longer possible.

4. *Palliative treatment* is given to relieve or diminish distressing symptoms such as pain, obstruction, pleural effusions, or hypercalcemia.

C. Treatment methods

1. *Combination chemotherapy* consists of two or more drugs (used effectively as single agents) administered simultaneously or in sequence to treat specific cancer and reduce the likelihood of drug resistance.

2. *Adjuvant chemotherapy* involves administering chemotherapeutic agents in combination with surgery or radiation therapy. This therapy may eradicate possible micrometastasis before it becomes clinically apparent.

D. Pharmacologic action

1. **Anticancer drugs directly or indirectly disrupt reproduction of cells by altering essential biochemical processes.**

2. Agents are classified according to their mechanism of action.

3. *Antimetabolites* inhibit cell reproduction by interfering with manufacture of protein; agents include:
   a. Methotrexate
   b. 5-fluorouracil (5FU)
   c. Cytosine arabinoside
   d. 6 mercaptopurine
   e. 6-thioguanine

4. *Alkylating agents* interfere with DNA replication; types include:
   a. Cyclophosphamide
   b. Thiotepa
   c. Mechlorethamine
   d. Chlorambucil
   e. Carmustine
   f. Lomustine
   g. Semustine
   h. Busulfan
   i. Phenylalanine mustard
   j. Cisplatin
   k. Decarbazine

      f.   Lymphocyte levels

      g.   Urinary creatinine levels

30. Provide refreshing mouth care before meals.

31. Serve high-protein and high-carbohydrate food; allow the client to choose foods, but guide his or her selection.

32. Present small portions attractively in a pleasant setting.

33. Ensure physical comfort, and encourage mealtime company.

34. Keep in mind that cancer or cancer treatment may contribute to altered taste and food preferences.

35. Assess the client's oral cavity daily, and report changes in sensation, appearance, or taste.

36. Provide instruction for an oral care regimen following meals and at bedtime.

37. Instruct the client to:

      a.   **Avoid lemon and glycerin products and all commercial mouthwashes; these promote drying and irritation.**

      b.   Gargle with a solution of baking soda and water (1 tsp in 500 mL) or salt ($\frac{1}{2}$ tsp), baking soda (1 tsp), and water (1000 mL).

      c.   Use a soft toothbrush or "toothette."

      d.   Remove dentures except for eating.

      e.   Avoid extremely hot or cold foods, spices, citrus juices.

      f.   Avoid smoking and alcohol intake.

      g.   Keep lips moist with K-Y Jelly or another water-based lip balm.

38. Instruct the client to report:

      a.   Any discomfort, areas of redness

      b.   Open lesions

      c.   Decreased tolerance to temperatures of food

39. Administer systemic or topical analgesics as prescribed.

40. Assist the client to cope with hair loss by:

      a.   Informing him or her if hair loss is expected and when

      b.   Explaining that the hair that regrows may differ in color or texture

      c.   Suggesting that occasional wig wearing before hair loss may ease the adjustment process and helping the client obtain a hairpiece before hair loss begins

      d.   Taking an honest, gentle, caring approach, encouraging client to express fears and feelings of loss

      e.   Realizing that hair loss may become so difficult that the client may refuse to accept treatment

      f.   Arranging for contact with another person who has experienced hair regrowth after chemotherapy

      g.   **Never communicating that hair loss is an insignificant problem compared to life-threatening alterna-**

tives; the client's emotional needs may be at least as great as physical needs

41. Advise a client with alopecia to:
    a. Use a mild, protein-based shampoo every 3 to 5 days, avoid excessive shampooing, rinse thoroughly, and gently pat hair dry
    b. Avoid using hair dryers, electric curlers, curling irons, hair clips, elastic bands, barrettes, bobby pins, hair spray, dye, and permanents—all of which may increase fragility of hair
    c. Sleep on a satin pillowcase to decrease hair trauma and tangles
    d. Avoid excessive brushing and combing of hair; comb only with a wide-tooth comb
    e. Wear a hairnet to minimize shedding of hair onto the bed or clothing
    f. Covering the head when outdoors to prevent body heat loss or sunburn

42. **Allow and encourage verbalization of anger, sadness, or resentment by the client and significant others.**

43. Convey sincere concern by listening, pointing out other attributes, appropriate touching to convey acceptance, and so forth.

44. Assess intensity and patterns of fatigue, and aggravating and alleviating factors.

45. Assess the impact of fatigue on the client's lifestyle.

46. Monitor laboratory values for anemia.

47. Help the client cope with fatigue by:
    a. Providing for rest periods during the day, especially before and after priority activities
    b. Helping him or her rearrange daily schedule and organize activities to conserve energy
    c. Teaching that fatigue is an expected side effect of chemotherapy that will resolve after treatment is completed
    d. Encouraging him or her to ask for assistance with necessary chores

48. Assess for pain and anxiety.

49. Assess for signs and symptoms of depression:
    a. Irritability
    b. Withdrawal
    c. Apathy
    d. Tearfulness
    e. Decreased ability to make decisions
    f. Impaired concentration or memory
    g. Increasing insomnia
    h. Suicidal ideas

50. Provide adequate protein and calorie intake; give dietary supplements as needed.
51. Encourage fluid intake of 3000 mL/day, unless contraindicated, to prevent accumulation of cellular waste products.
52. Administer blood products as prescribed.
53. Provide pain management as needed.
54. Assess the client's specific stressors.
55. Evaluate the client's perception of stressors and beliefs about their causes.
56. Determine available resources and support systems.
57. Provide for consistent, uninterrupted time with the client; encourage verbalization of concerns.
58. Design strategies; gather agency support to address concerns about equipment, prostheses, home care.
59. Assist the client in mastering self-care to the maximum level possible.
60. Explain the importance of staying involved in normal routines.
61. Encourage the client to generate good options for solving problems.
62. Identify unsuccessful coping behaviors, and make referrals to mental health professionals or clergy as indicated.

K. Evaluation
1. The client displays no evidence of infection from myelosuppression.
2. The client displays no evidence of bleeding from myelosuppression.
3. The client maintains sufficient nutritional intake to prevent dietary imbalance.
4. The client remains free of stomatitis.
5. The client demonstrates positive adaptation to body image changes related to alopecia.
6. The client alters activity pattern in response to changes in physical ability and energy level.
7. The client demonstrates appropriate coping mechanisms in adapting to the disease.
8. The client makes use of agency support as needed for home care.

IX. Bone marrow transplantation
A. Description and overview
1. This procedure involves aspirating bone marrow cells from a compatible donor and infusing them into the recipient.
2. Bone marrow transplantation is a complex therapy with a high risk of complications.
3. Types of transplantation include:
   a. Autologous: The marrow donor is the recipient; mar-

row is harvested during a period of disease remission, treated, and stored for later infusion.

    b.   Syngeneic: The marrow donor is the recipient's identical twin.

    c.   Allogeneic: The marrow donor is a family member whose HLA type matches that of the recipient.

B.   Objectives

    1.   Cure

    2.   Complete marrow recovery within 6 to 8 weeks

    3.   Proliferation of donor cells in marrow, leading to release of functional blood cells into circulation

C.   Indications

    1.   Acute lymphoblastic leukemias

    2.   Acute myelogenous leukemias

    3.   Lymphomas

D.   Nursing diagnoses

    1.   Fatigue

    2.   Fear

    3.   Risk for Infection

    4.   Altered Nutrition: Less than body requirements

    5.   Pain

    6.   Social Isolation

E.   Planning and implementation

    1.   Ensure thorough pretransplantation preparation, including:

        a.   Complete histocompatibility studies of all possible donors and the recipient

        b.   Thorough assessment of recipient and donor to determine physical and psychosocial factors that may influence transplantation

        c.   Large doses of chemotherapy or radiation to the recipient to eradicate any viable marrow

    2.   Monitor for signs and symptoms of infection.

    3.   Assess for signs and symptoms of graft-versus-host (GVH) disease, a syndrome induced by donor T lymphocytes acting against host tissues (see Section III of Chapter 19, Hematologic Disorders, for more information on GVH disease).

    4.   Explain to the client that fatigue is a common effect of transplantation and does not indicate disease exacerbation. Teach energy conservation measures, and encourage adequate rest.

    5.   **Instruct the client to:**

        a.   **Avoid physical injury and aspirin-containing products.**

        b.   **Promptly report signs of hemorrhage or infection.**

        c.   **Avoid parenteral injections if platelet count is depressed.**

    6.   Promote measures to reduce social isolation, including:

a. Frequent telephone calls
b. Television, radio, hobbies, other activities
c. Regular client–staff contact

F. Evaluation

1. The client exhibits no signs of infection, GVH disease, or hemorrhage.
2. The client verbalizes necessary precautions to prevent complications.
3. The client states energy conservation measures to reduce fatigue.
4. The client maintains adequate nutritional status.
5. The client interacts with others to prevent social isolation.

X. Promising approaches

A. Immunotherapy

1. This treatment uses the body's own immune mechanisms to combat and overcome cancer.
2. Through the administration of chemical or microbial agents, immunotherapy aims to challenge and induce mobilization of immune defenses.
3. The resultant delayed hypersensitivity response can be directed against cancer cells.
4. In *active immunotherapy,* the client is injected with antigen that stimulates development of antibodies; may be specific or nonspecific:
   a. Specific: The client is vaccinated with tumor-associated antigen to stimulate immune response.
   b. Nonspecific: Injected materials have no relationship to the tumor but increase the client's overall immune capacity.
5. *Passive immunotherapy* involves direct transfer of antitumor antibodies, immunologically competent lymphocytes, or immune lymphoid cells from a donor (a person cured of cancer or in remission) to a client with an active neoplasm; it provides short-term immunity.
6. *Adoptive immunotherapy* involves transferring passive immunity to a client, who later develops and maintains active immunity. Cells with antitumor reactivity to the client with cancer are administered; the client adopts the immunity from the cells and then incorporates it into his or her own immune system.
7. *Adjunctive immunotherapy* is a combination of the above immunotherapeutic approaches with other cancer modalities (surgery, radiation therapy, chemotherapy).

B. Biologic response modifiers (BRMs)

1. This therapy involves agents or treatment methods that have the ability to alter the immunologic relationship between tumor and host in a therapeutically beneficial way.

2. The goal is destruction or cessation of malignant growth.
3. The basis of BRM treatment lies in:
   a. Restoration
   b. Stimulation
   c. Augmentation of natural immune defenses
4. Types of BRMs include:
   a. Immunomodulating agents: Bacille Calmette-Guerin and *Corynebacterium parvum* (*C. Parvum*)
   b. Interferons
   c. Interleukins
   d. Monoclonal antibodies
   e. Lymphokines and cytokines

C. **Nursing considerations for investigational therapies**
1. Keep in mind that these approaches may be viewed as "last chance" efforts at cure.
2. When caring for a client receiving such therapy, be sure to gain familiarity with each agent given and potential adverse effects.
3. Careful documentation is essential for all aspects of data collection and nursing care.

Bibliography

American Cancer Society. (1992). *Cancer facts and figures.* Atlanta: American Cancer Society.

Baltzer, L., & Berkery, R. (1994). *Oncology pocket guide to chemotherapy.* St. Louis: C. V. Mosby.

Belcher, A. E. (1992). *Cancer nursing.* St. Louis: C. V. Mosby.

Bolander, V. R. (1994). *Sorensen & Luckmann's basic nursing: A physiologic approach.* (3rd ed.). Philadelphia: W. B. Saunders.

Clark, J., Queener, S., & Karb, V. (1990). *Pharmacologic basis of nursing practice* (4th ed.). St. Louis: C. V. Mosby.

DeVita, V. T., Jr., Hellman, S., & Rosenberg, S. A. (1995). *Important advances in oncology 1995.* Philadelphia: J. B. Lippincott.

Foley, J. F., Vose, M. D., & Armitage, J. O. (1994). *Current therapy in cancer.* Philadelphia: W. B. Saunders.

Hudak, C. M., & Gallo, B. M. (1994). *Critical care nursing: A holistic approach.* Philadelphia: J. B. Lippincott.

Nettina, S. (1996). *The Lippincott manual of nursing practice* (6th ed.). Philadelphia: Lippincott-Raven Publishers.

Phipps, W. J., Long, B. C., & Woods, N. F. (1994). *Medical-surgical nursing: Concepts and practice* (5th ed.). St. Louis: C. V. Mosby.

Porth, C. M. (1992). *Pathophysiology: Concepts of altered health states* (4th ed.). Philadelphia: J. B. Lippincott.

Smeltzer, S. C., & Bare, B. G. (1996). *Brunner & Suddarth's textbook of medical-surgical nursing* (8th ed.). Philadelphia: Lippincott-Raven Publishers.

STUDY QUESTIONS

1. Which of the major treatment modalities for cancer is the most frequently used?
   a. bone marrow transplantation
   b. chemotherapy
   c. radiation
   d. surgery

2. A fair-skinned, blonde client with a family history of dysplastic nevus syndrome has been advised that sun exposure greatly increases the risk for developing skin cancer. The client continues to sunbathe in the early afternoon. Which of the following nursing diagnoses is appropriate?
   a. Knowledge Deficit related to causes of skin cancer
   b. Dysfunctional Grieving
   c. Ineffective Denial
   d. Anxiety

3. A 28-year-old woman asks the nurse, "What can I do to make sure I don't get breast cancer like my mother and sister?" The nurse's best response would be
   a. "There is nothing you can do to make sure you don't get breast cancer."
   b. "You can detect the cancer early by doing self-breast exams monthly and having a mammogram every year."
   c. "You're frightened that you may get breast cancer like your mother and sister."
   d. "You should get a digital rectal examination every year and a yearly PAP test."

4. Which of the following factors are believed to contribute to between 80% and 90% of all cancers?
   a. environmental
   b. genetic
   c. socioeconomic
   d. geographic

5. The client diagnosed with a glioma of the brain asks the nurse to describe the kind of treatment that the client will undergo. The nurse should explain that the most likely treatment would be
   a. chemotherapy
   b. treatment for a benign lesion
   c. radiation therapy
   d. immunotherapy

6. Nursing interventions for a client receiving chemotherapy would include
   a. instructing the client not to remove marks placed on the skin by the radiation therapist and to decrease fluid intake during therapy
   b. instructing client to report any skin burns and to apply lotion to burned areas
   c. instructing the client to use a straight razor only when shaving and to self-administer IM injections with an 18-gauge needle
   d. instructing the client to avoid cuts, bruises, and trauma and to inspect the skin for bruises and tiny petechiae (red spots)

7. The nurse knows the client receiving radiation therapy understands the discharge teaching when the client states
   a. "I should gargle with Listerine daily."
   b. "I should eat foods low in protein and drink only cold beverages."
   c. "When I brush my teeth, I should brush vigorously and use a hard-bristle toothbrush."
   d. "I need to drink lots of fluids and avoid smoking."

8. When caring for a client receiving radiation therapy for a glioblastoma, the nurse should be alert for which of the following side effects?
   a. fatigue, nausea and vomiting, and headache
   b. fatigue, diarrhea, and stomatitis
   c. severe diarrhea and headache
   d. cystitis, diarrhea, and alopecia

9. A client receiving radiation therapy for painful prostatic metastasis of the lum-

bosacral spine states "I'm going to beat this disease." The nurse's best response would be

   a. "Once cancer gets into the bones, there is nothing to be done."

   b. "Many cancers are curable with radiation."

   c. "Have you considered trying a macrobiotic diet?"

   d. "You may obtain very good pain relief from the radiation."

10. Secondary cancer prevention refers to

   a. prevention of second malignancies

   b. detection and screening efforts to achieve early diagnosis and prompt intervention

   c. prevention of genetic cancer inheritance

   d. avoiding smoking and sun exposure

11. For early detection of colorectal cancer, the American Cancer Society's guidelines recommend

   a. digital rectal examination every year after age 40 and stool examination every year after age 50

   b. monthly testicular self-exams and yearly proctosigmoidoscopy after age 30

   c. having yearly physical exams and yearly kidney, ureter, and bladder (KUB) x-rays

   d. digital rectal exam yearly after age 25 and monitoring for changes in bladder habits

12. Which of the following statements about bone marrow transplantation is true?

   a. It is performed when cure is impossible.

   b. It is now fairly risk-free because of improved methods of marrow harvesting.

   c. It requires thorough physical and psychosocial assessment of both donor and recipient.

   d. The donor must always be a family member.

13. A client will be receiving aggressive chemotherapy for ovarian cancer. The plan of care for this client should include

   a. assigning a staff nurse to administer the chemotherapy

   b. checking laboratory values initially for reduced numbers of leukocytes, erythrocytes, and platelets

   c. putting the client in a private room and enforcing strict isolation

   d. communicating that hair loss is insignificant compared to potentially life-threatening complications

14. A client's lung tumor has been staged as T3, N1, M1. This indicates

   a. a measurable tumor with regional nodes and metastasis involved

   b. a well-differentiated tumor

   c. a tumor that cannot be treated

   d. the tumor markers

15. The family of a client receiving brachytherapy to the tongue asks the nurses how they can protect themselves when the client returns home. From this question, the nurse would determine that the family

   a. needs further instruction

   b. understands about brachytherapy

   c. has had no instruction

   d. cannot understand simple instructions

ANSWER KEY

1. *Correct response: d*
Surgery is the most frequently used major modality.
a. Bone marrow transplantation is not a major treatment modality.
b and c. Chemotherapy and radiation therapy are major modalities but not the most frequently used.
Comprehension/Safe care/Planning

2. *Correct response: c*
Though aware of the risk, the client still refuses to limit cancer risk activities.
a. The client understands the risk and preventive measures.
b and d. There is no evidence that the client is either anxious or grieving.
Knowledge/Psychosocial/Analysis (Dx)

3. *Correct response: b*
The American Cancer Society recommends monthly breast self-examinations and physical examinations every 3 years for women between ages 20 and 40. Mammograms are recommended yearly if there is a history of breast cancer in the family.
a. It is true that nothing can prevent breast cancer, but early detection provides an excellent chance of total recovery with no metastasis.
c. The client is asking for information; therapeutic responses are appropriate but not in this situation.
d. These are recommended for early detection of colon cancer and cervical cancer, respectively.
Knowledge/Health promotion/Planning

4. *Correct response: a*
Environmental factors are thought to contribute to 80% to 90% of all cancers.
b. Genetic factors combine with host mechanisms and environmental influences.
c and d. Socioeconomics and geographics are predisposing factors.
Comprehension/Safe care/Evaluation

5. *Correct response: b*
Gliomas are benign lesions.
a and c. Chemotherapy and radiation therapy are indicated only for neoplastic disease.
d. This scenario offers no evidence that the client's immune system is compromised.
Application/Physiologic/Implementation

6. *Correct response: d*
The client receiving chemotherapy is at risk for bleeding (decreased platelet count) and should avoid any activities that may cause bleeding. Ecchymoses (bruises) and petechiae are signs of bleeding.
a. Target marks are made on the skin when the client is receiving radiation therapy and fluid intake should be *increased* with chemotherapy.
b. Areas of redness occur after radiation therapy and lotion should not be applied. Do not refer to affected areas as burns.
c. Because clients receiving chemotherapy are prone to bleeding, they should use only electric razors, and IM injections should be avoided. If an injection is necessary, a small-gauge needle (21G) is recommended.
Application/Safe care/Implementation

7. *Correct response: d*
Increased fluid intake helps soothe irritated tissue and moisturize mucous membranes; smoking is an irritant.
a. Commercial mouthwashes contain alcohol and promote further drying of mucous membranes.
b. A high-protein, high-calorie diet is essential to facilitate healing of normal epithelial tissue.
c. RT may cause mouth ulcers; vigorous brushing is contraindicated.
Application/Health promotion/Implementation

8. **Correct response: a**
   Fatigue is an expected result of RT; nausea and vomiting are possible because of increased intracranial pressure resulting from brain irradiation.
   b, c, and d. Side effects of RT are directly related to the body site being irradiated. Brain irradiation would not result in diarrhea or stomatitis; headache is possible. Alopecia is expected.
   Analysis/Physiologic/Planning

9. **Correct response: d**
   The nurse should reinforce the positive effects of therapy for metastatic disease.
   a. Reclassification may occur from radiation to bony metastasis; the nurse should avoid destroying hope with negative responses.
   b. Metastatic disease dictates the goal of palliation.
   c. Macrobiotic diet is an unproved treatment method.
   Analysis/Psychosocial/Implementation

10. **Correct response: b**
    This answer is the definition of secondary cancer prevention.
    a. General cancer prevention measures apply to any malignancy.
    c. There is no known way to prevent genetic tendencies.
    d. Avoiding smoking and sun exposure are primary prevention measures.
    Application/Health promotion/ Implementation

11. **Correct response: a**
    The American Cancer Society (ACS) recommends a digital rectal examination every year after age 40, stool examinations for occult blood every year after age 50, and proctosigmoidoscopy every 3 to 5 years after age 50 following two normal annual examination findings for preventing colorectal cancer.
    b. Testicular self-exams are recommended to detect testicular abnor-

malities, and proctosigmoidoscopy is recommended regularly after *age 50* to detect colon disease.
    c. ACS recommends physical exams every 3 years from age 20 to 40; KUB is not used to detect colorectal cancer.
    d. ACS recommends yearly digital rectal exams after age 40; any change in bowel (not bladder) habits would suggest colorectal cancer.
    Knowledge/Health promotion/Planning

12. **Correct response: c**
    Thorough assessment of recipient and donor is required to determine physical and psychosocial factors that may influence bone marrow transplant.
    a. Cure is the singular goal of bone marrow transplant.
    b. Bone marrow transplant involves high risks.
    d. In autologous transplants, the marrow donor is also the recipient.
    Analysis/Health promotion/Assessment

13. **Correct response: b**
    Adequate counts must exist before therapy can begin.
    a. Only specially trained nurses should be involved in administering chemotherapy.
    c. Clients do not need to be in strict isolation when receiving chemotherapy but they should not be with clients who have infectious diseases.
    d. It is not productive to minimize emotional concerns.
    Application/Physiologic/Planning

14. **Correct response: a**
    Staging systems specify tumor characteristics, lymph node involvement, and evidence of metastasis.
    b. Grading, not staging, provides information about differentiation.
    c. Staging systems do not specify the treatability of tumors.
    d. Many malignancies are associated with specific cancer markers (labora-

tory values) that seem to indicate tumor progression or regression.
Analysis/Physiologic/Assessment

15. *Correct response: a*
This statement indicates that the family does not know that sealed sources placed in tissue in a container are removed before discharge; further instruction is indicated.
b, c, and d. The nurse should never jump to conclusions about a person's ability to understand information. A client and family members typically receive much information that is scary and completely foreign; reinforcement and clarification usually are necessary. Remember, these are not simple issues to people who are fearful and who have heard horrible "stories" about radiation.
Analysis/Safe care/Evaluation

Gerontologic Nursing

I. **Aging and older adults**
  A. Life span changes
  B. Stereotypes of older adults
  C. Modification of age-related changes
  D. Selected theories of aging
II. **Overview of gerontologic nursing**
  A. Health history
  B. Physical assessment
  C. Mental status examination
  D. Assessment of functional capacity
  E. Environmental assessment
  F. Special considerations for nursing intervention
  G. Psychosocial implications
III. **Dementias**
  A. Description
  B. Etiology and incidence
  C. Pathophysiology and management
  D. Assessment findings
  E. Nursing diagnoses
  F. Planning and implementation
  G. Evaluation
IV. **Osteoporosis**
  A. Description
  B. Etiology and incidence
  C. Pathophysiology and management
  D. Assessment findings
  E. Nursing diagnoses
  F. Planning and implementation
  G. Evaluation
V. **Pressure sores (decubitus ulcers)**
  A. Description
  B. Etiology and incidence
  C. Pathophysiology and management
  D. Assessment findings
  E. Nursing diagnoses
  F. Planning and implementation
  G. Evaluation

VI. **Falls**
  A. Etiology
  B. Pathophysiology and management
  C. Assessment findings
  D. Nursing diagnoses
  E. Planning and implementation
  F. Evaluation
VII. **Dehydration**
  A. Description
  B. Etiology and incidence
  C. Assessment findings
  D. Nursing diagnoses
  E. Planning and implementation
  F. Evaluation
VIII. **Constipation**
  A. Description
  B. Etiology and incidence
  C. Assessment findings
  D. Nursing diagnosis
  E. Planning and implementation
  F. Evaluation
IX. **Hearing deficit**
  A. Description
  B. Etiology and incidence
  C. Assessment findings
  D. Nursing diagnoses
  E. Planning and implementation
  F. Evaluation
X. **Visual deficit**
  A. Description
  B. Etiology, incidence, and pathophysiology
  C. Assessment findings
  D. Nursing diagnoses
  E. Planning and implementation
  F. Evaluation

Bibliography

Study questions

677

Note: This chapter is not meant to provide comprehensive coverage on the health of older adults. Other important health problems are presented elsewhere in this text; see particularly:

- ▶ Chapter 6, Respiratory Disorders (chronic obstructive lung disease, pneumonia)
- ▶ Chapter 8, Peripheral Vascular Disorders (hypertension)
- ▶ Chapter 9, Gastrointestinal Disorders (hiatal hernia)
- ▶ Chapter 10, Endocrine and Metabolic Disorders (diabetes mellitus)
- ▶ Chapter 14, Neurologic Disorders (cerebrovascular accident)
- ▶ Chapter 16, Musculoskeletal Disorders (osteoarthritis, fractures)
- ▶ Chapter 18, Renal and Urinary Disorders (incontinence)

I. Aging and older adults

A. Life span changes

1. Aging encompasses life span changes common to all people.
2. These changes involve biologic, social, and psychologic components.

B. Stereotypes of older adults

1. Refuting the stereotype of invariable, progressive physical and mental decline with aging, more than 80% of older adults live in the community.
2. The elderly population is heterogeneous and diverse.
3. Other inaccurate myths about older adults include:
   a. Most are inactive and unproductive.
   b. Most are abandoned by their families.
   c. Most have no sex life.
   d. Most are rigid and inflexible.

C. Modification of age-related changes

1. Age-related changes are modified by environment, heredity, and time-related pathologic events as well as race, ethnicity and culture.
2. A person's chronologic age is not always indicative of biologic age.

 3. Aging and disease are not synonymous; many pathologic changes can be treated and possibly reversed.

4. Certain reversible effects of disuse and physical deconditioning may result from prolonged bedrest and inactivity.

 5. The rate of aging may differ for various organ systems. Physiologic systemic changes that may be related to normal aging include:
   a. Cardiovascular system

   - ▶ Decreased cardiac output
   - ▶ Decreased heart rate response to stress
   - ▶ Decreased stroke volume
   - ▶ Increased blood pressure
   - ▶ Increased peripheral vascular resistance

b. Respiratory system

- ▶ Decreased vital capacity
- ▶ Decreased gas exchange and diffusing capacity
- ▶ Decreased cough efficiency
- ▶ Increased anteroposterior chest diameter

c. Integumentary system

- ▶ Diminished secretion of natural oils
- ▶ Decreased total body weight
- ▶ Decreased subcutaneous fat
- ▶ Increased body fat

d. Genitourinary system

- ▶ Decreased renal blood flow
- ▶ Reduced creatinine clearance
- ▶ Male: decreased bladder capacity, delayed voiding sensation, benign prostatic hyperplasia
- ▶ Female: decreased bladder capacity, relaxed perineal muscles

e. Gastrointestinal system

- ▶ Decreased basal metabolic rate
- ▶ Decreased salivation
- ▶ Difficulty swallowing food
- ▶ Delayed esophageal and gastric emptying
- ▶ Reduced gastrointestinal motility
- ▶ Delayed pancreatic insulin release

f. Musculoskeletal system

- ▶ Decreased bone and muscle mass
- ▶ Decreased deep tendon reflexes
- ▶ Decreased height
- ▶ Loss of muscle strength and size
- ▶ Degenerated joint cartilage

g. Nervous system

- ▶ Slowed reaction time
- ▶ Reduced cerebral circulation
- ▶ Increased confusion with physical illness and loss of environmental cues

h. Reproductive system

- ▶ Male: decreased size of penis and testes, slower sexual response
- ▶ Female: vaginal narrowing and decreased elasticity; decreased vaginal secretions, slower sexual response

        i.   Senses

- ► Vision: diminished ability to focus on close objects, decreased ability to distinguish colors, difficulty adjusting to changes in light intensity
- ► Hearing: decreased ability to hear high-frequency sounds
- ► Taste and smell: decreased ability to taste and smell

D.   **Selected theories of aging (not likely a single cause)**

    1.   Biologic theories include:

        a.   Cellular

        b.   Autoimmune

        c.   Neuroendocrine

    2.   Psychosocial theories encompass:

        a.   Disengagement

        b.   Activity

        c.   Continuity

        d.   Developmental stages

II. **Overview of gerontologic nursing**

    A.   **Health history**

    1.   **When obtaining a health history from an elderly adult, the nurse should determine the person's ability to hear and comprehend the questions and allow sufficient time for a response.**

    2.   The history should include the following parameters:

        a.   Previous illness

        b.   Lifestyle, including usual daily routine

        c.   Diet and fluid intake

        d.   Medication use

        e.   Sources of income, financial status

        f.   Social network

        g.   Presence of a confidant

        h.   Living arrangements

        i.   Personal perception of health status

        j.   Satisfaction with activity level

        k.   Available sources of healthcare and psychosocial support

    3.   The nurse should collect data in more than one session if the person shows signs of tiring.

    4.   The nurse should be alert for atypical disease presentation in elderly persons (e.g., painless myocardial infarction).

    B.   **Physical assessment**

    1.   **During physical assessment of an elderly person, the nurse should pay special attention to positioning, comfort, and mobility.**

  2. The nurse should compare findings on both sides of the body when norms for elderly persons are absent.

  3. Insufficient normative data commonly interfere with accurate evaluation of laboratory test results.

C. **Mental status examination**

  1. Altered mental status may be due to physical problems such as infection and heart failure.

  2. The client may feel threatened when the nurse assesses memory, orientation, reasoning, calculation ability, and judgment.

  3. To put the client at ease, the nurse should show kindness and empathy, and progress from simple to complex questions.

  4. A person with dementia may exhibit superficial social skills, creating a false impression of adequate mental function.

D. **Assessment of functional capacity**

  1. The nurse should evaluate activities of daily living (ADL) and instrumental activities of daily living (IADL; e.g., managing money, telephone use, shopping, use of transportation).

  2. Assessment findings will be influenced by pain, motivation, and environment, as well as by the client's functional ability.

  3. **A client's prior performance is a good predictor of current ability.**

E. **Environmental assessment**

  1. Assessment of the client's environment should cover:

   a. Cleanliness

   b. Temperature regulation

   c. State of repair

   d. Presence of smoke alarms

   e. Food storage and preparation facilities

   f. Safety features to reduce the risk of injury (e.g., adequate lighting, handrails, absence of throw rugs)

   g. Presence of stairs

   h. Medication storage

   i. Furniture with sharp edges or obstructed pathways

  2. This assessment also should evaluate the client's community for safety and for availability of:

   a. Public transportation

   b. Home health services

   c. Respite care

   d. Meals on Wheels

   e. Home maintenance assistance

   f. Senior centers

   g. Healthcare facilities

F. **Special considerations for nursing intervention**
1. Pay special attention to both functional status and specific medical problems.

2. **Emphasize client strengths; do not focus only on problems.**
3. **Always consider restorative potential or maintenance of function when setting goals for the client.**
4. Consider altered pharmacokinetics in the older adult when evaluating drug effects.
5. Recognize that the client may have increased susceptibility to disease due to:
   a. Impaired immunity
   b. Multiple disease states
   c. Chronic illness
6. Recognize the decreased adequacy of the body's response to stress.
7. Provide support and information to caregivers, family, and significant others; suggest self-help groups.
8. Establish mutually satisfactory means of communication, considering vision and hearing deficits.
9. Incorporate the multidisciplinary team into the care process.
10. Provide for continuity of care in unit transfers, among different levels of care, and by various service providers.
11. Recognize that Medicare and Medicaid legislation has a significant effect on care delivery and reimbursement of health professionals caring for older adults.

G. **Psychosocial implications**
1. Elderly persons are particularly susceptible to cumulative effects of loss and grief associated with:
   a. Social interactions: spouse, family, friends
   b. Self-concept: job, health
   c. Financial security: income, home, possessions
2. The elderly client may have difficulty coping with age-related lifestyle changes, leading to:
   a. Economic and psychologic stresses
   b. Feelings of loss of control and independence
3. The elderly client's coping ability may be overwhelmed quickly if past successful strategies are not encouraged.

III. **Dementias**
A. **Description: a group of chronic, progressive, organic mental disorders; the most common are Alzheimer's disease and multi-infarct dementia**
B. **Etiology and incidence**
1. The cause of Alzheimer's disease is unknown.

2. Multi-infarct dementia results from cerebrovascular disease producing multiple small cerebral infarctions.
3. Alzheimer's disease accounts for more than 50% of dementias and affects 2% to 4% of persons over age 65. Incidence increases with age, particularly after age 75.
4. Multi-infarct dementia accounts for about 15% of cases of dementia; incidence is greater in males than females, and onset generally is earlier than in Alzheimer's disease.

C. **Pathophysiology and management**
1. Alzheimer's disease is characterized by specific neurologic and biochemical changes, including:
   a. Neurofibrillary tangles, granulovacuolar degeneration of neurons, and senile or neuritic plaques, primarily in the cerebral cortex
   b. Brain atrophy, with widened cortical sulci and enlarged cerebral ventricles
   c. Decreased acetylcholine production
2. Typically of insidious onset, Alzheimer's disease produces multifaceted intellectual deficits (e.g., memory, abstract thought, judgment, and higher cortical functions) and personality and behavioral changes.
3. Pathologic changes in multi-infarct dementia include multiple areas of extensive localized softening, along with various changes in cerebral vessels.
4. Multi-infarct dementia is marked by an uneven decline in mental function due to cerebral damage. The pattern of deficits is patchy, depending on the areas of damage; some cognitive functions may be affected early, whereas others may remain relatively intact.
5. Management measures may focus on client safety.

D. **Assessment findings**
1. Clinical manifestations of Alzheimer's disease are highly variable and may include:
   a. Early, subtle changes such as forgetfulness, recent memory loss, and poor concentration, which the client may be able to hide
   b. Later, more overt signs of impaired cognition (e.g., severe memory loss and forgetfulness; inability to hold a conversation, think abstractly, or formulate concepts; poor hygiene and grooming and inappropriate dress; inability to perform IADLs)
   c. Behavioral changes, such as depression, anxiety, wandering, impulsive behavior, catastrophic reactions, imitation, emotional lability, and withdrawal
2. Common manifestations of multi-infarct dementia include:

        a.   Dizziness, headaches
        b.   Confusion
        c.   Patchy memory loss
        d.   Hallucinations, delusions
        e.   Focal neurologic signs (e.g., muscle weakness, dysreflexia, dysarthria)

   3.   Studies to evaluate dementias include:
        a.   Computed tomography (CT) scan
        b.   Electroencephalography (EEG)
        c.   Positron emission tomography (PET)
        d.   Blood chemistries

E.   **Nursing diagnoses**

   1.   Bowel Incontinence
   2.   Impaired Verbal Communication
   3.   Ineffective Family Coping: Compromised
   4.   Altered Health Maintenance
   5.   Impaired Home Maintenance Management
   6.   Risk for Injury
   7.   Impaired Physical Mobility
   8.   Altered Nutrition: Less than body requirements
   9.   Self Care Deficit: Bathing/Hygiene, Dressing/Grooming, Feeding, Toileting
   10.   Sleep Pattern Disturbance
   11.   Altered Thought Processes
   12.   Functional Urinary Incontinence
   13.   Risk for Violence
   14.   Risk for Caregiver Role Strain

F.   **Planning and implementation**

   1.   On admission:
        a.   Record the client's usual daily routine as well as words and behaviors used to communicate ADL needs; validate this information with a reliable informant in separate interview; chart words and techniques that "get through" to the client.

        b.   **Request that a family member or other person stay with the client if the client wanders or cannot be sent to diagnostic tests by himself or herself; avoid sedation and restraints whenever possible.**
        c.   Assign the client to a room that maximizes the potential for observation and is not next to an exit or stairwell (if the client is prone to wandering).
        d.   Orient the client to the room and the unit; mark the room and bedside area with familiar belongings.
        e.   Attach an ID bracelet; alert others to wandering (special clothing, care plan, posted notice).

2. Maximize effective communication by:

   a. Using short sentences, simple words, gestures, and written or pictorial cues, if needed; explain and repeat instructions unless this increases distress

   b. Maintaining a calm demeanor and a consistent approach

   c. Avoiding excessive questioning and confrontation

   d. Breaking down instructions into simple components

   e. Supporting the anxious or depressed client

   f. Attempting to analyze behavior for meaning

3. Maximize environmental safety by:

   a. Installing alarms on stairwells

   b. Instituting injury, fire, and poisoning precautions

   c. Providing adequate lighting in all rooms

   **d. Keeping the bed in low position or placing the mat-
   tress on the floor (Siderails may pose a hazard.)**

4. Intervene as necessary to manage evening agitation ("sun-
downing"): provide a night light, soft music, and supervision.

5. If indicated, create a limited-access, safe unit to obviate activity restriction and decrease the need for supervision.

6. Promote optimal functioning through:

   a. Fitting daily diagnostic and therapeutic procedures into
   the client's usual schedule as possible

   b. Assigning consistent caregivers

   c. Establishing a daily routine for care; maintaining the
   client's preadmission sleep–wake cycle if possible and
   desirable

   d. Providing a clock, calendar, and daily schedule in the
   room (but avoiding pressuring the client for accuracy)

   e. Prompting for ADLs with memory aids and verbal cues
   and encouraging performance within the limits of ability
   (avoiding pressure for performance, which could trigger
   catastrophic reaction)

   f. Focusing the client on simple, repetitive, and purposeful
   activities

   g. Monitoring for adverse effects of drug therapy

   h. Encouraging ambulation and other exercise

   i. Ensuring good grooming and personal hygiene

   j. Using distraction to alter undesirable behavior, break
   episodes of preservation, or remove from harm

   k. Intervening as necessary to calm an agitated client

   l. Limiting stimuli (e.g., noise, people, caffeine)

   m. Regularly assessing the skin, gums, teeth, and feet for
   breakdown and infection, and providing good skin and
   mouth care

   n. Maximizing opportunities for social interaction

        o.   Providing touch, respect, affection, praise, and the opportunity for choice

7. Optimize nutrition and fluid balance by:
   a. Monitoring food and fluid intake, noting increased or decreased hunger and thirst
   b. Reminding the client to eat regularly
   c. Providing small, frequent meals with high-calorie supplements if appropriate
   d. Matching food consistency to the client's chewing and swallowing ability

8. Optimize elimination by:
   a. Making sure the client knows where the bathroom is to encourage its use
   b. Monitoring bowel elimination patterns
   c. Preventing constipation
   d. Giving periodic reminders to urinate
   e. Scheduling toileting based on voiding pattern
   f. Providing protective pants as indicated

9. Provide discharge planning:
   a. **Begin discharge planning on the client's admission to the hospital.**
   b. Determine whether the client will be discharged to home alone, to live with family, or to a nursing home; evaluate whether independent living could be hazardous to the client.
   c. As indicated, assist the client's family in arranging for a nursing home, day care, or respite care.
   d. Refer the client and family to community agencies, legal and financial counseling, and disease-specific groups (e.g., the Alzheimer Disease and Related Disorder Association).
   e. Encourage regular healthcare following discharge.
   f. Document all client information on transfer forms to promote continuity of care.
   g. Teach home caregivers to assist the client with ADLs as needed and to provide any special care required.

G. Evaluation
1. The client demonstrates the ability to perform ADLs and IADLs to the maximum extent possible.
2. The client is included in social interactions with family, friends, and groups.
3. The client maintains adequate nutrition and hydration.
4. The client receives protection of rights and respect.
5. The client and family verbalize understanding of the disorder.
6. The client maintains adequate elimination patterns or control of incontinence as appropriate.

7. The client remains free from injury and infection.
8. The client receives analysis of words and behavior for meaning.
9. The client and family receive information about respite care, community services, and support organizations.
10. The client exhibits appropriate personal hygiene.
11. The caregiver verbalizes understanding of the cause of behavioral problems and methods of calming the client.
12. The caregiver maintains health and social contacts, using respite care when appropriate.

IV. Osteoporosis

A. Description: a disorder of bone metabolism making bones abnormally prone to fracture
B. Etiology and incidence
1. Osteoporosis may be iatrogenic or secondary to other disorders.
2. Predisposing factors include:
    a. Postmenopausal status
    b. Nutritional deficiency or malabsorption
    c. Catabolic hormone excess (e.g., Cushing's disease)
    d. Long-term corticosteroid use
    e. Prolonged immobilization
    f. Chronic disorders (e.g., liver disease)

3. **Osteoporosis affects approximately one fourth of all older adults; incidence is greatest in white females between ages 50 and 70.**
C. Pathophysiology and management
1. In osteoporosis, the rate of bone loss (resorption) exceeds bone formation, resulting in a decrease in total bone mass.
2. Bones affected by osteoporosis lose calcium and phosphate salts.
3. As a result, they become porous, brittle, and susceptible to fracture.
4. Osteoporosis primarily affects weight-bearing vertebrae; severe, advanced disease can affect ribs, long bones, and the skull.
5. Calcium replacement therapy helps some clients.
D. Assessment findings
1. Common clinical manifestations include:
    a. Fractures, particularly vertebral compression fractures, hip fractures, and long bone fractures
    b. Pain
    c. Visible deformity (e.g., kyphosis)
    d. Loss of height
    e. Constipation

2. Diagnostic evaluation includes:
    a. Radiographic and bone density studies showing loss of bone density, deformity
    b. Serum calcium, phosphorus, and alkaline phosphatase levels within normal ranges

E. **Nursing diagnoses**
    1. Constipation
    2. Risk for Injury
    3. Impaired Physical Mobility
    4. Pain

F. **Planning and implementation**
    1. Encourage regular, moderate exercise regimen (e.g., walking, swimming, aerobics).
    2. Teach knee flexion and muscle relaxing exercises.
    3. Instruct the client to perform range-of-motion exercises at least twice daily.
    4. Teach the client to move the trunk as a unit and maintain good posture and body mechanics.
    5. Encourage increased intake of foods high in calcium (e.g., milk, cheese, salmon, spinach, broccoli, rhubarb), vitamin D, fiber, and protein.

    6. Teach safety measures to prevent injury from falls.
    7. Use caution when turning, lifting, and transferring the client to prevent fracture.
    8. If indicated, apply a lumbosacral corset to promote spinal stability; avoid appliances that can decrease mobility.
    9. Instruct the client to sleep on a firm, nonsagging mattress.
    10. Teach the client about the disease process and prevention of progression.
    11. Administer medications as prescribed which may include:
        a. Nonnarcotic analgesics such as acetaminophen (Tylenol), aspirin, or ibuprofen (Motrin); as with any pain medication:

        ▶ **Assess pain level; assess client's condition and rule out complications requiring medical attention; give medication with food to minimize possible GI upset; assess effectiveness of drug 30 minutes after administration.**

        b. Stool softeners, such as docusate calcium (Surfak) and docusate sodium (Colace)

        ▶ **Instruct client that daily bowel movement is not necessary for normal bowel function.**
        ▶ **Advise client to aim for fluid intake of 2500 to 3000 mL daily and to increase dietary fiber intake.**

> ► Monitor bowel movements and keep daily record.
> ► Caution client to avoid laxative dependency.

    c.   Calcium (Os-cal) and vitamin D supplements to prevent calcium depletion

m ► Instruct client to take as directed because large doses over a long time may cause adverse effects, especially if the client has kidney disease.
      ► Adverse effects include GI distress, constipation, and renal calculi.

    d.   Estrogen (Premarin, Estrace, Estrovis) therapy in post-menopausal women

m ► Urge client to stop smoking, maintain desirable weight, and decrease cholesterol and triglyceride levels.
      ► Take drug with food.
      ► Notify physician of abnormal vaginal bleeding.

  G. **Evaluation**
1. The client maintains or improves mobility and physical function.
2. The client modifies lifestyle to include increased exercise, use of safety precautions, and independent ADLs within limitations of condition.
3. The client reports reduced discomfort and pain.
4. The client sustains no new fractures.
5. The client identifies and verbalizes plans to increase consumption of foods high in fiber, calcium, protein, and vitamin D.

V. **Pressure sores (decubitus ulcers)**
  A. **Description: localized areas of cellular necrosis on the skin and subcutaneous tissue**
  B. **Etiology and incidence**
1. As the name implies, pressure sores result from excessive pressure on body areas, particularly over bony prominences.
2. Older adults are especially susceptible due to:
    a.   Decreased skin thickness
    b.   Decreased vascularity of dermal layer, which slows tissue repair and healing capacity
3. Major risk factors include:
    a.   Decreased or limited activity, immobility
    b.   Malnutrition
    c.   Incontinence
    d.   Impaired circulation and sensation
    e.   Sensory deficits
    f.   Cognitive dysfunction

    4. Other risk factors from related conditions may include:
- a. Fever with diaphoresis
- b. Radiation therapy
- c. Anemia
- d. Dehydration

C. Pathophysiology and management

    1. Excessive pressure on the skin interrupts normal circulatory function by constricting cutaneous and subcutaneous blood vessels.

    2. Impaired circulation leads to tissue anoxia, necrosis, and ulceration.

    3. Ulcer severity depends on the intensity and duration of pressure.

    4. Ulcers are classified in four stages:
- a. Stage I: area with unresolved erythema, skin intact
- b. Stage II: blister, superficial skin break
- c. Stage III: involving the dermis through subcutaneous tissue with necrotic tissue, eschar, exudate
- d. Stage IV: involving subcutaneous tissue, fascia, and possibly muscle, joint, or bone with undermining sinus tract formation

    5. Necrotic tissue is susceptible to bacterial invasion and infection.

    6. A focus of management is prevention.

D. Assessment findings

    1. Pressure ulcers are marked by variable skin lesions, ranging from superficial erythema to small blisters or erosions to marked ulcerations.

    2. Signs of local infection may be apparent.

    3. Wound culture or biopsy may identify infective organisms and guide choice of antimicrobial therapy.

E. Nursing diagnoses

    1. Risk for Infection

    2. Pain

    3. Impaired Tissue Integrity

F. Planning and implementation

    1. Relieve pressure by:
- a. Turning the client at least every 2 hours
- b. Avoiding positioning the client on the ulcerated side
- c. Teaching wheelchair push-ups if appropriate
- d. Using pressure-relieving devices (e.g., egg crate mattress, convoluted foam, air-fluidized therapy) as necessary

    2. Prevent skin friction by:
- a. Using anatomic pads when necessary

    b.   Using a lift sheet to prevent dragging the client across the bed
3.   Prevent shearing force on the skin by:
    a.   Elevating the head of the bed 30 degrees when not contraindicated
    b.   Providing a footboard to prevent sliding down in bed
    c.   Helping the client maintain appropriate body position and alignment
4.   Keep skin clean and dry; if necessary, apply a fecal incontinence bag or external urine collection device.
5.   Apply pressure sore dressings according to lesion stage:
    a.   Stage I: transparent dressings
    b.   Stage II: transparent or hydrocolloid dressing
    c.   Stages III and IV: necrotic pressure ulcers must be debrided to create an area that will heal
6.   Avoid occlusive dressings.
7.   Use normal saline solution for dressing changes; avoid Betadine and Dakin's solution.
8.   Promote wound healing through:
    a.   Pressure relief
    b.   Nutritional support
    c.   Mechanical debridement with wet-to-dry dressing, if indicated
    d.   Preparation for surgical debridement, if indicated
    e.   Protection of the skin around ulcers
    f.   Administration of antibiotics or blood transfusions as prescribed
9.   Teach the client and family:
    a.   Measures to help prevent recurrence
    b.   Wound care and infection control measures
    c.   Sources of supplies and community resources

G. Evaluation
1.   The client exhibits resolution of pressure sores, as shown by:
    a.   Granulation tissue
    b.   No drainage or bleeding
    c.   Decrease in size and depth
    d.   Intact skin around ulcers
    e.   No maceration
2.   The client verbalizes understanding of measures to promote healing and prevent further damage.
3.   The client or caregiver correctly demonstrates wound care using occlusive dressing or other appropriate method.
4.   The client acknowledges the need for turning or pressure-relieving devices.

VI. Falls

    A. Etiology

        1. Falling results from the inability of the body's postural mechanism to sustain an upright position because of internal or external destabilization.

        2. Predisposing factors to falls in elderly clients include:

            a. Neuromuscular and cardiovascular problems

            b. Sensory deficits

            c. Environmental hazards

            d. Drug effects (e.g., diuretics, sedatives, hypnotics, cardiac glycosides, antiarrhythmics, antihypertensives)

    B. Pathophysiology and management

        1. A fall can produce various musculoskeletal traumas, including:

            a. Fractures, particularly hip fracture

            b. Dislocations

             c. Sprains

        2. It also can cause:

            a. Head injury

            b. Neurologic damage

            c. Tissue trauma

        3. A management focus involves prevention and ensuring a safe environment.

    C. Assessment findings

        1. Clinical manifestations of injury from falls may include:

            a. Pain

            b. Visible deformity

            c. Loss of movement

            d. Sensory changes

            e. Tissue damage (e.g., bruising, laceration, swelling)

        2. Diagnostic tests to evaluate damage due to falls include:

            a. Radiographs

            b. CT scans

    D. Nursing diagnoses

        1. Risk for Injury

        2. Impaired Physical Mobility

        3. Pain

        4. Self Care Deficit

        5. Risk for Impaired Skin Integrity

        6. Social Isolation

    E. Planning and implementation

        1. Provide appropriate emergency management, including:

            a. Wound care and repair

            b. Immobilization of affected limb

        c.   Hemorrhage control

        d.   Tetanus toxoid as prescribed

  2.   Institute preventive measures, such as:

        a.   Identifying a client at risk for falling

        b.   Observing the client frequently

        c.   Monitoring for side effects of drugs

        d.   Assessing for orthostatic hypotension

        e.   Taking safety precautions (e.g., keep bed in low position with siderails up; place call light within reach; provide a night light; apply a posey vest, seat belt, or restraints if necessary)

  3.   Provide follow-up care as necessary, which may include:

        a.   Limiting activity

        b.   Providing pain relief with prescribed medications and, if applicable, nonpharmacologic measures

        c.   Assessing for impaired circulation and nerve damage

        d.   Referring for radiographic and medical treatment

  4.   Develop a unit procedure for fall prevention and action plans to reduce the risk of injury.

  5.   **Teach the client about the importance of:**

        a.   **Safety precautions (e.g., wearing nonskid shoes, using adaptive devices, installing night lights, eliminating safety hazards)**

        b.   **Avoiding sudden or rapid position changes**

        c.   **Reporting falls and injuries promptly**

 F. **Evaluation**

  1.   The client exhibits diminished incidence of falling.

  2.   The client states the need for safety precautions to reduce the risk of falling.

  3.   The client identifies medications that affect balance.

  4.   The client calls for assistance as needed.

VII. **Dehydration**

 A. **Description: excessive loss of water from body tissues**

 B. **Etiology and incidence**

  1.   Dehydration may result from fluid volume depletion related to:

        a.   Marked decrease in water intake, enteral nutrition

        b.   Diminished sense of thirst

        c.   Age-related changes in body composition

        d.   Incontinence

        e.   Drug reactions

  2.   It also may be associated with medical problems such as:

        a.   Diabetes mellitus

        b.   Excessive fluid loss from fever, vomiting, or diarrhea

C. **Assessment findings**
1. Manifestations of dehydration include:
   a. Tented skin turgor
   b. Dry skin and mucous membranes, cracked lips and tongue
   c. Behavioral changes: delirium, apathy, confusion
   d. Oliguria
   e. Sunken cheeks, weight loss
   f. Hypotension
   g. Tachycardia
   h. Weakness
   i. Fever
2. Laboratory studies may reveal:
   a. Elevated blood urea nitrogen (BUN) level
   b. Elevated hematocrit value
   c. Elevated serum sodium level
   d. Elevated urine specific gravity

D. **Nursing diagnoses**
1. Activity Intolerance
2. Constipation
3. Fluid Volume Deficit
4. Altered Oral Mucous Membrane
5. Impaired Skin Integrity
6. Altered Thought Processes

E. **Planning and implementation**
1. Offer electrolyte supplements, as indicated, if the client is conscious.
2. Administer IV therapy as prescribed; monitor for fluid overload.
3. Measure intake and output; weigh daily.
4. Assess skin turgor and hydration of the buccal mucosa and tongue every shift.
5. Monitor vital signs.
6. Monitor laboratory study results.
7. Assess mental status and level of consciousness.
8. Teach the client about:
   a. The need for adequate fluid intake
   b. Effects of certain drugs on fluid balance (e.g., diuretics)
   c. Signs of dehydration to watch for and report
   d. The need to wear proper clothing and avoid excessive exposure to heat and sunlight

F. **Evaluation**
1. The client remains alert and oriented.
2. The client demonstrates the ability to drink adequate fluids.

    3. The client exhibits moist oral mucosa and tongue, elastic skin turgor.

    4. The client displays vital signs and laboratory study results within acceptable ranges.

    5. The client verbalizes understanding of the need to wear appropriate clothing and avoid excessive heat and sun exposure.

VIII. Constipation

A. Description: abnormal delay in defecation or infrequent passage of dry, hard stool

B. Etiology and incidence

    1. **An elderly client is at increased risk for constipation because of a tendency for decreased intake of roughage and fluids or decreased mobility.**

    2. Other contributing factors may include:

       a. Inability to recognize or neglecting the defecation urge

       b. Chronic enema or laxative use

       c. Neurologic degeneration

       d. Loss of abdominal muscle tone

       e. Environmental changes

       f. Emotional stress

       g. Effects of medication (e.g., narcotics, anticholinergics)

       h. Organic disorders (e.g., tumors, hypothyroidism, hemorrhoids)

C. Assessment findings

    1. The client may report infrequent defecation. (*Note:* Keep in mind that bowel regularity is quite subjective; what the client perceives as constipation may in fact be a normal elimination pattern.)

    2. Clinical manifestations of constipation may include:

       a. Abdominal distention and pain

       b. Absent or sluggish bowel sounds

       c. Stool-filled rectum on rectal examination

       d. Infrequent passage of dry, hard stool

D. Nursing diagnosis: Constipation

E. Planning and implementation

    1. **Encourage the client to:**

       a. **Increase roughage in diet unless contraindicated**

       b. **Increase fluid intake to greater than 2 L/day**

       c. **Perform regular, moderate exercise as possible**

    2. Establish a regular bowel evacuation schedule; provide privacy and assistance to the toilet or commode (if the client is able to use these) or with using a bedpan.

    3. Encourage ingestion of hot liquids after a large meal to stimulate gastrocolic reflex.

4. Teach the client about the causes and management of constipation.

 5. **As appropriate administer stool softeners (Surfak, Colace); bulk-forming agents (Metamucil, Effersylium); laxatives such as bisacodyl (Dulcolax, Ex-lax, Senokot); suppositories such as glycerin (Sani Supp); and enemas (Fleet). Monitor for side effects such as nausea, vomiting, diarrhea, and electrolyte imbalances.**

6. Keep in mind that severe constipation may lead to fecal impaction, which necessitates manual extraction of stool before initiating other treatments.

F. Evaluation

1. The client passes soft, formed stools regularly.
2. The client states an intention to incorporate methods to prevent constipation into daily routine.

IX. Hearing deficit

A. Description: hearing deficit associated with aging involves either sensorineural loss—presbycusis, progressive, and bilateral—or conductive loss (see Chapter 15, Eye, Ear, Nose, Sinus, and Throat Disorders, for more information)

B. Etiology and incidence

1. Presbycusis results from disturbances of the inner ear neural structures (e.g., cochlear nuclei, nerve pathways leading to the brain).
2. Conductive loss or transmission deafness results from disturbances of the sound transmission mechanism of the external or middle ear, which prevents sound waves from entering the inner ear. Older adults commonly suffer from conductive hearing loss due to impacted cerumen in the ear canal.

C. Assessment findings: See Chapter 15, Sections IX and X.

D. Nursing diagnoses

1. Impaired Verbal Communication
2. Sensory/Perceptual Alteration: Auditory
3. Social Isolation

E. Planning and implementation

 1. **Keep in mind that a hearing-impaired elderly client may be inaccurately labeled as demented because of impaired communication. Be sure to record the client's hearing deficit on the chart and care plan.**

2. Instruct the client in proper ear hygiene.
3. Work with the client to develop a means of communication that is effective and mutually satisfying (e.g., lip reading, writing).
4. When talking to the client, speak slowly and distinctly in a

low-pitched, clear voice; minimize background noise; and use nonverbal cues.

5. Instruct the client in the use and care of a hearing aid, if indicated.
6. Assist the client in obtaining assistive devices (e.g., amplifying mechanisms) as necessary.
7. Evaluate the impact of hearing loss on the client's lifestyle (social isolation) and safety.
8. Teach the client about environmental changes to promote independence and safety (e.g., installing a flashing light on the doorbell and telephone).

F. **Evaluation**
1. The client demonstrates effective communication using the technique or equipment of choice.
2. The client identifies potential safety hazards related to hearing loss.
3. The client maintains social contacts and avoids isolation.

X. Visual deficit

A. **Description: visual deficits commonly associated with aging include:**
1. Presbyopia: caused by thickening and hardening of the lens, which leads to decreased accommodation
2. Cataract: clouding or opacity of the normally transparent crystalline lens, which blurs vision and decreases visual acuity

B. **Etiology, incidence, and pathophysiology: See Chapter 15, Sections I through VII.**

C. **Assessment findings: See Chapter 15, Sections VI and VII.**

D. **Nursing diagnoses**
1. Sensory/Perceptual Alteration: Visual
2. Risk for Injury
3. Social Isolation

E. **Planning and implementation**
1. Encourage the use of magnifying eyeglasses as indicated.
2. Use large, bold letters for printed client education materials and signs. Avoid muted colors, especially in the blue and green spectrum; a sharp color contrast from background promotes readability.
3. **Protect the client from injury: keep paths clear of obstacles, provide adequate lighting, avoid glare.**
4. Identify yourself when approaching the client.
5. Insert a notation regarding the client's visual deficit in the care plan.
6. Keep the client's belongings and essential equipment in consistent locations within his or her visual field.

7. Help the client obtain assistive devices (e.g., magnifying lenses, large-print books) as necessary.
8. Teach the client the importance of annual eye examinations.
9. Encourage cataract extraction when visual deficit interferes with desired activities.
10. Following cataract extraction, help the client obtain special glasses or lenses and provide instruction regarding necessary adjustments to cope with altered depth perception, abnormal magnification, and loss of peripheral vision.

F. Evaluation
1. The client identifies potential safety hazards related to vision loss.
2. The client states an intention to modify lifestyle and environment as necessary to maximize functional abilities.
3. The client participates in desired social activities.
4. The client receives appropriate medical follow-up.

Bibliography

American Psychiatric Association. (1994). *Diagnostic and statistical manual of mental disorders* (DSMIV). Washington, DC: American Psychiatric Association.

Anderson, M. A., & Braun, J. (1995). *Caring for the elderly client.* Philadelphia: F. A. Davis.

Bolander, V. R. (1994). *Sorensen & Luckmann's basic nursing: A physiologic approach* (3rd ed.). Philadelphia: W. B. Saunders.

Carnevali, D., & Patrick, M. (1993). *Nursing management for the elderly* (3rd ed.). Philadelphia: J. B. Lippincott.

Clark, J., Queener, S., & Karb, V. (1990). *Pharmacologic basis of nursing practice* (4th ed.). St. Louis: C. V. Mosby.

Eliopoulos, C. (1993). *Gerontological nursing* (3rd ed.). Philadelphia: J. B. Lippincott.

Karch, A. (1996). *Lippincott's nursing drug guide.* Philadelphia: J. B. Lippincott.

Nettina, S. (1996). *The Lippincott manual of nursing practice* (6th ed.). Philadelphia: Lippincott-Raven Publishers.

Smeltzer, S. C., & Bare, B. G. (1996). *Brunner & Suddarth's textbook of medical-surgical nursing* (8th ed.). Philadelphia: Lippincott-Raven Publishers.

Springhouse Corporation. (1992). *Nursing student's guide to drugs.* Spring House, PA: Springhouse Corp.

Stanley, M., & Beare, P. G. (1994). *Gerontological nursing.* Philadelphia: F. A. Davis.

STUDY QUESTIONS

1. Which of the following statements about the aging process is correct?
   a. Age-related physiologic changes are distinct from those reflecting disease.
   b. Aging rate is consistent for various organ systems.
   c. A stereotype of progressive physical and mental decline is associated with aging.
   d. The effects of disuse and physical deconditioning caused by inactivity in the older adult are usually irreversible.

2. Which of the following likely would be the most successful approach when intervening for a client who has dementia and who will not sit and eat at mealtime?
   a. Demonstrate putting food in the mouth and eating. Have finger foods available so that the client can eat while pacing.
   b. Keep repeating the request to sit and eat until the client does so. Guide the client back into the chair when he or she rises.
   c. Restrain the client in the chair; place a tray in front of the client, and explain that it contains food.
   d. Question the client about preferred mealtimes and favorite foods; adapt foods and mealtimes to stated preferences.

3. Which of the following client statements would indicate successful learning regarding bowel management?
   a. "I will take a laxative every day."
   b. "I will walk two blocks once each week."
   c. "I will drink 2 quarts of fluid every day."
   d. "I will eat bran cereal once each week."

4. Which of the following would be an appropriate goal for a client with osteoporosis?

   a. Maintain a sedentary lifestyle.
   b. Demonstrate awareness of lifting safely.
   c. Verbalize knowledge of cure for the disease.
   d. Increase intake of dietary estrogen.

5. Which of the following is the most important consideration regarding history taking in elderly clients?
   a. Obtain information as quickly as possible, avoiding long interviews.
   b. Traditional historical information will provide adequate data.
   c. Adjust the method and pace of information gathering for sensory deficits and physical condition.
   d. Start the history with a mental status examination to validate reliability of informant.

6. A 76-year-old client has just been diagnosed with Alzheimer's disease. Discharge planning to a home-alone living situation for the client requires
   a. no community agency referrals because of the client's mild impairment (Discussing available services may provoke anxiety for the client and family members.)
   b. referrals for Meals on Wheels and adult care because of diagnosis of Alzheimer's disease; family respite needs to begin early
   c. arrangements for a visiting nurse to assess the home environment and link the client with appropriate community services
   d. discouraging home living and planning for posthospital nursing home admission because of the progressive decline expected with this diagnosis

7. Which of the following sets of assessment data would most likely lead the nurse to believe that a client's nursing diagnosis of Altered Thought Processes could be reversed?

a. depression, history of multiple strokes, known vitamin B deficiency
b. subdural hematoma, pneumonia, digoxin toxicity
c. brain tumor, intoxication, and dehydration
d. urinary tract infection, AIDS, history of head trauma

8. The nurse would know the client understands the discharge teaching concerning the estrogen replacement when the client states
a. "I should call my doctor if I start having any vaginal bleeding."
b. "This medication should be taken on an empty stomach so that it will absorb better."
c. "I should stop taking my medication if I notice that my feet are swelling."
d. "I do not need to quit smoking as long as I take my medication every day."

9. The nurse is completing an assessment of a 79-year-old client's environment for safety. Assessment data would include
a. public transportation and home health services
b. previous illness and fluid and diet intake
c. activities of daily living and instrumental activities of daily living
d. food storage, medication storage, and presence of smoke alarms

10. Physiologic changes that may be intrinsic to aging include
a. decreased cardiac output
b. decreased basal metabolic rate
c. increased pancreatic insulin release
d. increased creatinine clearance

11. Nursing interventions for preventing pressure sores include
a. turning the client every 8 hours
b. not using a lift sheet to move the client
c. using pressure-relieving devices
d. keeping the head of the bed flat at all times

12. Which of the following interventions would be appropriate to reduce the risk of constipation in a 79-year-old client hospitalized for a hip fracture?
a. Limit fluid intake to less than 2 L/day.
b. Avoid administering narcotic analgesics.
c. Perform range-of-motion exercises daily.
d. Administer daily enemas.

13. Which of the following nursing diagnoses would most likely lead the nurse to believe that a postmenopausal client is at risk for progressive osteoporosis?
a. Altered Nutrition: More than body requirements
b. Urinary Incontinence, Stress
c. Altered Patterns of Sexuality
d. Impaired Physical Mobility

14. Which of the following nursing interventions would be most appropriate to incorporate when working with a hearing-impaired client?
a. Provide nonverbal cues to augment communication.
b. Discourage reliance on amplifying devices.
c. Speak in a high-pitched voice.
d. Discourage attempts by the client to perform ear hygiene.

15. A client, aged 80, with a history of left hip fracture, is admitted with a 48-hour history of vomiting, diarrhea, and weight loss. Based on this information, the nurse should monitor the client closely for
a. hypokalemia
b. decreased serum creatinine level
c. hypertension
d. anasarca

16. Which of the following would represent the best evaluation criteria reflecting successful outcome of treatment for dehydration?
a. The client exhibits no signs or symptoms of CVA, arrhythmia, or hyperproteinemia.

b. The client exhibits no signs or symptoms of shock, circulatory overload, or hypokalemia.

c. The client exhibits no signs or symptoms of renal failure, pressure sores, or hypoproteinemia.

d. The client exhibits no signs or symptoms of congestive heart failure, polyuria, or hyperkalemia.

ANSWER KEY

702

1. **Correct response: c**
   Many stereotypes and myths about older adults alter our view of their capabilities.
   a. Aging changes are often difficult to distinguish from those reflecting disease.
   b. Aging rate can differ among various organ systems.
   d. Disuse and physical deconditioning effects are often reversible.
   Knowledge/Physiologic/Assessment

2. **Correct response: a**
   This approach provides nonverbal information and avoids questioning or explaining, which may not be understood or can be too stimulating.
   b, c, and d. Verbal instructions may not be understood or may be overstimulating. Food intake is possible without forcing the client to sit.
   Application/Physiologic/Implementation

3. **Correct response: c**
   Adequate fluid intake is essential for normal bowel function.
   a. Daily laxative use leads to physiologic dependence.
   b. Walking 2 blocks once a week is insufficient exercise.
   d. Fiber must be consumed daily to have a beneficial effect on bowel function.
   Comprehension/Physiologic/Evaluation

4. **Correct response: b**
   A client with osteoporosis is at risk for fracture; understanding of safe movement is essential.
   a. Regular, moderate exercise has a role in prevention and treatment of osteoporosis.
   c. There is no cure for osteoporosis.
   d. Estrogen cannot be ingested through the diet.
   Analysis/Health promotion/Planning

5. **Correct response: c**
   The rate and method of information exchange must be adjusted to enhance the client's ability to respond.
   a. A too-rapid pace could confuse the client and interfere with accurate data collection.
   b. Besides traditional health history information, history taking in elderly clients should include more detailed information in areas such as social supports, living arrangements, functional capacity, and drug-taking practices.
   d. Mental status examination is often perceived as threatening and thus should be done at the end of the assessment session.
   Comprehension/Psychosocial/Assessment

6. **Correct response: c**
   A visiting nurse can assess the appropriateness of home living and suggest modifications and referrals to enhance home care.
   a. The client and family need to be informed about available community services.
   b. This may not be appropriate; the family may want to provide some services in early stages to defer long-term expenses.
   d. Home living may be possible if hazards can be removed and necessary support systems provided.
   Application/Safe care/Planning

7. **Correct response: b**
   These problems are all potentially reversible causes of altered thought processes.
   a, c, and d. These responses all contain at least one cause of dementia; cognitive problems resulting from dementia do not have as high a likelihood of reversibility as do cognitive problems resulting from other causes.
   Analysis/Physiologic/Analysis (Dx)

8. Correct response: a
Vaginal bleeding is a sign of an adverse effect of this medication and should be reported to the client's physician immediately. The elderly woman would have gone through menopause during the 4th or 5th decade of life.

b. The estrogen replacement should be taken with food to decrease GI distress.

c. Edema of the feet is not an adverse side effect of estrogen replacement and the client should not stop taking the medication without notifying physician.

d. Clients should be encouraged to quit smoking because this makes them prone to emboli formation.

Comprehension/Health promotion/ Evaluation

9. Correct response: d
Assessment of the client's environment should include an assessment of the client's home: food storage and preparation facilities, medication storage, presence of smoke alarms, cleanliness, temperature regulation, state of repair, safety features to reduce the risk of injury.

a, b, and c. These are included in the assessment of the elderly client but are assessment of community resources, physical assessment, and assessment of functional capacities, respectively.

Knowledge/Psychosocial/Assessment

10. Correct response: b
Physiologic changes that may occur in elderly adults and that are not related to pathologic changes include decreased metabolic rate, gray hair, slowed reaction time, decreased tendon reflexes, delayed pancreatic insulin release, and body composition changes.

a. Cardiac output is decreased due to increased peripheral vascular resistance and decreased myocardial contraction.

c. The elderly client tends to have delayed pancreatic insulin release.

d. The elderly client tends to have decreased creatinine clearance which is indicative of renal disease.

Knowledge/Physiologic/Assessment

11. Correct response: c
Pressure on the skin can be minimized by using pressure-relieving devices such as convoluted foam mattresses and air-fluidized therapeutic devices.

a. The client should be turned every 2 hours.

b. A lift sheet should be used when moving a client to prevent dragging him or her across the bed and causing skin breakdown or raw areas.

d. The head of the bed should be elevated 30 degrees to prevent shearing force on the skin (unless contraindicated by pathologic condition).

Application/Health promotion/ Implementation

12. Correct response: b
A major side effect of narcotics and analgesics is constipation.

a. Fluid intake over 2 L/day is recommended to promote bowel function.

c. Range-of-motion exercise once each day is insufficient exercise.

d. Use of daily enemas fosters dependence.

Application/Health promotion/ Planning

13. Correct response: d
Weight-bearing exercise is important in the stabilization of osteoporosis.

a, b, and c. These nursing diagnoses do not represent risk factors for progression of osteoporosis.

Knowledge/Health promotion/ Analysis (Dx)

14. Correct response: a
Using nonverbal cues would facilitate communication with a hearing-impaired client.

b, c, and d. These interventions would discourage or hamper independence and facilitation of hearing.
Application/Psychosocial/Implementation

15. *Correct response: a*
As vomiting persists, fluid and essential electrolytes are lost, which may lead to circulatory failure.
b, c, and d. These problems are not specifically associated with this client's clinical profile.
Comprehension/Safe care/Assessment

16. *Correct response: b*
A client with inadequate treatment may develop shock. Aggressive fluid replacement may lead to circulatory overload and congestive heart failure. Inappropriate administration of potassium replacement may lead to either hypokalemia or hyperkalemia.
a, c, and d. These complications are not specifically associated with dehydration.
Analysis/Physiologic/Evaluation

Emergency Nursing

Note: This chapter covers emergency conditions not discussed elsewhere in this text. See appropriate chapters for information on these common emergency conditions:

▶ Chapter 7, Cardiovascular Disorders (cardiac arrest, myocardial infarction)
▶ Chapter 12, Immunologic Disorders (anaphylaxis)
▶ Chapter 13, Integumentary Disorders (burns)
▶ Chapter 14, Neurologic Disorders (head injuries, spinal cord injury)
▶ Chapter 16, Musculoskeletal Disorders (fractures)
▶ Chapter 20, Infectious Disorders (food poisoning)

I. Overview of emergency nursing
A. Roles and functions of emergency room nurse

1. Provide care to clients with urgent and critical physiologic or psychologic needs.
2. Understand that the perceptions of the ill or injured person or his or her family define a situation as an emergency.
3. Treat the client and family with understanding, and respect the anxiety they are experiencing. Keep in mind that emergency clients feel out of control because the suddenness of their problem leaves little or no time for coping and adjusting; also remember that family members or significant others need personal consideration.
4. Practice triage, a system for setting priorities of client care: steps in nursing process from assessment through evaluation conducted rapidly with emphasis on assessing and intervening to save life and limb (Table 23-1).

5. **The emergency room nurse requires advanced medical and surgical skills. Additional training and education may include advanced cardiac life support (ACLS), certified emergency room nurse (CEN), and advanced arrhythmia recognition.**

TABLE 23-1.
Priorities for Emergency Care

1. Assess respirations.
2. Ensure a patent airway, and ventilate if necessary.
3. Assess cardiovascular function.
4. Maintain adequate blood pressure.
5. Apply pressure to any bleeding sites.
6. Assess level of consciousness.
7. Reassess vital physical parameters continually.
8. Splint all suspected fractures.
9. Apply sterile dressings to wounds.

B. Practice settings
1. Emergency department
2. A mobile unit
3. Freestanding emergency unit
4. Suicide prevention center

II. Airway obstruction

A. Description and etiology
1. Airway obstruction refers to any mechanical impediment to oxygen delivery or absorption in the lungs.
2. Food is the most common cause of obstruction in a conscious person; the tongue, in an unconscious person.

B. Assessment findings
1. A client with *complete* airway obstruction is unable to breathe or speak, becomes cyanotic, and collapses.
2. A client with *incomplete* obstruction appears anxious, uses accessory muscles to breathe, may have stridor and flared nostrils, and usually is able to speak.

C. Nursing diagnosis: Ineffective Airway Clearance

D. Planning and implementation

1. **Keep in mind that airway obstruction takes priority over any other injury or emergency problem.**
2. In partial obstruction, instruct the conscious client to cough forcefully; if this does not dislodge the object, perform the abdominal thrust (Heimlich) maneuver.
3. In complete obstruction in a conscious client, immediately perform the Heimlich maneuver.
4. In partial or complete obstruction in an unconscious client, follow these steps:
   a. Position the client on his or her back.
   b. Use the head-tilt–chin-lift technique to open the airway. (Use the jaw thrust technique if cervical spine injury is suspected.)
   c. Attempt to ventilate the client.
   d. Perform the Heimlich maneuver.
   e. Perform a finger sweep.
   f. Attempt ventilation again.
   g. Chest thrusts may be used in advanced stages of pregnancy or in a markedly obese client.
   h. Continue until the obstruction is removed.
5. Methods for providing a patent airway include:
   a. oropharyngeal airway (insertion of a tubelike device over the back of the tongue into the lower posterior pharynx in a spontaneously breathing but unconscious client)

      b.   esophageal obturator airway (insertion of a tube through the mouth and advanced into the esophagus just below the bifurcation of the trachea in an unconscious client when endotracheal intubation is not possible; the proximal part of the tube has air holes at the level of the pharynx through which air or oxygen is delivered into the lungs)

      c.   endotracheal airway (insertion of an endotracheal tube into the mouth, via the vocal folds, and advanced to the trachea just above the bifurcation of the trachea in an unconscious client; the endotracheal cuff at the end of the tube is inflated to secure the tube)

      d.   tracheostomy (insertion of a tube into an opening in the trachea to bypass an upper airway obstruction, replace an endotracheal tube, or for long-term use of a ventilator)

      e.   cricothyroidotomy (a puncture or incision into the cricothyroid membrane to establish an emergency airway in a situation in which endotracheal intubation is not possible or contraindicated)

E. Evaluation

    1.   The client maintains a patent airway.

    2.   The client resumes spontaneous respirations.

III. **Near-drowning**

    A. **Description: the pathologic status of a person who has survived events that nearly led to drowning**

    B. **Assessment findings**

      1.   Near-drowning is commonly marked by:

         a.   Cyanosis

         b.   Pulmonary edema

         c.   Possible hypothermia

         d.   Possible cardiac arrest

      2.   Laboratory studies may reveal:

         a.   Severe hypoxia

         b.   Metabolic acidosis

    C. **Nursing diagnoses**

      1.   Ineffective Airway Clearance

      2.   Hypothermia

    D. **Planning and implementation**

      1.   Initiate vigorous, purposeful cardiopulmonary resuscitation (CPR).

      2.   Ventilate with 100% oxygen and positive end expiratory pressure.

      3.   Insert an IV line, a central venous line, an indwelling urinary catheter, or a nasogastric tube as ordered.

4. Initiate cardiac monitoring.
5. Begin internal rewarming (e.g., warm peritoneal dialysis, warm aerosol inhalation) and external rewarming (e.g., hyperthermia blanket) if necessary.
6. Monitor vital signs, level of consciousness, electrocardiogram (ECG) findings, central venous pressure (CVP), intake and output, arterial blood gas (ABG) values, and serum electrolyte levels.
7. Admit the client to the ICU.

E. **Evaluation**
1. The client resumes spontaneous respirations and pulse.
2. The client exhibits stable vital signs.
3. The client registers temperature above 97°F.
4. The client is alert and responsive.

IV. **Hemorrhage**
A. **Description: rapid, massive blood loss, either internally or externally**
B. **Etiology and pathophysiology**
1. Possible causes of hemorrhage include:
   a. External: penetrating trauma, lacerations
   b. Internal: blunt or penetrating trauma, blood dyscrasias, ruptured aortic aneurysm
2. Severe hemorrhage may result in hypovolemic shock from blood loss and necessitates immediate emergency intervention.
C. **Assessment findings**
1. Clinical manifestations of hemorrhage include:
   a. Obvious bleeding from wound or orifices
   b. Signs of internal bleeding (e.g., ecchymoses, occult or frank blood in urine or stool)
   c. Cold, moist, pale skin
   d. Apprehension
   e. Hypotension
   f. Tachycardia
   g. Oliguria
2. Guaiac testing of stool may detect occult blood.
D. **Nursing diagnosis: Fluid Volume Deficit**
E. **Planning and implementation**
1. Apply pressure over bleeding area or involved artery (external bleeding).
2. Elevate and immobilize the injured body part (external bleeding), and position the client supine.
3. Start a peripheral IV for blood replacement, and administer fluids, blood products as ordered.

   4. Apply medical antishock trousers (MAST) as indicated.
   5. Prepare the client for surgery, and continue to monitor vital signs, ABG levels, CVP, and level of consciousness.
   6. **Apply a tourniquet *only as a last resort* to stop bleeding.**
F. **Evaluation**
   1. The client shows no evidence of obvious bleeding.
   2. The client maintains vital signs, ABG levels, ECG waveforms, and urine output within normal ranges.

V. **Chest trauma**
A. **Description and etiology**
   1. Causes of blunt chest trauma include:
      a. Falls
      b. Blows
      c. Automobile accidents
   2. Common penetrating chest injuries include:
      a. Gunshot wounds
      b. Stab wounds
B. **Pathophysiology**
   1. Clients with blunt chest injuries require careful and complete assessment to detect hidden injuries such as:
      a. Tears of major blood vessels, causing internal hemorrhage
      b. Lung or heart contusions, which can develop into serious cardiorespiratory emergencies
   2. Clients with penetrating chest wounds usually require emergency nursing care that focuses on management of pneumothorax (accumulation of air in pleural space) that may partially or completely collapse the affected lung.
   3. Clients with pneumothorax are at risk for life-threatening tension pneumothorax.
C. **Assessment findings**
   1. Blunt chest trauma may be marked by:
      a. Tachypnea
      b. Stridor
      c. Cyanosis
      d. Assymmetric chest expansion
      e. Signs and symptoms of hypovolemia and shock
      f. Abrasions, bruises, and other signs of injury
   2. Penetrating chest trauma may produce:
      a. Dyspnea and tachycardia accompanied by sudden, sharp chest pain
      b. Diminished or absent breath sounds on the affected side
      c. Tympanic notes on chest percussion

      3. Tension pneumothorax may cause mediastinal shift and lead to:

         a. Shock

         b. Tracheal shifting from midline

         c. Severe respiratory distress

D. Nursing diagnoses

      1. Ineffective Breathing Pattern

      2. Decreased Cardiac Output

      3. Pain

E. Planning and implementation

      1. For a client with a blunt chest injury:

         a. Report abnormal findings immediately.

         b. Monitor vital signs, ECG, level of consciousness, ABG levels.

         c. Auscultate breath sounds, and assess for respiratory difficulty.

         d. Maintain airway, ventilation, and oxygenation if necessary.

         e. Treat shock as indicated.

         f. Prepare the client for surgery if necessary.

      2. For penetrating chest injury:

         a. Position the client in high-Fowler's position, and administer oxygen as necessary.

         b. Prepare the client for insertion of a chest tube as indicated.

         c. Monitor respirations, vital signs, level of consciousness, and ABG values.

F. Evaluation

      1. The client maintains vital signs, ABG values, and level of consciousness within normal ranges.

      2. The client maintains a patent airway and displays no evidence of tracheal shift.

VI. Abdominal trauma

A. Description and etiology

      1. Abdominal injuries may be:

         a. Blunt, due to falls, blows to the abdomen, or automobile accidents

         b. Penetrating (e.g., gunshot wounds, stab wounds)

      2. Clients with blunt abdominal wounds require careful and complete assessment because hidden injuries often are not easily detected.

B. Assessment findings

      1. Findings in a client sustaining abdominal injury may include:

         a. Visible bruises, lacerations, penetrating wounds, etc.

          b.   Abdominal distention, pain, tenderness
          c.   Absent or diminished bowel sounds
          d.   Hypotension and other signs of impending shock
    2. Guaiac testing of stool may detect occult blood.

C. **Nursing diagnoses**

    1. Risk for Fluid Volume Deficit
    2. Impaired Tissue Integrity

D. **Planning and implementation**

    1. Perform CPR if necessary.
    2. Maintain the client on bedrest with knees flexed (to decrease abdominal pain).
    3. **Instruct the client to lie still; explain that movement may dislodge the clot, causing hemorrhage.**
    4. Apply pressure to external bleeding wounds.
    5. Keep the client NPO.
    6. Insert a nasogastric tube, an IV catheter, and an indwelling urinary catheter as indicated.
    7. Cover any exposed viscera with sterile normal saline solution dressings.
    8. Administer prophylactic antibiotics and tetanus toxoid as directed.
    9. Monitor vital signs, CVP, and intake and output.
  10. Auscultate bowel sounds.
  11. Prepare the client for peritoneal lavage or surgery, if indicated.

E. **Evaluation**

    1. The client exhibits no signs of infection or abdominal distention.
    2. The client reports decreased pain.
    3. The client displays audible bowel sounds.
    4. The client maintains vital signs within normal ranges.

VII. **Poisoning with ingested agents**

  A. **Description: the condition resulting from accidental or deliberate ingestion of poisonous substances**

  B. **Etiology**

    1. Commonly ingested alkaline agents include:
        a.   Lye
        b.   Drain and oven cleaners
        c.   Bleach
        d.   Clinitest
    2. Acidic substances that may be ingested include:
        a.   Toilet bowl cleaners
        b.   Battery acid
        c.   Rust removers

C. **Assessment findings**
    1. Depending on the agent ingested, the client may experience:
        a. Burning pain in the mouth and throat
        b. Dysphagia
        c. Vomiting
        d. Drooling
        e. Respiratory distress
        f. Altered level of consciousness
    2. Possible laboratory studies include ABG, CBC, blood urea nitrogen (BUN), creatinine, and electrolyte levels.

D. **Nursing diagnoses**
    1. Ineffective Airway Clearance
    2. Pain
    3. Impaired Swallowing
    4. Impaired Tissue Integrity

E. **Planning and implementation**
    1. Open the airway, and provide ventilation and oxygenation if needed.
    2. Position the client on his or her side with the head down.
    3. Suction as needed to prevent aspiration of gastric contents into respiratory tract.
    4. Remove or inactivate poison before absorption occurs, through:
        a. Syrup of Ipecac—only for an alert client who has ingested a noncorrosive substance
        b. Gastric lavage
        c. Specific antidote to neutralize poisonous substance
        d. Milk or water for dilution if the client can swallow
    5. **Do *not* induce vomiting unless prescribed by physician.**
    6. Obtain a blood sample for analysis as ordered.
    7. Monitor neurologic status, noting:
        a. Seizure activity
        b. Mentation
        c. Central nervous system (CNS) depression
    8. Insert an indwelling urinary catheter, as ordered.
    9. Before discharge, provide the client or parents with poisoning prevention guidelines.
    10. Refer the client for psychiatric consultation if poisoning was a suicide attempt. (Admission to the hospital may be necessary.)

F. **Evaluation**
    1. The client exhibits moist mucous membrane.
    2. The client reports decreased pain and discomfort.
    3. The client states an interest in psychologic counseling if poisoning was a suicide attempt.

VIII. Substance abuse
   A. Description
   1. Substance abuse refers to misuse of specific substances intended to alter mood or behavior.
   2. Commonly abused substances include:
      a. Alcohol
      b. Narcotics
      c. Hallucinogens
      d. Amphetamines
      e. Barbiturates
      f. Aspirin
   3. Be aware that substance abusers often misuse more than one substance at the same time.

   B. Assessment findings
   1. Clinical manifestations of substance abuse vary widely, depending on the substance and the amount ingested.
   2. Common signs and symptoms include:
      a. Signs of CNS depression or stimulation
      b. Altered temperature (hypothermia or hyperthermia)
      c. Respiratory depression or tachypnea
      d. Hallucinations
      e. Seizure activity
      f. Abnormal pupil size and response
      g. Nausea and vomiting
      h. Altered renal function, marked by oliguria or polyuria, abnormal BUN, serum creatinine, and serum electrolyte levels
      i. Abnormal ABG values, indicating acidosis or alkalosis

   C. Nursing diagnoses
   1. Ineffective Breathing Pattern
   2. Sensory/Perceptual Alterations
   3. Risk for Violence

   D. Planning and implementation
   1. Treat the client suffering from drug overdose; focus on:
      a. Respiratory and cardiovascular support
      b. Elimination of drug(s) from the body
   2. Control airway, ventilation, and oxygenation. (Insertion of a cuffed endotracheal tube may be necessary.)
   3. Develop a supportive, empathic rapport, and attend the client at all times.
   4. Start IV fluid infusion as indicated.
   5. Remove ingested drug from the stomach with Ipecac or gastric lavage as ordered; prevent aspiration in a client with absent gag or cough reflexes by first intubating client.

6. Administer specific drug antidote; for example:
   a. Narcan for narcotic overdose
   b. Activated charcoal only after emesis or lavage
7. Assist with hemodialysis or peritoneal dialysis as indicated.
8. Treat hypothermia or hyperthermia as appropriate (see Sections IX and X).
9. Transfer an unconscious client to the ICU.
10. Arrange consultation with psychiatrist or drug or alcohol treatment program before discharge.

E. **Evaluation**
1. The client exhibits effective respirations.
2. The client maintains stable vital signs, ABG values, and ECG findings.
3. The client is alert and oriented.
4. The client maintains serum electrolytes, creatinine, BUN, and urinary output within normal ranges.

IX. Hypothermia and frostbite

A. **Description and etiology**
1. Hypothermia refers to abnormally low core body temperature (below 34.4°C or 94°F) resulting from exposure to cold environmental temperatures.
2. Frostbite involves damage to tissue and blood vessels due to exposure to extreme cold.

B. **Assessment findings**
1. Manifestations of hypothermia may include:
   a. Subnormal body temperature
   b. Altered level of consciousness: apathy, drowsiness, coma
   c. Weak or undetectable peripheral pulses
   d. Cardiac arrhythmias, possibly cardiac arrest
   e. Signs and symptoms of hypoxia and acidosis
2. In frostbite, the affected body part may be:
   a. Cold
   b. Hard
   c. White to bluish white
   d. Numb or painful
   e. Blistered
   f. Edematous

C. **Nursing diagnoses**
1. Hypothermia
2. Impaired Skin Integrity
3. Altered Tissue Perfusion

D. **Planning and implementation**
1. Initiate CPR if indicated.
2. Rewarm the client with:

          a.   Hyperthermia blanket (external)
          b.   Warmed humidified oxygen
          c.   Warmed IV fluids (internal)

3. Monitor vital signs, CVP, ECG, ABGs, intake and output.
4. Administer IV fluids and sodium bicarbonate as ordered.
5. For frostbite:
    a. Protect the affected area from injury; handle it gently, use a protective cradle if indicated, and maintain strict aseptic technique.
    b. Rewarm the body part (e.g., in a warm whirlpool).
    c. Elevate the body part.

E. **Evaluation**
1. The client maintains body temperature above 97°F.
2. The client maintains vital signs and ABG values within normal ranges.
3. The client is alert and oriented.
4. The client with frostbite maintains good skin integrity and exhibits palpable pulses in affected extremities.

X. **Hyperthermia (heat stroke)**
  A. **Description: abnormally high body temperature due to heat stress**
  B. **Etiology and pathophysiology**
1. Hyperthermia occurs when the body's heat-regulating mechanisms fail.
2. Risk factors include:
    a. Exposure to high humidity heat waves
    b. Age extremes
    c. Debilitating disease
    d. Impaired self-care ability
    e. Certain drugs (e.g., major tranquilizers, anticholinergics, diuretics, propranolol)
  C. **Assessment findings**
1. Common clinical manifestations of hyperthermia include:
    a. Hyperpyrexia
    b. Altered level of consciousness: confusion, delirium, or coma
    c. Hot, dry skin with absence of sweating
    d. Tachycardia
    e. Tachypnea
    f. Hypotension
    g. Possibly, vomiting and diarrhea
2. Laboratory studies may reveal grossly elevated SGOT, LDH, and CPK values.
  D. **Nursing diagnosis: Hyperthermia**

E.   Planning and implementation
1.   Reduce body temperature rapidly by:
     a.   Immersing the client in cool water
     b.   Sponging with cool water
     c.   Using a hypothermia blanket
     d.   Administering iced saline lavage
2.   Monitor vital signs, ECG findings, level of consciousness, CVP, and intake and output.
3.   Massage the client to promote circulation.
4.   Initiate IV fluids and oxygen therapy as indicated.
5.   Admit the client to the ICU.

F.   Evaluation
1.   The client maintains body temperature below 100°F.
2.   The client maintains vital signs, level of consciousness, ECG, and intake and output within normal parameters.

Bibliography

Bolander, V. R. (1994). *Sorensen & Luckmann's basic nursing: A physiologic approach* (3rd ed.). Philadelphia: W. B. Saunders.

Clark, J., Queener, S., & Karb, V. (1990). *Pharmacologic basis of nursing practice* (4th ed.). St. Louis: C. V. Mosby.

Hudak, C. M., & Gallo, B. M. (1994). *Critical care nursing: A holistic approach.* Philadelphia: J. B. Lippincott.

Nettina, S. (1996). *The Lippincott manual of nursing practice* (6th ed.). Philadelphia: Lippincott-Raven Publishers.

Smeltzer, S. C., & Bare, B. G. (1996). *Brunner & Suddarth's textbook of medical-surgical nursing* (8th ed.). Philadelphia: Lippincott-Raven Publishers.

Springhouse Corporation. (1992). *Nursing student's guide to drugs.* Spring House, PA: Springhouse Corp.

STUDY QUESTIONS

1. Which of the following statements describes why clients with emergencies are unique?
   a. The families of clients with emergencies are also in need of special attention.
   b. All the steps in the nursing process must be performed when caring for a client with an emergency.
   c. Emergency clients often feel an intense sense of anxiety because of the suddenness of the illness or injury.
   d. The psychosocial needs of clients with emergencies are necessarily neglected.

2. After rapid assessment, the nurse categorizes emergency clients by priority nursing diagnoses. Based on the following diagnoses, which client should be given priority attention?
   a. Risk for Trauma: a 14-year-old with a suspected fractured femur
   b. Risk for Suffocation: a 60-year-old with burns of the face and neck
   c. Impaired Skin Integrity: a 25-year-old with a lacerated finger
   d. Anxiety: a 50-year-old complaining of "feelings of panic"

3. Which of the following nursing interventions would be appropriate when planning care for the family of an emergency client?
   a. encouraging family members to be silent about their anxieties
   b. informing the family about the care the client is receiving only when the outcome is known
   c. discouraging any feelings of anger the family feels about the situation
   d. handling the family's feelings of denial by preparing the family for the reality of the client's condition

4. Nursing care of a client who has ingested a poison always includes which of the following nursing interventions?
   a. immediately administering an emetic to prevent further absorption of the poison
   b. placing the client in high-Fowler's position to facilitate respirations
   c. referring for psychiatric consultation before discharge
   d. performing ongoing assessment of neurologic and cardiorespiratory status

5. Symptoms of a partial airway obstruction include which of the following?
   a. stridor
   b. respiratory arrest
   c. inability to speak
   d. complete collapse

6. The emergency department nurse prepares to insert a nasogastric (NG) tube in a near-drowning victim. The purpose of the NG tube is to
   a. Obtain gastric contents for analysis.
   b. Establish a vehicle for medication administration.
   c. Prevent aspiration of any swallowed water.
   d. Establish a route for nutritional supplements.

7. Which of the following evaluation criteria represent successful resolution of internal bleeding?
   a. The client demonstrates an absence of hypertension and bradycardia.
   b. The client demonstrates an absence of hypotension and tachycardia.
   c. The client demonstrates an absence of pyrexia and flushing.
   d. The client demonstrates an absence of lethargy and drowsiness.

8. Which of the following nursing interventions would be appropriate for the client who has arrived in the emergency room with a head injury?
   a. Immobilize the spine.
   b. Place the client in modified Trendelenburg position.
   c. Restrain the client's arms.
   d. Infuse IV fluids rapidly.

9. A client comes to the emergency department complaining of chest pain and shortness of breath. The nurse repeatedly reassures the client and explains all procedures. The nurse's actions would be in response to which of the following nursing diagnoses?
   a. Self Esteem Disturbance
   b. Sensory/Perceptual Alteration
   c. Fear
   d. Altered Thought Processes

10. The nurse should use which of the following techniques to open the airway in a client with a suspected cervical spine injury?
   a. head tilt
   b. jaw thrust
   c. finger sweep
   d. Heimlich maneuver

11. Which of the following should the emergency nurse include in a teaching plan for the client with frostbite of the toes?
   a. Elevate the foot on pillows.
   b. Massage the foot with lotion.
   c. Apply lotion to toes daily.
   d. Walk briskly twice a day.

12. To evaluate the effectiveness of fluid replacement for the client in hemorrhagic shock, the emergency department nurse would look for a return to normal range of
   a. hemoglobin
   b. pulse rate
   c. temperature
   d. blood pressure

13. A 25-year-old client comes into the emergency department complaining of sudden shortness of breath after being hit accidentally in the right chest. Which of the following assessment findings would lead the nurse to suspect an emergency situation?
   a. an abrasion on the right chest wall
   b. right-sided chest pain
   c. tracheal shift to the left side
   d. anxiety

For additional questions, see
Lippincott's Self-Study Series Software
Available at your bookstore

ANSWER KEY

1. **Correct response: c**
   Clients with emergencies often have not had time to accept the traditional client role. This leads to a loss of control and increased anxiety and fear.
   a and b. These statements are true for all clients.
   d. This is an untrue statement.
   Knowledge/Psychosocial/Assessment

2. **Correct response: b**
   The nurse should always suspect an inhalation injury with facial burns. Inhalation injury may cause an airway obstruction. Maintaining a patent airway is always a first priority.
   a, c, and d. These all necessitate emergency care but are not prioritized before an airway obstruction.
   Analysis/Physiologic/Analysis (Dx)

3. **Correct response: d**
   The family's feeling of denial should be handled with understanding because denial may be the only way the family can deal with this unexpected emergency. The nurse must be honest with the family and prepare them for whatever may happen. False reassurance is not appropriate.
   a, b, and c. The nurse should encourage the family to verbalize their anxiety and anger and inform the family frequently of what is happening with their loved one.
   Comprehension/Health promotion/ Planning

4. **Correct response: d**
   A poisoning client needs careful monitoring to detect subtle changes in status, which can develop quickly.
   a. Induced vomiting is unsafe if the client has ingested a corrosive substance.
   b. High-Fowler's position is unsafe; rather, the client should be side-lying with head down to prevent aspiration in the event of vomiting.

   c. A psychiatric consultation is necessary only if the poisoning was a deliberate suicide attempt.
   Application/Safe care/Implementation

5. **Correct response: a**
   An incomplete airway obstruction often causes stridor.
   b, c, and d. These are signs of complete airway obstruction.
   Knowledge/Physiologic/Assessment

6. **Correct response: c**
   Near-drowning victims frequently swallow large amounts of water, which may be aspirated during resuscitation.
   a, c, and d. These measures would be unnecessary at this time.
   Comprehension/Safe care/Planning

7. **Correct response: b**
   Decreased blood pressure and tachycardia are cardinal signs of shock.
   a. Hypertension and bradycardia are not associated with shock.
   c. This is incorrect; the client's skin would be pale and cool.
   d. This is incorrect; shock is manifested by restlessness, not lethargy.
   Comprehension/Physiologic/Evaluation

8. **Correct response: a**
   A client with a head injury should be treated as a possible cervical spine injury until proven otherwise.
   b, c, and d. These measures would be unsafe because they may cause increased intracranial pressure.
   Analysis/Safe care/Implementation

9. **Correct response: c**
   Fear frequently occurs in the emergency client with chest pain because of the sense of experiencing a catastrophic event.
   a, b, and d. These answers are incorrect; this nurse's actions are not directed at these diagnoses.
   Analysis/Psychosocial/Analysis (Dx)

10. *Correct response: b*

The jaw thrust can be done without extending the neck and without causing further spinal injury.

a. The head tilt could possibly cause further spinal injury.

c and d. The finger sweep and Heimlich maneuver are used when a foreign object other than the tongue is thought to be obstructing the airway.

Application/Safe care/Implementation

11. *Correct response: a*

Elevating the part will prevent further swelling.

b, c, and d. These actions would cause further damage to the tissues.

Application/Health promotion/Planning

12. *Correct response: d*

Adequate fluid replacement expands the fluid volume in the intravascular space and will raise the blood pressure.

a. Hemoglobin measures red blood cell replacement, not overall fluid replacement.

b and c. Pulse rate and temperature are only indirectly related to fluid status.

Analysis/Physiologic/Evaluation

13. *Correct response: c*

A tracheal shift away from the affected side is indicative of mediastinal shift—a life-threatening complication if untreated.

a, b, and d. These findings would be expected, considering this client's history, but are not imminently life-threatening.

Analysis/Physiologic/Assessment

Perioperative Nursing

I. Perioperative nursing overview

A. General

1. The perioperative period encompasses a client's total surgical experience, including the preoperative, intraoperative, and postoperative phases.
2. Perioperative nursing refers to activities performed by the professional nurse during these phases.

B. Operative phases

1. The preoperative phase begins with the decision to perform surgery and ends with the client's transfer to the operating room (OR) table.
2. The intraoperative phase begins when the client is received in the OR and ends with his or her admission to the postanesthesia recovery room (PARR) or postanesthesia care unit (PACU).
3. The postoperative phase begins when the client is admitted to PARR or PACU and extends through follow-up home or clinic evaluation.

C. **Categories of surgery**
1. Optional surgery is done totally at the client's discretion (e.g., cosmetic surgery).
2. Elective surgery refers to procedures that are scheduled at the client's convenience (e.g., cyst removal).
3. Required surgery is warranted for conditions necessitating intervention within a few weeks (e.g., cataract surgery).
4. Urgent or imperative surgery is indicated for a problem requiring intervention within 24 to 48 hours (e.g., some cancers).
5. Emergency surgery describes procedures that must be done immediately to sustain life or maintain function (e.g., repair of a ruptured aortic aneurysm).

D. **Types of anesthesia**
1. General anesthesia refers to drug-induced depression of the central nervous system (CNS) that produces analgesia, amnesia, and unconsciousness (affects whole body); stages include:
   a. Stage I—beginning
   b. Stage II—excitement
   c. Stage III—surgical anesthesia
   d. Stage IV—danger
2. Regional anesthesia suspends sensation and motion in a body region or part; the client remains awake. Continuous monitoring is required in the event the block is not totally effective and the client experiences pain or reactions to blocking agents (e.g., nausea, cardiovascular collapse).
3. Regional anesthesia differs in terms of location and size of the anatomic area anesthetized and the volume and type of anesthetic agent used.

E. **General surgical considerations**
1. The client meets with the surgical team (e.g., surgeon, OR nurse, anesthesiologist, surgical technicians, surgical first assistants, radiographic or cardiovascular technicians) before surgery.
2. An anesthesiologist or nurse anesthetist makes a preoperative assessment to plan the type of anesthetic to be administered and to evaluate the client's physical status.
3. A professional registered OR nurse makes preoperative nursing assessments and documents the intraoperative client care plan.

4. **All persons in OR are required to don specific, clean attire, with the goal of "shedding" the outside environment. Specific clothing requirements are prescribed and standardized for all ORs.**
5. Hair must be completely covered; shoes have special covers; masks are worn at all times in the OR and are changed between operations or more often, if necessary.

6. Any personnel who harbor pathogenic organisms (e.g., those with colds or infections) must report themselves unable to be in the OR to protect the client from outside pathogens.

F. Principles of surgical asepsis
1. All items used in the OR must be sterile.
2. All personnel must perform a surgical scrub and wear a sterile mask, gown, and gloves.
3. Sterile, scrubbed personnel should touch only sterile items.
4. Sterile gown and sterile drapes have defined borders of sterility.
5. That which is used for one client must be discarded or, in some cases, resterilized.
6. The circulator and unsterile personnel must stay at the periphery of the sterile operating area in order not to contaminate the sterile area.
7. Sterile supplies are unwrapped and delivered by the circulator following specific standard protocol so as not to cause contamination.
8. The utmost caution and vigilance must be used when handling sterile fluids to prevent splashing or spillage.
9. OR personnel must practice strict universal precautions (blood and body substance isolation).

II. Preoperative period
A. Assessment
1. Identify any obvious risk factors for surgery-related complications, including:
   a. Age (The very young and old are at risk for increased stress from the surgical experience.)
   b. Nutritional status (Compromised nutritional status has a negative effect on recovery and wound healing.)
   c. Obesity (An obese client presents certain technical problems during surgery; is at greater risk for postoperative pulmonary complications such as hypoventilation and hypoxia; and is more likely to have coexisting cardiac, hepatic, biliary, endocrine, or metabolic problems that could complicate surgery.)
2. Assess respiratory status, including history of pulmonary problems, to identify risk factors for postoperative complications, such as:
   a. Dyspnea, complaints of shortness of breath
   b. Upper respiratory infection
   c. Cough, wheezing
   d. Copious mucus or expectorate
   e. Chest pain
   f. Clubbed fingers
   g. History of smoking

3. Assess cardiovascular status, noting:
   a. Blood pressure
   b. Pulse rate
   c. ECG tracings
   d. Presence and amplitude of peripheral pulses
4. Assess for and report evidence of fluid and electrolyte imbalance, including:
   a. Dehydration
   b. Hypovolemia
   c. Prolonged vomiting, diarrhea, or bleeding
   d. Abnormal serum potassium, sodium, magnesium, calcium, or pH level
5. Assess hepatic and renal function, noting:
   a. History of liver disease (e.g., cirrhosis, chronic alcoholism)
   b. Complaints of dysuria, oliguria or anuria, or urinary tract infections
   c. Urinalysis results
6. Examine the client's record for any endocrine or metabolic problems that could affect the client's response to surgery (e.g., poorly controlled diabetes mellitus).
7. Assess immunologic and hematologic function, noting:
   a. History of allergies
   b. Previous reactions to blood transfusion
   c. Immunosuppressed status
8. Assess neurologic function, noting:
   a. History of seizures or other neurologic disorders (e.g., Parkinson's disease, myasthenia gravis)
   b. Unsteady gait
   c. Unequal pupils
9. Evaluate medication history for drugs that could increase operative risk by affecting coagulation time or interacting with anesthetics, such as:
   a. Steroids
   b. Diuretics
   c. Phenothiazines
   d. Antidepressants
   e. Antibiotics
   f. Anticoagulants
10. Assess the client's and family's knowledge base to guide the preoperative teaching program.
11. Consider psychosocial factors that could affect the client's response to surgery, including:
   a. Anxiety and fear
   b. Defense mechanisms (e.g., regression, denial, intellectualization)
   c. Self-esteem and body image concerns

B. **Nursing diagnoses**
   1. Anxiety
   2. Body Image Disturbance
   3. Fear
   4. Knowledge Deficit
   5. Self Esteem Disturbance
C. **Planning and implementation**
   1. Teach the client:
      a. Deep-breathing and coughing exercises
      b. Relaxation techniques
      c. Postoperative exercises of extremities
      d. Turning and moving techniques
      e. Pain control techniques
      f. Incentive spirometry use
   2. Perform preoperative skin preparation as appropriate, which may include:
      a. Shaving the skin in and around the surgical area (*Note:* Shaving is somewhat controversial; generally, the longer the interval between shaving and surgery, the greater the risk of postoperative infection.)
      b. Using an electric razor or a depilatory cream as an alternative to a razor, if possible
      c. Having the client take a cleansing shower with antimicrobial scrub solution
   3. Provide gastrointestinal preparation as prescribed, which may include:
      a. Restricting solid food and fluid for 8 to 10 hours before surgery (to reduce the risk of aspiration)
      b. Posting an NPO sign at the client's bedside
      c. Administering an enema and inserting a nasogastric tube as prescribed

   𝕟 4. **Make sure the client or a responsible family member has provided informed consent for surgery. Verify that an operative permit is signed and witnessed, with informed consent based on understandable explanation from the surgeon about what will be done and the risks involved. Make sure that the client signs the permit if he or she is an emancipated minor or adult and is mentally competent to give valid consent. If these requirements cannot be met, a responsible relative or guardian should sign for the client. State laws govern situations when a relative or guardian is not available.**
   5. Perform standard preoperative procedures (using a checklist to ensure completeness, if desired):
      a. Take and record vital signs.

      b.   Verify any allergy, identification, or diabetic bands.

      c.   Validate NPO status.

      d.   Complete and record medical preoperative orders.

      e.   Remove all jewelry and nail polish.

      f.   Have the client void and don a clean hospital gown.

      g.   Remove dentures, eyeglasses, and hearing aids, or send labeled containers with the client to the OR for safe placement in case removal becomes necessary.

      h.   Administer preanesthetic medications, and instruct the client to stay in bed.

      i.   Document any client condition requiring OR staff attention (e.g., musculoskeletal or sensorineural problems).

 6.   Ensure safe transport of the client to the surgical suite (e.g., check for a stretcher with siderails, safety strap, and warm blankets).

  D.   Evaluation

      1.   The client demonstrates knowledge of postoperative exercises according to criteria.

      2.   The client states effects of preoperative medication.

      3.   The client uses relaxation techniques and imagery preoperatively and states the intention of using them postoperatively.

      4.   The client exhibits and reports decreased anxiety.

      5.   The client receives appropriate preoperative standards of care, as evidenced by a completed preoperative checklist.

      6.   The client verbalizes understanding of postoperative pain relief, including how to use devices such as client-controlled analgesia pumps if appropriate.

III.   Intraoperative period

  A.   Assessment

      1.   Classify the client's physical status for anesthesia:

         a.   No organic or systemic disturbance present

         b.   Mild disturbance (e.g., mild cardiac disease, mild diabetes mellitus)

         c.   Severe systemic disturbance (e.g., poorly controlled diabetes mellitus, pulmonary complications)

         d.   Life-threatening systemic disease (e.g., severe renal or cardiac disease)

         e.   Moribund—little chance of survival (e.g., ruptured aortic aneurysm)

      2.   **Assess the client's record for current signed consent; completed history and physical assessment record; recent laboratory and diagnostic reports; and evaluation of the client's overall physiologic, emotional, and psychologic status.**

      3.   **Specifically ask the client if he or she has any allergies.**

4. **Verify client identification and correct surgery scheduled.**
5. Assess for any special surgical considerations (e.g., locations where an electric grounding plate can be safely placed on the client, avoiding areas where metal or a prosthesis is present) and precautions (e.g., shielding with a lead apron if radiation is involved).
6. Assess the client's risk for accidental hypothermia or malignant hyperthermia during anesthesia administration and surgery. Be sure that antidotal supplies are readily available in an emergency.

B. Nursing diagnoses
1. Risk for Fluid Volume Deficit
2. Risk for Fluid Volume Excess
3. Hyperthermia
4. Hypothermia
5. Risk for Infection
6. Risk for Injury
7. Altered Tissue Perfusion
8. Risk for Decreased Cardiac Output
9. Risk for Impaired Gas Exchange

C. Planning and implementation
1. Ensure the client's safety in the OR; for example:
   a. Set room temperature and humidity to prevent hypothermia.
   b. Remove any potential contaminants.
   c. Curtail unnecessary room traffic.
   d. Keep room noise and talk at a minimum.
   e. Recheck electrical equipment for proper operation.
   f. Make sure that necessary equipment and supplies are available.
   g. Ensure that instruments, sutures, and dressings are ready.
   h. **Count and record sutures, needles, instruments, and sponges.**
   i. Make sure that staff call the client by name and provide individualized attention.
   j. Assist in transferring the client to the OR table.
   k. Cover the client with a warm blanket, and attach the safety strap.
   l. Remain at the client's side during anesthesia induction.
   m. Verify proper client positioning to protect nerves, circulation, respiration, and skin integrity.
   n. Ensure that newly requested items are quickly supplied to the anesthesia or scrub team by the circulating nurse.

2. Perform other actions as appropriate:

   a. **Act in the role of client advocate: provide privacy, protect from harm.**

   b. Follow established procedures and protocols.

   c. Document all OR care.

   d. Help coordinate health team activities.

   e. Promote ethical behaviors (e.g., respect, confidentiality).

   f. Monitor blood, fluid, and other drainage output.

D. Evaluation

1. The client remains free of any operative injury due to electrical, chemical, or physical hazards related to surgery.

2. The client maintains satisfactory body temperature between 96°F and 100°F on completion of surgery.

3. The client remains free of injury linked to positioning during surgery, as evidenced by no complaints of numbness, paralysis, or abrasions.

4. The client arrives safely in the recovery area and exhibits adequate respiratory effort and good skin color.

IV. Immediate postoperative period

A. Assessment

1. **Perform assessment immediately on the client's admission to the PARR or PACU to obtain baseline data.**

2. Position the client before assessment to ensure an adequate airway; most commonly, lateral Sims' position for an unconscious client unless contraindicated.

3. **Priorities for assessment include:**

   a. **Respiratory: airway patency, skin color**

   b. **Cardiovascular: vital signs**

4. The verbal report from the OR nurse and anesthesiologist or nurse-anesthetist to the PACU nurse should describe:

   a. The client's age and general condition

   b. Any intraoperative problems encountered

   c. Medical diagnosis, pathology

   d. Fluids administered, blood loss and replacement, tubings and drains present

   e. Specific individual problems or deficits: hearing, vision, and mental status; and any symptoms that might need to be immediately reported to the surgeon

B. Nursing diagnoses

1. Ineffective Airway Clearance

2. Ineffective Breathing Pattern

3. Risk for Fluid Volume Deficit

4. Risk for Infection

5. Impaired Physical Mobility

6. Pain
7. Impaired Tissue Integrity
8. Altered Tissue Perfusion: Cardiopulmonary and Peripheral
9. Altered Urinary Elimination

C. Planning and implementation

1. Document the client's condition on the recovery room scoring guide.
2. Assess at least every 15 minutes (or more frequently depending on the client's status):
    a. Airway
    b. Vital signs
    c. General appearance
    d. Level of consciousness and reflexes
    e. Pain level
    f. Urine output
    g. Intravenous or central line patency
    h. Drain or catheter patency
    i. Operative site and dressings for signs of hemorrhage or abnormal drainage
    j. Functioning of cardiac and O_2 monitors
3. Maintain airway patency and optimum respiratory function; position the client on side until he or she awakens, and administer oxygen as necessary.
4. Promote client comfort by administering prescribed analgesics which alter the client's pain level, for example, nonnarcotic analgesics such as acetaminophen (Tylenol); or narcotic analgesics such as acetaminophen with hydrocodone (Vicodin) or codeine (Tylenol 3), propoxyphene (Darvon), meperidine (Demerol), nalbuphine (Nubain), or morphine (Duramorph).

    a. **Be sure to assess the client's pain level on a pain scale denoting intensity and location.**
    b. **Be sure that pain is expected postoperative pain rather than a sign of complication.**
    c. **Administer analgesic agent, and institute safety precautions.**
    d. **Assess effectiveness of pain medication 30 minutes after delivery.**
    e. **Provide other comfort measures including repositioning and distraction.**
    f. **Encourage postoperative exercises as possible to prevent complications.**
5. Offer emotional support and reassurance.
6. Be alert for signs and symptoms of hypovolemic shock, a potential postoperative complication stemming from loss of blood and plasma during surgery.

D. **Evaluation (for discharge from recovery room)**
   1. The client performs deep breathing and coughing and exhibits clear lungs on auscultation.
   2. The client can lift his or her head off the pillow and hold it up.
   3. The client moves all extremities (unless contraindicated by surgery, physician's order, or previous physical condition).
   4. The client's dressings remain dry or have only light drainage apparent.
   5. The client's urinary output remains at least 30 mL/hour.
   6. The client maintains blood pressure and vital signs at stable levels and within normal ranges for the client's situation.
   7. The client reports pain relief with adequate dosages of pain medication.
   8. The client can be safely transferred to a clinical unit for further care.
   9. The client scores at least 7 out of 10 possible points on a postanesthesia scoring chart by the time of discharge to a clinical unit.

V. **Intermediate and extended postoperative periods**
   A. **Assessment**
   1. Perform a head-to-toe physical assessment on the client's admission to the clinical unit.
   2. Monitor overall condition and blood pressure, pulse, and respirations every 15 minutes for the first 2 hours, every 30 minutes for the next 2 hours, and, if stable, every 4 hours thereafter.
   3. Assess respiratory status, including:
      a. Rate, depth, and pattern
      b. Character of breath sounds
      c. Airway patency
   4. Assess circulatory status in extremities.
   5. Observe level of consciousness and responsiveness.
   6. Inspect surgical wounds, dressings, and drains; note signs of healing or infection, patency, and drainage characteristics.
   7. Assess comfort level, noting:
      a. Time of last pain medication
      b. Any current pain; its location, nature, and intensity
      c. Position of maximum comfort
      d. Complaints of nausea or vomiting
      e. Body temperature
      f. Constrictive or irritating casts, dressings, traction
   8. Evaluate urinary status, noting:
      a. Last voiding and amount
      b. Presence of indwelling catheter
   9. Explore psychosocial concerns related to such factors as:
      a. The nature of client's surgical diagnosis and prognosis

       b.   Available support systems

       c.   The client's need for rest and quiet

  10. Assess safety aspects, such as:

       a.   The need for side rails on the bed

       b.   Correct IV infusion rate

       c.   Splinting of IV site

       d.   Call bell kept within easy reach

       e.   Ambulation status and the need for assistance

       f.   Condition of all equipment

B. **Nursing diagnoses**

  1. Common nursing diagnoses applying to postsurgical clients include:

       a.   Ineffective Airway Clearance

       b.   Anxiety

       c.   Constipation

       d.   Risk for Fluid Volume Deficit

       e.   Risk for Infection

       f.   Risk for Injury

       g.   Impaired Physical Mobility

       h.   Altered Nutrition: Less than body requirements

       i.   Pain

       j.   Impaired Tissue Integrity

       k.   Altered Tissue Perfusion: Peripheral

       l.   Altered Urinary Elimination

  2. More individualized diagnoses addressing psychosocial concerns related to the client's particular condition and the nature of the surgery could include:

       a.   Body Image Disturbance

       b.   Hopelessness

       c.   Powerlessness

       d.   Spiritual Distress

C. **Planning and implementation**

  1. Promote lung expansion and help prevent atelectasis and pneumonia by:

       a.   Encouraging coughing, deep-breathing, and turning

       b.   Using an incentive spirometer, as indicated

       c.   Encouraging ambulation as tolerated

  2. Monitor for signs and symptoms of postoperative complications, including:

       a.   Hypovolemia

       b.   Hemorrhage

       c.   Pulmonary embolism

       d.   Allergic drug reactions

       e.   Cardiac arrhythmias

3. Provide appropriate pain relief measures, which may include:
   a. Prescribed analgesics, possibly client-controlled analgesia units
   b. Nonpharmacologic pain relief measures (e.g., relaxation, guided imagery)
4. Promote adequate fluid intake and monitor electrolyte balance.
5. Provide adequate nutrition; resume oral feeding as soon as gastric and bowel motility return, or provide IV hyperalimentation as indicated.
6. Auscultate for bowel sounds to detect the return of peristalsis. (Paralytic ileus may occur after abdominal or bowel surgery.)
7. As indicated, minimize abdominal distention resulting from decreased peristalsis (typically persisting 3 to 4 days postoperatively) through exercise, ambulation, decreased narcotic dosage, or rectal tube placement.
8. Assess for urinary retention after bladder catheter removal, particularly in clients who have undergone surgery involving the pelvic or rectal area. (See Chapter 18, Renal and Urinary Disorders)
9. Promote normal voiding patterns through such measures as:
   a. Providing privacy
   b. Running tap water or providing other stimuli to induce urination
   c. Increasing fluid intake
   d. Relieving pain
10. Assess for and report unrelieved nausea and vomiting; administer antiemetics as prescribed, and decrease the risk of aspirating vomitus through proper positioning.
11. Reduce the risk of nosocomial infection by maintaining medical and surgical asepsis. Classify the original surgical wound as clean, clean-contaminated, contaminated, or infected; observe for complications of a nonhealing wound. (See Chapter 20, Infectious Disorders)
12. Respond quickly to evisceration (rupture of wound with coils of intestines pushed out, preceded by a gush of serosanguineous fluid) by:
    a. Staying with and attempting to calm the client
    b. Positioning to decrease abdominal strain
    c. Applying moist, sterile saline dressings to cover exposed intestine
    d. Notifying the surgeon, who will need to perform reclosure surgery as soon as possible
13. Encourage movement and ambulation, as indicated. Have the client gradually increase exercise from lying, to sitting, to standing, to ambulating. Provide assistance and encouragement; maintain safety precautions.

14. Minimize the risk of deep vein thrombosis (DVT) by:
    a. Assessing for early signs (e.g., redness, swelling, tenderness along vein, positive Homans' sign)
    b. Applying elastic hose, applying a sequential compression device, or administering low-dose heparin, as prescribed
    c. Teaching measures to prevent vessel constriction (See Chapter 8, Peripheral Vascular Disorders)

15. Intervene as appropriate to prevent postoperative depression, disorientation, or psychosis; measures include:
    a. Providing preoperative teaching and information
    b. Orienting the client postoperatively
    c. Providing prescribed medication, close supervision, and consultation with mental health personnel as required

16. Teach the client and family members to assess for and report signs or symptoms of complications, such as:
    a. DVT
    b. Wound infection
    c. Wound dehiscence

17. Teach the client and family members about:
    a. Prescribed medications
    b. Treatments
    c. Diet
    d. Activity level
    e. Planned follow-up care

18. Discuss postoperative depression and ineffective coping with the client and family members; teach them about the grieving process and refer them to support groups as appropriate.

19. As necessary, refer the client and family to social services to arrange for such services as:
    a. Home care
    b. Meals on Wheels
    c. Visiting nurse
    d. Transportation assistance
    e. Special equipment (e.g., wheelchair, walker, oxygen equipment)

D. Evaluation

1. The client maintains optimum respiratory function, as evidenced by:
    a. Performing deep breathing exercises four times daily for the first 48 hours postoperatively
    b. Demonstrating clear breath sounds on auscultation
    c. Turning, exercising, and ambulating as instructed
    d. Coughing effectively to expectorate secretions and sputum

2. The client maintains optimum cardiovascular function, as evidenced by:

    a.   No signs or symptoms of cardiac arrhythmias
    b.   Good capillary refill and normal skin color
    c.   Normal body temperature and vital signs within acceptable ranges
    d.   No signs of hemorrhage or hematoma

3. The client reports adequate pain control.
4. The client maintains optimum fluid and electrolyte status.
5. The client maintains optimum nutritional status.
6. The client demonstrates optimum bowel elimination pattern.
7. The client demonstrates optimum urine elimination pattern.
8. The client displays optimum wound healing, as evidenced by:
   a. No abnormal wound drainage
   b. Afebrile state with normal white blood cell count
   c. Intact wound with no breakdown, redness, or signs of dehiscence or evisceration
9. The client attains optimum mobility and self-care ability by time of discharge.
10. The client exhibits optimum psychological functioning, as evidenced by:
    a. Absence of psychotic or disoriented behavior
    b. Ability to communicate needs to health care team
    c. Asking appropriate questions related to operation and sexual matters
    d. Reporting feelings of depression
    e. Appropriate eye contact
    f. Good grooming and personal hygiene (as ability allows)
11. The client or family members discuss assessment of potential complications and the importance of reporting symptoms.
12. The client or family members verbalize understanding of prescribed medications, diet, activity, and other therapies.
13. The client or family states appropriate arrangements made for home care.

Bibliography

Bolander, V. R. (1994). *Sorensen & Luckmann's basic nursing: A physiologic approach* (3rd ed.). Philadelphia: W. B. Saunders.

Burden, N. (1993). *Ambulatory surgical nursing.* Philadelphia: W. B. Saunders.

Carpenito, L. J. (1995). *Nursing diagnosis: Application to clinical practice* (6th ed.). Philadelphia: J. B. Lippincott.

Clark, J., Queener, S., & Karb, V. (1990). *Pharmacologic basis of nursing practice* (4th ed.). St. Louis: C. V. Mosby.

Dossey, B. M., Guzzetta, C. E., & Kenner, C. V. (1992). *Critical care nursing: Body-mind-spirit* (3rd ed.). Philadelphia: J. B. Lippincott.

Hudak, C. M., & Gallo, B. M. (1994). *Critical care nursing: A holistic approach.* Philadelphia: J. B. Lippincott.

Nettina, S. (1996). *The Lippincott manual of nursing practice* (6th ed.). Philadelphia: Lippincott-Raven Publishers.

Rothrock, J. C. (1995). *Perioperative nursing care planning* (2nd ed.). St. Louis: C. V. Mosby.

Scherer, J. C., & Timby, B. K. (1995). *Introductory Medical-Surgical Nursing* (6th ed.). Philadelphia: J. B. Lippincott.

Smeltzer, S. C., & Bare, B. G. (1996). *Brunner & Suddarth's textbook of medical-surgical nursing* (8th ed.). Philadelphia: Lippincott-Raven Publishers.

Watt-Watson, J. H., & Donovan, M. I. (1992). *Pain management: nursing perspective*. St. Louis: C. V. Mosby.

STUDY QUESTIONS

1. The female client confides to the OR nurse that she induces vomiting and takes laxatives daily. From this information, the nurse would suspect that the client is at specific risk for which of the following nursing diagnoses?
   a. Risk for Aspiration
   b. Risk for Fluid Volume Deficit
   c. Altered Tissue Perfusion: Peripheral
   d. Risk for Infection

2. The nurse notes that the ambient OR temperature is 68°F (20°C). What would be the most appropriate nursing diagnosis for the 70-year-old client who is undergoing abdominal surgery in this OR?
   a. Risk for Injury
   b. Altered Tissue Perfusion
   c. Risk for Altered Body Temperature
   d. Risk for Infection

3. For an unconscious client who was recently admitted to the PACU and who has no contraindication to movement, which of the following represents the most effective nursing intervention to promote adequate respiratory function?
   a. Place the client supine and perform jaw thrust maneuver.
   b. Turn the client every 10 minutes from side to side.
   c. Position the client on one side with a pillow at the back and with chin extended.
   d. Place the client prone to facilitate drainage of secretions.

4. Which of the following statements supports the evaluation that the client who had a radical perineal prostatectomy is coping positively with postoperative impotence?
   a. "The doctor told me about penile prostheses; I'm considering using one."
   b. "Cancer runs in my family; I feel doomed after this surgery."
   c. "I'm going right back to my teaching job and act like this didn't happen."
   d. "How many men my age have you cared for who've had this surgery?"

5. The nurse notes that the client scheduled for an emergency vaginal procedure (D&C) due to a spontaneous abortion is crying. The nurse's best response would be to
   a. Squeeze her hand and tell her, "There's nothing to be afraid of."
   b. Check her name band, and have the anesthesiologist give her a tranquilizer.
   c. Let her cry, and tell others to leave her alone until she is anesthetized.
   d. Stand by her side, and quietly ask her to describe what she is feeling.

6. The client is scheduled to have excess fat suctioned from the thighs for cosmetic reasons. When gathering preoperative assessment data, the nurse recognizes that this surgery is
   a. optional
   b. elective
   c. required
   d. urgent

7. The client signs the form, giving informed consent for surgery. After the physician leaves the room, the client asks the nurse, "When will this hotel bring me some food?" After the nurse confirms that the client is confused, the priority nursing action should be
   a. Report that the consent has been obtained from a confused client.
   b. Teach preoperative moving, coughing, and deep-breathing exercises.
   c. Insert a bladder catheter and evaluate output.
   d. Administer preoperative medication immediately.

8. Which of the following represents the most significant risk factor for postoperative physiologic complications?
   a. pregnancy
   b. hypertension

c. morbid obesity

d. age of 70 or older

9. Operating room personnel are required to wear specific, clean OR attire and cover hair and shoes. What is the rationale for this clothing?

   a. to promote a totally sterile environment

   b. to exclude the environment outside of surgery

   c. to provide uniforms that are non-static

   d. to isolate the client's diseases from OR staff

10. The OR nurse cautions the scrub team to be very quiet just as the client is receiving a general anesthetic. Evaluation of response to anesthesia at this point would demonstrate which of the following?

    a. The client has an increased risk of apnea.

    b. The client experiences noises as exaggerated in Stage I.

    c. The client may become excited and struggle.

    d. The client experiences an extension of time to get to Stage III.

11. Which of the following nursing interventions would be appropriate for a client who develops malignant hyperthermia crisis?

    a. Administer iced IV saline solution and dantrolene sodium.

    b. Begin monitoring heart rate and rhythm.

    c. Insert a bladder catheter with temperature probe.

    d. Type and crossmatch the client for whole blood administration.

12. The circulating nurse refuses to let the consulting surgeon come into an OR wearing a sterile gown that was worn in another surgery. This action is based primarily on

    a. value judgment

    b. critical thinking

    c. principles of asepsis

    d. assertiveness

13. A 60-year-old client has just had an abdominoperineal resection. Two hours postoperatively, the client's blood pressure drops from 126/78 mmHg to 102/68 mmHg and the pulse rate increases from 80 to 106 beats per minute. The client's skin is cool and pale. The nurse's best nursing action would be to:

    a. Notify the supervisor that the client is in moderate shock.

    b. Increase nasal oxygen flow rate to 8 L.

    c. Place the client in Trendelenburg position.

    d. Notify the surgeon, and ask for increased IV fluid rate.

14. A postoperative client is being discharged from PACU. The point score on the postanesthesia chart, indicating that the client has fulfilled minimal criteria for discharge, should be

    a. one point each in respiratory, circulatory, consciousness, color, and muscle activity, for a total of 5

    b. one point in at least three areas—respiratory, circulatory, consciousness—for a total of 3

    c. a total score for the five areas of 7 or above

    d. two points each in respiratory, circulatory, consciousness, color, and muscle activity, for a total of 10

15. A client who underwent abdominal surgery 36 hours ago has an increased temperature and pulse rate; shallow, rapid breathing; and bilateral adventitious lung sounds. Based on these data, which of the following priority nursing diagnoses would be most appropriate?

    a. Activity Intolerance

    b. Ineffective Airway Clearance

    c. Altered Tissue Perfusion: Cardiopulmonary

    d. Ineffective Individual Coping

16. A morbidly obese client who underwent a splenectomy 1 week ago has the wound staples removed. Two hours after staple removal, the nurse assesses

abdominal wound dehiscence. The most appropriate immediate nursing intervention would be

a. Place the client in a recumbent position, cover the wound with saline dressings, and call the surgeon immediately.

b. Leave client, stating that you will be right back with help.

c. Complete a head-to-toe assessment before calling the surgeon.

d. Place a sign on client's door to indicate drainage precaution status.

For additional questions, see
Lippincott's Self-Study Series Software
Available at your bookstore

ANSWER KEY

1. *Correct response: b*
This client is at risk for potassium imbalance (hypokalemia).
a. The client will not aspirate if the stomach is empty.
c and d. These answers do not relate directly to the question and are not specific to vomiting and purging.
Application/Safe care/Analysis (Dx)

2. *Correct response: c*
Elderly clients are very susceptible to accidental hypothermia from the environment. General anesthesia causes vasodilation, which will further aggravate the situation.
a. This is a possible diagnosis for all surgery clients but does not relate to this specific situation.
b. This is inaccurate—decreased fluid volume would stem from NPO status and bleeding.
d. This answer does not relate to the situation as presented.
Comprehension/Health promotion/
Analysis (Dx)

3. *Correct response: c*
This is the correct intervention until the client regains consciousness.
a. This intervention would be appropriate for a client with respiratory obstruction.
b. During the immediate postoperative period, turning every 10 minutes is inappropriate.
d. Postoperative clients are rarely, if ever, placed in the prone position.
Application/Physiologic/Planning

4. *Correct response: a*
Optimum psychosocial affect is manifested by the client asking or discussing matters related to sexuality. A penile prosthesis may be an appropriate alternative for an impotent man.
b. This response demonstrates possible depression.

c. This response demonstrates denial of feelings, which can lead to psychological problems over time.
d. This response does not address the problem specifically, although it may indicate the client's willingness to explore the problem further with the nurse.
Analysis/Psychosocial/Evaluation

5. *Correct response: d*
Therapeutic communication allows the client to express fear or grief.
a. This intervention is nontherapeutic and belittles the client's fear or emotion.
b. This intervention is nontherapeutic, because the nurse avoids the client's expression.
c. This intervention is nontherapeutic because the client would be left alone in an anxiety-producing environment.
Application/Psychosocial/Implementation

6. *Correct response: a*
Cosmetic surgeries, by definition, are most often optional.
b, c, and d. These answers are incorrect according to definitions in text.
Comprehension/Health promotion/
Assessment

7. *Correct response: a*
Legal consent must be obtained from a comprehending client or from a family member or guardian.
b. This would be inappropriate until the legality of the client's situation was assessed. If confusion makes the client unteachable, the nurse should report this also.
c. This usually would be done after the client was anesthetized to minimize pain. It is not a priority.
d. This would not be completed until the client's legal status was clear.
Analysis/Safe care/Planning

8. *Correct answer: c*
   Obese persons have been identified as carrying the greatest risk for complications during the intraoperative and postoperative phases.
   a, b, and d. Although pregnancy, hypertension, and advanced age are all risk factors, none is considered to be as significant a factor as obesity.
   Analysis/Health promotion/Assessment

9. *Correct answer: b*
   The main goal is to protect the client from infection by eliminating outside hazards of dust, pollutants, and so forth.
   a. A "total" sterile environment is impossible to achieve.
   c. Nonstatic clothes no longer are required, as nonexplosive gases are now used in the OR.
   d. The client is being protected from others.
   Comprehension/Health promotion/ Planning

10. *Correct answer: b*
    Hearing is extremely sensitive in Stage I, and noise reduction is important.
    a. Apnea will result from anesthetic drugs, but this is not a reason for quiet.
    c. The excitement stage is Stage II, not Stage I.
    d. The anesthetic, not noise, influences client transition to Stage III.
    Application/Physiologic/Evaluation

11. *Correct answer: a*
    Precise therapy is needed to decrease temperature and muscle rigidity. Supplies are usually kept in a special place; all OR nurses need to know the procedure and how to obtain needed supplies.
    b. A client always has the heart monitored for every surgery.
    c. Temperature is always monitored in the OR either by rectal, esophageal, or other route before surgery starts.

    d. Whole blood is not the therapy for malignant hyperthermia.
    Knowledge/Safe care/Implementation

12. *Correct answer: c*
    One principle of asepsis is the isolation of items for exclusive use for one client. Therefore, a sterile gown worn by a surgeon in another surgery must be left in that room.
    a, b, and d. These answers are incorrect; however, they are characteristics that certainly assist the nurse in enforcing strict principles of asepsis.
    Analysis/Physiologic/Assessment

13. *Correct answer: d*
    At this time the client could be showing early signs of hypovolemia and early shock and thus would require increased fluid. If symptoms should become more severe, the surgeon has already been alerted.
    a. This client is in early, not moderate, shock.
    b and c. These measures could be appropriate later but would not be critical actions early.
    Analysis/Physiologic/Implementation

14. *Correct answer: c*
    Seven points is the minimum score required for discharge from the PACU.
    a, b, and d. A client is not considered stable for discharge with a score below seven, and ten points are not necessary for discharge.
    Knowledge/Safe care/Evaluation

15. *Correct answer: b*
    Immediate nursing intervention could help prevent serious complications from atelectasis and pneumonia secondary to poor respiratory hygiene and immobility.
    a, c, and d. These measures would not be priority at this time.
    Application/Physiologic/ Analysis (Dx)

16. *Correct answer: a*

Appropriate intervention would involve protecting the protruding intestine, relieving abdominal pressure by positioning, and notifying the surgeon, who will schedule immediate surgery.

b, c, and d. None of these interventions would be appropriate for this client.

Application/Physiologic/Implementation

COMPREHENSIVE TEST—QUESTIONS

1. A group of nurse leaders has developed a system of interrelated and interdependent problem-solving steps based on the science of nursing. Which of the following best describes the result of their work?
   a. a framework for nursing practice called the nursing process
   b. a universal language for nurses known as a taxonomy of nursing diagnoses
   c. a definition of nursing focused on human responses to health problems
   d. a social policy statement for the nursing profession

2. Which of the following questions would be the most appropriate as part of the "role and relationship patterns" segment of the nursing health history?
   a. "What are your ideas about health?"
   b. "Do you have any problems with mobility?"
   c. "How would you describe your family's health?"
   d. "How would you describe your strengths and weaknesses?"

3. A 79-year-old client has pale, cold feet bilaterally, no hair tufts on toes, and a circumscribed 3-cm lesion on the plantar surface at the first metatarsal joint. Which of the following is the most likely source of the client's problem?
   a. insufficient venous circulation
   b. venous thrombosis
   c. expected age-related physiologic changes
   d. insufficient arterial circulation

4. An adult client has the following hematology and blood chemistry results.

   Hemoglobin: 15 mg/dL
   Hematocrit: 50%
   Serum sodium: 140 mEq/L
   Serum potassium: 4.5 mEq/L
   Serum cholesterol: 160 mg/100 mL
   Serum triglycerides: 100 mg/100 mL

   Which of the following statements about these findings is correct?
   a. Two results are below normal ranges.
   b. All results are within normal ranges.
   c. Three results are within normal ranges.
   d. One result is above normal range.

5. During a teaching session, the nurse discovers that the client wears a hearing aid and has difficulty with group discussions. Based on the nursing diagnosis Sensory/Perceptual Alteration: Auditory, modifications in the plan of care would most appropriately include which of the following?
   a. closed-circuit television
   b. computer-assisted instruction
   c. videotapes
   d. filmstrips

6. Which of the following behaviors would clue the nurse that the client is a tactile learner?
   a. After listening to the nurse's explanation on using home oxygen equipment, the client asks the nurse to write down the important information.
   b. The client reads printed instructions on home oxygen therapy carefully, underlining key points.
   c. The client picks up the oxygen tubing and begins attaching it to the oxygen cylinder before receiving teaching on the use of home oxygen equipment.
   d. The client listens to a discussion about using home oxygen equipment, asking questions to clarify certain steps.

7. In cellular injury, swelling of inflamed tissue results from

a. transient vasodilation followed by vasoconstriction
b. migration of white blood cells (WBCs) away from the site of injury
c. increased vascular permeability, with leakage of plasma fluids
d. irritation of nerve endings by fibrinogen

8. A client who has been receiving radiation therapy for breast cancer complains of dysphagia and skin texture changes at the radiation site. To help reduce the risk of complications and to enhance healing, the nurse would advise the client
   a. Apply heat to the radiation site to increase metabolic activity.
   b. Eat a diet high in protein and calories to optimize tissue repair.
   c. Apply cool packs to the radiation site to reduce swelling.
   d. Drink warm fluids frequently throughout the day to relieve discomfort on swallowing.

9. Pathologic cellular adaptation to excessive physiologic stress occurs to preserve cells. In evaluating this adaptive response in a client, which of the following findings would represent hyperplasia?
   a. The client displays an enlarged heart muscle on radiograph.
   b. The client displays loss of cell substance resulting in cell shrinkage.
   c. The client shows evidence of changes in epithelial cells from habitual smoking.
   d. The client demonstrates increase in breast size during pregnancy.

10. A client who was admitted with complaints of fatigue and muscle weakness takes 20 mg of furosemide daily for essential hypertension and has a serum potassium level of 2.8 mEq/L. Based on the physician's order for KCl 20 mEq in 100 mL D_5W over 2 hours, the nurse should take which of the following actions?

a. Teach the client about foods high in potassium.
b. Call the physician to clarify the order because KCl should be infused at a rate of 10 mEq every 2 hours.
c. Observe the ECG for peaked, narrow T waves.
d. Have laboratory results double-checked because low potassium levels commonly are hemolyzed.

11. A client is admitted with complaints of lethargy, confusion during the last few days, and loss of appetite with nausea and vomiting over the last 2 weeks. The client's ECG shows a shortened QT interval. Based on these data, the nurse would suspect that the client is experiencing
   a. hyponatremia
   b. hypermagnesemia
   c. hypercalcemia
   d. hyperkalemia

12. A client has severe diarrhea (passage of 15 explosive diarrheal stools in the past 10 hours) after eating fish last night. Which of the following group of abnormal laboratory values would the nurse expect?
   a. decreased blood urea nitrogen (BUN) and decreased hematocrit
   b. decreased BUN and increased hematocrit
   c. increased BUN and decreased hematocrit
   d. increased BUN and increased hematocrit

13. A client who is admitted in obvious respiratory distress is belligerent and confused as well. ABG values reveal pH of 7.55, PO_2 of 68, PCO_2 of 38, and HCO_3 of 29. Which of the following reasons would explain the client's behavior?
   a. The client is frightened by breathing difficulty.
   b. The client is experiencing metabolic alkalosis, which causes mental changes.

c. The client is experiencing respiratory acidosis, which causes mental changes.

d. The client is exhibiting typical behavior for someone in a respiratory crisis.

14. A client diagnosed with hypermagnesemia reports having a hiatal hernia and severe heartburn. The client reports taking antacids several times a day. Which of the following nursing diagnoses is appropriate?

a. Impaired Physical Mobility related to magnesium loss from bone

b. Knowledge Deficit related to the role of antacids in increasing serum magnesium levels

c. Sleep Pattern Disturbance related to neuromuscular irritability

d. Fluid Volume Excess related to magnesium retention

15. Pain described as sharp and prickling and occurring after a cut finger is transmitted over

a. the smallest unmyelinated type C nerve fibers

b. medium myelinated type A-gamma nerve fibers

c. the largest myelinated type A-alpha and beta nerve fibers

d. medium myelinated type A-delta nerve fibers

16. Which of the following nursing diagnoses would be appropriate for a client who "hates to bother the nurses" and so doesn't initially report intense pain when crutch-walking to the bathroom?

a. Powerlessness related to pain

b. Knowledge Deficit related to the need to call nurses

c. Fear related to pain

d. Self Care Deficit related to the need to call nurses

17. Which of the following nursing interventions would be appropriate for a very stoic client who refuses analgesics even when in severe pain?

a. Stay with the client, and hold his or her hand.

b. Use patient-controlled analgesia, transcutaneous electrical nerve stimulation (TENS), distraction, and as many psychologic interventions as the client will accept.

c. Insist on analgesia, administering it in food or fluid without the client's knowledge.

d. Do not provide pain relief measures until the client requests.

18. Which of the following steps should a client with periodic angina pain take *first* when pain occurs at home?

a. Take sublingual nitroglycerin and lie down.

b. Do mild breathing and range-of-motion exercises.

c. Take an extra long-lasting nitrate tablet.

d. Sit down and relax, using distraction and guided imagery.

19. A client with moderate to severe emphysema is admitted in acute respiratory distress. During the initial nursing assessment the client states that he continues to smoke regularly, mows the lawn weekly, and refuses to use oxygen in front of his friends. Which of the following nursing diagnoses would the nurse use to address these behaviors?

a. Anticipatory Grieving

b. Body Image Disturbance

c. Ineffective Denial

d. Impaired Social Interaction

20. Lung dysfunction impacts physical and mental performance because of the lungs' critical role in maintaining the body's acid–base balance. Specifically, the lung plays a primary role in controlling

a. arterial O_2 and blood urea

b. arterial CO_2 and cholesterol

c. arterial CO_2, serum albumin, and pH

d. arterial CO_2 and pH

21. In planning care of a client admitted to the thoracic ICU with pneumothorax, the nurse should recognize that an opening in the chest wall—whether due to a deliberate surgical intervention or to traumatic injury—causes the lung on that side to
   a. expand due to intake of atmospheric air
   b. collapse due to disturbed negative pressure in the pleural space
   c. expand due to altered lung pressures
   d. collapse due to disturbed positive pressure in the pleural space

22. The nurse detects premature ventricular contractions (PVCs) on the ECG of a client who had a mitral valve replacement 2 days ago. The nurse recognizes that PVCs may be dangerous because they
   a. significantly increase cardiac workload
   b. may lead to ventricular tachycardia or ventricular fibrillation
   c. are the most common cause of myocardial infarction
   d. decrease heart rate and blood pressure

23. A female client is diagnosed with unstable angina and is scheduled for coronary arteriography in the morning. The nurse finds her crying because fears she'll "have to cut back" on her activities and become a "burden" to her husband. Based on this information, which of the following nursing diagnoses would be most appropriate for this client?
   a. Impaired Verbal Communication
   b. Ineffective Family Coping: Compromised
   c. Knowledge Deficit
   d. Fear

24. Interventions to relieve discomfort associated with chronic arterial occlusive vascular disease are directed at
   a. improving venous return from the involved extremity
   b. avoiding narcotic analgesic drugs
   c. preventing edema in the extremities
   d. increasing circulation to the extremities

25. On assessing an older client, the nurse notes that the left leg is swollen and warm, with palpable pedal pulses; an open, wet ulcer above the medial malleolus; and thick, coarse, brown pigmented skin surrounding the ulcer. Based on these findings, the nurse likely would identify the probable cause of the ulcer as
   a. acute deep vein thrombosis
   b. chronic venous insufficiency
   c. chronic arterial insufficiency
   d. chronic lymphedema

26. In designing a nursing care plan for a client released from the emergency room after initial care for a penetrating foot injury, the most important advice the nurse could give would be
   a. Call the physician if red streaks appear on the foot or leg.
   b. Avoid crossing the legs at the knee or the ankle.
   c. Avoid smoking until the wound completely heals.
   d. Notify the physician immediately of warning signs of anaphylactic shock from the tetanus toxoid.

27. A nurse assesses a client 1 day after an above-the-knee amputation. During the assessment, the nurse notes a decrease in blood pressure, tachycardia, and tachypnea. The large bulky dressing on the stump has a 7-cm spot of red drainage at the distal portion. Which interpretation of these findings would be most appropriate?
   a. The client demonstrates normal response to recovery from general anesthetic.
   b. The client demonstrates an early response to pain and should be medicated with analgesic.
   c. The client demonstrates a response to excessive bleeding at

the stump and should be re-assessed at frequent intervals.

    d. The client demonstrates early signs of respiratory complications; vigorous deep breathing and coughing should be encouraged.

28. A client diagnosed with essential hypertension is started on an antihypertensive medication. The nurse inquires about the client's usual stressors and ways of dealing with them because

    a. The major cause of primary hypertension is excessive stress.

    b. Measures to reduce stress are part of any treatment regimen for hypertension.

    c. Asking the client to describe a personal stress level will help the client relax and foster a better nurse–client therapeutic relationship.

    d. Stress must be reduced before learning can occur.

29. Discharge instructions for the client who has a healing peptic ulcer include which of the following information about medication?

    a. Continue taking antacids on schedule even if symptoms subside.

    b. Take antacids with other medications.

    c. Avoid magnesium-containing antacids if a cardiac problem develops.

    d. Take antacids with meals.

30. In evaluating large intestinal function following an acute episode of ulcerative colitis, the nurse would assess for

    a. report of pain relief after eating

    b. evidence of adequate nutrient and vitamin absorption

    c. defecation of soft, formed stool

    d. absence of belching and acid reflux

31. When planning care for an adult with ulcerative colitis, the nurse should keep in mind that a common complication is

    a. anal fistula abscess

    b. ascites

    c. nausea and vomiting

    d. anorexia with weight loss

32. Diabetic ketoacidosis most commonly is precipitated by

    a. overeating

    b. infection

    c. a missed insulin dose

    d. psychologic stress

33. The nurse should advise a diabetic client with an open foot wound to

    a. Clean the foot, and observe for infection.

    b. Soak the foot daily, then bandage it.

    c. Clean the foot, and apply mercurochrome.

    d. Elevate the foot, and apply heat.

34. What emergency intervention may be necessary for the postoperative thyroidectomy client experiencing hemorrhage?

    a. intravenous calcium

    b. oral airway insertion

    c. tracheostomy

    d. intravenous thyroid hormone

35. A 16-year-old diabetic client exhibits the following behaviors: school truancy, five admissions for uncontrolled diabetes in the last 2 years, missed insulin injections, and isolation from friends. Which of the following nursing diagnoses would be most applicable for this client?

    a. Knowledge Deficit

    b. Altered Thought Processes

    c. Altered Nutrition: Less than body requirements

    d. Ineffective Individual Coping

36. Which of the following statements regarding impotence is correct?

    a. It almost always is caused by psychologic factors.

    b. It may be caused by a wide variety of vascular, neurologic, endocrine, and psychogenic causes, as well as by many medications.

c. It may be related to various dietary factors.

d. It occurs less frequently in elderly men.

37. A major complication of prostatectomy is hemorrhage due to

a. pressure on the incision

b. thrombosis

c. clots obstructing urinary drainage

d. infection

38. When teaching a client how to do a testicular self-examination, the nurse should advise him that

a. Tenderness is an early sign of testicular cancer.

b. The testes should feel smooth and oval, with no masses.

c. Masses are difficult to find, and prognosis for cancer cure is poor.

d. A firm, pea-sized lump may be normal.

39. When caring for a client who has undergone a hysterectomy, the nurse will perform urinary catheterization if the client cannot void within 8 hours postoperatively so as to prevent urinary retention. Catheterization is necessary because

a. Surgical manipulation in the area of the bladder may cause edema and nerve trauma, producing temporary atony.

b. The bladder often is removed with the uterus.

c. Infection invariably results from surgery, making voiding difficult.

d. Surgical menopause affects urinary function.

40. Which of the following statements regarding allergic dermatitis is correct?

a. Reaction to the allergen is immediate.

b. Contact dermatitis always results from a chemical irritant.

c. The effects of allergic dermatitis rarely progress beyond skin rash.

d. The range and intensity of reaction varies depending on the allergen.

41. A client with rheumatoid arthritis is worried about becoming unable to care for family members. The client realizes that the condition will continue to deteriorate. The nursing plan of care should begin with

a. teaching about the disease and its progression

b. making referrals to other healthcare team members as necessary

c. providing emotional support for the client and the family

d. assessing physical, psychosocial, and environmental needs

42. A client with multiple sclerosis fears inability to care for her children and becoming a burden to her family. Which nursing diagnosis is appropriate?

a. Knowledge Deficit of the disease process related to lack of exposure to information

b. Self Esteem Disturbance related to loss of independence

c. Ineffective Individual Coping related to possibility of joint deformities

d. Impaired Physical Mobility related to the progressive nature of the disease

43. A client diagnosed with an acute exacerbation of asthma is dyspneic, orthopneic, and irritable. The admission history has only been partially completed by the nurse from the previous shift. After the nursing supervisor notes that the history is incomplete, the nurse on duty's best course of action is

a. Wait or try to obtain the necessary information from the client's family.

b. Obtain the information from the client.

c. Have the nursing assistant get the necessary information from the client.

d. Obtain part of the history from the client now and the remainder later to let the client rest.

44. According to the criteria set by the American Burn Association, burn injuries involving second-degree burns over more than 25% of total body surface area (TBSA) in adults or 20% of TBSA in children and burn injuries involving third-degree burns over 10% or more of TBSA are classified as
   a. minor burn injuries
   b. moderate uncomplicated burn injuries
   c. major burn injuries
   d. full-thickness burn injuries

45. During initial assessment of a client with a major burn injury, the correct sequence of nursing interventions would be
   a. Eliminate the source of the burn, ensure airway patency, observe for and treat associated injuries, treat burn shock.
   b. Eliminate the source of the burn, ensure airway patency, cool the burn wound, apply topical antibiotic cream.
   c. Ensure airway patency, insert a nasogastric tube, insert a bladder catheter, start IV fluid infusion.
   d. Treat burn shock, ensure airway patency, put the client in isolation.

46. Using the Parkland formula (4 mL of lactated Ringer's solution/% TBSA burn/kg body weight/24 hours), the nurse would calculate fluid replacement for a 70-kg client with a 50% TBSA burn over 24 hours as
   a. 1400 mL
   b. 14,000 mL
   c. 6720 mL
   d. 700 mL

47. A parent of four young children is diagnosed with myasthenia gravis. As the client's symptoms of fatigue and decreased mobility progress, which of the following nursing diagnoses most likely would apply?
   a. Sensory/Perceptual Alteration: Gustatory
   b. Decreased Cardiac Output
   c. Altered Family Processes
   d. Altered Thought Processes

48. A client experiences constipation following a craniotomy. An evaluation criterion that would indicate this client's understanding of actions needed to achieve the goal of a regular defecation pattern (and avoiding straining at defecation) would be
   a. The client drinks adequate fluids and eats a fiber-free diet.
   b. The client drinks adequate fluids and asks for an enema.
   c. The client includes roughage in the diet and drinks adequate fluids.
   d. The client requests laxatives and includes roughage in the diet.

49. When ambulating a client who has undergone surgical removal of a protruded intervertebral lumbar disk, the nurse should take special care to
   a. Maintain proper body alignment; have the client wear well-fitting, skid-free walking shoes; and remove loose objects from the floor.
   b. Administer pain medication 15 minutes before ambulation.
   c. Maintain proper alignment, and provide a cane for the client to use.
   d. Provide prism glasses for the client.

50. A client sustained a moderate concussion in a motorcycle accident 1 day ago. Based on a current Glasgow Coma Scale score of 7, the nurse would include which of the following interventions in the nursing plan of care?
   a. decreasing noxious stimuli, monitoring vital signs and neurologic status carefully, and keeping the client on the back with the bed flat
   b. instituting a program of stimulation, monitoring vital signs and neurologic status carefully, elevating the head of the bed 60 degrees, and positioning the client

in a side-lying position with the body in alignment

c. encouraging the family to become involved in a stimulation program, decreasing monitoring at night so that the client can rest, and keeping the client in a prone position

d. decreasing noxious stimuli, monitoring vital signs and neurologic status carefully, elevating the head of the bed 30 degrees, and positioning the client on the side with the body in alignment

51. A client has a C5–6 vertebral dislocation and has been in skeletal traction for 2 days. The most important assessment parameter is correctness of traction and

a. amount of urine output

b. movement and sensation in the arms

c. movement, strength, and sensation in the toes and fingers

d. range of eye movement, and strength of corneal reflex

52. Administration of miotic medications to treat glaucoma results in which of the following vision alterations?

a. impaired near vision

b. increased sensitivity to light

c. impaired night vision

d. diplopia

53. Which of the following postoperative assessment findings would point to intraocular hemorrhage?

a. temperature elevation

b. diplopia

c. visual floaters

d. eye pain

54. A person who uses over-the-counter nasal decongestant drops and who reports unrelieved and worsening nasal congestion should be instructed to

a. Switch to a stronger dosage of the medication.

b. Discontinue the medication for a few weeks.

c. Continue taking the same medication, but use it more frequently.

d. Use a combination of medications for better relief.

55. The priority nursing diagnosis for the client with eardrum perforation would be

a. Knowledge Deficit regarding general ear care and hearing protection

b. Sensory/Perceptual Alteration: Auditory related to hearing loss

c. Risk for Injury related to infection

d. Pain related to vertigo, nausea, and vomiting

56. All the following nursing activities would be performed before a client is discharged following total laryngectomy. Which one would be most important?

a. referring to the Lost Chord Club for group support

b. providing a medical identification card explaining resuscitation needs for first-aid providers

c. teaching ways to prevent constipation since the Valsalva maneuver is no longer possible

d. discussing precautions to take when showering and shampooing

57. A client with multiple fractures is at increased risk for a fat embolism. When caring for such a client, the nurse should monitor for which early sign?

a. hematuria

b. mental confusion or restlessness

c. sudden temperature elevation

d. pallor and discoloration at the fracture site

58. When preparing a client for magnetic resonance imaging, the nurse should

a. Obtain informed consent, and administer prescribed preoperative medication.

b. Scrub the injection site for 15 minutes, using aseptic technique.

c. Remove any jewelry, and inquire about metal implants.

d. Assess for allergies to seafood or iodine-containing substances.

59. After receiving a long arm cast, a client complains of deep, throbbing elbow pain that is out of proportion to the injury. After noting diminished capillary refill in the fingers and cyanotic nailbeds, the nurse should plan to
  a. Notify the physician immediately, and prepare to bivalve the cast.
  b. Cut a "window" in the cast over the elbow area, and check for drainage or infection.
  c. Elevate the casted arm, apply ice packs, and assess every hour for symptom progression.
  d. Administer prescribed analgesics, and notify the physician.

60. In the immediate postoperative period following a below-the-knee amputation, the nurse typically would be most concerned with which of the following nursing diagnoses?
  a. Body Image Disturbance related to loss of body part
  b. Risk for Infection related to disruption in skin integrity
  c. Pain related to phantom sensation
  d. Risk for Altered Tissue Perfusion related to hemorrhage

61. Which of the following client behaviors would best indicate the client's acceptance of the loss of an amputated limb?
  a. looking at, touching, and caring for the residual limb
  b. inviting friends and family members to visit
  c. inquiring about methods to alleviate pain
  d. expressing the desire to go home and resume work

62. Portal hypertension results from which of the following pathophysiologic processes?
  a. obstructed blood flow from the GI tract to the liver
  b. diversion of ascitic fluid from the peritoneal cavity back to the venous system
  c. rupture of esophageal varices

  d. obstruction of bile flow through the common bile duct

63. Which of the following explanations best describes why the nursing diagnoses Altered Body Image and Self Esteem Disturbance may apply to a client with ascites?
  a. A grossly distended abdomen may make the client feel obese.
  b. Yellow-tinged skin may make the client feel self-conscious.
  c. Fecal incontinence may cause embarrassment.
  d. Muscle wasting may cause weakness and mobility problems.

64. When caring for a client after a large (2 to 3 L) paracentesis, the nurse should focus on monitoring for which of the following complications to ensure safe care?
  a. respiratory distress
  b. encephalopathy
  c. bleeding from the site
  d. vascular collapse

65. Which of the following represents the best evaluation criterion for assessing the effectiveness of treatment aimed at reducing aggravating factors related to cholecystitis?
  a. The client maintains intake and output within normal limits.
  b. The client reports no pain following a low-fat meal.
  c. The client maintains serum albumin within normal limits.
  d. The client displays improvement on ultrasonography.

66. When caring for a client with pancreatitis, why would the nurse expect to administer meperidine rather than morphine sulfate for pain analgesia?
  a. Meperidine provides more prolonged analgesia than morphine.
  b. Unlike meperidine, morphine causes spasms of the sphincter of Oddi.
  c. Meperidine is less addicting than morphine.

    d. Unlike meperidine, morphine may cause liver dysfunction.

67. When teaching a client about home peritoneal dialysis, the nurse should explain that the primary concept in prevention of peritonitis is to
    a. Consume a high-sodium diet.
    b. Increase the amount of dextrose in the dialysis solution.
    c. Maintain aseptic technique throughout the procedure.
    d. Add heparin to the dialysis solution.

68. The nurse should plan to check a client's internal arteriovenous (AV) fistula because bleeding after hemodialysis usually is related to
    a. excessive urea in blood
    b. heparin administration during dialysis
    c. increased platelet activity during dialysis
    d. increased hematocrit related to fluid removal during hemodialysis

69. Which of the following represents the most appropriate criterion for evaluating a client's management of elevated phosphate levels in chronic renal failure?
    a. The client eliminates dairy products from the diet.
    b. The client increases dietary calcium intake.
    c. The client takes iron supplements with meals.
    d. The client takes phosphate-binding medications with meals.

70. The spouse of a client with chronic renal failure confides to the nurse that the client has been confused, irritable, and paranoid and that, as a result, the spouse has been thinking of divorce. Based on this information, the nurse most likely would make which of the following diagnoses?
    a. Noncompliance with prescribed medication regimen
    b. Self Esteem Disturbance related to loss of kidney function

    c. Anxiety related to the dialysis procedure
    d. Altered Family Processes related to the effects of chronic renal failure

71. Which of the following statements regarding random donor platelet transfusion is correct?
    a. Platelets generally should be administered over 3 to 4 hours.
    b. Platelet transfusion is indicated only in clients who demonstrate active bleeding.
    c. Fever may affect the incremental platelet count after transfusion.
    d. An allergic reaction to platelet transfusion may include chills, hemoglobinuria, and hives.

72. A client received the first induction course of chemotherapy 10 days ago for treatment of acute myeloblastic leukemia. Complete blood count (CBC) results include WBC, 300/mm^3; Hgb, 10.4 g/dL; Hct, 31.5%; and platelet count, 35,000. The client has a temperature of 101.4°F and is complaining of fatigue and general malaise but denies any other symptoms. Based on these findings, the nurse's first intervention should be to
    a. Notify the physician immediately.
    b. Administer acetaminophen to decrease temperature and increase client comfort.
    c. Continue monitoring temperature every 4 hours, and notify the physician if the client develops any other symptoms of infection.
    d. Move the client to a semiprivate room farthest from the central activity of the nursing unit.

73. A client, aged 24, comes to the outpatient clinic complaining of feeling increasingly "tired and run down" over the last several weeks. A CBC is obtained; findings are WBC, 4,300/mm^3; Hgb, 6.0 g/dL; Hct, 25.3%; and platelet count, 175,000.

In planning care for this client the nurse should keep in mind which of the following principles?

a. This client will be very symptomatic because of the low hemoglobin level.

b. Hematocrit is consistently the best indicator of anemia because it is unaffected by the client's hydration status.

c. Pallor should be assessed on the palms of the hands.

d. Packed red blood cells should be transfused at a rapid rate because of the low level of hemoglobin.

74. Follow-up evaluation of a client with sickle cell anemia included discussion of self-care management to avoid crises. Which of the following practices would indicate the client's poor adjustment to lifestyle changes necessary to prevent crises?

a. The client demonstrates relaxation and guided imagery techniques.

b. The client avoids ingesting alcohol.

c. The client rests frequently to avoid fatigue.

d. The client participates in a regular program of strenuous exercise.

75. A client with symptomatic tuberculosis expresses concern about the future, especially the ability to work and to marry. Which of the following nursing diagnoses would best address the client's primary concerns?

a. Health Seeking Behaviors

b. Anticipatory Grieving

c. Ineffective Individual Coping

d. Self Esteem Disturbance

76. A client who recently received high-dose chemotherapy has a WBC count of $1000/mm^3$. How can the nurse best help protect the client during hospitalization?

a. Monitor closely for signs of infection.

b. Place the client in protective isolation.

c. Wash hands carefully before caring for the client.

d. Restrict all visitors.

77. Hearing loss resulting from a large amount of dry, hard wax in the ear canal would be classified as

a. conductive

b. perceptive

c. sensorineural

d. impacted

78. Which of the following data would lead the nurse to establish falling precautions for an elderly ambulatory hospital client being treated for congestive heart failure and depression?

a. use of cathartics

b. chronic depression

c. excessive diuresis

d. slow ambulation

79. Which of the following statements indicates that a 70-year-old stroke client with right lower paralysis understands ways to prevent pressure sores?

a. "I'll shift my weight while sitting in the wheelchair, and examine my right foot every day."

b. "I'll spend the day in a reclining chair, and apply lotion to my right leg every 4 hours."

c. "I'll wear my support stockings daily, and my daughter will give me a good back rub every night."

d. "I'll sit on an inflatable ring in my wheelchair and wear comfortable, nonskid shoes."

80. Which of the following would be the most appropriate goals of care for a hospitalized, terminally ill, cachectic 90-year-old client?

a. The client will verbalize that he or she is free of pain, not hungry, and happy to remain in bed.

b. The client will demonstrate effective coughing and deep-breathing exercises, ability to eat independently, and acceptance of diagnosis.

c. The client will be free of skin breakdown, demonstrate adequate nutritional intake, and be able to take part in desired activities.

   d. The client will exhibit no signs and symptoms of deep vein thrombosis, pneumonia, or urinary tract infection.

81. A 78-year-old confused and delirious client comes to the emergency department on a hot summer day. The client's skin feels warm, but not sweaty. The client's spouse tells the nurse that the client takes "water pills" for high blood pressure. Based on this information, which of the following nursing diagnoses would be most appropriate?

   a. Hyperthermia
   b. Altered Thought Processes
   c. Ineffective Thermoregulation
   d. Ineffective Breathing Pattern

82. Which of the following is the appropriate route for administering small doses of narcotics to a client with a major burn?

   a. intravenous
   b. intramuscular
   c. subcutaneous
   d. oral

83. After an automobile accident, the client is admitted to the emergency room complaining of abdominal discomfort. The nurse instructs the client to lie down on a stretcher. The primary rationale for this action is to

   a. decrease abdominal pain
   b. decrease the risk of dislodging an intra-abdominal clot
   c. facilitate peristalsis
   d. decrease the risk of peritoneal infection

84. A client who was stung by a bee complains of shortness of breath and has hives on the face and neck. The expected outcome of an epinephrine injection would be

   a. easier breathing
   b. diminished pain at the sting site
   c. drowsiness
   d. increased itching

85. For a client scheduled for surgery, the nurse should begin preoperative teaching by

   a. assessing the client's knowledge base related to the surgical procedure and its expected outcome
   b. identifying standardized teaching plans to ensure consistency
   c. describing the risks of the surgical procedure
   d. having the client read printed instructional materials

86. Postoperative teaching for the client scheduled for a vaginal hysterectomy would focus on

   a. pelvic muscle strengthening exercises
   b. turning in bed, deep-breathing, and arm and leg exercises
   c. availability of support systems (e.g., psychologist, clergy)
   d. how to use a bedpan and call light

87. The 1-day postoperative client who had a partial thyroidectomy has hypotension, tachycardia, tachypnea, swelling around the dressing, and whispered speech. Based on these findings, the nurse notifies the physician because

   a. The client is exhibiting signs and symptoms of pulmonary embolism.
   b. The client is exhibiting signs and symptoms of internal bleeding.
   c. The client is exhibiting signs and symptoms of septic shock.
   d. The client is exhibiting signs and symptoms of electrolyte imbalances common in thyroidectomy clients.

88. Two days after cholecystectomy a client complains of upper abdominal pain and a sensation of bloating after eating solid food. Vital signs are stable, bowel sounds are hypoactive, and abdominal distention is evident. Which of the following nursing actions would be appropriate?

   a. Apply a hyperthermia pad.

b. Administer an antiemetic.

c. Insert a rectal tube.

d. Administer a narcotic analgesic.

89. Twelve hours after a near drowning, the client becomes anxious, tachypneic, and complains of dyspnea. The nurse suspects adult respiratory distress syndrome (ARDS) and administers 8 L/min oxygen by nasal cannula. The nurse would expect arterial blood gas values to show which of the following?

a. Decreased oxygen (below 60 mmHg) level

b. Increased oxygen (above 100 mmHg) level

c. Normal carbon dioxide (35–45 mmHg) level

d. Normal oxygen (80–100 mmHg) level

90. The client has a hemothorax secondary to a gunshot wound and chest tubes are inserted. Five hours after chest tube insertion the nurse would expect which of the following in the water-seal chamber of the Pleur Evac suction apparatus?

a. Vigorous bubbling

b. Fluctuation with breathing

c. Bloody drainage

d. No fluctuation

91. A 48-year-old client complains of chest pain. Signs and symptoms that further support a diagnosis of a myocardial infarction would include

a. jugular vein distention and hepatomegaly

b. fever and petechiae over the chest area

c. nausea and vomiting and cool, clammy, pale skin

d. pericardial friction rub and absent apical pulse

92. A client diagnosed with congestive heart failure is placed on digoxin 0.125 mg PO every day. A nursing intervention for this medication is

a. Do not administer if radial pulse is less than 60.

b. Hold medication if digoxin level is 1.4 ng/mL.

c. Administer if apical pulse is 84.

d. Administer if potassium level is 3.1 mEq/L.

93. The nurse knows that the client with a permanent pacemaker understands instructions concerning pacemaker failure when the client states

a. "If I should feel light-headed I should stop what I am doing and take a nitroglycerin."

b. "I should check my incision and notify the physician if it appears infected."

c. "I should take my pulse daily and it should be irregular after I have completed my 2-mile walk."

d. "If I have episodes of dizziness, weakness, and irregular pulse, I should call my doctor."

94. A client is admitted with the diagnosis of cholelithiasis. The nurse would expect to assess which of the following signs and symptoms?

a. cramping pain in right upper quadrant after a high-fat meal and nausea and vomiting

b. abdominal tenderness with back pain and hepatomegaly

c. right lower quadrant pain at McBurney's point and elevated temperature

d. acute epigastric gain after eating a spicy meal and belching

95. The client is diagnosed with peptic ulcer disease and is placed on an antacid (Maalox). The nurse understands the purpose of this medication is to

a. decrease the production of hydrochloric acid

b. neutralize gastric acidity

c. coat the stomach mucosa

d. increase the production of pepsin

96. The client is having excessive diarrhea secondary to ulcerative colitis. Which of the following signs and symptoms

would require the nurse to notify the physician?

a. moist mucous membranes and serum sodium level of 137 mEq/L

b. intake equaling output for 8 hours and serum calcium level of 9 mg/dL

c. negative Trousseau's sign and serum magnesium level of 2.0 mEq/L

d. Tented skin turgor and serum potassium level of 3.1 mEq/L

97. Teaching for the client with a hiatal hernia would include

a. Consume a low-fiber diet.

b. Recline after meals.

c. Avoid bending and lifting.

d. Eat three large meals a day.

98. The nurse and client would identify which of the following outcomes for the client diagnosed with a sexually transmitted disease (STD)? The client

a. demonstrates increased lymphadenopathy

b. reports decreased sexual activity

c. reports decreased pain and discharge

d. chooses sex partner(s) who do not need treatment

99. The nurse knows that the client with Crohn's disease understands the teaching concerning the medication prednisone when the client states

a. "I should take this medication after each loose stool."

b. "If I start getting a round moonface I should quit taking the medication immediately."

c. "I should not stop this medication abruptly; I should follow directions to reduce the dose gradually."

d. "I will have to stay on this medication the rest of my life to prevent a flare-up of my condition."

100. A client is admitted for a transient ischemic attack (TIA). The client's family asks the nurse, "We don't know what is going on; what is a TIA?" The nurse's best response would be

a. "I think you should ask the doctor; would you like me to call her?"

b. "The blood supply to the brain has decreased and permanent brain damage has occurred."

c. "A TIA is a temporary interruption of blood flow to the brain, but symptoms are temporary."

d. "TIA means transient ischemic attack."

101. The nurse would assess which of the following signs and symptoms in the client whose serum potassium level is 3.0 mEq/L?

a. anorexia, fatigue, and muscle cramping

b. tetany, positive Chvostek's sign, and seizures

c. hot, flushed skin, diaphoresis, and hypotension

d. headache, drowsiness, and tachypnea

102. The nurse would assess which of the following signs and symptoms in the client diagnosed with appendicitis?

a. anorexia and dull left-lower quadrant pain

b. abdominal distention and diarrhea

c. steatorrhea and weight loss

d. pain at McBurney's point and low-grade fever

103. The client has just had a seizure that was witnessed by a family member. Which of the following questions would be most important for the nurse to ask the family member concerning the seizure activity?

a. "Why didn't you call for the nurse sooner?"

b. "How do you feel after seeing your loved one have a seizure?"

c. "Can you tell me how long the seizure lasted?"

d. "Did you say something to upset your twin?"

104. The nurse knows the client understands the teaching concerning a femoral cardiac catheterization when the client states
- **a.** "I will be asleep during this procedure so I won't feel anything."
- **b.** "After the procedure, I will be able to walk to the bathroom with assistance."
- **c.** "When the doctor puts the dye in I may feel a hot flushed feeling and some chest discomfort."
- **d.** "I will have to keep my arm perfectly straight after the procedure."

105. Teaching for the client taking sublingual nitroglycerin for angina would include
- **a.** instructing the client to take the nitroglycerin around the clock
- **b.** explaining to the client that a subsequent headache indicates that the medication is not effective
- **c.** instructing the client to put the tablet on the tongue and swallow after the tablet dissolves
- **d.** teaching the client to take a tablet every 5 minutes (for up to 3 times) when chest pain occurs; then if chest pain does not stop, go to the hospital

106. The nurse understands the pathophysiology of a sigmoid colostomy when he or she tells the client that the stool from the colostomy should be
- **a.** liquid
- **b.** semisoft
- **c.** formed
- **d.** pastelike

107. The client is on warfarin sodium (Coumadin) and has blood drawn for PT/PTT study. The client's PT is 24, PTT is 39, and the control is PT 12.9/PTT 37 seconds. Based on this information, the nurse would
- **a.** Hold the medication and assess for bleeding.
- **b.** Administer the medication as ordered.
- **c.** Prepare to administer protamine sulfate.
- **d.** Notify the physician immediately.

108. On the first postoperative day after abdominal surgery, the client complains of severe abdominal pain: "8" on a scale of 1 to 10. The nurse should
- **a.** Medicate the client as soon as possible.
- **b.** Help the client with guided imagery.
- **c.** Have the client turn, cough, and deep-breathe.
- **d.** Rule out complications and then medicate if assessment findings are within normal limits.

109. Which of the following signs and symptoms would the nurse assess for the client diagnosed with chronic open-angle glaucoma?
- **a.** Gradual loss of peripheral vision
- **b.** Cloudy-appearing lens
- **c.** No pain or eye redness
- **d.** Complaints of floating spots

110. When teaching about general ear care, the nurse should instruct the client to
- **a.** Avoid chewing gum or sucking on hard candy when flying in airplanes.
- **b.** Insert only cotton swabs into the ear.
- **c.** Blow the nose with mouth and both nostrils closed.
- **d.** Protect hearing by wearing ear muffs or plugs around loud noises.

111. The nurse is aware that one of the earliest and most predominant signs distinguishing intrinsic from extrinsic laryngeal cancer is
- **a.** throat pain when drinking hot liquids
- **b.** foul-smelling breath
- **c.** persistent hoarseness
- **d.** hemoptysis

112. The client with a fractured femur is placed in skeletal traction. Nursing interventions for this client would include

a. removing the traction every 2 hours and turning the client to a prone position

b. assessing any pin sites for signs of irritation or infection

c. not using a bedboard under the client's mattress

d. cleansing pin sites with tincture of benzoin

113. In a client diagnosed with liver failure secondary to cirrhosis of the liver, the nurse would assess which of the following signs indicating portal hypertension?

a. fluid wave on abdominal percussion

b. dark, frothy urine

c. clay-colored stools

d. flapping tremors of hands

114. A client is diagnosed with renal calculi. Nursing interventions to help prevent stone recurrence would include

a. encouraging fluid intake to 1000 mL daily

b. explaining the need for decreased physical activity

c. encouraging dietary modification based on the stone's composition

d. teaching the client to care for ileal conduit

For additional questions, see
Lippincott's Self-Study Series Software
Available at your bookstore

Answer Sheet for Comprehensive Exam

With a pencil, blacken the circle under the option you have chosen for your correct answer.

	A	B	C	D			A	B	C	D			A	B	C	D
1.	○	○	○	○	21.		○	○	○	○	41.		○	○	○	○
2.	○	○	○	○	22.		○	○	○	○	42.		○	○	○	○
3.	○	○	○	○	23.		○	○	○	○	43.		○	○	○	○
4.	○	○	○	○	24.		○	○	○	○	44.		○	○	○	○
5.	○	○	○	○	25.		○	○	○	○	45.		○	○	○	○
6.	○	○	○	○	26.		○	○	○	○	46.		○	○	○	○
7.	○	○	○	○	27.		○	○	○	○	47.		○	○	○	○
8.	○	○	○	○	28.		○	○	○	○	48.		○	○	○	○
9.	○	○	○	○	29.		○	○	○	○	49.		○	○	○	○
10.	○	○	○	○	30.		○	○	○	○	50.		○	○	○	○
11.	○	○	○	○	31.		○	○	○	○	51.		○	○	○	○
12.	○	○	○	○	32.		○	○	○	○	52.		○	○	○	○
13.	○	○	○	○	33.		○	○	○	○	53.		○	○	○	○
14.	○	○	○	○	34.		○	○	○	○	54.		○	○	○	○
15.	○	○	○	○	35.		○	○	○	○	55.		○	○	○	○
16.	○	○	○	○	36.		○	○	○	○	56.		○	○	○	○
17.	○	○	○	○	37.		○	○	○	○	57.		○	○	○	○
18.	○	○	○	○	38.		○	○	○	○	58.		○	○	○	○
19.	○	○	○	○	39.		○	○	○	○	59.		○	○	○	○
20.	○	○	○	○	40.		○	○	○	○	60.		○	○	○	○

Comprehensive Test—Answer Key

	A	B	C	D			A	B	C	D			A	B	C	D
61.	○	○	○	○		79.	○	○	○	○		97.	○	○	○	○
62.	○	○	○	○		80.	○	○	○	○		98.	○	○	○	○
63.	○	○	○	○		81.	○	○	○	○		99.	○	○	○	○
64.	○	○	○	○		82.	○	○	○	○		100.	○	○	○	○
65.	○	○	○	○		83.	○	○	○	○		101.	○	○	○	○
66.	○	○	○	○		84.	○	○	○	○		102.	○	○	○	○
67.	○	○	○	○		85.	○	○	○	○		103.	○	○	○	○
68.	○	○	○	○		86.	○	○	○	○		104.	○	○	○	○
69.	○	○	○	○		87.	○	○	○	○		105.	○	○	○	○
70.	○	○	○	○		88.	○	○	○	○		106.	○	○	○	○
71.	○	○	○	○		89.	○	○	○	○		107.	○	○	○	○
72.	○	○	○	○		90.	○	○	○	○		108.	○	○	○	○
73.	○	○	○	○		91.	○	○	○	○		109.	○	○	○	○
74.	○	○	○	○		92.	○	○	○	○		110.	○	○	○	○
75.	○	○	○	○		93.	○	○	○	○		111.	○	○	○	○
76.	○	○	○	○		94.	○	○	○	○		112.	○	○	○	○
77.	○	○	○	○		95.	○	○	○	○		113.	○	○	○	○
78.	○	○	○	○		96.	○	○	○	○		114.	○	○	○	○

COMPREHENSIVE TEST—ANSWER KEY

1. **Correct response: a**
   This is the definition of the nursing process.
   b. This describes the work of the North American Nursing Diagnosis Association (NANDA).
   c and d. These are not definitions of nursing process but are self-explanatory.
   Comprehension/NA/NA

2. **Correct response: d**
   This question assesses self-concept, one of the factors associated with "role and relationship patterns."
   a. This is a part of the assessment associated with "health promotion and protection patterns."
   b and c. These are associated with the "health and illness patterns" segment.
   Application/Psychosocial/Assessment

3. **Correct response: d**
   Along with the signs described, other indications of arterial insufficiency include delayed capillary refill in toenails; thin, shiny skin of the lower extremities; and diminished or absent pulses.
   a and b. These signs are not associated with insufficient venous circulation or venous thrombosis.
   c. Normal age-related changes do not include lesions on the feet.
   Analysis/Physiologic/Assessment

4. **Correct response: b**
   All results are at about midnormal ranges.
   a, c, and d. No results are above or below normal ranges.
   Analysis/Physiologic/Assessment

5. **Correct response: b**
   Given this client's hearing deficit, computer-assisted instruction may be the most effective teaching tool.
   a, c, and d. These would not ac-

commodate the client's hearing deficit as well as the computer.
   Application/Physiologic/Evaluation

6. **Correct response: c**
   By putting together the equipment without waiting for instructions, this client demonstrates that he or she is primarily a tactile learner.
   a and b. These behaviors demonstrate a visual pattern of learning.
   d. This behavior demonstrates an auditory pattern of learning.
   Analysis/Health promotion/Assessment

7. **Correct response: c**
   Tissue swelling results from increased vascular permeability and leakage of plasma fluids.
   a. Increased vascular permeability results from transient vasoconstriction followed by vasodilation.
   b. White blood cells migrate to the site of injury.
   d. Nerve-ending irritation by chemical mediators (e.g., as histamine) results in pain.
   Comprehension/Physiologic/Assessment

8. **Correct response: b**
   A well-balanced diet high in protein and calories promotes tissue repair.
   a and c. Either heat or cold applied to the radiation site could impair healing by destroying enzymes and causing vasoconstriction, respectively.
   d. Warm fluids would increase rather than decrease esophageal discomfort.
   Analysis/Health promotion/ Implementation

9. **Correct response: d**
   Hyperplasia involves an increase in the number of cells in an organ or tissue, often related to hormonal influences.
   a, b, and c. These represent hyper-

trophy, atrophy, and metaplasia, respectively.
Application/Physiologic/Evaluation

10. *Correct response: a*
Because furosemide is a diuretic that commonly causes potassium depletion, the client should eat foods high in potassium.
b. The stated rate of KCl infusion is correct (10 mEq/hour).
c. Hyperkalemia will manifest as peaked, narrow T waves on ECG.
d. Hyperkalemia—not hypokalemia—can result from hemolysis.
Analysis/Health promotion/Planning

11. *Correct response: c*
These assessment data most strongly suggest hypercalcemia.
a and b. Although the client's symptoms could also suggest either hyponatremia or hypermagnesemia, the ECG changes clearly point to calcium imbalance.
d. Hyperkalemia is marked by muscle weakness and paresthesias.
Comprehension/Physiologic/Assessment

12. *Correct response: d*
Due to increased loss of water and electrolytes from diarrhea, this client likely would develop fluid volume deficit (FVD). Laboratory values diagnostic of FVD include increased blood urea nitrogen (BUN) and hematocrit.
a, b, and c. These findings are not consistent with the scenario.
Analysis/Physiologic/Evaluation

13. *Correct response: b*
Metabolic alkalosis is marked by pH above 7.45 and HCO_3 above 26 mEq/L.
a. Nothing in the scenario indicates that fright is accounting for the client's behavior.
c. In acidosis, pH is below 7.35.
d. The nurse should not assume that such behavior would be expected in response to a respiratory crisis; such an assumption could cause

the nurse to ignore the underlying physiologic cause.
Application/Psychosocial/Implementation

14. *Correct response: b*
Because many antacids contain magnesium, indiscriminate antacid use may contribute to high magnesium levels.
a. Immobility leads to loss of calcium from bones, not magnesium.
c. Neuromuscular irritability causing sleep disturbance is a symptom of hypomagnesemia.
d. Fluid volume excess results from retention of sodium, not magnesium.
Application/Safe care/Analysis (Dx)

15. *Correct response: d*
A-delta fibers transmit pain faster than type C and therefore deliver the first sharp sensations.
a. C-fiber activation produces persistent, dull, aching pain.
b and c. Type A-alpha, beta, and gamma fibers transmit touch, pressure, heat, cold, and movement much faster.
Comprehension/Physiologic/Assessment

16. *Correct response: d*
This diagnosis would alert other nurses to the possibility that the client may attempt to crutch-walk without assistance and fall.
a, b, and c. No information in this scenario suggests any of these diagnoses.
Analysis/Safe care/Analysis (Dx)

17. *Correct response: b*
These are noninvasive interventions that most persons will accept.
a. This would not be sufficient.
c. This would violate the client's rights.
d. This would avoid attempting to meet the client's needs.
Application/Psychosocial/Planning

18. **Correct response: a**
Anginal pain decreases with rest and the improved coronary circulation provided by sublingual nitroglycerin.
   b. These measures will increase myocardial oxygen demand and exacerbate pain.
   c. These tablets do not provide immediate symptom relief.
   d. These measures will not improve coronary circulation.
Analysis/Health promotion/
Implementation

19. **Correct response: c**
Continuation of behaviors detrimental to health are usually a sign of ineffective denial.
   a. Grieving over loss of health (rather than anticipatory) is very likely a part of this client's emotional response, but it would not lead to this self-destructive behavior.
   b and d. This scenario offers no evidence that the client is experiencing disturbance of either body image or social interaction.
Application/Psychosocial/Analysis (Dx)

20. **Correct response: d**
CO_2 and H_2O, in differing concentrations, react to form carbonic acid (H_2CO), which in turn dissociates to form bicarbonate (HCO_3) and hydrogen (H^+) ions. This reaction determines the pH of arterial blood and the acid–base balance of the human body. CO_2 is blown off or conserved by the lungs as one variable in keeping this balance.
   a. Although the lungs do control O_2 intake, O_2 is not a primary mediator in acid–base balance.
   b. The mechanism for cholesterol control is not in the lungs.
   c. Urea and albumin are affected by the kidneys.
Application/Physiologic/Assessment

21. **Correct response: b**
Any opening in the chest causes pneumothorax (collapsed lung). As the pleura is incised or penetrated, atmospheric air rushes into the pleural space, which normally maintains a negative pressure to provide for lung expansion. Disruption of this negative pressure causes the lung to collapse.
   a. The lung will collapse, not expand, if any penetration of the pleura is made.
   c. Lung expansion is controlled by both lung pressure and intrapleural pressure. However, if intrapleural pressure is disturbed, the lung will collapse.
   d. Pressure in the intrapleural space is negative.
Analysis/Physiologic/Planning

22. **Correct response: b**
PVCs can lead to lethal arrhythmias because they indicate ventricular irritability.
   a, c, and d. These actions are not characteristic of PVCs.
Comprehension/Physiologic/Assessment

23. **Correct response: d**
The client is expressing fear over the uncertainty surrounding her future.
   a and b. No information in this scenario would point to either of these diagnoses.
   c. The client may have a knowledge deficit, but more assessment would be needed to confirm this.
Analysis/Psychosocial/Analysis (Dx)

24. **Correct response: d**
Improving circulation decreases ischemia, the basic cause of pain in arterial occlusive disorders.
   a. Venous return is not involved in the mechanism causing pain in arterial occlusive disorders.
   b. Narcotic pain medication may be necessary in combination with other measures.
   c. Edema is not the mechanism causing discomfort.
Comprehension/Physiologic/
Implementation

25. *Correct response: b*
Chronic venous stasis causes chronically swollen legs; thick, coarse, brown-pigmented skin; and non-painful, wet ulcers on the ankles.
  a. Ulcers do not form rapidly enough to appear with acute deep vein thrombosis.
  c. Ulcers associated with chronic arterial insufficiency are marked by muscle atrophy; thin skin; dry, painful ulcers; and diminished or absent pedal pulses.
  d. Ulcers rarely develop in lymphedema.
Analysis/Physiologic/Assessment

26. *Correct response: a*
Red streaking indicates lymphangitis and spread of infection.
  b. Although not crossing the legs will help promote venous return, edema of the foot does not represent as serious a threat to health as does increasing infection.
  c. Although avoiding smoking is an important health consideration, it will not affect health status as immediately as infection will.
  d. Anaphylactic reaction to tetanus toxoid usually occurs immediately after administration, while the client is in the healthcare setting.
Application/Health promotion/Planning

27. *Correct response: c*
Blood pressure, pulse, and respiratory changes, along with blood on the dressing, are consistent with bleeding, one of the most common postamputation complications.
  a. Recovery from anesthesia usually is accompanied by a return to baseline vital signs, which are not known in this case.
  b. Although pain can be a factor in vital sign changes, the question does not address the client's pain perception.
  d. Respiratory atelectasis after surgery often is accompanied by temperature elevation; although deep breathing is appropriate, vigorous deep breathing and coughing is not.
Analysis/Safe care/Evaluation

28. *Correct response: b*
Stress reduction represents one aspect of blood pressure control.
  a. A single major cause of primary hypertension remains unknown.
  c. The nurse's active listening skills and client acceptance are essential to a therapeutic nurse–client relationship; the client's comfort level may or may not be significant.
  d. Stress may or may not interfere with learning. Most important to education in this case are the client's understanding of the problem and treatment alternatives and the client's active involvement in the therapeutic regimen.
Application/Psychosocial/Analysis (Dx)

29. *Correct response: a*
Antacids decrease acidity and should be continued even in the absence of symptoms.
  b and d. Antacids should be taken 1 hour before or 2 hours after meals for best results and should not be given with medications (which can alter the acid content and thus absorption of the drug).
  c. Sodium, not magnesium, content is of concern for cardiac clients.
Application/Health promotion/Implementation

30. *Correct response: c*
Primary large bowel functions include absorption of water and elimination of feces.
  a. Relief of pain after ingestion of food is a sign of duodenal ulcer.
  b. The small bowel is primarily responsible for the absorption of nutrients.
  d. Belching and reflux are symptoms of hiatal hernia.
Analysis/Physiologic/Evaluation

31. Correct response: d
Anorexia and weight loss are common complications of ulcerative colitis.
a. Anal involvement is rare; an anal fistula or abscess is common with Crohn's disease.
b and c. Neither ascites nor nausea and vomiting would be expected with this diagnosis.
Application/Psychosocial/Planning

32. Correct response: b
Infection, causing increased stress hormones, insulin resistance, and increased insulin need, is the most frequent cause of diabetic ketoacidosis (DKA).
a, c, and d. Overeating, missing a single insulin dose, or psychologic stress may increase blood glucose levels but will not cause DKA.
Comprehension/Physiologic/Assessment

33. Correct response: a
The open area should be cleaned with plain soap and water and observed for any signs of infection.
b. Soaking the foot is not advised because of the increased potential for injury.
c. Mercurochrome or any iodine product is not advised because of its potential to damage tissue.
d. Applying heat also can increase the risk of tissue damage.
Application/Safe care/Implementation

34. Correct response: c
Hemorrhage in the postoperative thyroidectomy client may cause compression of the trachea, necessitating emergency tracheostomy to maintain an airway.
a and d. Calcium and thyroid hormone replacement may be needed but are not related to hemorrhage.
b. Insertion of an oral airway would not be sufficient for this client.
Analysis/Physiologic/Planning

35. Correct response: d
The inability to continue usual social patterns is a sign of ineffective coping.
a, b, and c. None of these nursing diagnoses account for the antisocial and self-destructive behaviors described.
Analysis/Psychosocial/Analysis (Dx)

36. Correct response: b
Impotence can result from various psychological and physiologic problems.
a. Psychological factors are not the only contributing factors to impotence.
c. Although dietary factors conceivably could play a part in a physiologic disorder leading to impotence, they are not of primary consideration.
d. Incidence of impotence increases with age.
Knowledge/Health promotion/Planning

37. Correct response: c
Clots that obstruct urinary drainage and cause urinary retention can lead to hemorrhage from the prostatic bed, given its high vascularity.
a. Pressure on the incision may cause pain, but not usually hemorrhage.
b and d. Thrombosis and infection are not usually associated with hemorrhage.
Knowledge/Physiologic/Assessment

38. Correct response: b
The testes normally feel smooth and oval, with no masses.
a. Tenderness or pain is not a common early symptom of testicular cancer.
c. Testicular masses generally are easy to detect.
d. With early detection and treatment, prognosis generally is fair to good.
Application/Health promotion/Implementation

39. *Correct response: a*
Surgical manipulation in the area around the bladder may cause nerve trauma and edema, which can affect voiding.
b, c, and d. These statements are simply not correct.
Analysis/Safe care/Implementation

40. *Correct response: d*
The allergen determines the nature of the dermatitis.
a. Onset of reactions can range from immediate to as long as 21 days after exposure.
b. The dermatitis may be due to primary irritants or allergic sensitizers.
c. The inflammation may range from redness to ulcerations and is dependent on many factors.
Comprehension/Physiologic/Assessment

41. *Correct response: d*
Assessment is the first step in nursing care for all clients.
a, b, and c. Although these all are important interventions for a client with rheumatoid arthritis, none of them can be effective without a thorough assessment of individual needs.
Application/Health promotion/ Implementation

42. *Correct response: b*
This client is expressing doubts about her ability to continue in her current role.
a, c, and d. Although these other diagnoses could be appropriate, they are not related to the client's comments.
Analysis/Psychosocial/Analysis (Dx)

43. *Correct response: a*
Acute dyspnea will interfere with the client's ability to talk, and answering questions will tire the client unnecessarily. Thus, the nurse would best wait until the client can breathe easier or try to obtain the information from family members.

b, c, and d. None of these would be the best approach to obtaining health history information for this client.
Analysis/Safe care/Planning

44. *Correct response: c*
Major burn injuries are defined as those involving second-degree burns over more than 25% TBSA in adults or 20% of TBSA in children, or those involving third-degree burns over 10% of TBSA or more in any client.
a. Minor burn injury involves second-degree burns over less than 15% of TBSA, or less than 10% of TBSA in children.
b. Moderate uncomplicated burn injury is defined as second-degree burns over 15% to 25% of TBSA in adults or 10% to 20% of TBSA in children, or third-degree burns over more than 10% of TBSA without involvement of special care areas.
d. Full-thickness burn injury involves the epidermis, dermis, and underlying subcutaneous tissue.
Comprehension/Physiologic/Assessment

45. *Correct response: a*
The appropriate sequence of nursing actions for clients with major burn injuries is eliminate the source of the burn, ensure airway patency, assess for and treat associated injuries, and treat burn shock.
b, c, and d. The other actions may be appropriate during care of such a client, but response *a* represents the correct sequence for initial assessment.
Analysis/Safe care/Implementation

46. *Correct response: b*
14,000 mL is the correct number.
a, c, and d. None of the other fluid replacement amounts would be adequate.
Application/Health promotion/ Evaluation

47. *Correct response: c*
In myasthenia gravis, severe fatigue can significantly alter family processes.

a. Myasthenia gravis can entail changes that affect eating (e.g., increased salivation with difficulty swallowing and chewing) but is not associated with altered taste.

b. Cardiac output changes are not directly related to myasthenia gravis.

d. Myasthenia gravis is not associated with altered thought processes except indirectly as related to fatigue.

Analysis/Psychosocial/Analysis (Dx)

48. *Correct response: c*
Ensuring adequate fluid and dietary fiber intake is the first step in preventing or easing constipation.

a, b, and d. Before resorting to a laxative or enema, fluids and dietary modifications should be tried.

Comprehension/Physiologic/Evaluation

49. *Correct response: a*
Proper alignment will reduce pain and protect the surgical site; well-fitting shoes help prevent slipping and sudden, jerky movements; removing objects also improves safety.

b. Not all clients require pain medication.

c. A cane would be needed only if the client had suffered foot drop.

d. Prism glasses are not appropriate.

Application/Health promotion/Planning

50. *Correct response: d*
The autonomic nervous system is very labile; noxious stimuli would tend to increase intracranial pressure. Elevating the head of the bed assists in venous return and in breathing. Positioning on the side helps facilitate breathing; frequent monitoring is needed to detect any adverse changes so that therapy can be implemented immediately.

a, b, and c. None of these sets of interventions would be appropriate for this client.

Analysis/Safe care/Implementation

51. *Correct response: c*
Traction is needed to keep vertebrae in alignment because vertebral movement could damage the cord. Both fingers and toes need to be assessed because changes may indicate the need for immediate medical intervention.

a, b, and d. None of these sets of parameters would be appropriate for this client.

Application/Physiologic/Assessment

52. *Correct response: c*
Miotics cause pupil constriction, impairing night vision.

a. Near vision impairment can result from mydriatics.

b and d. Increased sensitivity to light and double vision result when one eye is aphakic (without lens) and the other is phakic (with lens), not as an effect of medication.

Application/Physiologic/Evaluation

53. *Correct response: d*
Postoperative eye pain is indicative of increased intraocular pressure or hemorrhage.

a. Slight temperature elevation would be expected postoperatively as a manifestation of the inflammatory response.

b. Double vision results when one eye has a lens and the other does not.

c. Floaters are symptoms of retinal detachment.

Comprehension/Physiologic/Assessment

54. *Correct response: b*
Prolonged use of decongestant drops (3 to 5 days) can lead to rebound congestion, which is relieved by discontinuing the medication for 2 or 3 weeks.

a, c, and d. Continuing the medica-

tion or increasing the dose would worsen this phenomenon.
Analysis/Safe care/Implementation

55. Correct response: c
The eardrum separates the external ear from the middle ear. Perforation increases susceptibility to suppurative otitis media and necessitates special ear care.
a, b, and d. The client may or may not experience hearing loss or pain and should receive general ear care instruction, but the priority concern with perforation is infection.
Analysis/Physiologic/Analysis (Dx)

56. Correct response: d
With a permanent tracheostomy, the airway must be protected from water and particulate matter.
a. Referral to support groups is important but not essential for safety.
b and c. Although the client should carry medical identification for special needs and should receive an explanation regarding loss of strength with Valsalva maneuver, these interventions are not essential for self-care safety in activities of daily living.
Application/Health promotion/Planning

57. Correct response: b
Mental disturbances such as confusion, irritability, restlessness, disorientation, stupor, or coma are often the first sign of systemic fat embolism. These symptoms are caused by hypoxemia and may begin subtly with rapid advancement of respiratory, cardiovascular, and other systemic symptoms depending on where the embolus lodges.
a, c, and d. These signs and symptoms are not associated with fat embolism.
Comprehension/Physiologic/Assessment

58. Correct response: c
A client undergoing magnetic resonance imaging (MRI) is exposed to a magnetic field approximately 15,000 times greater than the earth's magnetic field. It is therefore very important to remove all metal objects and assess for electrically, magnetically, or mechanically activated implants such as pacemakers, clips, staples, or shrapnel.
a. Because MRI is not an invasive procedure, it does not require informed consent.
b and d. MRI involves no injections or contrast media.
Application/Safe care/Implementation

59. Correct response: a
The client's symptoms suggest compartment syndrome, a condition caused by either a decrease in compartment size or an increase in compartment contents. In such cases, the nurse should notify the physician immediately and prepare for releasing the constriction by bivalving the cast, cutting dressings, or performing a fasciotomy.
b, c, and d. This client needs *immediate* relief of pressure inside the cast; none of these interventions would be appropriate.
Analysis/Physiologic/Planning

60. Correct response: d
Hemorrhage from a loosened ligature is the most threatening complication in the immediate postoperative period following limb amputation. The client should be monitored very closely during this period for any signs or symptoms of bleeding either from the operative site or in the suction drainage. A large tourniquet should be kept at the bedside to apply in the event of hemorrhage.
a, b, and c. Although these other nursing diagnoses also may be applicable during the postoperative period, none are of as much concern as the potential for hemorrhage.
Application/Health promotion/ Analysis (Dx)

61. *Correct response: a*
A client undergoing limb amputation typically experiences altered body image and must learn to accept the loss and a new image. It is important for the nurse to work closely with the client, build a trusting relationship, and encourage the client to look at, feel, and care for the residual limb. Once the client can do these tasks, he or she is on the way to accepting the loss and beginning to build a new self-image.
b, c, and d. Although these nursing diagnoses could apply to a client recovering from amputation, Altered Body Image applies to virtually all such clients.
Analysis/Psychosocial/Evaluation

62. *Correct response: a*
Obstructed blood flow is the cause of portal hypertension.
b. Ascites results from portal hypertension; it is not a cause.
c. Esophageal varices are a result of portal hypertension, not a cause.
d. Obstruction of bile flow would lead to jaundice, not portal hypertension.
Comprehension/Physiologic/Assessment

63. *Correct response: a*
Clients commonly associate a distended abdomen with obesity, resulting in a body image alteration.
b. Ascites does not cause jaundice, although they commonly occur together.
c. Fecal incontinence is not generally associated with ascites.
d. Muscle wasting does not result from ascites.
Analysis/Psychosocial/Analysis (Dx)

64. *Correct response: d*
The removal of large amounts of ascites may lead to acute fluid shifts and hypotension.
a. Respiratory distress is not usually associated with this procedure.

b. Paracentesis does not affect ammonia level or alter protein status.
c. Bleeding from the site may occur, but it is not the most important side effect to monitor for.
Application/Safe care/Implementation

65. *Correct response: b*
History of pain following a high-fat meal may lead the nurse to advise the client to avoid this type of dietary intake.
a. Intake and output does not provide information regarding the aggravating factors of the disorder.
c and d. These criteria do provide important information about the disorder but do not provide keys to aggravating factors.
Application/Health promotion/Evaluation

66. *Correct response: b*
Morphine causes spasm of the sphincter of Oddi (at the end of the pancreatic duct), which may aggravate pancreatitis.
a. Meperidine is actually somewhat shorter acting than morphine.
c. Both drugs are potentially addictive.
d. Morphine use is not associated with liver dysfunction.
Analysis/Physiologic/Planning

67. *Correct response: c*
Aseptic technique is essential in all aspects of peritoneal dialysis procedure to prevent microorganisms from invading the peritoneal cavity.
a. Sodium intake is not related to peritonitis.
b. Dextrose in dialysis solution is related to fluid removal; it is an excellent medium for bacterial growth.
d. Heparin helps prevent fibrin clots in the catheter.
Application/Physiologic/Implementation

68. *Correct response: b*
Heparin is added to dialyzer blood to

prevent clotting in the dialyzer; the client's blood becomes anticoagulated and bleeding may occur.

a. Urea level usually is decreased after dialysis and is not related to bleeding.

c. Dialysis does not affect platelet activity.

d. Increased hematocrit would not contribute to bleeding.

Analysis/Safe care/Planning

69. Correct response: d
Phosphate-binding medications bind with phosphate in food and prevent its absorption.

a. Dairy products are an excellent source of HBV protein and calcium.

b. Dietary calcium has no effect on phosphate levels.

c. Iron intake has no effect on phosphate levels.

Application/Health promotion/ Evaluation

70. Correct response: d
This client's symptoms are disrupting the marital relationship.

a, b, and c. Nothing in this scenario would lead the nurse to formulate any of these diagnoses.

Analysis/Psychosocial/Analysis (Dx)

71. Correct response: c
Fever and infection may decrease the incremental count after transfusion.

a. Platelets should be administered as rapidly as tolerated by the client.

b. Platelets may be transfused in selected instances to prevent bleeding.

d. Hemoglobinuria is indicative of a hemolytic transfusion reaction (lysis of RBCs).

Comprehension/Health promotion/ Assessment

72. Correct response: a
Fever and infection in a severely neutropenic client (neutrophils less than 500/mm^3) can be rapidly fatal if

broad-spectrum antibiotic therapy is not instituted quickly.

b. This is incorrect because it would not be the immediate intervention.

c. Once the physician is notified, the client should be monitored frequently.

d. The client should be in a private room. (The location of the room should not compromise frequent monitoring.)

Analysis/Physiologic/Implementation

73. Correct response: c
Color changes are best assessed where capillary beds are superficial and pigmentation is minimal.

a. A client may experience few symptoms if the onset of anemia has been gradual and there is adequate cardiopulmonary compensation.

b. Hematocrit can be affected by hydration (plasma volume) as well as RBC size.

d. Too-rapid infusion of packed RBCs in a client with compensated anemia may produce circulatory overload.

Comprehension/Physiologic/Planning

74. Correct response: d
Strenuous physical activity is contraindicated because the physiologic stress can precipitate crises.

a. Relaxation and other techniques would be encouraged to control emotional stress, which can precipitate crises.

b and c. Ingestion of alcohol and fatigue are both precipitating factors for crises.

Application/Psychosocial/Evaluation

75. Correct response: a
The concerns expressed show an interest in finding answers to maximize abilities in the future, which is characteristic of health-seeking behavior.

b. Although anticipatory grieving may occur, it is not evident from this scenario.

c and d. The scenario offers no evidence to indicate that the client is coping ineffectively or has a disturbed self-concept.
Analysis/Psychosocial/Analysis (Dx)

76. **Correct response: c**
The most important measure to decrease the risk from nosocomial exogenous organisms is proper handwashing.
    a. Observing for signs of infection is important, but prevention takes precedence over detection.
    b. Isolation may be done in some institutions, but handwashing is most important.
    d. Family members who are ill should certainly stay away; however, close family who practice good handwashing and wear protective garb can help sustain the client through this difficult time.
Application/Safe care/Implementation

77. **Correct response: a**
Impacted cerumen is a leading cause of conductive hearing loss.
    b and c. Perceptive and sensorineural hearing loss involve the middle or inner ear.
    d. "Impacted" is not a type of hearing loss.
Comprehension/Psychosocial/Analysis (Dx)

78. **Correct response: c**
Volume depletion from diuretic use may increase a client's risk of falling.
    a. Cathartics may cause problems with elimination, but unless the client abuses them, leading to electrolyte imbalance, they would not increase the risk of falling.
    b and d. Chronic depression and slow ambulation would not be indications for fall precautions.
Analysis/Physiologic/Assessment

79. **Correct response: a**
Regular position changes and weight shifts can help prevent pressure sores. The skin of the affected extremity needs to be visually inspected because altered sensation likely is present.
    b. Regular position changes are important. Lotion can exacerbate skin breakdown.
    c. These measures will not prevent pressure sores.
    d. Sitting on an inflatable ring can impair tissue perfusion.
Application/Health promotion/Evaluation

80. **Correct response: c**
Cachectic older adults are malnourished and at risk for skin breakdown; goals should incorporate these factors. In addition, the nurse should encourage dying clients to participate in desired activities rather than just focus on disease treatment and prevention.
    a, b, and d. These interventions are not as applicable as those described in response c.
Analysis/Physiologic/Planning

81. **Correct response: a**
This client's history and signs and symptoms are consistent with hyperthermia. There is no evidence that respiratory function has changed although this could be a later consequence of unresolved hyperthermia.
    b, c, and d. These all would be appropriate diagnoses based on the information presented in this scenario.
Application/Physiologic/Analysis (Dx)

82. **Correct response: a**
IV is the most appropriate route for this client.
    b, c, and d. A client with major burns is in shock and therefore has poor peripheral circulation needed for absorption of IM or subcutaneous medication. Clients with severe burns commonly develop paralytic ileus and are NPO and cannot take oral medication.
Analysis/Physiologic/Planning

83. *Correct response: b*
Activity may dislodge a clot and start hemorrhage.
   a. Decreasing abdominal pain should result from this action, but it is not the primary reason for bedrest in this situation.
   c. Immobility will not facilitate peristalsis.
   d. Immobility will not decrease the potential for infection.
Analysis/Safe care/Implementation

84. *Correct response: a*
Epinephrine acts as a bronchodilator and will relieve dyspnea.
   b, c, and d. The action of epinephrine will not diminish pain, cause drowsiness, or increase itching.
Application/Health promotion/Evaluation

85. *Correct response: a*
Many fears related to surgery are based on inadequate or inappropriate information. Assessing the client's knowledge and identifying misconceptions allows the nurse to tailor the teaching plan to the client's specific needs.
   b. All teaching should be individualized based on the client's particular needs.
   c. Explaining any risks related to surgery is the physician's responsibility.
   d. Written materials only supplement preoperative teaching and do not supplant interactive sessions.
Comprehension/Psychosocial/Assessment

86. *Correct response: b*
Turning, extremity exercises, and deep breathing are important to postoperative recovery.
   a. Kegel exercises would not be appropriate at this time and would be done only by medical orders.
   c. Availability of support systems is not as high a priority as physiologic integrity according to Maslow's Hierarchy of Needs; teaching should be focused on the highest priority.
   d. Teaching the use of a bedpan and call light are part of the client's initial orientation to the unit.
Analysis/Health promotion/Planning

87. *Correct response: b*
Signs of hypovolemic shock and edema suggest internal bleeding.
   a. Pulmonary embolism is marked by chest pain and hemoptysis, among other signs and symptoms.
   c. This scenario presents no information to suggest septic shock.
   d. A client undergoing partial thyroidectomy would not have had all parathyroids disrupted and would not likely experience electrolyte imbalance.
Analysis/Physiologic/Evaluation

88. *Correct response: c*
The client is experiencing postoperative flatus and difficulty in expelling gas, which is common at this stage of recovery.
   a. A hyperthermia pad will not help the client expel gas.
   b. The client is not experiencing nausea or vomiting; thus, an antiemetic would be inappropriate.
   d. Narcotics will decrease peristalsis and lead to increased abdominal distention.
Application/Physiologic/Implementation

89. *Correct response: a*
The cardinal sign of ARDS is decreased oxygen (below 60 mmHg) with a high flow rate of oxygen.
   b, c, and d. These are not expected in ARDS. The CO_2 level would be increased.
Comprehension/Physiologic/Planning

90. *Correct response: b*
Five hours after chest tube insertion there should be fluctuation with inspiration and expiration. This should

continue until the lung has fully expanded.

  a. The nurse would suspect an air leak with vigorous bubbling.

  c. Bloody drainage would be in the drainage chamber, not the waterseal chamber.

  d. If there is no fluctuation at this time, the nurse should assess for kinks or clots in the tubing.

Knowledge/Safe care/Evaluation

91. *Correct response: c*
Common clinical manifestations of a myocardial infarction include radiating chest pain; diaphoresis; cool, clammy, pale skin; nausea and vomiting; dyspnea with or without crackles; syncope; and restlessness.

  a, b, and d. These clinical manifestations represent congestive heart failure, endocarditis, and pericarditis, respectively.

Application/Physiologic/Assessment

92. *Correct response: c*
Digoxin should not be administered if the apical pulse is less than 60. Hold the medication and notify physician before administering digoxin.

  a. Assess the apical pulse only, *not* the radial pulse.

  b. Normal digoxin level is 0.5–2 ng/mL.

  d. Decreased potassium level can increase digoxin toxicity, so do not administer digoxin if potassium level is low (normal, 3.5–5.5 mEq/L).

Knowledge/Safe care/Planning

93. *Correct response: d*
If there is pacemaker failure, the client will exhibit the signs and symptoms that required seeking medical attention in the first place (dizziness, weakness, irregular pulse).

  a, b, and c. If the client feels lightheaded the physician should be notified. Signs of infection should be reported, but infection would

not cause the pacemaker to fail. Irregular pulse rate should be reported to the physician immediately.

Comprehension/Health promotion/ Evaluation

94. *Correct response: a*
Possible clinical manifestations of cholelithiasis include episodic cramping pain in the right upper abdominal quadrant after a high-fat meal, with pain radiating to the right shoulder; nausea and vomiting; fat intolerance; fever; and leukocytosis.

  b, c, and d. These are clinical manifestations of liver failure, appendicitis, and peptic ulcer, respectively.

Application/Physiologic/Assessment

95. *Correct response: b*
Antacids are given for acute epigastric pain secondary to peptic ulcer. The antacid neutralizes the gastric pH to prevent erosion of the mucosal lining.

  a. Histamine (H_2) receptor antagonists (cimetidine, famotidine) decrease the stimulus for hydrochloric acid production.

  c. Cytoprotective agents produce an ulcer-adherent complex that hastens healing by coating the mucosal lining.

  d. Pepsin is an enzyme and is not affected by antacids.

Knowledge/Safe care/Evaluation

96. *Correct response: d*
Tented skin turgor and hypokalemia (normal potassium level of 3.5–5.5 mEq/L) are indicative of fluid volume deficit secondary to diarrhea, requiring medical intervention.

  a, b, and c. All of the data is normal and would not require any intervention.

Application/Physiologic/Planning

97. *Correct response: c*
Client teaching should include decreasing activities dealing with

Valsalva's maneuver (bending, lifting heavy objects, straining, constipation).
a, b, and d. The nurse should encourage eating a high-fiber diet to decrease constipation; sitting up for at least 2 hours after eating; and eating small, frequent, bland meals, respectively.
Application/Health promotion/Implementation

98. *Correct response: c*
Evaluation criteria for a client with a sexually transmitted disease (STD) would include the outcome goal: the client reports decreased pain and discharge.
a, b, and d. The client should have decreased lymphadenopathy, must abstain from sexual activity, and should make sure sexual partners get treatment.
Analysis/Safe care/Evaluation

99. *Correct response: c*
Prednisone therapy must be decreased gradually to prevent an adrenal crisis. After prolonged prednisone therapy, adrenal insufficiency may develop if medication is stopped abruptly.
a, b, and d. Prednisone is taken daily. Moon-face is a side-effect of therapy but not a cause for stopping the medication. Prednisone is ordered for acute exacerbations of Crohn's disease; long-term prednisone therapy will suppress the adrenal gland.
Comprehension/Health promotion/Evaluation

100. *Correct response: c*
In a TIA, temporary interruption of blood flow (lasting from seconds to hours) produces transient neurologic deficits that clear completely within 12 to 24 hours. This response is easy for a layperson to understand.
a. This response is inappropriate; the nurse can explain what TIA means.

b. This is the explanation for a cerebral vascular accident (CVA).
d. This is the definition of TIA and not helpful to the client's family.
Knowledge/Psychosocial/Implementation

101. *Correct response: a*
Common clinical manifestations of hypokalemia (potassium level <3.6 mEq/L) are anorexia, fatigue, muscle weakness, paresthesia, ECG changes.
b, c, and d. These are clinical manifestations of hypocalcemia, hypermagnesemia, and metabolic acidosis, respectively.
Knowledge/Physiologic/Assessment

102. *Correct response: d*
The clinical manifestations of appendicitis are acute abdominal pain, usually in the right lower quadrant (McBurney's point); rebound tenderness; nausea and vomiting; and low-grade fever.
a, b, and c. These are not associated with appendicitis.
Knowledge/Physiologic/Assessment

103. *Correct response: c*
It would be most important for the nurse to assess how long the seizure lasted, which body parts were affected, and whether the client noticed an aura.
a and d. These questions are condescending and not appropriate for assessing seizure activity.
b. This may be appropriate at a later time, but it is not priority and is not concerned with seizure activity.
Comprehension/Physiologic/Assessment

104. *Correct response: c*
The client may experience these symptoms during a cardiac catheterization and should be informed of this.
a. The client is awake during the procedure.
b. The client will be on strict bedrest for 8 to 12 hours after the procedure to prevent arterial bleeding.

d. A femoral cardiac catheterization requires the client to keep the leg straight; a brachial cardiac catheterization requires the client to keep the arm straight.

Comprehension/Health promotion/ Implementation

105. *Correct response: d*

When the client has chest pain, the client should stop activity; place a nitroglycerin tablet under the tongue every 5 minutes, for up to 3 times; and, if pain remains unrelieved, go to the hospital because continuing pain may indicate a myocardial infarction.

a. Sublingual nitroglycerin is for acute chest pain and is not taken on a regular basis.

b. A headache is a common side effect of sublingual nitroglycerin and means the medication is effective.

c. Sublingual nitroglycerin should be placed under tongue; the tablet should not be swallowed.

Application/Health promotion/ Implementation

106. *Correct response: c*

During a sigmoid colostomy, the rectum and part of the descending colon is removed. Enough of the colon is left so that the stool formed is the same consistency as that eliminated through the rectum prior to surgery.

a, b, and d. These are incorrect and would occur with colostomies higher than the descending colon.

Knowledge/Physiologic/Assessment

107. *Correct response: b*

When a client is on warfarin (Coumadin) the PT should be 1.5–2.5 times the control. A PT of 24 is therapeutic and the medication should be administered as ordered.

a, c, and d. These are incorrect. The antidote for warfarin is aquamephyton (vitamin K).

Comprehension/Safe care/Evaluation

108. *Correct response: d*

The nurse must realize that pain may indicate a postoperative complication. This must be ruled out before administering a pain medication.

a. The nurse must not medicate without first assessing the client for complications.

b and c. Pain is expected 1 day after surgery in this client and pain medication should be given liberally. Turning, coughing, and deep breathing should be performed after the client receives pain medication.

Application/Physiologic/Implementation

109. *Correct response: a*

Clinical manifestations of chronic open-angle glaucoma include no early symptoms, blurred vision, diminished accommodation, gradual loss of peripheral vision (tunnel vision), mild aching of the eyes, and halos around light with elevated intraocular pressure.

b and c. These are clinical manifestations of cataracts.

d. This is a sign of retinal detachment.

Knowledge/Physiologic/Assessment

110. *Correct response: d*

The nurse should instruct the client to protect ears from loud noises, which can injure eardrums and cause hearing loss.

a. The client should chew gum or suck hard candy when flying. Doing so opens the eustachian tubes and allows air into the middle ear.

b. The client should not insert any object smaller than a finger into the ear and never beyond the extent of the visible ear.

c. The client should blow the nose with mouth and nostrils open to prevent forcing contaminated material into the middle ear.

Knowledge/Health promotion/ Implementation

111. *Correct response: c*

Persistent hoarseness is the earliest and most predominant sign of intrinsic laryngeal cancer; there is no early hoarseness with the extrinsic type.

a. This is a sign seen primarily in extrinsic laryngeal cancer.

b and d. These are late symptoms with both types of laryngeal cancer.

Knowledge/Physiologic/Assessment

112. *Correct response: b*

During skeletal traction a Kirschner wire or Steinman pin may be inserted through the bone; these sites should remain infection free. Infection could lead to osteomyelitis.

a. Skeletal traction weights should be removed only when ordered by the physician or in an emergency.

c. A bedboard should be placed under the mattress to ensure extra firm support.

d. Tincture of benzoin is not used to cleanse wound sites; it is a barrier substance used to prevent skin breakdown, for example from adhesive tape or Steri-Strips.

Application/Safe care/Implementation

113. *Correct response: a*

Clinical manifestations of portal hypertension include shifting dullness or fluid wave on abdominal percussion, caput medusae, enlarged palpable spleen, and bruits.

b and c. These are clinical manifestations of jaundice.

d. This is a sign of hepatic encephalopathy.

Knowledge/Physiologic/Assessment

114. *Correct response: c*

Nursing measures to prevent stone recurrence include dietary modification (calcium, uric acid), increasing fluid intake to between 3 and 4 L daily, promoting increased physical activity, and monitoring urine pH.

a. Fluid intake should be between 3 and 4 L daily.

b. Physical activity should be increased.

d. An ileal conduit is performed when the bladder must be removed because of trauma or cancer.

Application/Health promotion/Implementation

Index

Page numbers followed by *f* indicate figures; those followed by *t* indicate tabular material.

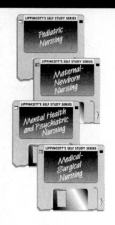
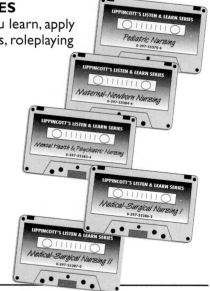
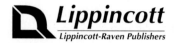